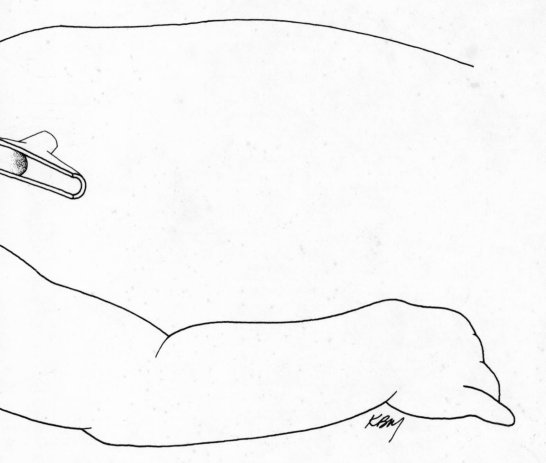

Anesthesia for infants and children

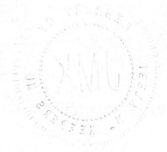

Anesthesia for infants and children

ROBERT M. SMITH, M.D., F.F.A.R.C.S. Ireland (Hon.)

Anesthesiologist, The Children's Hospital Medical Center,
Boston, Massachusetts

FOURTH EDITION

with 308 illustrations

The C. V. Mosby Company

ST. LOUIS • TORONTO • LONDON   1980

Fourth edition

Copyright © 1980 by The C. V. Mosby Company

All rights reserved. No part of this book may be reproduced in any manner without written permission of the publisher.

Previous editions copyrighted 1959, 1963, 1968

Printed in the United States of America

The C. V. Mosby Company
11830 Westline Industrial Drive, St. Louis, Missouri 63141

Library of Congress Cataloging in Publication Data

Smith, Robert Moors, 1912-
    Anesthesia for infants and children.

    Bibliography: p.
    Includes index.
    1. Pediatric anesthesia. I. Title.
[DNLM: 1. Anesthesia—In infancy and childhood.
WO440 S658a]
RD139.S6 1979   617'.96   79-18284
ISBN 0-8016-4699-5

GW/VH/VH 9 8 7 6 5 4   03/D/066

Contributors

ROBERT J. BERKOWITZ, D.D.S.

Assistant Professor of Pedodontics, University of Pennsylvania School of Dental Medicine; Director of Pedodontic Residency Program, The Children's Hospital of Philadelphia, Philadelphia, Pennsylvania

CHARLES D. COOK, M.D.

Professor and Chairman, Department of Pediatrics, State University of New York, Downstate Medical Center; Pediatrician-In-Chief, Kings County and State University Hospitals, Brooklyn, New York

DAVID R. COOK, M.D.

Associate Professor of Anesthesiology, University of Pittsburgh School of Medicine; Director, Department of Anesthesia, Children's Hospital of Pittsburgh, Pittsburgh, Pennsylvania

KATHRYN E. McGOLDRICK, M.D.

Clinical Instructor in Anesthesia, Harvard Medical School; Assistant Anesthesiologist, Massachusetts Eye and Ear Infirmary, Boston, Massachusetts

ETSURO K. MOTOYAMA, M.D.

Professor of Anesthesiology and Pediatrics, University of Pittsburgh School of Medicine, Pittsburgh, Pennsylvania; formerly Director of Pediatric Anesthesia and Pediatric Pulmonology, Yale–New Haven Medical Center, New Haven, Connecticut

TAE H. OH, M.D.

Associate Professor of Anesthesiology and Child Health and Development, George Washington University School of Medicine; Attending Anesthesiologist, The Children's Hospital National Medical Center, Washington, D.C.

MARK C. ROGERS, M.D.

Assistant Professor of Anesthesiology and Pediatrics, Johns Hopkins Medical School; Director, Pediatric Intensive Care Unit, Johns Hopkins Hospital, Baltimore, Maryland

To my wife

Margaret Louise Smith

and to 200,000 brave young patients
about whom this book is written

Preface

The fourth edition of this book has been prepared with the same intention as previous editions—to present a comprehensive study of the clinical management of pediatric patients for the use of practitioners at all levels of experience. A definite attempt has been made to offer information in some depth concerning concepts behind various approaches to anesthetic management but at the same time to keep the material in a form that is easily available for immediate clinical application. References have been selected to include those of either historic or scientific value, and many that have held only temporary interest have been eliminated. Chapters have been grouped in three sections to place emphasis first on general considerations of a biologic and technical nature, second on actual anesthetic management of specific clinical problems, and third on aspects of support, postoperative care, and complications.

Although there has been continued progress in the field of pediatric anesthesia, emphasis is not placed on what is new but on what is believed to be of most importance in carrying infants and children through their surgical exposure. Pediatric anesthesia has attained some degree of maturity, and our experience at The Children's Hospital Medical Center during the past 30 years, involving over 200,000 patients, is used as the basis of evaluation of anesthetic technics and underlying theory.

An attempt has been made throughout this edition, through text and illustrations, to show that the child is an individual human being rather than a pathologic specimen or a statistic. Care of the awake child is an important aspect of anesthesiology but one that has been seriously neglected. Greater accomplishments of surgery make this more evident. More complicated operations on sicker children have extended the stress of the operative period into many days of postoperative recovery involving a variety of intensely distressing experiences while few, if any, advances have been made in reduction of such stress.

It may be surprising to find so much of the material in this book devoted to the details of the operative surgery. This is intentional, since a great many of the operations performed on infants and children are unfamiliar in adult surgery, and it is absolutely essential for the pediatric anesthesiologist to know the type and extent of the operative procedure that the surgeon is planning to do.

This edition has been completely rewritten. Drs. Charles D. Cook and Etsuro K. Motoyama have once again contributed a most valuable chapter on respiratory physiology, and Dr. Motoyama, in association with Drs. David R. Cook and Tae H. Oh, has compiled a new chapter combining the management of respiratory insufficiency and intensive care. Drs. Mark C. Rogers, Kathryn E. McGoldrick, and Robert J. Berkowitz are largely responsible for the chapters on anesthesia for cardiac, ophthalmic, and dental surgery, respectively. These additional contributors have broadened the aspects of specialized areas appreciably and added much to the accuracy of the information.

Once again I owe great appreciation to many individuals who have contributed in a variety of ways. My associates in anesthesia have certainly provided me with excellent service, much advice, and great freedom to work. Numerous secretaries and critics have aided in preparing material and culling out errors. I am particularly thankful that my wife has remained loyal in spite of the several years of lost weekends.

Robert M. Smith

Contents

PART ONE

THEORETICAL AND TECHNICAL CONSIDERATIONS

CHAPTER 1

Basic concepts and changing forces

If one considers 1930 to be the approximate beginning of pediatric anesthesia, a review of the subsequent 50 years shows that the basic goals of patient safety and relief of suffering have endured, but numerous forces have altered our approach to these goals.

Anesthetic technics have evolved, as have the skills of those using and teaching them, so that high-risk patients can be brought through most operative procedures using any one of several anesthetic methods. More concern is now directed toward the development of monitoring and supportive measures than toward new anesthetic technics. In monitoring, measurement is the essential factor, and the degree to which one is able to measure the child's responses during operation is a fair indication of the progress of pediatric anesthesia.

At the same time, the responsibilities of the anesthesiologist have been extended beyond the operating room, carrying him into the recovery room, nursing divisions, and intensive care areas, where he is concerned with both surgical and nonsurgical patients. Resuscitative technics, prolonged ventilatory support, and use of elaborate mechanical and physiologic instrumentation are now essential elements of anesthesiology.

The forces acting on the distribution of patients are complex and contradictory. The age range of pediatric surgical patients has undergone considerable fluctuation in recent years. The prime surgical targets were once 6- to 10-year-olds, younger children having been considered excessive risks. Attention then shifted to the neonate, and methods were developed for repair of tracheoesophageal fistula and other life-threatening congenital anomalies. Interest in teenage patients has been stimulated recently by recognition of the problems of adolescence, by longer survival of children with self-limiting diseases such as Down's syndrome, cystic fibrosis, and leukemia, and by extension of insurance benefits to cover them.

There is also an evolutionary force affecting the type of operation performed at any one center. Young surgeons rapidly learn the operations laboriously developed by their predecessors and then move out to the suburbs and intercept the patients before they reach the major hospital. Thus, survival of major teaching hospitals depends on continued development of newer procedures. Presently, our goal at the Children's Hospital Medical Center is less concerned with the standardized repair of neonatal defects; attention is focused on kidney transplants, repair of advanced scoliosis, and new approaches to congenital cardiac lesions and malignant disease.

Although the high cost of major urban hospitals is driving many patients away, this trend is being countered by development of outpatient medical and surgical clinics as well as day-care facilities, which have numerous advantages.

Another force bringing pediatric patients back to the city is regionalization of medical care. With present communication and transportation, it is unreasonable to attempt complicated high-risk procedures in hospitals that do not have both equipment and personnel who are equal to the task. Equipment is often extravagantly provided in suburban communities, but it is rarely possible to staff these hospitals on a 24-hour basis with personnel of required excellence.

The effect of these forces on the individual who accepts the responsibility of providing anesthesia for pediatric patients must be recognized. The "complete" pediatric anesthesiologist needs a variety of talents. A thorough medical training is essential, and basic experience in pediatrics and neonatology is most advantageous. The pediatric anesthesiologist should strive for continued excellence in his own and related pediatric and surgical areas and should attempt to cultivate an unattainable combination of attributes that include the ability to comfort fearful children, to encourage the fainthearted and suppress the wild, to deal with equally distraught parents and grandparents, and to mollify harassed surgeons.

It may be important for the anesthesiologist to be ready to accept extreme-risk patients in the hope that he will be able to provide a final chance with every advantage of professional and technical skill currently available.

It is essential that the pediatric anesthesiologist be aware that he is working at all times as a member of a team, all of whom are working for precisely the same goal. There are times when he must insist on his own way, but many other times when he can bend to others' reasoning. He should be fussy and meticulous yet have unbounded enthusiasm and try to see things as a child sees them. He should love children, but may not lose his heart to them.*

*As yet, no such individual has been discovered.

Fundamental differences

The reason for undertaking a special study of pediatric anesthesia is that children and especially infants differ sharply from adult patients. Many of the important differences, however, are not the most obvious. Although the most apparent contrast in the neonate is his size, immature enzymatic activity probably could prove a greater problem to an uninformed anesthetist.

Differences of anatomic structure related to actual size and proportion have been fairly well worked out, although electron microscopy is opening vast new areas in cellular structure that should be of great significance. Recognition of physiologic differences relating both to general metabolism and to function of various organ systems is of great practical value to the anesthesiologist, and investigation continues to be active here.

In the field of pediatric pathology, much remains to be learned in such areas as immunology, genetics, organ transplantation, and cancer. In gross pathology, the variances between child and adult seem relatively clearcut and often quite striking (omphalocele, conjoined twins) and need little more than enumeration to be appreciated. Major differences exist both in the types of lesions seen in infants and children and in the altered response of the young to illness.

Rapid development has occurred in the field of pediatric pharmacology, which has recently become alive with important new concepts and information and is justly establishing itself as one of the fundamental building blocks of pediatric anesthesia (Weiss and others, 1960; Done, 1964).

Another aspect that now demands greater attention is the psychologic factor—not because of new revelations in this field, but because of the growing gap between it and progress in other fields as well as the growing awareness of both lay and professional observers that emotional experiences of the hospitalized child may be shattering. The psychologic factor is discussed first to focus attention on this imbalance.

PSYCHOLOGIC DIFFERENCES

From a scientific standpoint it is difficult to measure psychologic or emotional differences. It is generally agreed, however, that the infant has minimal emotional response at birth but thereafter his development proceeds rapidly. Between 1 and 2 years of age his cognitive development outstrips his ability to express himself, and he becomes emotionally hypersensitive (Jackson, 1951). This state is partially relieved with the onset of speech, but he remains highly impressionable throughout childhood. The gradual reduction of psychologic fragility appears to reverse itself in many adolescents before resuming a more gradual decline, making the entire slope much like that of basal metabolism (p. 22).

The emotional response of the infant and small child is characteristically an unrestrained, all-or-none reaction. Complete lack of self-control, and the small child's increased

5

rate of metabolism, render sedative drugs ineffective until given in relatively high dosage. A child's attempt to cooperate in spite of opposite preferences usually does not appear much before school age, and without sedation he must be won by seduction rather than persuasion.

A second widely accepted generalization is that the emotional experiences of childhood leave much deeper and more lasting impressions than those of the adult and may have a seriously upsetting effect on the child's psychologic development (Levy, 1945; Cassell, 1965).

Figures from studies made over a span of several years are impressive. Eckenhoff (1953) reported that 15% of 50 children undergoing tonsillectomy showed later emotional disturbance, and Rosen and Brueton (1970) found that 50% of 52 children appeared to have been "disturbed" by similar exposure. It is reasonable to review some of the experiences that may seem commonplace to hospital personnel but may have an upsetting influence on children who are not only more impressionable but are also on the receiving end of these traumatic factors. The list below does not enumerate all of the varieties of distress involved but demonstrates a wide range of unpleasant sensations. Uncomprehending exposure to any combination of these insults should give a 3-year-old a lasting impression of life in the hospital.

DISTRESSING EXPERIENCES OF HOSPITALIZED CHILDREN

Physical pain

  Needles
  Postoperative wounds
  Chest tubes
  Dressing changes

Discomfort

  Dizziness, nausea
  Examination of ears, throat, rectum
  Arterial or intravenous infusions
  Nasogastric or urethral drainage
  Prolonged tracheal intubation, tracheostomy
  Mechanical ventilators
  Postoperative tracheal suctioning

Emotional stress

  Separation from parents
  Unpleasant smells, tastes:
    Vomitus, dressings, medicines, anesthetics

Unpleasant sounds:
  Screaming fellow patients
  Clattering instruments
Disturbing sights:
  Masked, gowned personnel
  Bleeding, disfigured, crippled, comatose, and moribund comrades
  Events associated with "cardiac arrest" in the next bed

Some of the great advances in supportive care and monitoring may actually increase the child's emotional problems. Now, in addition to the once feared oxygen tent, patients are subjected to prolonged mechanical ventilator therapy, tracheostomy, tracheal and gastric intubation and suction, traction apparatus, chest tubes, and other apparatus of unknown psychologic effect (Kiely, 1974). There is wide variation in the degree of distress such situations cause; some children give way to frenzied uncontrol, whereas others show only mild interest in the same situation. There must be more effort made in recognizing those children who are more easily alarmed and in overcoming their underlying disturbances (Mason, 1965; Bothe and Galdston, 1972) (see Chapter 4).

DIFFERENCES IN RESPONSE TO PHARMACOLOGIC AGENTS

The extent of the difference between infant, child, and adult in response to drugs was not recognized until quite recently. Before 1960 the chief concern in pediatric pharmacology was to find a formula by which to convert adult dosages to pediatric dosages. However, the rapid succession of the thalidomide tragedy, fatal chloramphenicol poisonings, and sulfonamide deaths, all traced to unsuspected prenatal and neonatal responses to standard drugs, brought sudden realization of the problem and initiated intense activity. Within 5 years, work by Weiss and associates (1960), Nyhan (1961), Silverman (1962), Yaffe (1962), Done (1964), Shirkey (1965), and others had laid the groundwork for the new field of pediatric pharmacology and related areas of pediatric toxicology and pharmacogenetics.

The first lesson learned from the unexpected fatalities was that *dosages for neonates cannot be calculated from adult schedules by any single factor.* For older children, formulas have been tried on the basis of age, weight, body surface area, and, for liquids, ml/100 calories metabolized (see Appendix). Actually none is reliable, and Nyhan (1968) commented that one might as well go by age, since that is the simplest.

Pharmacokinetics

The rapid development of pediatric pharmacology has been aided by application of pharmacokinetic methods by which mathematical methods are used to relate drug dosage, pharmacologic effects, and time (Jusko, 1972). The variables that determine the level and duration of drug concentration include (1) the dose and form of the drug, (2) its uptake or absorption, (3) its concentration and distribution, (4) the specific action of the drug at the receptor site, and (5) its metabolism or biotransformation and excretion (Azarnoff, 1973). Pharmacokinetic constants at each age level include plasma-protein binding, biologic half-life, coefficient of distribution, and rate of elimination (Sereni and Principi, 1968); patient variables include age, genetic factors, disease, and environment. Gustafson and Coursin (1968) list seven different age levels at which particular pharmacologic reactions are seen (Table 2-1). Although many unexpected responses are encountered daily, the systematic investigation of progressive phases of numerous agents has uncovered the mechanism of many irregular drug actions.

The alterations noticed consist first of change in the principal action of the drug in respect to its speed of onset, intensity or effectiveness, and duration of action and second of the incidence or frequency and the severity of side effects.

Several hundred drugs have already been shown to have different effects in patients of different ages, and more are certain to be

Table 2-1. Developmental stages of pharmacologic responses

Stage	Drug	Effect
First trimester of pregnancy	Thalidomide Anticancer drugs—aminopterin Androgens Antithyroid agents	Teratogenic, abortion Death Masculinization Fetal goiter
Last trimester of pregnancy	Thiouracil Radioactive iron Narcotics	Abnormal organ growth, enzyme induction Congenital goiter Withdrawal symptoms
Immediate pre-partum period	Analgesics Sulfonamide Novobiocin Reserpine Vitamin K	Depression Hemolytic anemia Enzyme inhibition Nasal congestion Kernicterus
Lactation period	Bromides Steroids Contraceptives Phenobarbital—phenytoin	Methemoglobinemia
Neonatal period	Antibiotics Narcotics Anesthetics	Toxicity or varied sensitivity
Infancy-3 yr	Salicylates Phenytoin	Salicylate acidosis Gingival hyperplasia
Adolescence	Vitamin A Anovulatory agents used for acne	Pseudotumor cerebri Metabolic disturbances

Data from Gustafson, S. R., and Coursin, D. B.: The pediatric patient, Philadelphia, 1968, J. B. Lippincott Co.

found. The anesthesiologist cannot know them all but should be aware of the situation, know the mechanisms involved, and be able to apply pharmacokinetic methods in evaluation of new agents.

The principal differences in the child's handling of drugs can be related to each phase of a drug's passage through his body.

Uptake or absorption. Drugs may enter the body by inhalation, ingestion, or injection. Difference in uptake or absorption is seen in the premature infant's delayed uptake of sulfonamide and the neonate's delayed uptake of riboflavin from the gastrointestinal tract, but more important response alterations are seen with inhaled agents.

Kety's classic measurement of uptake of gases (1951) has enabled anesthesiologists to contribute much to pharmacologic evolution. Using Kety's principles, Salanitre and Rackow (1969) reported the uptake of inhaled agents to be significantly more rapid in infants than in children and more rapid in children than in adults (Fig. 2-1). The difference was attributed to relatively greater cardiac output and alveolar ventilation* in the younger subject and to an increased percentage of richly perfused visceral tissues. Eger and associates (1971) confirmed this work using models and suggested additional factors; they also noted that although these findings suggest more rapid induction of infants, the higher concentration of agent required by younger patients reduces this advantage (p. 10).

The solubility of inhalation agents is of practical interest in anesthesia. The uptake of less soluble anesthetics (nitrous oxide, cyclopropane) is more rapid in both adults and infants than that of more soluble anesthetics such as ether and methoxyflurane. In the presence of right-to-left shunts, as in tetralogy of Fallot, uptake is delayed, the difference being greater with less soluble agents; thus, the resultant prolongation of cyclopropane induction would be relatively greater than the prolongation of ether induc-

*That infants have relatively greater alveolar ventilation now appears controversial (p. 16).

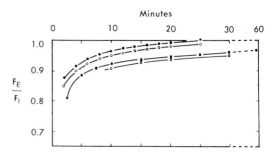

Fig. 2-1. Pulmonary equilibration curves with nitrous oxide. *Solid circles,* infants aged 0 to 6 months; *open circles,* children aged 1 to 5 years; *solid squares,* adults breathing nitrous oxide, 10% in oxygen; *open squares,* adults breathing nitrous oxide, 70% in oxygen. (From Salanitre, E., and Rackow, H.: Anesthesiology **30:**388, 1969.)

tion (Eger, 1974; Eger and Severinghaus, 1964) (Fig. 2-2).

Distribution of drugs. Among several differences related to distribution of drugs, decreased plasma protein concentration of the neonate and greater competition for protein binding sites, especially of plasma albumin, are significant. Displacement of bilirubin from binding sites by sulfonamides, vitamin K, salicylates, and caffeine and sodium benzoate is known to cause accumulation of free bilirubin with resultant development of kernicterus.

Increased permeability of membranes, particularly the placental and blood-brain barrier, in the fetus and neonate allows more rapid penetration of many agents, especially those in a free molecular, nonionic form with a high partition coefficient, such as thiopental (Mirken, 1975). Another factor allowing increased cerebral penetration is the neonate's lack of myelination. Distribution of antibiotics and several barbiturates is facilitated in proportion to this deficiency.

A child's response to drugs that are distributed to body fluids is altered with considerable changes in the ratio of extracellular fluid volume (ECV) to total body water (TBW). Thus, although the dose-response relationship of children to succinylcholine is still unsettled (Stead, 1955; Lim and others, 1964; Walts and Dillon, 1969), many are convinced that the child's reputed increased

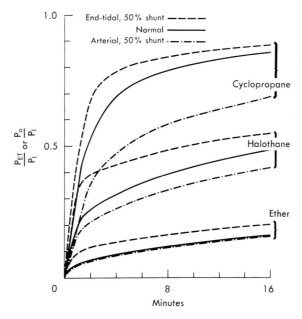

Fig. 2-2. When no ventilation-perfusion abnormalities exist, the alveolar (P_A or P_{ET}) and arterial (P_a) anesthetic partial pressures increase together *(continuous lines)* toward the inspired partial pressure (P_I). When 50% of the cardiac output is shunted through the lungs, the rate of rise of the end-tidal partial pressure *(dashed lines)* is accelerated while the rate of rise of the arterial partial pressure *(dot-dashed lines)* is retarded. The greatest retardation is found with the least soluble anesthetic, cyclopropane. (From Eger, E. I. II: Anesthetic uptake and action, Baltimore, 1974, The Williams & Wilkins Co. © 1974, Edmond I. Eger II, M.D.)

tolerance to succinylcholine is related to his ECV/TBW ratio, which is highest at birth and decreases throughout childhood (Cook, 1974; Ecobichon and Stephens, 1973).

Receptor site. Although differences in receptor site sensitivity are not clearly defined, it is known that infants are definitely less resistant to bilirubin toxicity than are adults. Nyhan and Lampert (1965) stated that many responses suggesting increased sensitivity in neonates are actually due to increased drug concentration caused by immature metabolism or excretion.

In general, neonates do show more tendency toward toxicity, but in relation to anesthetic agents, most observations suggest that young patients require a greater drug concentration to achieve the same response. It is obvious that infants are less affected by nitrous oxide and ethylene than are adults. Deming (1952) demonstrated that infants require a higher blood concentration of cyclo-

propane than adults for the same clinical effect (17 mg/dl vs 12 mg/dl). Reynolds (1966) found similarly increased requirements of halothane in infants, and Nicodemus and associates (1969) found that the mean effective dose (ED_{50}) of halothane in infants 0 to 6 months old averaged 1.20% as compared with 0.94% in adults. Gregory and associates (1969) showed that the minimum alveolar concentration (MAC) of halothane was a factor of age from birth throughout life, varying from 1.08 at birth to 0.64 in advanced age (Fig. 2-3).

Metabolism or biotransformation. In the metabolism or biotransformation of drugs, a host of material has already been uncovered by enzymologists, anesthesiologists, and electron microscopists, and the surface has barely been scratched. The processes of detoxification and degradation by conjugation, oxidation, reduction, and hydrolysis all involve enzyme activity that infants less than 3

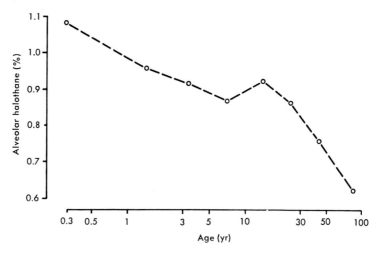

Fig. 2-3. Halothane MAC *(vertical axis)* constantly decreases with age, with the possible exception of a slight increase at puberty. (From Gregory, G. A., Eger, E. I. II, and Munson, E. S.: Anesthesiology **30:** 488, 1969.)

months old may not produce and that may be dangerously reduced or overproduced at other stages of development.

Deficient glucuronyl transferase, which is essential for *conjugative glucuronidation* of chloramphenicol, was found to be the cause of many infant deaths (Weiss and others, 1960). Bilirubin toxicity and increased sensitivity of infants to sulfisoxazole (Gantrisin), morphine, acetanilid, thyroxine, and steroids also have been traced to the same deficiency. Glucuronyl transferase does not reach normal levels until 1 month after birth, and the level of uridine diphosphogalactose dehydrogenase, also essential for glucuronidation, is low until 2 months of age.

Sulfonamide and isoniazide (INH) toxicity in infants has been explained by a deficiency of coenzyme A, a conjugative enzyme essential in acetylation of these drugs.

Oxidative metabolism, carried on in the lungs and other areas but chiefly accomplished by hepatic microsomes, is an area of great interest at all age levels. Pediatricians have found that microsomal enzymes, deficient for 4 to 8 weeks after birth, metabolize amphetamines, chlorpromazine, steroids, and other agents; anesthesiologists are finding this area to be the focal point for clues to halogen toxicity and malignant hyperthermia (Holaday and others, 1970; Van

Dyke and Wood, 1973; Britt and others, 1973). Of special importance to pediatric anesthesia is the possible explanation for the child's apparent freedom from hepatic toxicity following halothane anesthesia.

Reductive metabolism activated by reductases found in several parts of the body (Goldstein and others, 1968) is involved in conversion of chloral hydrate to trichlorethanol and also in the metabolism of several antibiotics, including the potentially lethal chloramphenicol.

Hydrolysis, chiefly of amines and esters, accounts for the metabolism of local anesthetic agents as well as succinylcholine. The hydrolysis of succinyldicholine to succinylmonocholine and then to succinic acid and choline has been explored extensively, and it is well known that prolonged apneic response may be caused by ineffective pseudocholinesterase due to either reduced tissue concentration or genetic defect (Lehmann and Ryan, 1956; Kalow, 1962).

Altered response to a drug may be caused by change in the rate of excretion via the biliary system or kidneys, a delay producing prolonged and/or toxic effects. At birth this is evident especially in reduction of renal clearance and concentrating power, these deficiencies being more pronounced in premature or sick infants (p. 25). Silverio and

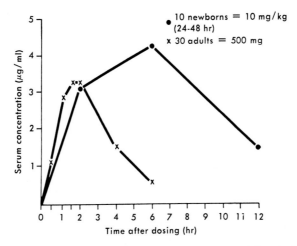

Fig. 2-4. Mean serum levels of anhydrous ampicillin in newborns and adults, single oral doses. (From Silverio, J., and Poole, J. W.: Pediatrics **51:**578, 1973. Copyright American Academy of Pediatrics 1973.)

Poole (1973) demonstrated the infant's susceptibility to ampicillin toxicity and explained it on the basis of delayed renal clearance (Fig. 2-4).

In his investigation of succinylcholine, Levy (1970) also found evidence of increased pharmacologic effect secondary to delayed renal excretion. The prolonged effect of succinylcholine in three infants (Walts and Dillon, 1969) was subjected to pharmacokinetic analysis by applying the excretion formula:

$$t = \frac{2.7}{k} (\log A^\circ - \log A_{min})$$

where

    t = duration of excretion
    2.7 = conversion factor $\log^{10}$ to natural log
    k = elimination rate constant
    A° = dose
    A_{min} = minimum effective dose

Since succinylcholine is eliminated by first order kinetics, Levy was able to deduce that delayed excretion caused the prolonged effect in two of the three infants described.

The response of the newborn to d-tubocurarine was first thought to be one of increased sensitivity (Stead, 1955), but later evidence of Long and Bachman (1967) suggested a normal dose response, with pro-

longed effect due in part, at least, to immature renal function.

Drug interactions

The response of a patient to a drug may be altered at any stage by interaction with another endogenous or exogenous agent. Halothane and epinephrine interaction, digitalis and curare interaction, droperidol-epinephrine antagonism, and curare-antibiotic responses are well known.

Altered drug responses may be caused by change in pH and solubility or by competition for binding sites and blockage of drug effect. In addition, many agents are known to cause inhibition or acceleration (induction) of microsomal drug-metabolizing enzyme systems (Conney, 1967). Soyka (1972) noted that inducers are of three types: small organic molecules (alcohol, phenobarbital), chlorinated hydrocarbons (chloral hydrate, phenytoin), and polycyclic hydrocarbons (carcinogens 3-Mc and 3,4 benzpyrene).

Increased phenytoin toxicity has been ascribed to enzyme induction by phenobarbital, pentobarbital, and halothane (Karlin and Kutt, 1970). In view of the many children undergoing neurosurgery who have been receiving chronic barbiturate and phenytoin therapy, this has important overtones. Also, the demonstration by Harrison and Smith

(1973) of the extreme toxicity of fluroxene in animals pretreated with pentobarbital is alarming.

Although enzyme inhibitors have aroused less concern than inductors, Yaffe (1962) lists several, including anticoagulants, methylphenidate, and phenyramidol, and has shown that novobiocin reduces glucuronyl transferase activity in infancy.

Pharmacogenetic drug responses

Several anesthetic agents and other drugs have been found to cause altered responses because of hereditary defects (Cohen and Weber, 1972; Brown and others, 1975). The prolonged apnea that occurs after succinylcholine administration in patients with abnormal pseudocholinesterase is well known (Kalow, 1962; Whittaker, 1970). Increased barbiturate effect shown by patients with porphyria (Jackson, 1973), sensitivity to phenylephrine in dysautonomia (Dancis and Smith, 1970), and abnormal response to muscle relaxants in patients with myoneural disorders (Cohen, 1966) are also well documented. Although the role of halothane in initiating malignant hyperthermia in susceptible individuals is not at all clear, the presence of hereditary factor is widely suspected (Britt, 1974). The management of these and similar disorders is discussed in other sections of this book.

ANATOMIC AND PHYSIOLOGIC DIFFERENCES
Size

The most striking contrast between child and adult is in size, but the degree of difference and the variation even within the pediatric age group are hard to appreciate. The contrast between a 2-pound infant and an overgrown 200-pound youth is even more impressive when it is stated that by weight the 200-pound boy is 100 times or 10,000% the size of the baby. In size comparisons it makes considerable difference whether one uses weight, height, or body surface area as the basis of comparison. As pointed out by Harris (1957) a normal 7-pound newborn is $1/3.3$ the size of an adult in length, but $1/9$ adult size in body surface area and $1/21$ adult size in weight (Fig. 2-5).

Of the body measurements, surface area is probably the most significant since it closely parallels variations in basal metabolic activity

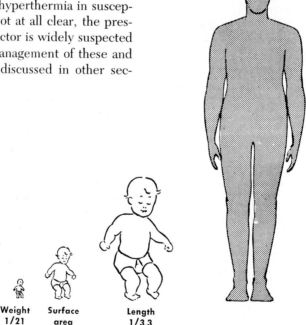

Weight   Surface   Length
1/21   area   1/3.3
         1/9

Fig. 2-5. Proportions of newborn to adult with respect to weight, surface area, and length. (From Harris, J. S.: Ann. N.Y. Acad. Sci. **66:**966, 1957.)

measured in calories per hour per square meter. For this reason, surface area is believed a better criterion than age or weight in judging basal fluid and nutritional requirements. For clinical use this practice appears somewhat difficult, but reference to the nomogram of Talbot and associates (Fig. 2-6) facilitates the procedure considerably. In general, the smaller the patient, the greater the relative surface area of the body. At birth the body surface averages 0.2 m², whereas in the adult it averages 1.75 m². A table of average weight, height, and surface area is presented for reference (Table 2-2).

Proportion or relative size

Less obvious than the difference in overall size is the difference in proportion or relative size of body structures in the pediatric group. This is especially important in regard to the head, which is large and bulky at birth and proceeds to outgrow all other areas throughout early infancy (Fig. 2-7), leading to the *most common mistake of the inexperienced pediatric anesthetist, who invariably underestimates the size of airway and mask.*

The infant's neck is so short that it appears nonexistent, the chin often meeting the chest at the level of the second rib. The chest is relatively small, the abdomen is protuberant and weakly muscled, and the arms and legs are short and poorly developed. Such disproportions are of special consequence when they involve respiratory exchange, as many of them do.

Poor development of bodily support by bone and muscle may combine with disproportion to create problems for the child. Some of these problems become especially evident when children are positioned for operation. In the prone position the shoulders are too small to give adequate support in spite of attempts to build them up with padding. If the child is made to sit up for a pneumoencephalogram, the neck is a very weak stem for the heavy head.

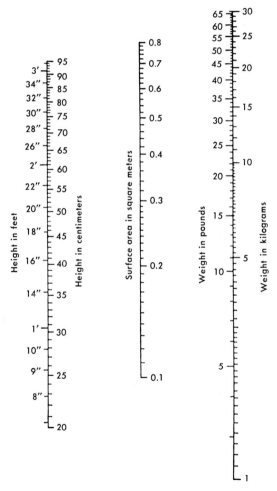

Fig. 2-6. Body surface area nomogram for infants and young children. (Reprinted by permission of the publishers and The Commonwealth Fund, from Talbot, N. B., Sobel, F. H., McArthur, J. W., and Crawford, J. D.: Functional endocrinology from birth through adolescence, Cambridge, Mass., Harvard University Press; copyright, 1952, by The Commonwealth Fund.)

Table 2-2. Relationship of body surface area to age, weight, and height

Age	Height (in)	Weight (lb)	Surface area of body (m²)
Newborn	20	6.6	0.20
3 mo	21	11.0	0.25
1 yr	31	22.0	0.45
3 yr	38	32.0	0.62
6 yr	48	46.0	0.80
9 yr	53	66.0	1.05
15 yr	63	110.0	1.50
Adult	68	154.0	1.75

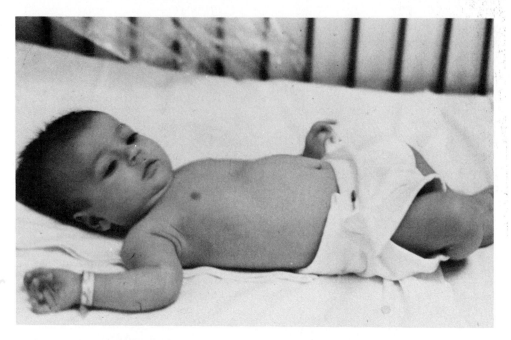

Fig. 2-7. A normal infant has a large head, narrow shoulders and chest, and a large abdomen.

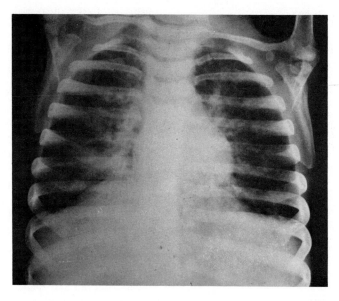

Fig. 2-8. The structure of the infant thorax is relatively weak, and expansion is reduced by horizontally positioned ribs. (From Harris, G. B., and Wittenborg, M. H.: Int. Anesthesiol. Clin. **1**:53, 1962.)

The thoracic cage of the infant consists of a classic combination of structural handicaps. The thorax is small, and the sternum is soft, affording an unstable base for the ribs. In the premature infant the sternum may be deeply retracted with each inspiration. The ribs of the infant are horizontally positioned, reducing the bucket-handle motion on which thoracic respiration depends (Fig. 2-8). The diaphragm rides high, and its motion is embarrassed by the characteristically large abdomen of healthy babies. Intercostal muscles

Table 2-3. Dimensions of respiratory tract components in children

Age	Lung volume (ml)	Alveolar surface area (cm²)	Tracheal length (cords to carina) (cm)	Tracheal diameter (mm)
Birth	100	16,000	4.0	6.0
3 mo	150	16,250	4.0	6.8
6 mo	230	57,000	4.2	7.2
1 yr	400		4.3	7.8
18 mo	470	111,000	4.5	8.8
2 yr	500	184,000	5.0	9.5
3 yr	550	236,000	5.3	
4 yr	600		5.4	11.0
5 yr	700		5.6	
6 yr	800		5.7	

From Hall, J. E.: The physiology of respiration in infants and young children, Proc. R. Soc. Med. **48**:761, 1955.

of normal respiration are poorly developed, and accessory muscles appear to give relatively little assistance in times of need. Although exchange has been shown to be efficient under normal conditions (Cook and others, 1957), these factors make it extremely difficult to meet increased demands imposed by illness or surgery.

The upper respiratory tract in children is predisposed to obstruction because of the narrow nasal passages and glottis. Abundant secretions and a large tongue may be expected, and hypertrophied tonsils and adenoids and other pathologic lesions are often superimposed.

There are important differences in the structural relationships in the airway of the infant as compared with the adult. As noted by Eckenhoff (1951), the larynx of the newborn is more cephalad, the rima glottidis lying opposite the interspace of the fourth and fifth vertebrae. In addition, the vocal cords slant upward and backward because of approximation of the hyoid to the thyroid cartilage. The structure of the epiglottis is characteristically narrow and omega-shaped (Ω) (see Fig. 8-7), and the loose areolar tissue of the glottis makes it especially susceptible to the formation of edema simply as a result of overhydration.

The actual dimensions of the respiratory tract are of importance. The findings of Engel (1947) were summarized and tabulated by Hall (1955), as shown in Table 2-3. Further details are given in Chapters 3 and 8.

Eckenhoff (1951) has emphasized Engel's finding that the narrowest area of the upper respiratory tract may be at the cricoid ring rather than at the rima glottidis (Fig. 2-9). Since the cricoid forms an enclosed ring, it is the only nonexpansile structure of the upper airway. Like Eckenhoff and Colgan and Keats (1957), I have encountered several situations where an endotracheal tube that passed the vocal cords would not pass through the cricoid ring. Nearly all of these cases occurred in children who had several congenital anomalies, especially those involving craniofacial dysostosis (Crouzon's disease and Apert's syndrome).

Details of the anatomic structure of the lower respiratory tract more closely related to physiology are described in Chapter 3. Among many important features, two that have been of special interest to pediatric anesthesiologists are the relationship of anatomic dead space to the size of the growing child and the proportion of alveolar surface area to body surface area. The relationship of anatomic dead space to lean body weight has been widely accepted as being the same throughout normal development. This relationship is 1 ml of dead space per pound of body weight. The relationship of alveolar surface area to body surface area has been less easily determined, and different views have been entertained. Belief that infants had proportionately greater alveolar surface area and greater alveolar ventilation was accepted by some and used as an explanation for more

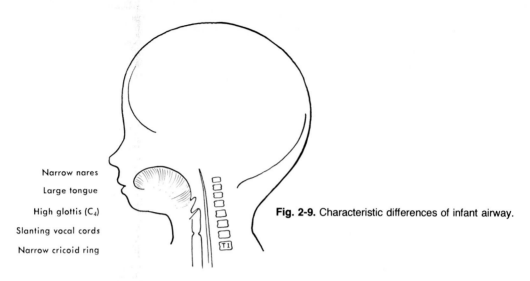

Narrow nares

Large tongue

High glottis (C₄)

Slanting vocal cords

Narrow cricoid ring

Fig. 2-9. Characteristic differences of infant airway.

rapid uptake of gaseous anesthetics. However, work of Dunnill (1962) and of Hogg and associates (1970) gives more conclusive evidence that the relationship of air-tissue interface to body surface area remains the same throughout the period of growth.

Central and autonomic nervous systems

Tremendous differences between infant, child, and adult obviously are seen in the responses of the central nervous system. Anatomic differences are easily recognized but not easy to interpret.

The brain of the neonate is relatively large, weighing 350 grams (as compared with 1350 grams in the adult). The external aspect shows obvious lack of development of cortical sulci (Arey, 1944), and the cellular structure shows very meager distribution of functioning elements, even when compared with an infant only 6 months old (Conel, 1939).

The myelination of nerve tracts has been studied carefully, because it was formerly believed that function depended on myelination (McGraw, 1943; Langworthy, 1933). Although this view is now questioned, function and myelination are known to be closely associated in many areas. Myelination of sensory nerve tracts of the spine is complete at birth, whereas that of the motor nerve tracts is not complete until the child is about 2

years old (Thomas, 1952). In the fiber tracts of the brain, myelination progresses more slowly, gradually extending through the connecting areas of the midbrain and the reticular system. It is believed that the process continues until middle life.

Of some interest to those using spinal anesthesia in infants is consideration of the level to which the spinal cord extends in the dural sheath. At birth it extends to the third lumbar vertebra, and by the time the child is 1 year old the cord has assumed its permanent position, ending at the first lumbar vertebra (Gray, 1973).

Hassan and Williams (1973) injected radiopaque material into the epidural space of neonates and found that it extended to L-4; the material then filled the inferior vena cava and the pelvic and hepatic veins, thus demonstrating an easy route of escape for drugs intended for epidural use in infants.

From a functional standpoint, a characteristic of infant physiology is variability and lack of control, as seen in respiration, muscular activity, and temperature regulation. Much of this instability may be traced to inadequate neurologic function, the result of either incomplete anatomic development of nerve pathways or lack of functional experience in neuromuscular coordination (Nelson and others, 1975).

At what age is an infant able to feel pain?

This is a matter of considerable practical interest to the anesthesiologist, and controversy still exists as to whether a neonate needs anesthesia, be it for circumcision or craniotomy (Weiss, 1968; Smith and Smith, 1972). Anatomically, sensory organs are present, and stimuli can be carried to the thalamus and will initiate motor retraction responses. Corticothalamic association is poorly developed, however, and the neonate probably simulates the lobotomized patient who may state that he feels pain but shows no displeasure. McGraw (1943), investigating the infant's reaction to noxious stimuli, found that some neonates showed no response at all to pinprick and, when stimulated by electric current, required twice as much current as infants 1 month old. In the light of present uncertainty, it is generally agreed that anesthesia should be provided for surgical patients of all ages but should not be undertaken by unskilled personnel.

In contrast to the central nervous system, the infant's autonomic nervous system is extremely well developed at birth. As noted by Dekaban (1959), "at 1 day of age the infant can yawn, sneeze and cough as well as a college senior." The question of vagal and sympathetic preponderance has been discussed. Although bradycardia is easily evoked by vagal stimulation, the increased peripheral vasoconstrictive tone that infants are believed to maintain suggests effective sympathetic activity.

The activity of baroreceptors has been studied in infancy (Moss and others, 1968), and normal responses have generally been obtained from birth onward, though duration of response may be limited.

There is evidence that rapid fatigability of nervous response is a characteristic of the child's general reaction. This may explain the child's short bursts of activity, his increased need of sleep, and his decreased tolerance to respiratory obstruction.

Respiratory physiology

It is of maximum importance for the anesthesiologist to be familiar with the role of respiratory function in oxygen uptake, carbon dioxide release, and acid-base and temperature control as well as the inhalation of anesthetics. Respiration in the child and especially in the infant shows remarkable variations and presents the anesthesiologist with innumerable problems. For a complete discussion of respiratory physiology in children, see Chapter 3.

Cardiovascular system

The infant starts life with a relatively large heart—30 grams in a 2500-gram neonate as compared with 300 grams in a 70-kg adult. X-ray studies show that the infant's heart is as wide as it is high, takes up half the lateral diameter of the chest, and appears considerably larger on expiration than on inspiration. Blood volume is approximately 85 ml/kg as compared with 65 ml/kg in adult males. The blood volume of a 2500-gram newborn would thus be 212.5 ml.

Immediately after birth, the cardiovascular system begins a series of complex changes that, although less extensive than those of respiration, do not end for several years. Born with a relative fluid overload (both extravascular and blood volume) and faced with sudden changes in pulmonary perfusion and pressure-volume-flow dynamics, even normal infants are subject to cardiac failure, which brings high mortality in neonates with congenital cardiac lesions (Nadas and Fyler, 1972).

The early closure of a ductus arteriosus, foramen ovale, and sinus venosus reduces the large initial alveolar-arterial oxygen gradient, but more subtle changes remain that are of interest to the anesthesiologist.

Heart rate and rhythm. "The younger the child, the faster the heart rate" is a commonly accepted rule in pediatrics. In a newborn, for instance, average heart rates are about 120 per minute with upper limits of normal at about 170 per minute (Table 2-4). This rate gradually decreases, so that by 4 years of age the average heart rate is under 100 per minute and by 10 years is 90 per minute. The anesthesiologist concerned with children, however, should be aware that slow heart rates, particularly in neonates, are more to

Table 2-4. Average pulse rate at different ages

Age	Lower limits of normal	Average	Upper limits of normal
Newborn	70	120	170
1-11 mo	80	120	160
2 yr	80	110	130
4 yr	80	100	120
6 yr	75	100	115
8 yr	70	90	110
10 yr	70	90	110

From Kaplan, S.: The cardiovascular system. In Nelson, W. B., editor: Textbook of pediatrics, ed. 7, Philadelphia, 1959, W. B. Saunders Co., p. 821.

Table 2-5. Normal blood pressure for various ages (Adapted from data in the literature. Figures have been rounded off to nearest decimal place.)

Ages	Mean systolic ±2 S.D.	Mean diastolic ±2 S.D.
Newborn	80 ± 16	46 ± 16
6 mos-1 year	89 ± 29	60 ± 10*
1 year	96 ± 30	66 ± 25*
2 years	99 ± 25	64 ± 25*
3 years	100 ± 25	67 ± 23*
4 years	99 ± 20	65 ± 20*
5-6 years	94 ± 14	55 ± 9
6-7 years	100 ± 15	56 ± 8
7-8 years	102 ± 15	56 ± 8
8-9 years	105 ± 16	57 ± 9
9-10 years	107 ± 16	57 ± 9
10-11 years	111 ± 17	58 ± 10
11-12 years	113 ± 18	59 ± 10
12-13 years	115 ± 19	59 ± 10
13-14 years	118 ± 19	60 ± 10

From Nadas, A. S., and Fyler, D. C.: Pediatric cardiology, ed. 3, Philadelphia, 1972, W. B. Saunders Co.
*In this study the point of muffling was taken as the diastolic pressure.

be feared than tachyarrhythmias. The newborn is said to have a predominance of vagal tone, and although this is a subject of some controversy, it is true that vagal stimulation in newborns results in very slow heart rates with low cardiac output. These bradyarrhythmias are precipitated by micturition, defecation, and surgical stimulation of vagal responses. In particular, tracheal intubation of the newborn may result in profound bradycardia, which the anesthesiologist must be prepared to correct with atropine. The sinus arrhythmias commonly seen in children are of little concern but do indicate absence of vagal inhibition in preoperative patients.

After atropinization, an infant's heart rate may increase to 170 to 190 before induction. This represents almost complete vagal release, and more atropine or the effect of subsequent anesthesia rarely results in further increase. Rates of 200 to 230 occasionally may be seen in infants without evident complications.

When children do develop tachyarrhythmia, most commonly it is paroxysmal atrial tachycardia. Unlike adults, however, the rates are very rapid, up to 400 per minute, and the young infant is capable of conducting this rapid rate from atrium to ventricle at a 1:1 ratio. The presence of such a fast heart rate, though often idiopathic, should suggest the possible presence of the Wolff-Parkinson-White syndrome or thyrotoxicosis. As shown by electrocardiograph, mild right ventricular

preponderance is normal until the child is about 6 months old.

Blood pressure. A child's blood pressure is slightly less than an adult's. At birth the systolic pressure is usually between 75 and 85 mm Hg and rises 5 to 10 mm Hg within 2 weeks (Nadas and Fyler, 1972). Table 2-5 shows average blood pressures for children. Diastolic pressures average 30% below systolic. Although the blood pressure of infants has been difficult to measure by standard methods, recently developed noninvasive technics are accurate and practical (p. 199).

The observation of blood pressure is actually of greater importance in infants than in adults, since there is less margin for error and infants develop both shock and overhydration more readily. Central venous pressure also is low at birth and gradually increases during early childhood (Fig. 2-10).

Myocardial contractility. The ability of the heart to contract is dependent both on the intrinsic properties of the cardiac muscle and on the ability of the autonomic nervous system to elicit from the heart a higher degree

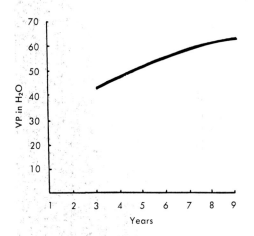

Fig. 2-10. Central venous pressure shows gradual increase during childhood. (From Burch, G. E.: A primer of venous pressure, Philadelphia, 1950, Lea & Febiger.)

of contractility at a given end-diastolic volume. Recent work has suggested that the newborn heart is not fully innervated with sympathetic fibers at birth and that, as such, it may not be as prepared to undergo stress as is the heart of a healthy adult (Friedman and others, 1968). This subject is not entirely clarified but should be kept in mind when dealing with neonates.

Congenital heart disease. The anesthesiologist's most frequent cause of concern in relation to the cardiovascular system in children is associated with congenital heart lesions. The response of the abnormal heart will be discussed in Chapter 16. It should be pointed out at this juncture, however, that any time there is a communication between the systemic and pulmonary circuits, as in an atrial or ventricular septal defect or with a patent ductus arteriosus, the key determinant of the physiology is the relationship between the pulmonary artery resistance and the systemic vascular resistance. Whether there is a right-to-left shunt and consequent cyanosis or a left-to-right shunt and resultant heart failure is not dependent on the size or location of the hole. Rather, it is dependent on the resistance to blood flow to the pulmonary artery or to the systemic vasculature. At birth, the pulmonary resistance is very high, but it de-

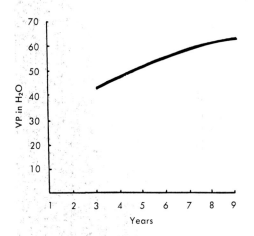 creases exponentially over the first month or two of life (Rudolph, 1961). It may rise, however, with the stress of surgery or with pulmonary problems after anesthesia, and an anesthesiologist should be aware of the dynamic nature of all cardiac shunts.

Red blood cells, hemoglobin, and oxygen transport. The fact that there is a reduction of the hemoglobin level between 3 months and 3 years of life is well known (Fig. 2-11) and has been the source of a long-standing dispute between surgeon and anesthesiologist concerning the safe minimum level for a patient undergoing anesthesia. The reason for the so-called anemia has never been determined. Iron deficiency and rapid growth have been ruled out, and more recently Card and Brain (1973) proposed hyperphosphatemia with resultant elevation of 2,3-diphosphoglycerate (2,3-DPG) level as the cause, although this was countered with the possibility that the increase in 2,3-DPG could also be the result of the anemia.

Whatever the cause, the changing relationships of the oxygen dissociation curve with age are important. During gestation, cord blood has greater affinity for oxygen than maternal blood. Fetal hemoglobin (HbF) differs in many respects from adult hemoglobin (HbA); it is more soluble and has appreciably less than the normal level of 2,3-DPG (Cooper and Hoagland, 1972; Nathan and Oski, 1974).

The resultant reduction of P_{50} and the shift to the left of the oxyhemoglobin dissociation curve were described by Morse and associates (1950). The changing proportions of HbF and HbA (Fig. 2-12) are paralleled by a shift to the right of the dissociation curve, which approximates the adult position ($P_{50} = 27$ mm Hg) at 4 to 6 months (Oski, 1973) and progresses considerably past it by 6 to 8 months. Oski (1973a) demonstrated that the elevated adenosine triphosphate (ATP) and 2,3-DPG levels persist throughout childhood and compensate so well for the reduced hemoglobin concentration that the oxygen delivery from 8 months to 18 years is practically unchanged (Table 2-6). The point is also made that anemia must be judged by its

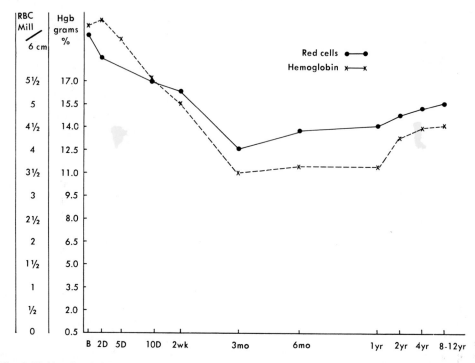

Fig. 2-11. Usual variation in hemoglobin and red blood cell count during infancy and childhood. (From Kaplan, S.: The cardiovascular system. In Nelson, W. E., editor: Textbook of pediatrics, ed. 7, Philadelphia, 1959, W. B. Saunders Co.)

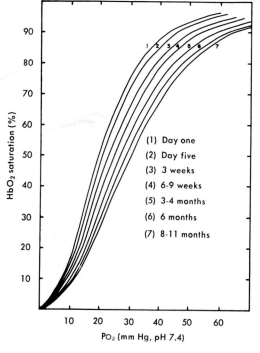

(1) Day one
(2) Day five
(3) 3 weeks
(4) 6-9 weeks
(5) 3-4 months
(6) 6 months
(7) 8-11 months

Fig. 2-12. Oxyhemoglobin equilibrium curve of blood from normal term infants at different postnatal ages. The P_{50} on day 1 is 19.4 ± 1.8 mm Hg and has shifted to 30.3 ± 0.7 at age 11 months (normal adults = 27.0 − 1.1 mm Hg). (From Oski, F. A.: Pediatrics **51:** 494, 1973. Copyright American Academy of Pediatrics 1973.)

20

Table 2-6. Oxygen unloading changes with age

Age	P_{50} (mm Hg)	Percent saturation at venous oxygen tension of 40 mm Hg	Hemoglobin (g/100 ml)	Oxygen unloaded* (ml/100 ml)
1 day	19.4	87	17.2	1.84
3 weeks	22.7	80	13.0	2.61
6-9 weeks	24.4	77	11.0	2.65
3-4 months	26.5	73	10.5	3.10
6 months	27.8	69	11.3	3.94
8-11 months	30.0	65	11.8	4.74
5-8 years	29.0†	67	12.6	4.73
9-12 years	27.9†	69	13.4	4.67
Adult	27.0	71	15.0	4.92

From Oski, F. A.: Designation of anemia on a functional basis, J. Pediatr. **83**:353, 1973.
*Assumes arterial oxygen saturation of 95%.
†Derived from data of Card and Brain; remainder of P_{50} as previously reported.

effect rather than by the number of red cells present. Because of compensatory factors, tissue hypoxia as evidenced by increased cardiac output, tachycardia, or elevated lactate/pyruvate ratio is rarely observed until hemoglobin concentration falls below 6 g/dl.

Energy metabolism

The rate of metabolic activity or oxygen consumption sets the patterns for many of the child's reactions to everyday life as well as to anesthesia, surgery, illness, and medical therapy. This pattern in the child is one of increased basal activity plus the capacity for further elevation in response to various stimuli.

Studies by Lewis and associates (1943) and Lee and Iliff (1956) at the University of Colorado have resulted in curves in which the maximal point is reached between 6 and 18 months of age (Fig. 2-13). The highest point in their mean curves for both boys and girls is approximately 58 calories/hr/m^2. After the first peak there is a gradual fall in metabolic rate until puberty is approached. Immediately before puberty there may be a definite rise in metabolic activity, with a postpubertal fall, but this deflection is not marked and may occur at any time between 11 and 15 years of age. A composite of several individual curves will consequently show a plateau effect instead of a prepubertal peak.

Basal oxygen requirements of the newborn are estimated to be approximately 6 ml/kg/min, and those of the adult 4 ml/kg/min (Cross and others, 1957). Considerable attention has been called to the correlation of basal oxygen consumption and surface area. Although it is true that surface area is a better guide to basal metabolic energy than age, height, or weight, it must be remembered that the child is seldom at basal conditions. Fever increases the oxygen requirement 7% per degree of temperature elevation, illness and emotion add further need, and muscular activity may raise it an additional 300% to 400%. The situation fluctuates widely from day to day and from moment to moment, depending on the state of health or the state of mind of the child. This characteristic variability makes it practically impossible to gauge body needs by any fixed measurement of age, weight, or even body surface, since none of these factors changes with temperature, shock, or excitement. In general, it may be assumed that during childhood relatively larger doses of sedatives will be required in view of elevated basal metabolism, but fluid and nutritional needs must be estimated very largely on a short-term basis, with greatest reliance on changing clinical signs.

Liver

Under normal circumstances the liver is the source of many of the infant's characteristically different responses to drugs, foods,

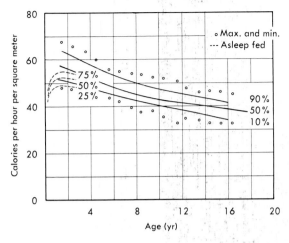

Fig. 2-13. Basal metabolic activity in boys from birth to 21 years of age. Broken lines indicate studies on infants fed and asleep; solid lines show studies done on children in a fasting, awake condition. (Unpublished graph courtesy Dr. Alberta Iliff, Child Research Council, University of Colorado School of Medicine, Denver, Colo.)

and foreign substances. As already described in detail, there is great diversity in the maturation of enzyme systems, with resultant inability to metabolize such compounds as bilirubin and chloramphenicol for several weeks after birth.

In the application of standard liver function tests to infants, Yudkin and Gellis (1949) found sulfobromophthalein sodium (Bromsulphalein) excretion to be delayed at birth but found no measurable difference in other functions.

During most of life, the profusion of metabolic processes that are continually in progress in the liver make it the seat of greatest oxygen demand and greatest heat production. As shown by Holliday (1971), however, the brain is the site of greatest oxygen utilization until the infant is approximately 3 months old.

The response of the liver to infection is rather remarkable. Children of school age have an extremely high incidence of infectious hepatitis (both A and B), with very low mortality. However, children appear to be almost totally immune to halothane hepatitis, if there is such an entity.

In relation to anesthesia and surgery, the liver poses tremendous problems. Whether for excision of cysts or tumors, for repair of ruptured liver, or for transplantation, most hepatic surgery involves the danger of profuse and/or uncontrollable hemorrhage (see Chapter 17).

Kidney

Respiratory and cardiac adjustments may appear dramatic at the moment of birth, but those of kidney function and fluid metabolism are of fundamental and increasing importance. Expanding interest in this field has brought forth voluminous literature and considerable confusion. Several disputed areas are of immediate practical concern to anesthesiologists, especially maturation of the infant kidney, related hazards of overyhydration and underhydration, the infant's sodium tolerance, and the possible danger of rapid changes in serum osmolality.

Although much uncertainty exists concerning the development of the kidney, important anatomic and physiologic data have been obtained. Pioneer work of Darrow and Yannet (1935), McCance (1950), and Barnett and Vesterdahl (1953), descriptions of the functional development of the kidney by Rubin and associates (1949), Edelmann (1967), and McCrory (1972), and discussions of total body fluids by Holliday and Segar (1957) and Metcoff (1968) stand out as especially valuable.

These and other sources are drawn on freely in the following paragraphs and in greater detail in Chapter 25.

The question of renal maturation. Great emphasis has been placed on establishing the age at which the child's kidneys should be considered "mature." Some uncertainty has come from the fact that answers to this question have varied from the first week of life to the twentieth year. Much of the confusion could be resolved by defining the term *mature*, which obviously has been used with widely different intent but which at this point may be divided into anatomic and functional aspects.

Anatomic maturation. Gross comparison of the neonatal and adult kidneys shows the combined weight of both infant kidneys to be 20 to 30 grams and of both adult kidneys to be 300 grams. Although the neonate's kidney contains the full number of glomeruli (1 to 1.25 million per kidney), Fetterman and associates (1965) have shown that the individual glomerulus continues to grow; the mean diameter at birth is 110 mm and 20 years later is 280 mm.

Nephrons show pronounced lack of uniformity at birth. Juxtamedullary glomeruli develop before cortical glomeruli, producing a heterogeneity that persists until the child is 12 to 14 years old. Because of the more rapid development of glomeruli as compared with corresponding proximal tubules, a condition of glomerulotubular imbalance is produced, the glomeruli remaining dominant throughout childhood and adolescence.

It can be seen that the kidneys do not attain their final fixed internal structural relationships and external growth until the body is full grown. Anatomic maturity may be judged on this basis, on cytologic development, or on other factors. The popular concept appears to be that the kidney is anatomically mature by 2 weeks after birth, when nephrons and vasculature are completely formed, although they have not assumed their final size or proportion.

Functional maturation. Most of the confusion about renal immaturity has concerned function. Numerous measurements of discrete functions of the kidney have been carried out. According to tests originally used, which were devised for the adult kidney, the neonatal kidney did poorly, and the concept was firmly established that the infant kidney was immature (McCance, 1950). The specific features most often termed immature have been (1) inability to excrete large water loads rapidly, (2) inability to excrete sodium loads, (3) inability to concentrate urine, (4) inability to excrete excess acid, and (5) reduced glomerular permeability. Although the existence of these deficiencies is still being asserted in authoritative texts, each of the impugned functions has been reevaluated and its significance questioned, reduced, or eliminated. Before accepting traditional concepts, one must bear in mind these considerations:

1. Most evaluations of renal function in infants vary widely with different standards of reference (see below).
2. Many values of renal function suggesting reduced efficiency at birth can be partially explained by unfavorable conditions associated with neonatal existence, such as lower blood pressure, high fluid intake, and low urea-producing content of diet.
3. Any concept of incompetence of infant kidneys must be weighed against their obvious adequacy in meeting the particular demands placed on them.
4. Although the capability of the normal infant's kidney probably has been underrated, the highly variable performance of the neonatal kidney suggests danger of exaggerated disturbance in the presence of acute or chronic illness.

Difficulty in finding a suitable standard of reference has been a major problem in evaluating infant renal function, especially when one compares it with the function of the adult kidney. Standards employed have included body surface area, body weight, age, total body water, and kidney size. Although the best standard for one function may be relatively poor for another, an attempt has been made to find a single standard by which to evaluate all. Comparison on the basis of 1.73 m² body surface area (BSA) as suggested by

Table 2-7. Comparison of renal function in infants and children with that in adults. All values are corrected to 1.73 m² SA

Age*	Number of cases	GFR (C$_{IN}$) ml/min	Percent of adult	C$_{PAH}$ ml/min	Percent of adult	Tm$_{PAH}$ mg/min	Percent of adult	Tm$_{GLUCOSE}$ mg/min	Percent of adult
Newborn	43	26 ± 1.7	21	88 ± 4.2	13				
3 days old	26	36 ± 3.9	30	134 ± 14.3	24				
1-2 weeks	6	54 ± 8.0	44						
P: 1-2 weeks	6	50 ± 10.0	40	154 ± 34	24	13 ± 6	17	70.6 ± 19.6	19
P: 1-2 months	9					16.1 ± 5.2	20	105.3 ± 27.2	28
2-4 months	9	56 ± 10.0	44	234 ± 50	36	24 ± 15	30	170 ± 5‡	45
P: 2-5 months	6	68 ± 21.0	55	222 ± 60	34	51 ± 20 M†	64		
6 months-1 year	6	77 ± 14.0	62	352 ± 73	54	66 ± 19 M	82		
1-3 years	6	96 ± 22.0	77	537 ± 122	80	65 ± 24 M	81		
3-8 years	8	131 ± 26	105	659 ± 115	101	77 ± 20 M	96		
8-14 years	13	120 ± 20	96	631 ± 98	96				
20-40 years									
Male		125 ± 19	100	655 ± 98	100	80 ± 12	100	375 ± 56	100
Female		110 ± 17	100	570 ± 86	100	77 ± 11	100	303 ± 45	100

From Rubin, M. I., Bruck, E., and Rapoport, M.: Maturation of renal function in childhood; clearance studies, J. Clin. Invest. **28:**1144, 1949.
*P, prematurely born.
†M, mannitol used to measure GFR.
‡Two observations.

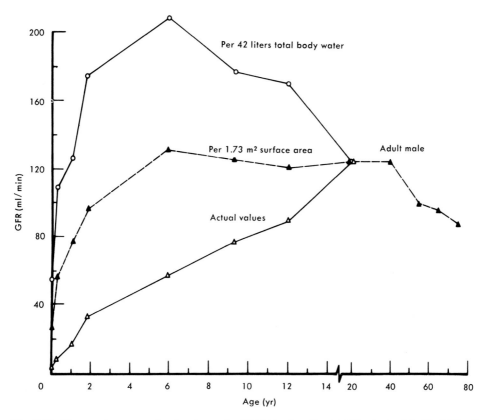

Fig. 2-14. Changes in mean value for glomerular filtration rate with age (△), when related to 1.73 m² surface area (▲) and when related to 42 liters of body water (○). (From McCrory, W. W.: Developmental nephrology, Cambridge, 1972, Harvard University Press.)

Rubin and associates (1949) and shown in Table 2-7 has been favored by many, and McCrory (1972) even stated, "it is now the custom to express all measurements of renal function by correcting values to 1.73 m² BSA." However, one still finds other methods in use. An example of the problem is seen in Fig. 2-14, which shows, in assessment of glomerular filtration, how much the result depends on the standard employed.

The important function of glomerular filtration has been found by all tests to be reduced at birth. This has been explained by Gruskin and associates (1968) and by Assali and associates (1968) as being due to increased resistance of afferent renal arteries; this resistance is reversed by vasodilation shortly after birth.

Although reduced efficiency in water excretion could be explained by decreased glo-

merular filtration, other factors involved include cardiac output, blood pressure, and hormonal influences (antidiuretic hormone and aldosterone).

Janovski and associates (1965) and Edelmann and associates (1966) have shown that when the neonate is presented with a testing load of water, he can excrete it but requires a significantly longer time to do it. Although it is conceded that a 6-week-old infant manages a high intake of fluid remarkably well, it was nicely shown in the work of Ames (1953) that this function develops rapidly but at birth is definitely reduced (Fig. 2-15). All this would seem to imply that there is a greater risk of overhydration for at least 2 weeks after birth.

Our understanding of the infant's ability to control sodium excretion has been confused by misinterpretation of investigative find-

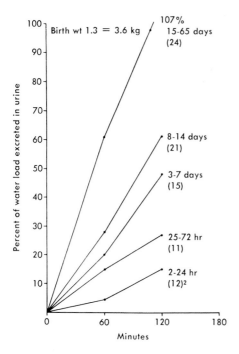

Fig. 2-15. Comparison of water excreted by various age groups following intravenous administration of 2.5% glucose, 30 ml/kg body weight, given at approximately −10 to 0 min. Figures in parentheses indicate the number of patients in each group. (From Ames, R. G.: Pediatrics **12**:272, 1953. Copyright American Academy of Pediatrics 1953.)

ings, by interplay between antidiuretic hormone, aldosterone, and the kidneys, and by intrarenal sodium-potassium exchange.

The studies of Dean and McCance (1949), using salt loads equivalent to those used with adults, implied that infants do not tolerate salt. Clinical errors involving serious consequences of saline overdosage confirmed the concept and led to strict limitation of saline solution during the operative period.

Subsequent investigation by Giebisch (1969), Edelmann (1967), and Greenberg and associates (1967), using modified methods of evaluation, indicated that the infant kidney is able to respond to moderate changes in sodium ingestion and that 6-day-old infants react normally to exogenous aldosterone. McLean and Paulsen (1958) and Bennett and associates (1971) have further reported that during the stress of the operative period, infants tend to lose rather than retain sodium. The ability of the neonate to excrete initial excess

sodium is also used as evidence of early renal competence.

In McCrory's detailed discussion of this problem (1972), he concluded that except for relatively low glomerular filtration rate (GFR), the newborn kidney function appears adequate for excretion of usual sodium requirements. He also stated that infants retain excess sodium, with resultant danger of acute expansion of extracellular fluid (ECF) volume, edema, and hypernatremia.

The neonate can dilute urine to 50 mOsm/kg, thereby equalling the adult. Under usual circumstances his concentrating power is markedly restricted, a maximum of 400 mOsm/kg, comparing poorly with the 1200 mOsm/kg attained by the adult. Part of the difference can be explained by lack of urea-forming solids in the infant diet. Any reduction of concentrating power reduces the infant's ability to retain fluids in the face of dehydration. It is extremely fortunate that in spite of the small infant's decreased protection against development of dehydration, renal failure, so lethal to adults, very rarely occurs in children.

Limited excretion of excess acid, due to either reduced bicarbonate resorption or failure to secrete hydrogen ions, has been thought to be a weakness of the infant, but in both cases the fault appears to be due to environmental or adaptive factors, with little significant hazard to the child.

There is definite reduction of glomerular permeability at birth; the infant allows passage of dextran molecules with a molecular weight of no more than 15,000, whereas passage of those having a molecular weight of 50,000 is possible in the adult. Similar limitation of excretion of various therapeutic agents, including ampicillin and other antibiotics, is of importance.

Measurements of renal blood flow (RBF) and tubular resorption of glucose and phosphate suggest varying degrees of immaturity depending on the standard employed for evaluation, but levels similar to those of adults are usually attained between 3 months and 2 years of age.

After their investigation of the situation,

Strauss and associates (1965) concluded that there were so many variables that it was impossible to generalize about renal function in the neonate. Although this view is justified, it seems possible to pick out several tendencies that appear to predominate.

The infant kidney seems to show definite functional limitations for the first 2 to 4 weeks of life, during which time the margin for error in therapy is reduced. After this period, normal infants tolerate a considerably wider range of therapeutic assault, but infants with any form of renal impairment will continue to be easy prey to injudicious treatment. Therapeutic aspects of fluid therapy are discussed in Chapter 25. To specify any single point at which the kidney should be termed mature, without more exact definition of the term, does not seem reasonable.

External controlling factors that affect renal function, notably aldosterone and antidiuretic hormone (ADH), though present at birth, play somewhat unpredictable roles in neonatal fluid balance.

Threatened with large amounts of sodium or water, infants seem to tolerate salt and actually have difficulty in retaining it, possibly as a manifestation of inappropriate ADH stimulation. Overhydration is more difficult for the neonate to survive, however, because of renal vascular resistance that prevents glomerular exposure and promotes hypervolemia.

Fluid and electrolyte metabolism

Among the essential differences between adult and child, that of total fluid metabolism is of primary importance. This subject is discussed in detail in Chapter 25. Fluid requirement follows a pattern similar to that of oxygen requirement, being minimal at birth, accelerating rapidly to a maximum between 9 and 18 months of age, and then gradually receding throughout childhood and adult life. The increased rate of fluid metabolism that exists throughout childhood plays a large part in causing the greater danger of both dehydration and fluid excess.

The tendency to generalize about the fluid requirements of patients of different age

groups has led to acceptance of dangerous concepts. Because of the rapid changes that occur and the variation in their time of appearance, as well as the unknown influences of different diseases, *a highly individualized approach must be employed in all problems of fluid management.*

Metabolic response to anesthesia and surgery

The child's metabolic response to anesthesia and surgery has been said to differ in several respects from that of the adult, but the varied conditions of separate investigations have led to some confusion. Bunker and associates (1952) found that infants and dogs developed slight metabolic acidosis during ether anesthesia, whereas adults did not. Graff and associates (1964) and Reynolds (1966) found no acidosis, possibly because they used nonrebreathing technics.

Extensive studies of carbohydrate metabolism show that adults develop hyperglycemia, increases in glucogenic hormones, plasma insulin, adrenalin, cortisol, and growth hormone, and lactic acidemia (Oyama, 1973) in response to ether, but show none of these effects with halothane or thiopental relaxant mixtures. Watson (1972) measured blood glucose in children more than 2 years old and found no increase during nitrous oxide relaxant technics, nor did Clarke (1970) and Black and Rea (1964) using methoxyflurane. Patients were not subjected to significant stresses in any of these studies.

The metabolic reaction of infants during and after surgery has been measured by meticulous procedures but again with varied results. Rickham (1957) was convinced by his work that neonates showed less potassium loss after surgery than adults, as well as decreased incidence of ileus and shortened catabolic phase. McLean and Paulsen (1958) observed the primary difference to be absence of water or sodium retention. Knutrud (1965), repeating the investigations of Rickham with a more extensive plan, was unable to find any real difference in the infant's potassium response when compared with that of the adult.

Many pediatric surgeons have upheld the concept that the infant is a better surgical risk in the first 48 hours of life than in the next 51 weeks (Rickham, 1957; Gross, 1953). Most authors give credit to maternal steroids for this supposed advantage. Although it is obviously better to operate on seriously ill neonates at once, there are several reasons why a normal child should be stronger when a month old than at birth. Kidneys can perform more effectively, liver enzymes have become more active, the danger of respiratory distress syndrome is past, the dangers of retrolental fibroplasia and intracranial hemorrhage are reduced or eliminated, and cardiac lesions, if present, are less apt to be unrecognized.

In several thousand operations at The Children's Hospital Medical Center on patients under 1 year old, survival rates show no support for the concept of reduced viability of older infants. In relation to this, one could point to the apparent reduction of stamina in infants of caesarean birth. Unstressed by labor, their mothers undoubtedly provided them with less steroid.

In the responses of glucose-insulin-epinephrine(or norepinephrine)-glucagon, the infant has a lower fasting blood glucose level, and at birth the adrenal gland produces little or no epinephrine, the entire catechol output consisting of norepinephrine (West and others, 1951) that is produced by the organs of Zuckerkandl along the sympathetic chain. Adrenals are oversized at birth but have little functional use (Lanman, 1953; Klein, 1954).

Although preoperative restriction of food and fluid has been criticized, measurement by Watson (1972) of fasting blood glucose level before operation in children 2 years and over showed hypoglycemic levels to be rare. Smith and Chandra (1973) found similar results in infants under 2 years.

Increasing evidence of the importance of fatty acid metabolism led Talbert and associates (1967) to study the response of infants to surgical stress by measurement of fatty acids and catecholamines. They found that plasma free fatty acids were consistently increased following the minor stress of bilateral inguinal herniorrhaphy, whereas neither epinephrine nor norepinephrine increased significantly. This greater sensitivity of fatty acid concentration as a measure of stress is also seen in adults.

Filler and Das (1971) implanted a pH electrode in muscle to study reactions of infants during operation and recovery. Results show that changes at tissue levels are more rapid and more intense than is suggested by serum levels.

Specific disorders of metabolic response to anesthesia are of considerable concern, especially those of malignant hyperthermia (p. 593) and potassium flux (p. 258).

The foregoing observations can be summarized as follows. From a strictly metabolic point of view, the young infant does not appear to show clearly defined differences from the adult. Immature kidneys and enzyme systems alter response to stress and drugs. The neonate does not develop his own steroids for several weeks, and his sympathetic nervous system response is chiefly activated by norepinephrine rather than epinephrine (West and others, 1951).

Temperature regulation

The regulation of body heat is another function that has exaggerated responses during childhood. Temperature regulation is of special interest at present for several reasons: (1) loss of body temperature is a constant concern during routine infant surgery (Roe, 1966; Smith, 1973), (2) induced profound hypothermia has become an integral part of cardiac surgery in neonates (Mohri and others, 1969), and (3) in older children, especially those with preexisting fever or in overheated environments, there is danger of hyperthermic reactions (see Chapter 26).

During fetal existence, body temperature is maintained approximately 0.5° C above that of the mother (Adamsons and Towell, 1965). At birth it is normal for the infant's rectal temperature to fall when conditions are ideal, which are believed to be a room temperature of 32° to 34° C, relative humidity of 50%, and air velocity not greater than 5 cm/sec.

At birth the infant is homeothermic and possesses a number of heat-controlling mechanisms. His normal heat production or basal metabolic activity, measured and expressed in oxygen consumption, is 6 ml of O_2/kg/min. Heat loss, like that of older persons, occurs chiefly through radiation and convection, each of which accounts for approximately 50% of the total. Under usual circumstances, heat loss through conduction is almost negligible in humans. The importance of radiant heat loss is rather striking. An infant lying uncovered in a room heated to 85° F will lose heat by radiation to a black wall 15 feet distant (Silverman, 1962).

Neonatal response to cold stress. When exposed to a cool environment, infants lose heat rapidly because of greater surface area and lack of protective subcutaneous tissue. The protective mechanism of vasoconstriction is present from birth, but shivering, although it has been observed, is seldom an effective heat-producing mechanism. Two possible mechanisms for nonshivering thermogenesis have been discovered in the neonate. In 1957 Moore and Underwood suggested that norepinephrine could be a factor in neonatal thermogenesis. It has been known that norepinephrine plays a more important role than epinephrine in neonatal life. Stern and associates (1965) showed that catechol response in neonates exposed to

cold consisted chiefly of norepinephrine release (Fig. 2-16), but the mechanism by which it increases heat production has not been completely defined. It may involve acceleration of carbohydrate and lipid metabolism, increased cardiovascular work, or increased neuromuscular activity. The catecholamines appear to be intimately involved in temperature regulation at all ages. In older persons, it has been observed that shivering is inhibited by anesthetic agents that stimulate catechol excretion but that it is prominent with agents such as thiopental and halothane, which do not evoke adrenocortical response. Injection of epinephrine or norepinephrine into the cerebral ventricles reduces body temperature, whereas administration of 5-hydroxytryptamine raises the temperature, probably by action on hypothalamic thermoregulation centers (Feldberg and Myers, 1964).

The second heat-producing mechanism in neonates is thought to exist in the brown adipose tissue known to have an essential role in hibernating animals. Johansson (1959), Joel (1965), and Aherne and Hull (1964) demonstrated that infants possess a specialized layer of adipose tissue distributed along the spine, nape of the neck, axillae, and perirenal area and that it has an increased vascular, nervous, and mitochondrial content, which in turn holds a high concentration of norepi-

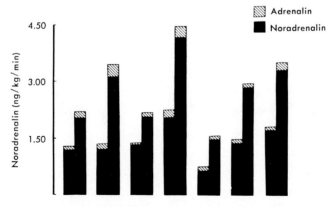

Fig. 2-16. Mechanism of infant response to cold. Chart shows urinary catecholamine levels of infants at normal temperature, paired with response after cooling. Note that norepinephrine (noradrenalin) is a major factor at normal temperature and plays a predominant role in response to cooling. (From Stern, L., Lees, M. H., and Leduc, J.: Pediatrics **36**:367, 1965. Copyright American Academy of Pediatrics 1965.)

nephrine (Fig. 2-17). This tissue has a high oxygen requirement and is believed to play an important part in heat production in the newborn.

In studying the thermal factors that influence the neonate, Adamsons and Towell (1965) found that rectal temperature and oxygen consumption have no correlation (Fig. 2-18). An infant with a rectal temperature of 36° C might have the same oxygen consumption if the temperature rose to 38° C. On the other hand, a very close correlation was found between oxygen consumption and the difference between rectal temperature and

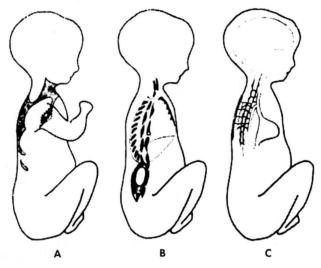

Fig. 2-17. Brown adipose tissue in superficial, **A,** and deep, **B,** sites in the newborn. **C,** Diagrammatic representation of venous drainage from the interscapular pad. (From Aherne, W., and Hull, D.: Proc. R. Soc. Med. **57:**1172, 1964.)

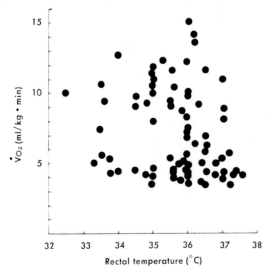

Fig. 2-18. Relationship of oxygen requirement to rectal temperature. Complete lack of correlation is obvious. (From Adamsons, K., Jr., Gandy, G. M., and James, L. S.: J. Pediatr. **66:**495, 1965.)

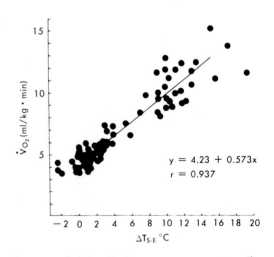

$$y = 4.23 + 0.573x$$
$$r = 0.937$$

Fig. 2-19. Relationship between oxygen consumption and the temperature gradient between skin temperature and environment of mature human newborns with varying deep body and skin temperatures. (From Adamsons, K., Jr., Gandy, G. M., and James, L. S.: J. Pediatr. **66:**495, 1965.)

skin temperature, suggesting that peripheral receptors have much to do with body temperature control, actually more than the hypothalamic centers (Fig. 2-19).

Using gradient calorimetry, Benzinger (1969) has produced conflicting evidence that suggests that sweating and vasodilation are stimulated not by skin temperature but by temperature of blood reaching an anterior thalamic center and that cooling is caused by inhibitory responses travelling from skin to a posterior thalamic center.

Employing similar methods, Ryan and associates (1973) measured total body oxygen consumption in hypothermic infants under halothane anesthesia. Their finding of a twofold increase in oxygen utilization at lower temperatures is an interesting departure from traditional concepts. Although infants were known to lose heat readily during anesthesia and operation, it had been commonly believed that anesthesia would prevent increased oxygen demand during initial cooling.

Older children show greater tendency toward hyperthermic responses during anesthesia. While less frequently seen than the hypothermia of infants, it signifies the presence of a pathologic rather than a physiologic response and carries greater mortality. The management of hyperthermia is discussed in Chapter 26.

PATHOLOGIC DIFFERENCES

In pediatrics as elsewhere, pathology is inseparably related to anatomy and physiology, as the terms histopathology and pathophysiology imply. The addition of growth and growth disturbances increases the complexity of the approaches involved. Special activity in these areas is currently focused on sorting out chromosomal disorders with the hope of early diagnosis or prevention, on controlling neoplastic disease, and on developing immunologic technics for disease prevention and tissue transplantation. Although discussion of these aspects is not possible here, all carry important practical applications and deserve individual inquiry.

For the anesthesiologist, the many important differences seen in pediatric pathology may be divided into (1) conditions that are seen predominantly in infancy and childhood, and (2) differences in the characteristic response of the young to illness and disease.

Lesions confined to infancy and childhood

Many pathologic entities that are incompatible with life are known only to pathologists and neonatologists, but others that are fatal in childhood are also known by pediatricians. Extreme prematurity, in itself a type of pathologic condition, absence of vital organs, and combinations of multiple severe defects of brain, heart, intestine, or kidney contribute heavily to the high mortality of the newborn. After one loses a battle to save the life of a small infant, a list of the autopsy findings such as those shown below impresses one with not only the futility but the misdirection of such efforts.

AUTOPSY FINDINGS IN A REPRESENTATIVE NEONATAL DEATH (ONE INFANT)

Left diaphragmatic hernia via foramen of Bochdalek associated with hypoplasia of left lung and left main bronchus
Imperforate anus with rectourethral fistula
Horseshoe kidney
Tetralogy of Fallot
Ventricular septal defect
Patent ductus arteriosus
Atrial septal defect, secundum
Bicuspid pulmonary valve
Agenesis of gallbladder and cystic duct
Solitary hepatic cyst
Urethral obstruction
Low birth weight (2.2 kg)
Bilateral hydrocele
Testicular hypoplasia
Acute renal tubular necrosis
Early neuronal necrosis of pons, cerebellum, and mesencephalon

During infancy and childhood, the pathologic conditions vary from the common hypertrophied tonsils, club feet, and strabismus to the less familiar mucopolysaccharidoses and gastroschisis or the relatively rare cri du chat syndrome. To those working in pediatric centers it soon becomes evident that the number of "rare defects" is infinite. Hecht and Lovrien (1970) list 200 diseases related to heredity alone. Thus, although a single syndrome may be seen only once or twice in a lifetime, there is such an endless variety that three or four different ones may appear on the operating schedule each day. One learns to recognize a few by name and should have recourse to information concerning others. In this regard, it is good to have at hand not only standard pediatric texts but those of a more specific nature such as *Pathology of the Fetus and the Infant* by Potter and Craig (1975), *Congenital Malformations* by Warkany (1971), and the very helpful text by Katz and Kadis entitled *Anesthesia and Uncommon Diseases* (1973).

Although any attempt even to classify the important pediatric diseases would be futile here, a few that have particular importance to the anesthesiologist are listed below. These include not only such defects as the Pierre Robin and Treacher Collins syndromes, in which the threat of airway obstruction is obvious, but those such as Turner's, Marfan's, Hurler's, and Wilson's syndromes that carry, in addition to an obvious external defect, a more significant, ominous, underlying lesion of heart, kidneys, or other organs.

PATHOLOGIC LESIONS CHARACTERISTIC OF CHILDREN

Prematurity

Congenital anomalies
Harelip, cleft palate
Pierre Robin syndrome
Treacher Collins syndrome
Choanal atresia
Esophageal atresia
Diaphragmatic hernia
Omphalocele
Hirschsprung's disease
Cystic hygroma
Sacrococcygeal teratoma
Imperforate anus
Prune belly
Double ureters
Myelomeningocele
Encephalocele

Inborn errors of lipid, carbohydrate, and amino acid metabolism

Growth disorders
Arachnodactyly
Spondylolisthesis

Osteogenesis imperfecta
Craniosynostosis
Chondrodystrophy
Hunter-Hurler syndrome

Tumors, hormonal disorders, and diseases of endocrine and autonomic nervous systems
Wilms' tumor
Neuroblastoma
Adrenogenital syndrome
Fanconi syndrome
Niemann-Pick disease
Familial dysautonomia

Not only may one be ignorant of the significance of an unusual syndrome, but in children there is an increased possibility of overlooking its presence completely. If the complicating disease is directly related to the intended operation, as it would be in removal of nasal polyps from a child with cystic fibrosis, its presence could hardly be missed. However, if a child who is scheduled for an orthodontic procedure has a totally unrelated condition such as adrenogenital syndrome or dysautonomia, the greater problem could easily go unrecognized by both surgeon and anesthetist.

It should be emphasized that although exotic eponyms may worry the unsophisticated anesthetist, even in the most erudite surroundings a runny nose, loose teeth, large tonsils, full stomach, and slightly low hematocrit are the most troublesome pathologic lesions encountered in pediatric surgical patients.

Characteristic response of children to illness

Clement Smith (1976) pointed out that newborns have poorly defined responses to insult or illness. In the presence of pneumonia or peritonitis they may show little reaction in the way of temperature elevation or leukocytosis. This view does not imply that infants are particularly weak but that their response is different. We have already presented the surgeon's opinion that the neonate tolerates surgery better than the older infant.

The typical pattern of response to illness reverses itself as infants grow in strength and activity; an exaggerated reaction to infection and disease becomes apparent in rapid temperature elevation, leukocytosis, and high pulse and respiratory rates, with increased incidence of vomiting, convulsions, and similar manifestations. These rapid and extreme fluctuations are characteristic of most infants over 1 month old.

The intensity of many individual diseases differs in relation to the patient's age and metabolic activity. Neoplastic lesions that grow slowly in adults may spread with alarming speed in children; on the other hand, sacrococcygeal teratomas are usually benign if removed before the third month of the child's life, whereas those removed at later dates are increasingly malignant (Gross, 1953). The severity and complications of childhood diabetes are far greater than when the disease develops later in life. Age seems to play a strange part in the incidence of postoperative tracheitis, which occurs with extreme rarity in neonates and adults but with some frequency in children between 1 and 10 years of age. Another age-related disparity is seen in relation to body fluids. Children become dehydrated much more rapidly than adults, but they rarely develop renal failure, a leading cause of operative morbidity in the adult.

BIBLIOGRAPHY

Adamsons, K., and Towell, M.: Thermal homeostasis in the fetus and newborn, Anesthesiology **26**:531, 1965.

Aherne, W., and Hull, D.: Section of pediatrics; site of heat production in the newborn infant, Proc. R. Soc. Med. **57**:1172, 1964.

Ames, R. G.: Urinary water excretion and neurohypophyseal function in full term and premature infants shortly after birth, Pediatrics **12**:272, 1953.

Aranda, J. B., Saheb, N., Stern, L., and Avery, M. E.: Arterial oxygen tension and retinal vasoconstriction in newborn infants, Am. J. Dis. Child. **122**:189, 1971.

Arey, L. B.: Developmental anatomy, Philadelphia, 1944, W. B. Saunders Co.

Assali, N. S., Bekey, G. A., and Morrison, L. W.: Fetal and neonatal circulation. In Assali, N. S., editor: Biology of gestation, vol. 2, New York, 1968, Academic Press, Inc., p. 51.

Azarnoff, D. L.: Use of pharmacokinetic principles in therapy, N. Engl. J. Med. **289**:635, 1973.

Barnett, H. L., and Vesterdahl, J.: The physiologic and clinical significance of immaturity of kidney function in young infants, J. Pediatr. **42**:99, 1953.

Bennett, E. J., Bowyer, D. E., and Jenkins, M. T.: Studies in aldosterone excretion of the neonate undergoing anesthesia and surgery, Anesth. Analg. (Cleve.) **50**:638, 1971.

Benzinger, J. H.: Clinical temperature; new physiological basis, J.A.M.A. **209**:1200, 1969.

Black, G. W., and Rea, J. L.: Effects of methoxyflurane (Penthrane) anaesthesia in children, Br. J. Anaesth. **36**:26, 1964.

Bothe, A., and Gladston, R.: The child's loss of consciousness; a psychiatric view of pediatric anesthesia, Pediatrics **50**:252, 1972.

Britt, B. A.: Malignant hyperthermia; a pharmacogenetic disease of skeletal and cardiac muscle, editorial, N. Engl. J. Med. **290**:1140, 1974.

Britt, B. A., and Kalow, W.: Malignant hyperthermia; aetiology unknown, Can. Anaesth. Soc. J. **17**:316, 1970.

Britt, B. A., Kalow, W., Gordon, A., and others: Malignant hyperthermia; an investigation of five patients, Can. Anaesth. Soc. J. **20**:431, 1973.

Brown, B. R., Jr., Watson, P. D., and Taussig, L. M.: Congenital metabolic disease of pediatric patients; anesthetic implications, Anesthesiology **43**:197, 1975.

Bunker, J. P., Brewster, W. R., Smith, R. M., and Beecher, H. K.: Metabolic effects of anesthesia in man. III. Acid-base balance in infants and children during anesthesia, J. Appl. Physiol. **5**:233, 1952.

Card, R. T., and Brain, M. C.: The "anemia" of childhood; evidence for a physiologic response to hyperphosphatemia, N. Engl. J. Med. **288**:388, 1973.

Cassell, S. E.: The psychologic responses of children to hospitalization and illness, Springfield, Ill., 1965, Charles C Thomas, Publisher.

Clark, R. E., Orkin, I. R., and Rovenstine, E. A.: Body temperature studies in anesthetized man; effect of environmental temperature, humidity, and anesthesia system, J.A.M.A. **154**:311, 1954.

Clarke, R. S. J.: The hyperglycaemic response to different types of surgery and anaesthesia, Br. J. Anaesth. **42**:45, 1970.

Cohen, E. N.: Patients with altered sensitivity. In Foldes, F. F., editor: Muscle relaxants, Philadelphia, 1966, F. A. Davis Co.

Cohen, S. N., and Weber, W. W.: Pharmacogenetics. In Symposium on pediatric pharmacology, Pediatr. Clin. North Am. **19**:31, 1972.

Colgan, F. J., and Keats, A. S.: Subglottic stenosis; a cause of difficult intubation, Anesthesiology **18**:265, 1957.

Conel, J. L.: The postnatal development of the human cerebral cortex, Cambridge, 1939, Harvard University Press.

Conney, A. H.: Pharmacological implications of microsomal enzyme induction, Pharmacol. Rev. **19**:317, 1967.

Cook, C. D., Sutherland, J. M., Segal, S., and others: Studies of respiratory physiology in the newborn infant. III. Measurements of mechanics of respiration, J. Clin. Invest. **36**:440, 1957.

Cook, D. R.: Neonatal pharmacology; a review, Anesth. Analg. (Cleve.) 53:544, 1974.

Cooper, H. A., and Hoagland, H. C.: Subject review; fetal hemoglobin, Mayo Clin. Proc. 47:402, 1972.

Cross, K. W.: Respiratory control in the neonatal period. In Cold Spring Harbor Symposia on Quantitative Biology. Vol. 19: The mammalian fetus; physiological aspects of development, New York, 1954, The Biological Laboratory.

Cross, K. W., Tizard, J. P. M., and Trythall, D. A. H.: The gaseous metabolism of the newborn infant, Acta Paediatr. 46:265, 1957.

Dancis, J., and Smith, A. A.: Familial dysautonomia, J. Pediatr. 77:174, 1970.

Darrow, D. C., Cook, R. E., and Segar, W. E.: Water and electrolyte metabolism in infants fed cow's milk mixtures during heat stress, Pediatrics 14:602, 1954.

Darrow, D. C., and Yannet, H.: Changes in the distribution of body water accompanying increase and decrease in extracellular electrolyte, J. Clin. Invest. 14:266, 1935.

Davies, D. F., and Shock, N. W.: Age changes in glomerular filtration rate, effective renal plasma flow and tubular secretory capacity in adult males, J. Clin. Invest. 29:496, 1950.

Dawkins, M. J. R., and Scopes, J. W.: Non-shivering thermogenesis in the human newborn infant, Nature 206:201, 1965.

Dean, R. F. A., and McCance, R. A.: Renal responses of infants and adults to administration of hypertonic solutions of sodium chloride and urea, J. Physiol. (Lond.) 109:81, 1949.

Dekaban, A.: Neurology of infancy, Baltimore, 1959, The Williams & Wilkins Co.

Deming, M. V.: Agents and techniques for induction of anesthesia in infants and young children, Anesth. Analg. (Cleve.) 31:113, 1952.

Done, A. K.: Developmental pharmacology, Clin. Pharmacol. Ther. 5:432, 1964.

Dunnill, M. S.: Postnatal growth of the lung, Thorax 17:329, 1962.

Eckenhoff, J.: Some anatomic considerations of the infant larynx influencing endotracheal anesthesia, Anesthesiology 12:401, 1951.

Eckenhoff, J.: Relationship of anesthesia to postoperative personality changes in children, Am. J. Dis. Child. 86:587, 1953.

Ecobichon, D. J., and Stephens, D. S.: Perinatal development of human blood esterases, Clin. Pharmacol. Ther. 14:44, 1973.

Edelmann, C. M., Jr.: Maturation of the neonatal kidney. In Proceedings of the Third International Congress on Nephrology, vol. 1, Washington, 1966, Basel, 1967, S. Karger.

Edelmann, C. M., Jr.: Pediatric nephrology, Pediatrics 51:854, 1973.

Edelmann, C. M., Jr., Barnett, H. L., and Stark, H.: Effect of urea on concentration of urinary nonurea solute in premature infants, J. Appl. Physiol. 21:1021, 1966.

Edelmann, C. M., Jr., and Spitzer, A.: The maturing kidney; a modern view of well-balanced infants with imbalanced nephrons, J. Pediatr. 75:509, 1969.

Eger, E. I.: A mathematical model of uptake and distribution. In Papper, E. M., and Kitz, R. J.: Uptake and distribution of anesthetic agents, New York, 1963, McGraw-Hill Book Co.

Eger, E. I.: Anesthetic uptake and action, Baltimore, 1974, The Williams and Wilkins Co.

Eger, E. I., Bahlman, S. H., and Munson, E. S.: The effect of age on the rate of increase of alveolar anesthetic concentration, Anesthesiology 35:365, 1971.

Eger, E. I., and Severinghaus, J. W.: Effect of uneven pulmonary shunt distribution of blood and gas on induction with inhalation anesthetics, Anesthesiology 25:620, 1964.

Engel, S.: The child's lung, ed. 2, London, 1962, Edward Arnold, Publishers, Ltd. (ed. 1 published in 1947).

Feldberg, W., and Myers, R. D.: Effects on temperature of amines injected into the cerebral ventricles; a new concept of temperature regulation, J. Physiol. (Lond.) 173:266, 1964.

Fetterman, G. H., Shuplock, N. A., Philipp, F. J., and Gregg, H. S.: The growth and maturation of human glomeruli and proximal convolutions from term to adulthood; studies by microdissections, Pediatrics 35:601, 1965.

Filler, R. M., and Das, J. B.: Muscle surface pH; a new parameter in monitoring of the critically ill child, Pediatrics 47:880, 1971.

Finberg, L.: Dehydration secondary to diarrhea. In Smith, C. A., editor: The critically ill child, ed. 2, Philadelphia, 1976, W. B. Saunders Co.

Friedman, W. F., Pool, P., Jacobowitz, D., and others: Sympathetic innervation of the developing rabbit heart, Circ. Res. 23:25, 1968.

Friis-Hansen, B. J.: Changes in body water compartments during growth, Acta Paediatr. Scand. (Suppl.) 110:1, 1957.

Friis-Hansen, B. J., Holaday, M., Stapleton, T., and Wallace, W. M.: Total body water in children, Pediatrics 7:321, 1951.

Giebisch, G.: Functional organization of proximal and distal tubular electrolyte transport, Nephron 6:260, 1969.

Glaser, G. H.: The neurological status of the newborn; neuromuscular and electroencephalographic activity, Yale J. Biol. Med. 32:173, 1959.

Goldstein, A., Aronow, L., and Kalman, S. M.: Principles of drug action; the basis of pharmacology, New York, 1968, Harper & Row, Publishers, Inc.

Graff, T. D., Holzman, R. S., and Benson, D. W.: Acid-base balance in infants during halothane anesthesia with the use of an adult circle absorption system, Anesth. Analg. (Cleve.) 43:583, 1964.

Gray, H.: Anatomy of the human body, ed. 29, Philadelphia, 1973, Lea & Febiger.

Greenberg, A. J., McNamara, H., and McCrory, W. W.: Renal tubular response to aldosterone in normal infants and children with adrenal disorders, J. Clin. Endocrinol. Metab. 27:1197, 1967.

Gregory, G. A., Eger, E. I., and Munson, E. S.: The relationship between age and halothane requirement in man, Anesthesiology 30:488, 1969.

Gross, R. E.: Surgery of infancy and childhood, Philadelphia, 1953, W. B. Saunders Co.

Grupe, W. E.: The kidney. In Klaus, M. H., and Fanaroff, A. A., editors: Care of the high-risk infant, Philadelphia, 1973, W. B. Saunders Co.

Gruskin, A. B., Edelmann, C. M., Jr., and Yuan, S.: Maturational changes in renal blood flow in piglets, Fed. Proc. 27:630, 1968.

Gustafson, S. R., and Coursin, D. B.: The pediatric patient, Philadelphia, 1968, J. B. Lippincott Co.

Hall, J. E.: The physiology of respiration in infants and young children, Proc. R. Soc. Med. 48:761, 1955.

Harris, J. S.: Special pediatric problems in fluid and electrolyte therapy in surgery, Ann. N.Y. Acad. Sci. 66:966, 1957.

Harrison, G. G., and Smith, J. S.: Massive lethal hepatic necrosis in rats anesthetized with fluroxene after microsomal enzyme induction, Anesthesiology 39:619, 1973.

Hassan, S. Z., and Williams, J. R.: Spread of radiopaque solution in the epidural space of human neonate, J. Reprod. Med. 10:31, 1973.

Hecht, F., and Lovrien, E. W.: Genetic diagnosis in the newborn; a part of preventive medicine, Pediatr. Clin. North Am. 17:1039, 1970.

Hogg, J. C., Williams, J., Richardson, J. B., and others: Age as a factor in the distribution of lower airway conductance and in the pathologic anatomy of obstructive lung disease, N. Engl. J. Med. 202:1283, 1970.

Hogg, S., and Renwick, W.: Hyperpyrexia during anaesthesia, Can. Anaesth. Soc. J. 13:429, 1966.

Holaday, D. A., Rudofsky, S., and Treuhaft, P. S.: The metabolic degradation of methoxyflurane in man, Anesthesiology 33:579, 1970.

Holliday, M. A.: Metabolic rate and organ size during growth from infancy to maturity and during late gestation and early infancy, Pediatrics 47:169, 1971.

Holliday, M. A., and Segar, W. E.: The maintenance need for water in parenteral fluid therapy, Pediatrics 19:823, 1957.

Hsia, D. Y., Dowben, R. M., and Riabov, S.: Inhibitors of glucuronyl transferase in the newborn, Ann. N.Y. Acad. Sci. 111:326, 1963.

Hunt, A. D.: On the hospitalization of children; an historical approach, Pediatrics 54:542, 1974.

Hunt, E. E., Jr.: The developmental genetics of man. In Falkner, F., editor: Human development, Philadelphia, 1966, W. B. Saunders Co.

Jackson, K.: Psychological preparation as a method of reducing emotional trauma of anesthesia in children, Anesthesiology 12:293, 1951.

Jackson, K., Winkley, B., Faust, O. A., and others: Behavior changes indicating emotional trauma in tonsillectomized children; final report, Pediatrics 12:23, 1953.

Jackson, S. H.: Genetic and metabolic disease. In Katz, J., and Kadis, L. B., editors: Anesthesia and uncommon diseases, Philadelphia, 1973, W. B. Saunders Co.

James. L. S., Weisbrot, I. M., Prince, C. F., and others: The acid-base status of human infants in relation to birth asphyxia and the onset of respiration, J. Pediatr. 33:379, 1958.

Janovski, M., Martinek, J., and Stanincova, F.: Antidiuretic activity in the plasma of human infants after a load of sodium chloride, Acta Paediatr. Scand. 54:543, 1965.

Joel, C. D.: The physiological role of brown adipose tissue. In Renold, A. E., and Cahill, G. F., section editors: Handbook of physiology, vol. 5, Washington, D.C., 1965, American Physiological Society.

Johansson, B.: Brown fat; a review, Metabolism 8:221, 1959.

Jusko, W. J.: Pharmacokinetic principles in pediatric problems, Pediatr. Clin. North Am. 19:81, 1972.

Kalow, W.: Pharmacogenetics; heredity and response to drugs, Philadelphia, 1962, W. B. Saunders Co.

Karlin, J. M., and Kutt, H.: Acute diphenylhydantoin intoxication following halothane anesthesia, J. Pediatr. 76:941, 1970.

Katz, J., and Kadis, L. B.: Anesthesia and uncommon diseases, Philadelphia, 1973, W. B. Saunders Co.

Kety, S. K.: Exchange of inert gases at lungs and tissues, Pharmacol. Rev. 3:1, 1951.

Kiely, N. F.: Psychiatric aspects of critical care, Crit. Care Med. 2:139, 1974.

Kissane, J. M., and Smith, M. G.: Pathology of infancy and childhood, St. Louis, 1967, The C. V. Mosby Co.

Klein, R.: Neonatal adrenal physiology, Pediatr. Clin. North Am. 1:321, 1954.

Knutrud, O.: The water and electrolyte metabolism in the newborn child after major surgery, Oslo, 1965, Universitetsforlaget.

Langworthy, O. R.: Development of behavior patterns and myelinization of the nervous system in the human fetus and infant, Contrib. Embryol. 24:3, 1933.

Lanman, J. T.: Function of adrenal cortex in premature infants without recognized disease. I. Pediatrics 11:120, 1953.

Lee, V. A., and Iliff, A.: The energy of infants and young children during postprandial sleep, Pediatrics 18:739, 1956.

Lehmann, H., and Ryan, E.: The familial incidence of low pseudocholinesterase level, Lancet 2:124, 1956.

Levy, D. M.: Psychic trauma of operations in children, Am. J. Dis. Child. 69:7, 1945.

Levy, G.: Pharmacologic intelligence; pharmacokinetics of succinylcholine in newborns, Anesthesiology 32:551, 1970.

Lewis, O. J.: The development of blood vessels of the metanephros, J. Anat. 92:84, 1954.

Lewis, R. C., Duval, A. M., and Iliff, A.: Standards for the basal metabolism of children from 2 to 15 years of age inclusive, J. Pediatr. 23:1, 1943.

Lim, H. S., Davenport, H. T., and Robson, J. G.: The

response of infants and children to muscle relaxants, Anesthesiology **25**:161, 1964.

Lipton, E. L., Steinschneider, A., and Richmond, J. G.: Autonomic nervous system in early life, N. Engl. J. Med. **273**:147, 1965.

Long, G., and Bachman, L.: Neuromuscular blockage by *d*-tubocurarine in children, Anesthesiology **28**:723, 1967.

Mason, E. A.: The hospitalized child; his emotional needs, N. Engl. J. Med. **272**:406, 1965.

McCance, R. A.: Renal physiology in infancy, Am. J. Med. **9**:229, 1950.

McCance, R. A., Naylor, N. J. B., and Widdowson, E. M.: The response of infants to a large dose of water, Arch. Dis. Child. **29**:104, 1954.

McCance, R. A., and Widdowson, E. M.: The correct physiological basis on which to compare infant and adult renal function, Lancet **11**:860, 1952.

McCrory, W. W.: Developmental nephrology, Cambridge, Mass., 1972, The Commonwealth Fund, Harvard University Press.

McGraw, M. B.: The neuromuscular maturation of the human infant, New York, 1943, Columbia University Press.

McLean, E. C., and Paulsen, E. P.: The response of the newborn to major surgery; urinary electrolyte, nitrogen, and water losses, Am. J. Dis. Child. **96**:473, 1958.

Metcoff, J.: The regulation of the body fluids. In Cooke, R. E., editor: The biologic basis of pediatric practice, New York, 1968, McGraw-Hill Book Co.

Mirkin, B. L.: Perinatal pharmacology, Anesthesiology **43**:156, 1975.

Mohri, H., Dillard, D. H., and Merendino, K. A.: Hypothermia; halothane anesthesia and the safe period of total circulatory arrest, Surgery **72**:349, 1969.

Moore, R. E., and Underwood, M. C.: Possible role of noradrenaline in control of heat production in the newborn mammal, Am. J. Physiol. **190**:240, 1957.

Morse, M., Cassels, D. E., and Holder, M.: The position of the oxygen dissociation curve of blood in normal children and adults, J. Clin. Invest. **29**:1091, 1950.

Moss, A. J., Emmanouilides, G. C., Monset-Couchard, M., and Marcan, B.: Vascular responses to postural changes in normal newborn infants, Pediatrics **42**:250, 1968.

Moya, F., and Thorndike, S.: The effects of drugs used in labor on the fetus and newborn, Clin. Pharmacol. Ther. **5**:628, 1965.

Nadas, A. S., and Fyler, D. C.: Pediatric cardiology, ed. 3, Philadelphia, 1972, W. B. Saunders Co.

Nathan, D. G., and Oski, F. A.: Hematology of infancy and childhood, Philadelphia, 1974, W. B. Saunders Co.

Nelson, W. E., Vaughan, V. C. III, and McKay, R. J., Jr., editors: Nelson textbook of pediatrics, ed. 10, Philadelphia, 1975, W. B. Saunders Co.

Nicodemus, H. F., Nassiri-Rahimi, C., Bachman, L., and Smith, T. C.: Median effective doses (ED_{50}) of

halothane in adults and children, Anesthesiology **31**:344, 1969.

Nyhan, W. L.: Toxicity of drugs in the neonatal period, J. Pediatr. **59**:1, 1961.

Nyhan, W. L.: Pharmacogenetics. In Shirkey, H. C., editor: Pediatric therapy, ed. 2, St. Louis, 1968, The C. V. Mosby Co.

Nyhan, W. L., and Lampert, F.: Response of fetus and newborn to drugs, Anesthesiology **26**:487, 1965.

Oski, F. A.: Designation of anemia on a functional basis, J. Pediatr. **83**:353, 1973.

Oski, F. A.: The unique fetal red cell and its function, Pediatrics **51**:494, 1973a.

Oyama, T.: Endocrine responses to anaesthetic agents, Br. J. Anaesth. **45**:276, 1973.

Paine, R. S.: Detection of neurologic abnormalities in young infants, Int. Anesthesiol. Clin. **1**:1, 1962.

Potter, E. L., and Craig, J. M.: Pathology of the fetus and the infant, ed. 3, Chicago, 1975, Year Book Medical Publishers, Inc.

Reynolds, R. N.: Acid-base equilibrium during cyclopropane anesthesia and operation in infants, Anesthesiology **27**:127, 1966.

Rickham, P. P.: The metabolic response to neonatal surgery, Cambridge, 1957, Harvard University Press.

Roe, C. F., Santulli, T. V., and Blair, C. S.: Heat loss in infants during general anesthesia and operations, J. Pediatr. Surg. **1**:266, 1966.

Rosen, M., and Brueton, M.: Emotional disturbances in children having tonsillectomy and adenoidectomy aged 5-6 years, Excerpta Medica Foundation, 1970, p. 686.

Rowe, M. O.: Physiologic monitoring in surgical pediatrics. In Gans, S. L., editor: Surgical pediatrics, New York, 1973, Grune & Stratton.

Rubin, M. I., Bruck, E., and Rapoport, M.: Maturation of renal function in childhood; clearance studies, J. Clin. Invest. **28**:1144, 1949.

Rudolph, A. M.: Normal and abnormal respiration in children, Thirty-seventh Ross Conference on Pediatric Research, Columbus, Ohio, 1961.

Ryan, J. F., Wilson, J. R., Goudsouzian, N. G., and Jasinska, M. T.: Oxygen consumption as a measure of thermoregulation in children, American Society of Anesthesiologists, San Francisco, October 11, 1973.

Salanitre, E., and Rackow, H.: The pulmonary exchange of nitrous oxide and halothane in infants and children, Anesthesiology **30**:388, 1969.

Scopes, J. W.: Metabolic rate and temperature control in the human body, Br. Med. Bull. **22**:88, 1966.

Searles, P. W., and Seymour, D. G.: Body temperature variation and effects during surgery, anesthesia and hypothermia, Anesth. Analg. (Cleve.) **36**:50, 1957.

Sereni, F., and Principi, N.: Developmental pharmacology, Annu. Rev. Pharmacol. **8**:453, 1968.

Shirkey, H. C.: Drug dosage for infants and children, J.A.M.A. **193**:443, 1965.

Shwachman, H., and Khaw, K. T.: Cystic fibrosis. In Shirkey, H. C., editor: Pediatric therapy, ed. 5, St. Louis, 1976, The C. V. Mosby Co.

Silverio, J., and Poole, J. W.: Serum ampicillin after oral administration to newborn, Pediatrics 51:578, 1973.

Silverman, W. A.: Sulfonamides in the neonate. In May, C. D., editor: Perinatal pharmacology, report of Forty-first Ross Laboratories Conference on Pediatric Research, Columbus, Ohio, 1962.

Simmons, M. A., Adcock, E. W., Bard, H., and others: Hypernatremia and intracranial hemorrhage in neonates, N. Engl. J. Med. 270:704, 1964.

Smith, C. A.: The physiology of the newborn infant, ed. 3, Springfield, Ill., 1959, Charles C Thomas, Publisher.

Smith, C. A., and Nelson, N.: Physiology of the newborn infant, ed. 4, Springfield, Ill., 1976, Charles C Thomas, Publisher.

Smith, P. C., and Smith, N. T.: Anaesthetic management of a very premature infant, Br. J. Anaesth. 44:736, 1972.

Smith, R. M.: Temperature monitoring and regulation. In Gans, S. L., editor: Surgical pediatrics, New York, 1973, Grune & Stratton.

Smith, R. M., and Chandra, P.: Unpublished data, 1973.

Soyka, L. F.: Clinical pharmacology of digoxins, Pediatr. Clin. North Am. 19:241, 1972.

Stanbury, J. B., Wyngaarden, J. B., and Frederickson, D. S.: The metabolic basis of inherited disease, New York, 1960, McGraw-Hill Book Co.

Stead, A. L.: The response of the newborn infant to muscle relaxants, Br. J. Anaesth. 27:124, 1955.

Stephen, C. R., Dent, S. J., Hall, K. D., and others: Body temperature regulation during anesthesia in infants and children, J.A.M.A. 174:1579, 1960.

Stern, L., Lees, M. H., and Leduc, J.: Temperature, oxygen and catecholamine excretion in newborn infants, Pediatrics 36:367, 1965.

Strauss, J., Adamsons, K., Jr., and James, L. W.: Renal function of normal full-term infants in the first hours of extra-uterine life, Am. J. Obstet. Gynecol. 91:286, 1965.

Talbert, J. L., Karmen, A., Graystone, J. E., and others: Assessment of infant's response to stress, Surgery 61:626, 1967.

Talbot, N. G., Sobel, E. H., McArthur, J. W., and Crawford, J. D.: Functional endocrinology from birth through adolescence, Cambridge, 1952, Harvard University Press.

Thomas, A.: Etudes neurologiques sur le nouveau-né et le jeune nourrison, Paris, 1952, Masson et Cie editeurs.

Van Dyke, R. A., and Wood, C. L.: Metabolism of methoxyflurane; release of inorganic fluoride in human and rat hepatic enzymes, Anesthesiology 39:613, 1973.

Walts, L. F., and Dillon, J. B.: The response of newborns to succinylcholine and d-tubocurarine, Anesthesiology 31:35, 1969.

Ward, R.: Porphyria and its relation to anesthesia, Anesthesiology 26:212, 1965.

Warkany, J.: Congenital malformations; notes and comments, Chicago, 1971, Year Book Medical Publishers, Inc.

Watson, B. G.: Blood glucose levels in children during surgery, Br. J. Anaesth. 44:712, 1972.

Way, W. L., Costley, E. C., and Leong Way, E.: Respiratory sensitivity of the newborn infant to meperidine and morphine, Clin. Pharmacol. Ther. 6:454, 1965.

Weiss, C.: Does circumcision of the newborn require an anesthetic? Clin. Pediatr. (Phila.) 7:128, 1968.

Weiss, C. F., Glazka, A. J., and Weston, J. K.: Chloramphenicol in the newborn infant, N. Engl. J. Med. 262:787, 1960.

West, G. B., Shepard, D. M., and Hunter, R. B.: Adrenalin and noradrenalin concentrations in adrenal glands at different ages and in some diseases, Lancet 2:966, 1951.

Whittaker, M.: Genetic aspects of succinylcholine sensitivity, Anesthesiology 32:143, 1970.

Yaffe, S. J.: Strain variation in drug response. In May, C. D., editor: Perinatal pharmacology; report of Forty-first Ross Conference on Pediatric Research, Columbus, Ohio, 1962.

Yudkin, S., and Gellis, S.: Liver function in newborn infants, Arch. Dis. Child. 24:12, 1949.

CHAPTER 3

Respiratory physiology

ETSURO K. MOTOYAMA and CHARLES D. COOK

More than any other speciality of medicine, anesthesiology is intimately concerned with the physiology of respiration. This is apparent not only when general anesthesia is used but also when regional anesthesia and preanesthetic medication are used. In the patient subjected to general anesthesia there is usually partial, and at times complete, interference with the control of breathing, necessitating regulation of ventilation by the anesthesiologist for the maintenance of adequate oxygenation and normal acid-base balance (PCO_2 and pH). In addition, such factors as loss of the cough reflex and sigh mechanism, encroachment of airway patency due to the positioning of the patient, secretions, laryngospasm, or reduction of the resting lung volume (functional residual capacity [FRC]), commonly seen under general anesthesia, interfere with normal ventilatory function and pulmonary gas exchange, partic-

ularly in small infants. Postoperative management of ventilation is also an important task for the anesthesiologist. Many anesthesiologists are currently assuming the responsibilities of the acute care specialist and coordinator in the intensive care unit, since they are most appropriately trained to take care of acute cardiopulmonary problems in critically ill patients.

This chapter, together with Chapter 27, presents some of the practical aspects of respiratory physiology and their application to anesthesia in infants and children and to certain pulmonary diseases seen in the pediatric age group. Also included are brief reviews of prenatal and postnatal lung development and of neonatal respiratory adaptation. Such knowledge is important for proper management of infants and children with respiratory insufficiency or of those undergoing anesthesia and surgery. Although there are many similarities between the ventilation of infants and children and that of adults, there are both quantitative and qualitative differences between the two.

The respiratory system is made up of the respiratory centers in the brainstem, the central and peripheral chemoreceptors, the phrenic and intercostal (efferent) and vagal (afferent) nerves, the thoracic cage (including the musculature of the chest and abdomen and the abdominal contents), the upper and lower air passages, the lungs, and the pulmonary vascular system. The following headings suggest the functional subdivisions of the respiratory system:

1. Control of breathing
2. Lung volumes
3. Mechanics of breathing
4. Ventilation
5. Gas diffusion
6. Pulmonary circulation
7. Ventilation-perfusion relationships
8. Oxygen transport
9. Surface activity and lung function
10. Ciliary activity

The principal desired result of these functions in all age groups is to maintain the oxygen and carbon dioxide equilibrium in the body. The lungs also contribute importantly to the regulation of acid-base balance. The maintenance of a stable body temperature (by loss of water through the lungs), although occasionally important, is, on the whole, a secondary function. The nonrespiratory function of the lungs, although important, is not discussed in this chapter.

CONTROL OF BREATHING

The mechanism that regulates and maintains pulmonary gas exchange is remarkably efficient. In a normal individual the level of arterial P_{CO_2} is maintained within a very narrow range when O_2 demand and CO_2 production vary greatly during exercise and rest. This is achieved by a precise matching of the level of ventilation to the output of CO_2. The control of breathing can be divided into neural and chemical controls, although they are interrelated intimately.

Neural control

Under normal circumstances, pulmonary ventilation is maintained with rhythmic contraction and relaxation of respiratory muscles. According to the classic concept of the respiratory control mechanism, the neurons in the medullary inspiratory center possess tonic activity that is periodically inhibited by the excitement of neurons in the adjacent expiratory center. Expiratory neurons were thought to be driven by afferent vagal impulses from the pulmonary stretch receptors and by a group of neurons in the pontine pneumotaxic center. These neurons were thought to be capable of periodic spontane-

ous discharge and of driving rhythmic respiration in the absence of vagal activity (Pitts, 1946). The pontine apneustic center was considered as the site of the inspiratory tonicity as well as rhythmic inhibition by the pneumotaxic center and the vagus. These theories of respiratory control, which had been accepted for a number of years, were based on the experiments in which the brainstem was transected at various levels.

More recently, the development of microelectrode techniques and the direct measurement of action potentials from single neurons in the intact brainstem has dramatically improved the understanding of control of breathing. It is now evident that respiratory neurons in the medulla have inherent rhythmicity even when they are separated from the higher levels of the brainstem; such "pacemaker" neurons have not been found in the pontine pneumotaxic center. Instead, it appears that medullary respiratory neurons drive pontine respiratory neurons (Hukuhara, 1974). Probably the pneumotaxic center plays a secondary role to modify the inspiratory off-switch mechanism (von Euler and Trippenbach, 1975; Gautier and Bertrand, 1975).

In the cat, respiratory neurons are concentrated in two areas near the level of the obex. The dorsal respiratory group (DRG) is located in the vicinity of the nucleus tractus solitarius and contains inspiratory cells; the ventral respiratory group (VRG) is associated with the nucleus ambiguus and the nucleus retroambigualis and consists of both inspiratory and expiratory cells (Mitchell and Burger, 1975). Inspiratory and expiratory neurons are interconnected with reciprocal negative feedback pathways so that the excitation of one group of neurons results in the inhibition of the other and vice versa (Burns, 1963). Recent studies, however, have indicated that inspiratory neurons inhibit expiratory neurons during inspiration but the reverse is not the case during expiration (Mitchell and Herbert, 1974).

Respiratory neurons receive a wealth of excitatory inputs from central (cortical, hypothalamic) and peripheral (vagal, glossopharyngeal, and spinal) sources. In addition, sufficient traffic of activities in the nonrespiratory systems surrounding respiratory neurons appears important for the maintenance of spontaneous rhythmic discharge (Burns, 1963).

Neural regulation of respiration has been reviewed by Mitchell and Burger (1975); their work should be consulted for further details.

Chemical control

Regulation of alveolar ventilation and maintenance of normal arterial P_{CO_2}, pH, and P_{O_2} are the principal functions of the medullary and peripheral chemoreceptors (Mitchell, 1966; Leusen, 1972).

The medullary, or central, chemoreceptors, located near the surface of the ventrolateral medulla, are anatomically separated from the medullary respiratory center. They respond to changes in hydrogen ion concentration in the adjacent cerebrospinal fluid (CSF) rather than to changes in arterial P_{CO_2} or pH (Pappenheimer and others, 1965). Since carbon dioxide rapidly passes through the blood-brain barrier into the CSF, which has poor buffering capacity, the medullary chemoreceptors are readily stimulated by respiratory acidemia. In contrast, ventilatory responses of the medullary chemoreceptors to acute metabolic acidemia and alkalemia are limited, because changes in the hydrogen ion concentration in arterial blood are not rapidly transmitted to the CSF. In chronic acid-base disturbances, the pH of CSF (and presumably interstitial fluid) surrounding the medullary chemoreceptors is generally maintained close to the normal value of about 7.3 regardless of arterial pH (Mitchell and others, 1965). Ventilation under these circumstances becomes more dependent on the hypoxic response of peripheral chemoreceptors.

Peripheral chemoreceptors, particularly the carotid bodies, located near the bifurcation of the common carotid artery, react rapidly to changes in Pa_{CO_2} and pH and contribute to the respiratory drive, which amounts to about 15% at rest (Severinghaus, 1972).

The carotid bodies are perfused with extremely high levels of blood flow and respond rapidly to an oscillating Pa_{CO_2} rather than a constant Pa_{CO_2} at the same mean values (Dutton and others, 1964; Fenner and others, 1968). This mechanism may in part be responsible for hyperventilation during exercise.

The primary role of peripheral chemoreceptors is their response to changes in arterial P_{O_2}. Moderate to severe hypoxemia (i.e., Pa_{O_2} <60 torr) results in a significant increase in ventilation in all ages (Dripps and Comroe, 1947), except in newborn (particularly premature) infants, whose ventilation is decreased (Cross and Oppé, 1952). Peripheral chemoreceptors are also in part responsible for hyperventilation in hypotensive patients. Absence of respiratory stimulation in hypoxemic states, such as moderate to severe anemia and carbon monoxide poisoning, is because Pa_{O_2} in the carotid bodies, in spite of a decrease in O_2 content, is maintained near normal levels and the chemoreceptors are therefore not stimulated.

In acute hypoxemia, the ventilatory response via the peripheral chemoreceptors is partially opposed by hypocapnia, which depresses the medullary chemoreceptors. When a hypoxic environment persists for a few days, for example during an ascent to high altitude, ventilation increases further as CSF bicarbonate decreases and CSF pH returns toward normal (Severinghaus and others, 1963). However, more recent studies (Foster and others, 1975; Bureau and Bouverot, 1975) demonstrated that the return of CSF pH toward normal is incomplete and that the secondary increase in ventilation precedes the changes in CSF pH, indicating that some other mechanisms are involved. In chronic hypoxemia lasting for a number of years, the carotid bodies, which initially exhibit little adaptation to hypoxemia, gradually lose their hypoxic response. In high-altitude natives, the blunted response of carotid chemoreceptors to hypoxemia takes 10 to 15 years to develop and is sustained thereafter (Sørensen and Severinghaus, 1968; Lahiri and others, 1976). In cyanotic heart diseases, the hypoxic response is lost much sooner but returns after surgical correction of the right-to-left shunts (Edelman and others, 1970).

In patients who have chronic respiratory insufficiency with hypercapnia, hypoxemic stimulation of the peripheral chemoreceptors provides the primary impulse to the respiratory center. If these patients are given excessive levels of oxygen, the stimulus of hypoxemia is removed, ventilation decreases or ceases, PCO_2 is further increased, patients become comatose (CO_2 narcosis), and death may follow unless ventilation is supported. Rather than oxygen therapy, such patients need their effective ventilation increased artificially with or without added inspired oxygen. Tracheostomy will decrease the dead space and, in some cases, may increase the effective ventilation (alveolar ventilation) enough to maintain spontaneous ventilation.

The graphic demonstration of relations between the alveolar or arterial PCO_2 vs minute ventilation ($\dot{V}_E/PCO_2$) is commonly known as the CO_2 response curve, which normally reflects the response of the chemoreceptors and respiratory center to CO_2. The CO_2 response curve is a useful means to evaluate the chemical control of breathing, provided that the mechanical properties of the respiratory system including the neuromuscular transmission, respiratory muscles, thorax, and lung are intact. In normal individuals, ventilation increases more or less linearly as the inspired concentration of CO_2 increases up to 9% to 10%, above which ventilation starts to decrease (Dripps and Comroe, 1947). Under hypoxic conditions, CO_2 response is potentiated, resulting in a shift to the left of the CO_2 response curve (Fig. 3-1) (Nielsen and Smith, 1951). In comparison,

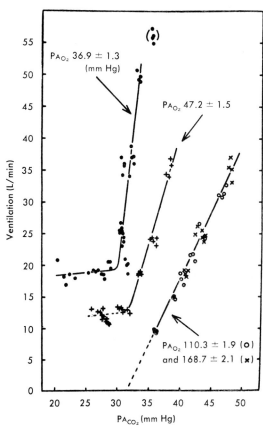

Fig. 3-1. Effect of acute hypoxemia on the ventilatory response to carbon dioxide (steady state) in one subject. Inspired oxygen was adjusted in each experiment to keep alveolar oxygen tension (PA_{O_2}) constant at the level as indicated. (From Nielsen, M., and Smith, H.: Acta Physiol. Scand. **24**:293, 1951.)

anesthetics, narcotics, and barbiturates in general depress the medullary chemoreceptors and, by decreasing the slope, shift the CO_2 response curve to the right in a progressive manner as the anesthetic concentration increases (Munson and others, 1966).

A shift to the right of the CO_2 response curve in an awake human may be caused by decreased chemoreceptor sensitivity to CO_2, as seen in patients whose carotid bodies had been destroyed (Wade and others, 1970). It may also be caused by lung disease and resultant mechanical failure to increase ventilation in spite of intact neuronal response to CO_2. In the latter it has been difficult to separate the neuronal component from the mechanical failure of the lungs and thorax, since both factors often coexist in patients with chronic lung diseases (Guz and others, 1970). More recently, Whitelaw and associates (1975) have demonstrated that the negative mouth pressure generated by inspiratory effort against airway occlusion at FRC (occlusion pressure) correlates well with neuronal (phrenic) discharges but is uninfluenced by mechanical properties of the lungs and thorax. Thus, the occlusion pressure is a useful means to evaluate the ventilatory drive clinically.

As mentioned previously, hypoxemia potentiates the chemical drive and increases the slope of the CO_2 response curve ($\dot{V}_E/P_{CO_2}$). Such a change has been interpreted as "a multiplicative effect" of the stimulus, whereas a parallel shift of the curve has been considered "an additive effect." This analysis may be useful for descriptive purposes, but it is misleading. Since ventilation is the product of tidal volume and frequency ($\dot{V}_E = V_T \times f$), an additive effect on its components could result in a change in the slope of the CO_2 response curve. Obviously the response to CO_2 of tidal volume and frequency should be examined separately to understand the effect of various respiratory stimulants and depressants.

Milic-Emili and Grunstein (1976) have proposed that ventilatory response to CO_2 be analyzed in terms of the mean inspiratory flow ($\overline{V}_I = V_T/T_I$, where T_I is the inspiratory time) and in terms of the ratio of inspiratory time to total ventilatory cycle duration (T_I/T_{TOT}). Since the tidal volume is equal to $\overline{V}_I \times T_I$ and respiratory frequency is $1/T_{TOT}$, ventilation can be expressed as:

$$\dot{V}_E = V_T \times f = \overline{V}_I \times T_I/T_{TOT}$$

The advantage of analyzing the ventilatory response in this fashion is that $\overline{V}$ is an index of inspiratory drive, which is independent of the timing element. The tidal volume, on the other hand, is time dependent, since it is $\overline{V} \times T_I$. The second parameter, T_I/T_{TOT}, is a dimensionless index of effective respiratory timing that is determined by the vagal afferent and/or central inspiratory off-switch mechanism (Bradley and others, 1975). From this equation it is apparent that in respiratory disease or under anesthesia, changes in pulmonary ventilation may be due to a change in $\dot{V}_I$ and/or T_I/T_{TOT}. A reduction in T_I/T_{TOT} indicates that the relative duration of inspiration decreased or that expiration increased. Such a reduction in T_I/T_{TOT} ratio may be due to changes in central or peripheral mechanisms. In contrast, a reduction in $\overline{V}_I$ may indicate a decrease in central (bulbopontine) inspiratory drive or neuromuscular transmission or an increase in inspiratory impedance (i.e., increased flow resistance and/or decreased compliance). By relating the mouth occlusion pressure to $\overline{V}_I$, it is now possible clinically to determine whether changes in the mechanics of the respiratory system contribute to the reduction in $\overline{V}$ (Milic-Emili, 1977). Derenne and associates (1976) analyzed the timing component of ventilation in humans under methoxyflurane anesthesia and found that the CO_2 response of ventilation and tidal volume were decreased. This decrease was due to a reduction in $\dot{V}_I$ (or V_T/T_I) while the timing component (T_I/T_{TOT}) was unchanged. Furthermore, the decrease in $\overline{V}_I$ was not due to a decrease in central inspiratory drive but to an increase in impedance of respiratory drive, since the occlusion pressure at 0.1 second ($P_{0.1}$) did not decrease in comparison with that in awake subjects (Fig. 3-2). These results indicated that the main cause for the decrease in ven-

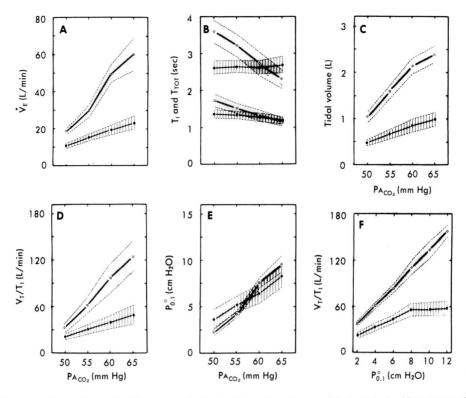

Fig. 3-2. Comparison of subjects anesthetized with methoxyflurane *(filled circles)* with a group of normal conscious subjects *(open circles)*. At each level of PA_{CO_2} the values (for instance of $\dot{V}_E$) from the regression lines of each subject were averaged to give a single point. Band has the width of one standard error of the mean. **A,** Ventilatory response; **B,** changes in T_I and T_{TOT} with CO_2; **C,** tidal volume response; **D,** inspiratory flow rate response; **E,** occlusion pressure response; **F,** V_T/T_I plotted against occlusion pressure ($P^0_{0.1}$). (From Derenne, J. P., Couture, J., Iscoe, S., and others: J. Appl. Physiol. **40:**805, 1976.)

tilation under light methoxyflurane anesthesia was not due to central depression or neuromuscular blockade but was the result of stiffening of the respiratory apparatus.

CO_2 response may be completely lost in patients with various central nervous system dysfunctions (Ondine's curse; Severinghaus and Mitchell, 1962). In the awake state, these patients have chronic hypoventilation but can breathe on command. During sleep they further hypoventilate or become apneic to the point of CO_2 narcosis and death unless mechanically ventilated or unless a phrenic pacemaker is installed (Glenn and others, 1973).

Lung receptors

There are a number of receptors in the upper airways and lungs that are sensitive to mechanical and chemical stimulation and influence ventilation as well as other nonrespiratory functions. There are three major types of lung receptors: the pulmonary stretch receptors, the irritant receptors, and the J-receptors. The functions of the lung receptors have been reviewed by Widdicombe (1974) and Paintal (1973).

Pulmonary stretch receptors. Pulmonary stretch receptors lie within the submucosal smooth muscle in the membranous posterior wall of the trachea and central airways (Bartlett and others, 1976). They are activated by the distension of the airways during lung inflation and inhibit inspiratory activity (Hering-Breuer inflation reflex). This reflex also produces dilation of the upper airways from the larynx to the bronchi. Furthermore, it is thought to be responsible for accelerated heart rate and systemic vasoconstriction observed with moderate lung inflation (Widdicombe, 1974). These effects are abolished by bilateral vagotomy.

Studies by Clark and von Euler (1972) have demonstrated the importance of the inflation reflex in adjusting the pattern of ventilation in the cat and human. In the cat anesthetized with pentobarbital, inspiratory time decreases as tidal volume increases with hypercapnia, indicating the presence of the inflation reflex in the normal tidal volume range. They demonstrated an inverse hyperbolic relation between the tidal volume and inspiratory time. In the adult human, inspiratory time is independent of tidal volume until the latter increases to about twice the normal tidal volume, when the inflation reflex appears. However, in the newborn, particularly in the premature infant, the inflation reflex is present in the eupneic range for a few months (Olinsky and others, 1974).

Apnea, frequently observed in patients at the end of surgery and anesthesia with the endotracheal tube cuff still inflated, may be related to the inflation reflex, since the trachea has a high concentration of stretch receptors (Bartlett and others, 1976). In these patients, deflation of the cuff promptly restores the rhythmic ventilation.

Irritant receptors. Inhalation of irritant gases (diethylether, halothane), smoke, and dust particles stimulates the irritant receptors, located on the epithelial surface of large and small airways, and causes reflex hyperpnea and constriction of the larynx and bronchi (Mills and others, 1970). The irritant receptors are also stimulated by histamine-induced bronchoconstriction, pulmonary congestion, microemboli, and atelectasis as well as hyperinflation of the lungs. In contrast to the stretch receptors, the irritant receptors adapt rapidly to large lung inflation, distortion, or deflation. Since they are stimulated by deflation of the lung and produce hyperpnea, the irritant receptors are considered to play an important role in the Hering-Breuer deflation reflex (Sellick and Widdicombe, 1970). This reflex, if it exists in humans, may

account in part for increased respiratory drive when the lung volume is abnormally decreased, as in respiratory distress syndrome of the newborn and in pneumothorax.

When the vagal conduction is partially blocked by cold, inflation of the lung produces prolonged contraction of the diaphragm instead of inspiratory inhibition from the inflation reflex. This reflex, the paradoxical reflex of Head, is most likely mediated by the irritant receptors and may be related to the complementary cycle of respiration, or "sigh mechanism," that functions to reaerate parts of the lung that have collapsed during quite shallow breathing due to increased surface force (Mead and Collier, 1959). In the newborn, inflation of the lung initiates gasping. This mechanism was considered to be analogous to the paradoxical reflex and may help to inflate unaerated portions of the newborn lung (Cross and others, 1960). In addition, the paradoxical reflex is often observed in the newborn period when the infants are mechanically ventilated (Motoyama, unpublished observation). This reflex may be an important reason why the patient's inspiratory drive can easily be synchronized with the control mode of a mechanical ventilator. A similar phenomenon has been observed in adult patients sedated with narcotics and on a ventilator.

J-receptors. Extensive studies by Paintal (1973) have demonstrated the presence of receptors supposedly located near the pulmonary capillary or alveolar wall (juxtapulmonary capillary receptors). These receptors are innervated by slow-conducting nonmyelinated vagal afferent fibers. They are stimulated by pulmonary congestion, pulmonary edema, pulmonary microemboli, and irritant gases such as halothane and cause apnea followed by rapid shallow breathing, hypotension, and bradycardia. All these responses are abolished by bilateral vagotomy. The J-receptors also produce severe reflex contraction of the laryngeal muscles, which may be responsible for the infrequent but severe laryngospasm observed during halothane anesthesia.

When irritant gases or particles are inhaled, there is a tightness or distressing sensation in the chest probably due to the activation of lung receptors. They may thus contribute to the sensation of dyspnea in lung congestion, atelectasis, and pulmonary edema. Bilateral vagal block in patients with lung disease abolished dyspneic sensation, and breath-holding time increased (Noble and others, 1970).

Control of breathing in perinatal and early postnatal periods

Given this general background on the control of breathing, we can now look into the adaptation of breathing at birth and what peculiarities and differences there are in the control mechanism in infants and children.

Based on early observations it had been believed that there was some inhibitory mechanism in utero and that the fetus did not normally make respiratory movements (Barcroft, 1946). Recent studies, however, have established that fetal lambs exhibit rhythmical as well as irregular respiratory movements associated with excursion of amniotic liquid in and out of the trachea (Dawes, 1973). Such fetal respiratory movements are stimulated by mild hypercapnia and acidemia, but they are abolished by mild hypoxemia and general anesthesia. Similar breathinglike movements have been confirmed in the human fetus using the ultrasound scanning technique (Boddy and Robinson, 1971). Thus, the respiratory center and chemoreceptors are apparently functional and active in utero to a certain extent. It is difficult, though, to compare their activities and sensitivities quantitatively with those in the newborn period, when the "breathing" changes from liquid to air. Burns (1963) has proposed the influence of other sensory impulses on the medullary respiratory center rhythmicity. The lack of other stimuli, such as thermal or tactile, in the fetus may in part be responsible for relative suppression of respiratory movements before birth (Harned and Ferreiro, 1973). Conversely, a rise in incubator air temperature can cause apnea in the premature newborn (Perlstein and others, 1970). Absence of oscillating changes

in Pa_{CO_2}, which stimulates the carotid chemoreceptors, together with relatively low Pa_{O_2} of the fetus (20 to 30 torr) may be among the additional factors.

During normal labor and vaginal delivery, the human fetus goes through a period of severe hypoxemia, hypercapnia, and acidemia. Such chemical changes appear to be the principal factors in the onset of breathing at birth. In full-term fetal lambs, severe hypoxemia stimulates fetal gasping and ventilation even after total peripheral chemodenervation, although hypercapnia, acting via the peripheral chemoreceptors, has a stimulatory effect on the degree of hypoxemia for the initiation of fetal gasping. Medullary chemoreceptors in the fetus do not respond to increased CO_2 and have little influence on the onset of gasping (Chernick and others, 1975). The mechanisms leading to the onset of breathing have recently been reviewed by Purves (1974). Once the rhythmical breathing of the newborn has begun, ventilation is adjusted to achieve a lower Pa_{CO_2} (Fig. 3-3, Table 3-1) than is found in older children and adults. Although this difference remains to be elucidated, it most likely represents a poor buffering capacity in the neonate and a ventilatory compensation for metabolic acidosis. The Pa_{CO_2} of the infant approximates

Table 3-1. Normal blood-gas values

	Po₂ (torr)	So₂ (%)	Pco₂ (torr)	pH
Pregnant women at term (artery)	88*	96	32	7.40
Umbilical vein	31	72*	42	7.35
Umbilical artery	19	38*	51	7.29
1 hour of life (artery)	62	95	28	7.36
24 hours of life (artery)	68	94	29	7.37
Child and adult (artery)	99	97	41	7.40

Compiled from data from Crawford, J. S.: Am. J. Obstet. Gynecol. **93**:37, 1965; Quilligan, E. H., Katigbak, E., Nowacek, C., and others: Am. J. Obstet. Gynecol. **90**:1343, 1964; Oh, W., Arcilla, R. A., Lind, J., and others: Acta Paediatr. Scand. **55**:593, 1966; Nelson, N. M., Prod'hom, L. S., Cherry, R. B., and others: Pediatrics **30**:963, 1962; and Nelson, N. M., Prod'hom, L. S., Cherry, R. B., and others: J. Appl. Physiol. **18**:534, 1963.
*Estimated values.

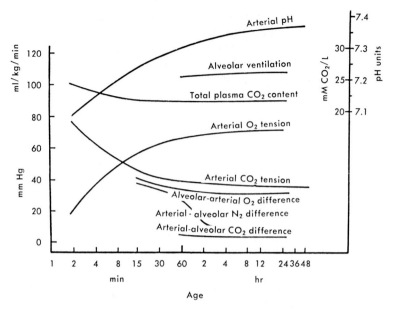

Fig. 3-3. Postnatal changes in arterial blood gases. (From Nelson, N. M.: Respiration and circulation after birth. In Smith, C. A., and Nelson, N. M., editors: The physiology of the newborn infant, ed. 4, Springfield, Ill., 1976, Charles C Thomas, Publisher, p. 229.)

the adult level within a few weeks after birth (Nelson, 1976).

Ventilatory response of the newborn to hypoxic and hyperoxic mixtures has been studied (Miller and Behrle, 1954; Rigatto and others, 1975). When 15% oxygen was administered, there was a transient increase in ventilation in both premature and full-term newborns that was followed by a sustained decrease in ventilation. Sixteen days after birth, however, hypoxemia induced sustained hyperventilation as in older individuals, primarily by increasing V_T. When 100% oxygen was given, there was a transient decrease in ventilation followed by sustained hyperventilation. This ventilatory response to oxygen is different from that of the adult, in whom a sustained decrease in ventilation was observed followed by little or no increase in ventilation (Dripps and Comroe, 1947).

Another difference in the control of breathing between newborn, especially premature, infants and older individuals is the tendency of the newborn to breathe irregularly (Fig. 3-4). The pH of arterialized capillary blood during irregular breathing is slightly alkalotic and the P_{CO_2} slightly lower than that of regular breathers. In contrast, preterm infants breathing periodically are hypoventilating, and administration of oxygen often abolishes irregular and periodic breathing (Avery and Fletcher, 1974). These findings suggest that hypoxia may be a primary event leading to periodic or irregular breathing and apnea (Rigatto and Brady, 1972). A possible basis for this phenomenon is that the medullary respiratory centers in these newborns are not yet fully matured. The sudden infant death syndrome may be related to this immaturity of the respiratory control mechanism (Steinschneider, 1972). Irregular or periodic breathing and inability to sustain ventilation under hypoxemic conditions in early postnatal periods are of particular clinical importance for anesthesiologists. In this age group, residual anesthesia or sedation, mild hypothermia, airway obstruction, atelectasis, and their combinations during the postanesthetic period tend to provoke irregular breathing and apnea without warning.

The response of infants to inspired CO_2 has

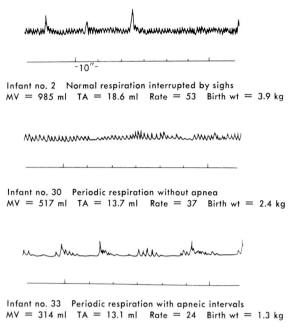

Infant no. 2   Normal respiration interrupted by sighs
MV = 985 ml   TA = 18.6 ml   Rate = 53   Birth wt = 3.9 kg

Infant no. 30   Periodic respiration without apnea
MV = 517 ml   TA = 13.7 ml   Rate = 37   Birth wt = 2.4 kg

Infant no. 33   Periodic respiration with apneic intervals
MV = 314 ml   TA = 13.1 ml   Rate = 24   Birth wt = 1.3 kg

Fig. 3-4. Body plethysmograph-spirometer tracings illustrating types of breathing in normal newborn infants. *MV,* minute volume; *TA,* tidal air. (From Cook, C. D. In Gordon, B. L., editor: Clinical cardiopulmonary physiology, ed. 2, New York, 1960, Grune & Stratton, Inc., p. 507. By permission.)

been studied. Avery and associates (1963) found that the ventilation of infants at a given alveolar P_{CO_2} was greater than that of adults but that the rate of change in ventilation per unit body weight was not different. Greater ventilation at a given P_{CO_2} is probably related to higher CO_2 production and a limited buffering capacity in infants. For a more critical comparison, it is apparent that the ventilatory response to CO_2 should be analyzed in terms of tidal volume and frequency or the central drive and timing component (Milic-Emili and Grunstein, 1976), since the frequency response to CO_2 in the newborn is known to be different (Olinski and others, 1974).

Summary

There has been dramatic progress in the understanding of neuronal and chemical control of breathing in recent years. Although such information is still limited during the perinatal and early postnatal periods, it is apparent that in most respects the control of breathing in infants and children resembles that in adults. However, newborns tend to regulate gas exchange to effect a lower Pa_{CO_2}, probably as an adjustment to metabolic acidosis. In addition, infants maintain ventilation poorly under hypoxemic conditions and have a tendency toward irregular breathing, which may be based on "immaturity" of the respiratory center and its inability to react to lack of oxygen.

LUNG VOLUMES

During the early postnatal years, maturation and growth of the lungs continue at a rapid pace with respect to an increase in bronchiolar generations and alveolar number as well as alveolar size. During this period, the lung volume of infants as compared with body size is not any larger than that in older children and young adults. Since the metabolic rate of the infant is nearly twice as high as that of the adult, ventilatory requirement per unit lung volume in infants is greatly increased. Thus, infants seem to have far less

47

Table 3-2. Normal values for lung functions for persons of various ages

Age	1 wk	1 yr	3 yr	5 yr	8 yr	12 yr	♂ 15 yr	♂ 21 yr	♀ 21 yr
Height (cm)	48	75	96	109	130	150	170	174	162
Weight (lb)	6.5	22	32	40	58	85	125	160	125
FRC (ml)	75*	(263)	(532)	660	1174	1855	2800	3030	2350
VC (ml)	100†	(475)	(910)	1100	1855	2830	4300	4620	3380
$\dot{V}_E$ (ml/min)	550	(1775)	(2460)	(2600)	(3240)	(4150)	5030	6000	5030
V_T (ml)	17	(78)	(112)	(130)	(180)	(260)	360	500	420
f (frequency)	30	(24)	(22)	(20)	(18)	16	14	12	12
$\dot{V}_A$ (ml/min)	385	(1245)	(1760)	(1800)	(2195)	(2790)	3070	4140	3530
V_D (ml)	7.5	21	37	49	75	105	141	150	126
C_I (ml/cm H_2O)	5	(16)	(32)	44	71	91	130	163	130
Peak flow rates (L/min)	10			136	231	325	437	457	365
R (cm H_2O/L/sec)	29‡	(13)	(10)	8	6	5	3	2	2
$D_{L_{CO}}$ (ml/mm Hg/min)§				11	15	20	27	28	24
Cardiac output (L/min)	(0.9)	1.9	2.7	3.2	4.4	5.7	(7.0)	(7.6)	(7.2)
Lung weight (g)	49	120	166	211	290	470	640	730	

Compiled from data in Cook, C. D., Cherry, R. B., O'Brien, D., and others: J. Clin. Invest. **34**:975, 1955; Cook, C. D., Sutherland, J. M., Segal, S., and others: J. Clin. Invest. **36**:440, 1957; Comroe, J. H., Jr., and others: The lung, Chicago, 1962, Year Book Medical Publishers, Inc.; Bucci, G., Cook, C. D., and Barrie, H.: J. Pediatr. **58**:820, 1961; Murray, A. B., and Cook, C. D.: J. Pediatr. **62**:186, 1963; Cook, C. D., and Hamann, J. F.: J. Pediatr. **59**:710, 1961; Long, E. C., and Hull, W. E.: Pediatrics **27**:373, 1961; and Koch, G.: Respir. Physiol. **4**:168, 1968.
*Supine.
†Crying vital capacity.
‡Nose breathing.
§Single breath technique.
Parentheses, interpolated values.

reserve in lung surface area. Normal values for lung volumes and function for persons of various ages are compiled in Table 3-2 for the purposes of comparison.

To understand pulmonary ventilation and some of the respiratory abnormalities encountered in infants and children, it is useful to review the subdivisions of the lungs as shown in Fig. 3-5. In normal children and adolescents these lung volumes are related to body size, especially height (Cook and Hamann, 1961) (Table 3-2). Although the data on newborn and small infants are incomplete, it appears that in most instances the relative sizes of the lung compartments are approximately constant from infancy through young adulthood. However, in the immediate postnatal period the FRC is relatively low, gradually increasing during the first 24 to 48 hours of life. In the premature infant with marginal amounts of pulmonary surfactant in the alveolar lining layer (see below),

there is a tendency for areas of atelectasis to persist for a few days to a few weeks.

Polgar and Promadhat (1971) have compiled most of the published data on pulmonary function tests in children, and their book should be consulted for details of the techniques and the results of the studies performed in normal infants and children. Graphs and formulas for predicting normal lung volumes for boys and girls of various sizes are shown in Fig. 3-6 and Table 3-3 together with the standard errors.

The limits of these lung volumes are imposed by both the thorax and the lungs themselves. Total lung capacity (TLC) is the largest lung volume allowed by the strength of the respiratory muscles stretching the thorax and lungs, and the residual volume (RV) is the amount of air remaining after forced expiration. In open chest surgery or pneumothorax, the lungs may collapse still further, particularly if high concentrations of oxygen

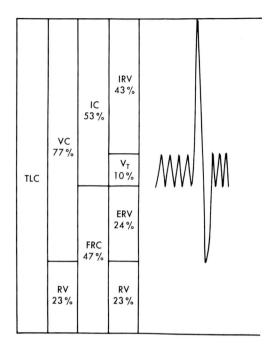

Fig. 3-5. Lung subdivisions: *TLC,* total lung capacity; *VC,* vital capacity; *FRC,* functional residual capacity; *IC,* inspiratory capacity; *IRV,* inspiratory reserve volume; *RV,* residual volume; *ERV,* expiratory reserve volume; *V_T,* tidal volume.

have been used and the trapped oxygen is taken up by the pulmonary circulation.

As can be seen from Fig. 3-5, in the person with a normal ventilatory system the volume reserve is great. However, in patients with abnormalities, the range between tidal volume needed for metabolic requirements and the vital capacity (VC) may be very limited.

The resting lung volume, or FRC, is determined by the balance between a number of different forces: the thoracic structures tend to expand the lungs while the lungs themselves tend to collapse. For the upright position, the balance point in the resting state (FRC or end-expiratory position) is reached in older children and adults when the pressure in the interpleural space is approximately -5 cm H_2O (in newborns the end-expiratory pressure is -1 or -2 cm H_2O). In this connection it is worth noting that negative pressure surrounding the lungs is the same, with respect to lung expansion, as positive pressure within the airways; thus, the net transpulmonary pressure represents the force expanding or contracting the lungs. In contrast, negative intrathoracic pressure

has quite a different effect from positive airway pressure with respect to pulmonary circulation.

Anesthesia, surgery, abdominal distension, and disease may all alter the lung volumes. The prone or supine patient has a smaller FRC than the standing or sitting patient because the abdominal contents shift. FRC is further decreased under general anesthesia with or without muscle relaxants (Westbrook and others, 1973). Such a decrease in FRC may result in the closure of small airways, uneven distribution of ventilation, ventilation–pulmonary perfusion imbalance, and hypoxemia as discussed in the following sections. In certain conditions, such as the respiratory distress syndrome of the newborn, in which the lung resists expansion, the FRC is further reduced. When the air passages are narrowed as in asthma or cystic fibrosis, there will be air trapping on expiration and FRC will be increased.

The importance of the air that remains in the lungs at the end of normal expiration is often overlooked. This FRC serves as a buffer that minimizes cyclic changes in Pco_2

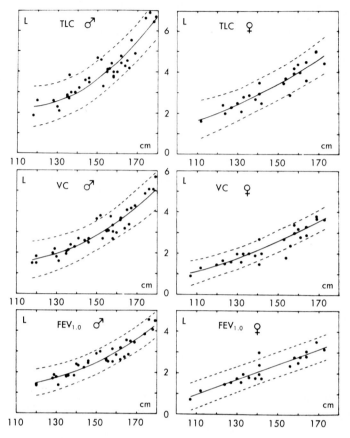

Fig. 3-6. Total lung capacity (TLC), vital capacity (VC), and forced expiratory volume at 1.0 second (FEV$_{1.0}$) in relation to body height in boys and girls. The drawn lines are regression equations (Table 3-3); 95% confidence limits are indicated by dashed lines. (From Zapletal, A., Motoyama, E. K., van de Woestijne, K. P., and others: J. Appl. Physiol. **26:**308, 1969.)

Table 3-3. Normal values for lung volumes (L) in relation to body height (cm)

y		N	a*	b*	c*	130 cm	150 cm	170 cm
TLC	♂	37	+15.1397	−0.22713	+0.001002	2.55 ± 0.51	3.62 ± 0.46	5.49 ± 0.47
	♀	24	+ 1.7592	−0.03394	+0.000300	2.41 ± 0.40	3.41 ± 0.40	4.66 ± 0.42
VC	♂	39	+ 7.9942	−0.12509	+0.000605	1.96 ± 0.40	2.85 ± 0.35	4.21 ± 0.43
	♀	26	+ 0.1694	−0.01217	+0.000189	1.78 ± 0.27	2.60 ± 0.25	3.56 ± 0.27
FRC	♂	37	+ 9.3716	−0.14152	+0.000602	1.15 ± 0.36	1.70 ± 0.34	2.71 ± 0.36
	♀	24	− 2.1776	+0.02556	0	1.11 ± 0.27	1.66 ± 0.25	2.17 ± 0.28
RV	♂	37	− 1.0519	+0.01270	0	0.60 ± 0.27	0.85 ± 0.26	1.11 ± 0.29
	♀	24	− 0.8046	+0.01092	0	0.61 ± 0.23	0.83 ± 0.22	1.05 ± 0.24
FEV$_{1.0}$	♂	33	+ 6.6314	−0.10261	+0.000499	1.73 ± 0.31	2.47 ± 0.29	3.61 ± 0.32
	♀	21	− 3.0378	+0.03640	0	1.69 ± 0.30	2.42 ± 0.29	3.15 ± 0.30

From Zapletal, A., Motoyama, E. K., van de Woestijne, K. P., and others: Maximum expiratory flow-volume curves and airway conductance in children and adolescents, J. Appl. Physiol. **26:**308, 1969.
*a, b, c = coefficients in regression equations of the type $y = a + bx + cx^2$, where y is the measurement and x is height in cm. N = number of observations. Data for height 130, 150, and 170 cm are predicted values ± standard error.

and PO_2 of the blood during each breath. In addition, the fact that air normally remains in the lungs throughout the respiratory cycle means that relatively few of the alveoli collapse. If air were completely exhaled with each expiration, all alveoli would collapse and have to be reexpanded again with inspiration, and large surface forces would have to be overcome with each breath. Although collapse does not occur during normal breathing, with the initiation of ventilation at birth and with open chest surgery unusually high pressures are necessary for expansion of the lung to its normal volume. Transpulmonary pressure of 4 to 6 cm H_2O is, under normal conditions, enough to effect an adequate tidal volume, but 15 to 25 cm H_2O (and occasionally even more) is necessary for initial expansion or reexpansion of collapsed lungs.

Summary

It appears that the lung volumes of normal infants are smaller functionally than those of older individuals. The subdivisions of the lung volumes, on the other hand, are similar in proportion during postnatal growth and development. These volumes are the result of a balance between the elastic forces of thoracic structures and the elastic characteristics of the lungs. A variety of conditions, including prematurity and anesthesia, may influence these factors and alter the lung volumes. The air remaining in the lungs at the end of expiration minimizes the changes in blood gases during the respiratory cycle; this remaining air also reduces the surface forces that must be overcome during ventilation.

MECHANICS OF BREATHING

To ventilate the lungs the respiratory muscles must overcome certain opposing forces within the lungs themselves. These forces can best be considered under two main headings: elastic and resistive* properties.

*The term *resistive* is used to include tissue viscosity and airflow resistive factors. Since these cannot easily be separated and since airflow resistance is clinically the most important, the term *flow resistance* will be used throughout.

Elastic properties

When the lungs are expanded, elastic recoil tends to contract the lungs spontaneously. This elastic force is fairly constant over the range of normal tidal volume but it increases at the extremes of deflation or inflation (Fig. 3-7). Elastic properties of the lungs are measured and expressed as lung compliance (C_l) in units of volume changes per units of pressure changes. Thus, $C_l = \dfrac{\Delta V}{\Delta P}$, where ΔV is usually the tidal volume and ΔP is the change in transpulmonary pressure (the difference between the airway and pleural pressures) necessary to produce the tidal volume. These measurements are made at points of no flow, i.e., at the extremes of tidal volume when there is no flow-resistive component (static compliance). As is apparent in Fig. 3-7, lung compliance may vary with changes in the midposition of the tidal ventilation without any inherent alterations in the elastic characteristics of the lungs. Therefore, a more accurate description of the elastic properties of the lungs is provided by measuring the pressure-volume relationship over the entire range of TLC.

In normal individuals, lung compliance measured during the respiratory cycle (i.e., the dynamic compliance) is approximately the same during quiet breathing as the static compliance. When there is airway obstruction, however, the ventilation of some of the lung units may be functionally decreased, resulting in a decreased dynamic compliance while the static compliance is relatively unaffected. This difference between the static and dynamic compliance is increased with increasing respiratory frequency (frequency dependence of compliance) and is a sign of airway obstruction (Woolcock and others, 1969).

When the lungs are stretched, energy is stored up and is released when the lungs return to their original size. In this way, quiet normal expiration is the result of the elastic recoil of the lungs and chest wall and involves little or no additional work. The situation in the infant and the anesthetized patient may be somewhat different, since

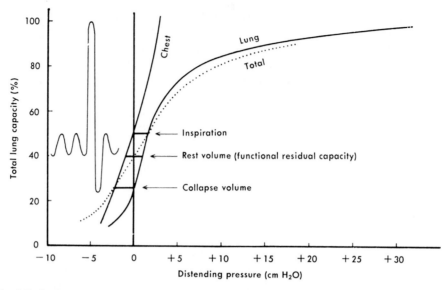

Fig. 3-7. Static pressure-volume diagram of the neonatal respiratory system. A normal spirogram is shown for volume orientation. Distending pressure on the abscissa represents transpulmonary pressure, or the difference between atmospheric and interpleural pressures. NOTE: (1) the chest wall is extremely compliant (high slope); (2) the lung compliance decreases (low slope) at extremes of lung volume; and (3) the functional residual capacity is relatively low. (From Nelson, N. M.: Pediatr. Clin. North Am. **13**:769, 1966.)

expiration may have an active phase, as discussed later.

To consider volume-pressure relations from another point of view, a normal tidal volume may be obtained by using transpulmonary pressures of approximately 4 to 6 cm H_2O in persons of all sizes, provided that the lungs are normal and normally expanded initially. The total transthoracopulmonary pressure necessary to ventilate the lungs in a closed chest is, in the adult, approximately twice the required transpulmonary pressure, since the thoracic structures must also be expanded. The chest wall is extremely compliant in the newborn, and it therefore requires by itself almost no force for expansion (Fig. 3-7). The combined compliance of chest wall* and lung, or the compliance of the total respiratory system (C_{rs}), is expressed as $1/C_{rs} = 1/C_l + 1/C_w$, where C_l is lung compliance and C_w is chest wall compliance.

*Chest wall includes intrathoracic and extrapulmonary structures: rib cage, diaphragm, abdominal contents, and abdominal wall, i.e., all the extrapulmonary structures that participate in breathing movements.

Lung compliance in normal individuals of different sizes, in general, is directly proportional to lung size (Table 3-2). When compliance is compared per unit of lung volume (e.g., FRC, VC, or TLC), lung compliance becomes similar for all sizes. Recent studies, however, indicate that lung compliance is relatively high (static recoil pressure is low) in healthy infants, resembling that of old persons with the loss of elastic recoil (Motoyama, 1977). Such a characteristic of infants' lungs may, at least in part, account for the high incidence of small airway diseases in this age group.

During postnatal development, lung compliance gradually decreases (elastic recoil increases), reaching the lowest values (the highest elastic recoil) between the ages of 16 and 20 years when the functional maturation of the lungs is completed (Motoyama, 1977; Zapletal, Misur, and Sammanek, 1971).

Chest wall compliance is also high in the newborn and decreases with age. It may be measured in the anesthetized and paralyzed patient or the trained subject by measuring the compliance of the total respiratory system (i.e., volume change vs airway pressure change) and subtracting that of the lungs alone (Butler and Smith, 1957).

Besides the lungs and chest wall, the air passages themselves have a compliance that may be important. With deep inspiration the air passages of normal persons increase in size, whereas on forced expiration they decrease to a point at which airway closure and air trapping may take place. Closing volume is the lung volume above RV at which dependent lung zones (i.e., lower lung segments in the upright position) cease to ventilate, presumably because of the closure of small airways. Closing capacity is the sum of closing volume and RV. Whether this closure is anatomic or merely the result of dynamic compression and reduction in flow (see the maximum expiratory flow-volume curve below) is controversial (Hughes and others, 1970; Hyatt and others, 1973). Since the patency of small airways depends in part on the elastic recoil of the lungs, closing capacity as percent of TLC is relatively high in young children (Mansell and others, 1972) and would be even higher, at least theoretically, in infants. Closing capacity increases with aging as well as with small airway disease such as chronic bronchitis due to smoking and emphysema in adults.

Lung compliance is reduced in most situations in which lung volume is decreased (e.g., removal of lung tissue, atelectasis, intrapulmonary tumors), although it is normal when corrected for lung volumes. Compliance is also decreased when surface forces are increased (as in the respiratory distress syndrome) or elastic recoil is abnormally elevated (interstitial pulmonary fibrosis).

Emphysema is associated with a loss of elasticity and therefore an abnormal elevation in compliance. Chest wall compliance decreases with such conditions as scleroderma, kyphoscoliosis, and ankylosing spondylitis involving the thoracic structures.

Flow-resistive properties

The resistive properties of the lungs include tissue viscous resistance (resistance of the tissues themselves to deformation) and resistance to the flow of air within the air passages. In contrast to compliance, which can be measured only at points of no flow (e.g., at the extremes of tidal volume or during interrupted ventilation), flow resistance is present only when the lungs (or the air within them) are in motion.

Airflow resistance (R) is expressed as a unit pressure (P) per unit flow ($\dot{V}$) (cm H_2O/L/sec) and, assuming a laminar flow, is related to the length (l) and radius (r) of a tube and the viscosity of the gas (η) as shown in Poiseuille's law:

$$R = \frac{8 l \eta}{\pi \, r^4}$$

It is apparent from the equation that the most important factor influencing flow resistance is the change in the radius of air passages, since it is inversely proportional to r^4.* Therefore, it is reasonable to suppose that infants with their small air passages have higher absolute resistance than do larger children and adults (Table 3-2). From this relationship it also might be expected that relatively small amounts of bronchiolar inflammation or secretions would lead to relatively greater degrees of obstruction in infants than in older persons (Fig. 3-8). One such example may be the severe and often life-threatening obstruction of upper airways seen only in infants and young children with acute epiglottitis and subglottic croup (laryngotracheobronchitis).

Based on Rohrer's earlier work (1915), it was believed that peripheral airways with small calibers were the major contributors to the total airway resistance. More recently, however, Weibel (1963) has proved in his elegant studies of airway morphometry that the total cross-sectional area for each generation of airways increases dramatically toward the periphery (Fig. 3-9). Indeed, about two thirds of the total airway resistance exists between the airway opening and the trachea, and most of the remaining resistance is in the large central airways. Contribution of the air-

*Flow resistance is related to $1/r^5$ when turbulence is present.

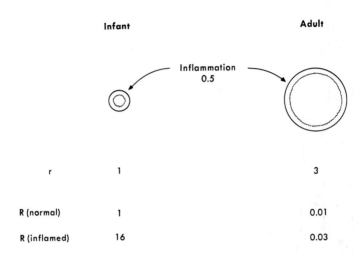

Fig. 3-8. Effect of inflammation on airway resistance in infants and adults. *r*, radius of an air passage; *R*, flow resistance.

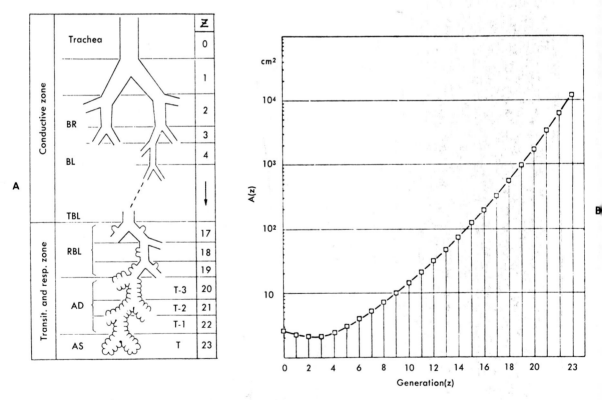

Fig. 3-9. A, Diagrammatic representation of the sequence of elements in the conductive and transitory zones of the airways. *z*, the order of generation of branching; *T*, the terminal generation. **B,** Total airway cross-sectional area, *A(z)*, in each generation, *z*. (From Weibel, E. R.: Morphometry of the human lung, New York, 1963, Academic Press, Inc., pp. 111, 138.)

ways smaller than a few millimeters in diameter is only about 10% of the total (Macklem and Mead, 1967).

These findings have important clinical implications. If the peripheral airways contribute so little to the total airway resistance, disease processes involving small airways, such as emphysema in adults and cystic fibrosis in children, would not be detectable by measurement of the total airway resistance. For instance, complete obstruction of every peripheral airway would increase the total airway resistance only by 10%, an increase within the usual variations in measurements. For this reason, the peripheral airways have been called the lungs' "quiet zone" (Mead, 1970). Apparently, the measurement of total airway resistance is not a sensitive clinical test for detecting small airway obstructions.

During quiet breathing, pleural pressure remains subatmospheric, whereas during forced expiration, pleural pressure increases considerably above atmospheric pressure and, in turn, increases alveolar pressure. The resultant pressure gradient between the alveoli and the airway opening (atmospheric) produces the expiratory flow. In the periphery of the lung this pressure within the airways is higher than the pleural pressure because of elastic recoil of the lung. By comparison, in major intrathoracic airways, the pressure within the lumen is near atmospheric and is lower than the surrounding pleural pressure. At some point along the airways the pressure within the airway lumen should equal the pleural pressure surrounding the airway (equal pressure point, EPP) (Mead and others, 1967). During forced expiration, the airway between EPP and the trachea is dynamically compressed, and the flow rates consequently become independent of effort (i.e., any additional expiratory effort or pressure does not increase flow). Under these circumstances, the maximum expiratory flow rate ($\dot{V}_{max}$) is determined by the flow resistance of the upstream segment between the alveoli and EPP (R_{us}) and the elastic recoil pressure of the lung ($P_{st(l)}$) as follows:

$$\dot{V}_{max} = \frac{P_{st(l)}}{R_{us}}$$

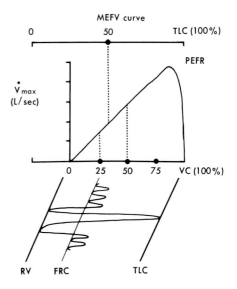

Fig. 3-10. A schematic drawing of maximum expiratory flow-volume (MEFV) curve as compared with a more conventional spirogram.

The maximum expiratory flow-volume (MEFV) curve obtained during forced expiration relates maximum expiratory flow rates to corresponding lung volumes (Fig. 3-10). Clinically, the measurement of $\dot{V}_{max}$ is an extremely sensitive test to detect lower airway obstruction, since it eliminates the component of the upper airway resistance between the mouth and EPP (Zapletal, Motoyama, Gibson, and Bouhuys, 1971).

Airway resistance decreases with the growth of the size of the body as well as the lungs. Between 6 and 18 years of age there is a linear correlation between airway conductance (reciprocal of resistance) and height (Zapletal and others, 1969) (Fig. 3-11). Information on airway dynamics in children less than 6 years of age is limited. However, airway conductance, normalized for lung volumes, appears disproportionately high (resistance is low) in the newborn (Polgar, 1967).

Based on studies of autopsy lungs, Hogg and associates (1970) reported that airway conductance of peripheral airways in children less than 6 years of age was disproportionately low (i.e., resistance was high).

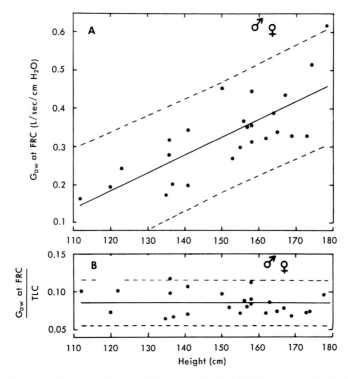

Fig. 3-11. A, Airway conductance (G_{aw}) at FRC vs standing height in boys and girls. **B,** The same data with conductance expressed in terms of TLC/sec/cm H_2O. The drawn lines are regression equations; 95% confidence limits are indicated by dashed lines. G_{aw} at FRC = $-0.3819 + 0.00472 \times$ height (cm). (From Zapletal, A., Motoyama, E. K., van de Woestijne, K. P., and others: J. Appl. Physiol. **26:**308, 1969.)

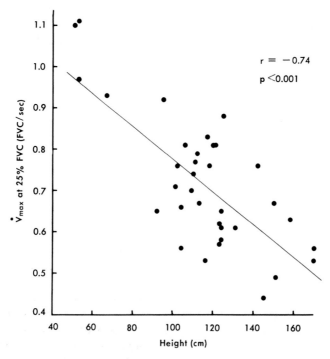

Fig. 3-12. Maximum expiratory flow rate ($\dot{V}_{max}$) at 25% forced vital capacity (FVC) from deflation flow-volume curves vs height in anesthetized boys and girls. $\dot{V}_{max}$ is expressed in FVC units/sec to normalize for lung size. (From Motoyama, E. K.: Pediatr. Res. **11:**220, 1977.)

With oral airway

Average ΔPes = 6 cm H_2O

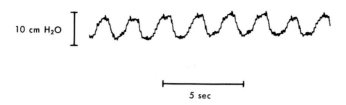

10 cm H_2O

5 sec

Without oral airway

Average ΔPes = 12 cm H_2O

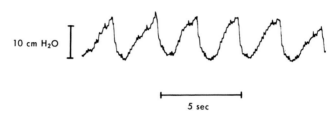

10 cm H_2O

5 sec

Fig. 3-13. Intraesophageal pressure changes (ΔPes) indicating low airway resistance with proper use of oral airway *(top)* and increased resistance due to inadequate neck and mandible extension without oral airway *(bottom)*.

These authors postulated that the diameter of small airways at the same generation was disproportionately smaller in infants than in older children and adults. Although this theory is attractive to explain clinical pictures of frequent and severe lower airway disease in infants, it is in conflict with the data of Polgar (1967) on airway conductance from normal newborns. In addition, MEFV curves obtained from anesthetized infants and children have shown that maximum expiratory flow rate, normalized for body size, is disproportionately higher in infants and decreases with growth, indicating that lower airway resistance is lower, rather than higher, in early postnatal years (Motoyama, 1977) (Fig. 3-12).

Resistance may be increased when air passages are narrowed from bronchospasm (e.g., asthma), from secretions or inflammations (e.g., bronchiolitis and croup), from foreign bodies, or from pressure (e.g., vascular rings, mediastinal tumors, or tuberculous nodes). Resistance may also be increased during anesthesia because of improper maintenance of the airway (Fig. 3-13) or high resistance of the external apparatus. All of these factors will increase the work of breathing. Under such circumstances a relatively large tidal volume and low respiratory rate will be most efficient in relation to the work of breathing as well as to ventilation itself.

The flow resistance of individual parts of the lung will influence their ventilation. If extreme narrowing exists, only small amounts of new air will enter the air spaces below with each respiratory cycle, resulting in uneven distribution of ventilation and ventilation-perfusion imbalance, as discussed later.

Lung compliance and flow resistance can

be measured by simultaneously measuring changes in flow, volume, and interpleural pressure (Fig. 3-14). Fortunately intraesophageal pressure changes are good indices of interpleural pressure changes, although in the supine position the weight of the mediastinum on the esophagus produces artifacts that are difficult to evaluate.

Summary

In absolute terms, lung compliance is directly related to body or lung size. In relative terms, however, lung compliance is relatively higher in infants and young children than in older children and young adults. In normal lungs, compliance is highest in the tidal volume range; it is reduced at both extremes of lung volume. When a healthy adult patient is ventilated artificially, about one half of the pressure required is to expand the lungs and the other half is to expand the chest wall. In contrast, the chest wall in infants is extremely compliant and requires little pressure to expand. In normal lungs the majority of airway resistance exists in large central airways; contribution of small airways is only a fraction of the total flow resistance. Flow resistance in absolute terms is largest in persons with the smallest air passages; thus, small infants are more prone to airway obstruction of upper and lower airways. When lung volumes are taken into account, there is controversy as to whether airway resistance is relatively higher or lower in infants in comparison with older individuals.

VENTILATION

Ventilation involves the movement of air in and out of the lungs. The diaphragm is the most important muscle for normal inspiration, although the intercostal and accessory respiratory muscles aid in a maximal inspiratory effort. Quiet expiration results from the elastic recoil of the lungs and chest wall and the relaxation of the diaphragm. The expiration of a newborn, even when resting or asleep, appears active rather than passive as in the older child and adult. A similar active expiration has been observed in anesthetized children (Motoyama and Cook) and adults (Freund and others, 1964), but the mechanism is unknown. Forced expiration is accomplished with the aid of the spinal flexors, the intercostal, and especially the abdominal muscles.

Tidal volume (V_T) is the amount of air

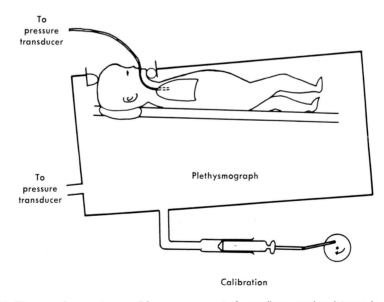

To pressure transducer

To pressure transducer

Plethysmograph

Calibration

Fig. 3-14. Diagram of apparatus used for measurement of compliance and resistance in newborns. Intraesophageal catheter is shown in place. Pressure changes in body-plethysmograph were used to measure flow and tidal volume changes.

moved into or out of the lungs with each breath. Minute volume ($\dot{V}_E$) is the amount of air breathed in or out in a minute, i.e., $\dot{V}_E = V_T \times f$ (frequency).

Frequency of quiet breathing decreases as a person increases in age. The exact basis for this change in the rate of breathing with age is not known but may be related to the work of breathing. It has been suggested that individuals often tend to adjust their respiratory rate and tidal volumes so that their ventilatory needs are accomplished with a minimum of work (McIlroy and others, 1954). The relatively high rate for newborns (average, 34 breaths per minute) as compared with adults (average, 12 per minute) at least is consistent with this minimum work concept (Cook and others, 1957) (Fig. 3-15). However, Mead (1960) has presented data indicating that respiration in the normal resting state is adjusted so that there is a minimum average force required of the respiratory muscles; he postulated that the principal site of the sensory end of the control mecha-

nism may be in the lungs. In certain situations the minimum work of breathing and minimum average force required would occur at the same frequency of respiration, but this would not invariably be true.

Only part of the minute volume is effective in gas exchange, i.e., the alveolar ventilation ($\dot{V}_A$), whereas part merely ventilates the respiratory dead space. If the minute noneffective ventilation ($\dot{V}_E - \dot{V}_A$) is divided by the frequency, one obtains the calculated physiologic respiratory dead space. In the normal person the physiologic and anatomic dead spaces are approximately the same. Since the air passages are compliant structures, the size of the dead space correlates closely with the degree of lung expansion. When airway obstruction and emphysema are present, dead space increases. However, physiologic dead space is influenced more importantly by the evenness of distribution of gas within the lungs and by the perfusion of the alveoli. Thus, when there is uneven ventilation of the lungs (as in asthma or cystic

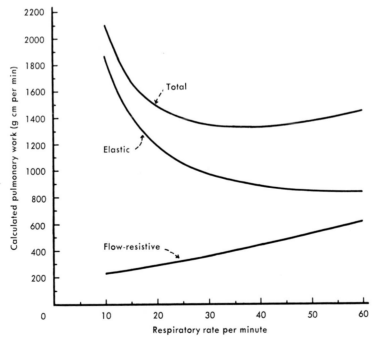

Fig. 3-15. Calculated pulmonary work in newborns vs respiratory rate. The theoretical minimum work of respiration occurs at a rate of 37 per minute. Observed resting respiratory rates were 38. (From Cook, C. D., Sutherland, J. M., Segal, S., and others: J. Clin. Invest. **36:**440, 1957.)

fibrosis) or the blood supply to various areas of the lungs decreases (as with pulmonary emboli), there will be increases in the physiologic dead space.

Although the anatomic dead space represents an inefficient part of the respiratory tract in respect to gas exchange, it does have some important functions; on inspiration, gas is humidified and warmed in the respiratory dead space. These functions are compromised when patients are intubated or tracheostomized.

A useful approximation of the dead space in a normal person results from the fact that it can be expressed as 1 ml for each pound of normal body weight (Radford and others, 1954). A more exact estimate of the anatomic dead space may be obtained in children and young adults from its relation to body height (Hart and others, 1963). Although the calculations are based on the not entirely accurate assumption that there is no diffusion of gas from dead space to alveoli, the importance of changes in respiratory dead space can be appreciated from the estimated compensation adjustments shown in Table 3-4. The figures also suggest that, from the ventilatory point of view, it is inefficient to increase total ventilation by increases in rate; it is most effective to increase tidal volume to compensate for dead space changes or increased ventilatory requirements.

The V_D/V_T ratio is approximately constant

Table 3-4. Calculated adjustments in a 2.5-kg infant secondary to changes in respiratory dead space

	Dead space		
	5 ml	**10 ml**	**10 ml**
Tidal volume	15 ml	15 ml	19.7 ml
Minute volume	510 ml	990 ml	670 ml
Rate per minute	34	66	34
Alveolar ventilation	330 ml	330 ml*	330 ml*

*These calculations are based on the assumption that gas would not diffuse from the dead space to the alveoli. Actually some diffusion does occur so that with very rapid ventilation patients can survive even when their dead space approaches their tidal volume or vice versa.

(0.3) from infancy to adulthood (Table 3-2). However, an absolute increase in dead space, whether due to respiratory abnormalities or external apparatus, is much more critical to the infant than to the adult because of the infant's small tidal volume and the relatively larger volume of dead space added.

Alveolar ventilation ($\dot{V}_A$) or the minute effective ventilation may be expressed in terms of the CO_2 in the peripheral arterial blood. Thus, we have the equation:

$$\dot{V}_A = \frac{(P_B - 47) \times \dot{V}_{CO_2}}{Pa_{CO_2}}$$

where

$$\begin{aligned}
\dot{V}_{CO_2} &= CO_2 \text{ production per minute} \\
Pa_{CO_2} &= \text{arterial } CO_2 \text{ tension} \\
P_B - 47 &= \text{barometric pressure minus water} \\
&\quad \text{vapor tension at } 37° \text{ C}
\end{aligned}$$

The difference between minute volume and alveolar ventilation ($\dot{V}_E - \dot{V}_A$) is the wasted ventilation due to physiologic dead space. Perhaps the concept of $\dot{V}_A$ is easier to understand if one considers it similar in some way to the renal clearance of a substance; in the lungs, CO_2 is the substance being cleared. It can be seen that if $\dot{V}_{CO_2}$ remains constant when $\dot{V}_A$ is halved, Pa_{CO_2} will double. As is apparent in Table 3-4, measurement of $\dot{V}_A$ provides a far better index of the efficacy of ventilation than measurement of $\dot{V}_E$. $\dot{V}_E$ may be very large, but, if it is composed mostly of ineffective ventilation, $\dot{V}_A$ may not be adequate.

Alveolar ventilation is considerably higher per unit of lung volume in the normal infant than in the adult. This would be expected since the oxygen consumption is also higher per unit of lung volume or body weight (Cook and others, 1955).

Ventilation in any area of the lungs is influenced by the flow resistance (R, expressed as $P/\dot{V}$, cm H_2O/ml/sec) and compliance (C, expressed as V/P, ml/cm H_2O) of that particular area. The product of resistance and compliance (RC), or the time constant (expressed as a unit of time), is similar for the various areas of a normal lung. In diseased lungs, as in asthma, pneumonia, and cystic fibrosis, the time constant becomes abnormal in affected areas and is associated with uneven distribution of ventilation. The distribution of ventilation may be studied by measuring the nitrogen washout curve; this involves breathing 100% O_2 and measuring the decline of the concentration of alveolar N_2, an inert gas, in successive expirations. Nitrogen concentration for both normal children and adults is less than 2.5% after 7 minutes of oxygen breathing. This value is increased in patients with an uneven distribution of ventilation, since the elimination of nitrogen from poorly ventilated areas is prolonged. In addition, by using xenon and a gamma camera, scintigraphic information can be obtained that can provide useful data on regional distribution of ventilation (Ball and others, 1962; Goodrich and others, 1972).

It is a common practice for anesthesiologists to manually or mechanically control the ventilation of the patient during anesthesia, since most of the anesthetic techniques used today produce a reduction or cessation of spontaneous ventilation. What information is available for aiding the proper maintenance of ventilation during anesthesia? One may estimate the patient's ventilatory requirements from his size. This has been done by Radford and associates (1954), and their nomogram (Fig. 3-16) has proved useful, provided that the patient has a normal cardiopulmonary system and that there is no increase in physiologic dead space and/or shunting of blood. Since anesthetized patients tend to develop atelectasis and shunting (and an increase in physiologic dead space) because of the absence of "sigh mechanism" and a decrease in FRC, it is necessary to hyperinflate the lungs periodically as well as to increase the tidal volume above the predicted values. One should also take the mechanical dead space and "internal compliance" of anesthetic equipment into consider-

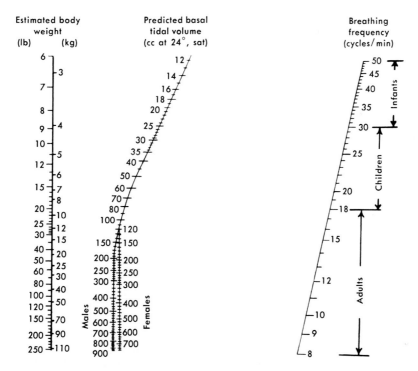

Fig. 3-16. Nomogram for predicted basal tidal volume. Corrections to be applied: add 10% if subject is awake; add 9% for each degree centigrade of fever; add 8% for each 1000 meters of altitude above sea level. Add the dead space of the anesthetic apparatus. (From Radford, E. P., Jr., Ferris, B. J., Jr., and Kriet, B. C.: N. Engl. J. Med. **251**:877, 1954.)

ation for the proper estimation of the patient's ventilatory requirement (see Chapter 27). Physiologic dead space is further increased in patients in the intensive care unit with acute respiratory insufficiency. In these patients it is practical to start with a tidal volume of 15 ml/kg or roughly twice as much as that predicted from the nomogram. A proper adjustment of ventilation can be made with the measurement of arterial P_{CO_2} and P_{O_2} as a guide.

Summary

Ventilation is made up of effective and dead space ventilation. Except in early infancy where it is relatively higher, it is very similar for all ages when compared on the basis of lung or body size. Absolute changes in dead space or ventilation are relatively more critical in smaller persons. In the monitoring of respiration, the measurement of alveolar ventilation is more useful than total ventilation. Changes in Pa_{CO_2} reflect changes in alveolar ventilation. Changes in the regional time constants (RC) in diseased lungs are associated with uneven ventilation. Nitrogen washout curve has been used as one standard test for uneven ventilation. More recently the lung scan with xenon and a gamma camera has provided useful information on the distribution of ventilation.

GAS DIFFUSION

The ultimate purpose of pulmonary ventilation is to allow diffusion of O_2 through the alveolar epithelial lining, basement membrane, and capillary endothelial wall into the plasma and red cells and diffusion of CO_2 in the opposite direction. As is apparent on electron micrographs of lung tissue (Fig. 3-25), the distance for gases to diffuse between the alveolar space and capillary lumen is extremely small, about 0.3 μ in humans (Weibel, 1973). Since these processes apparently follow the physical laws of diffusion without any active participation on the part of the lung tissue, pressure gradients must exist or gas exchange will not occur. On the other hand, if the gradient is increased because of changes of gas tensions either within

the alveoli or in the blood, the exchange of gas will be more rapid. Furthermore, since the blood P_{O_2} affects the blood P_{CO_2}, changes in one moiety will produce changes in the diffusion of the other. Carbon dioxide diffuses approximately 20 times faster than oxygen in a gas-liquid environment. Therefore, the impairment of CO_2 diffusion does not become apparent in clinical situations until extremely severe disease is present.

Pulmonary gas diffusion is another example of the similarities between pediatric and adult respiratory physiology, since it is relatively constant for all ages when size is taken into consideration (Bucci and others, 1961; Stahlman and Meece, 1957).

Although diffusion of gases within the lung is necessary for survival, comparatively few conditions occurring in children affect diffusion per se. Diffusing capacity is decreased in the "alveolar capillary block syndrome" (Bates, 1962). This decrease was considered to be primarily due to increased thickness of alveolar-capillary membranes, but it is now believed that uneven distribution of ventilation with resulting ventilation-perfusion imbalance is the more important cause of arterial oxygen desaturation (Finley and others, 1962). Anemia is also associated with a decreased diffusing capacity. This is in part explained by the decrease in the ability of blood to carry the inspired gases. Patients with congenital heart disease and left-to-right shunts frequently have an increased diffusing capacity secondary to increased blood volume and flow in the lungs (Bucci and Cook, 1961). Conversely, diffusing capacity may be reduced when the pulmonary blood flow is markedly decreased, as in pulmonic stenosis.

The diffusing capacity of the lungs may be measured with a foreign gas, carbon monoxide, used in small concentrations (0.3% or less) or by varying the concentration of inspired oxygen (Forster, 1957). In general, these techniques are useful for research and, in a few instances of respiratory insufficiency, as diagnostic aids.

PULMONARY CIRCULATION

In prenatal life, pulmonary vascular resistance is high, and the major portion of right ventricular output runs parallel to the left ventricular outflow, bypassing the lungs and flowing into the descending aorta through the ductus arteriosus. With the onset of ventilation at birth, there is a sudden fall in the pulmonary vascular resistance and an increase in the blood flow through the lungs that enables the organism to exchange oxygen and carbon dioxide and sustain independent existence. The principal factors that control this vital adjustment in vascular re-

sistance are the chemical changes (i.e., changes in P_{O_2} and P_{CO_2} or pH) in the environment of the pulmonary vessels (Cook and others, 1963). An increase in P_{O_2} also produces constriction and subsequent closure of the ductus arteriosus. The pulmonary arterial pressure, which is slightly higher than the pressure in the ascending aorta in the fetus (Assali and Morris, 1964), shows some decrease at birth and continues to decrease with a concomitant rise in systemic blood pressure until it approaches the adult level within the first year of life (Fig. 3-17) (Rudolph, 1970). If the lungs do not expand

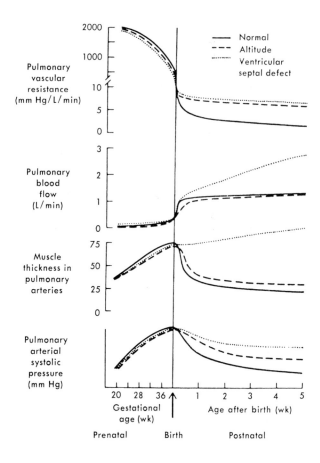

Fig. 3-17. Schematic representation of fetal and postnatal changes in pulmonary vascular resistance, pulmonary blood flow, thickness of smooth muscle in the medial layer of pulmonary arteries, and pulmonary arterial systolic pressure. At birth, the pulmonary vascular resistance in normal infants falls rapidly in response to a rise in blood oxygen tension; it falls more slowly in infants born at high altitude or with a ventricular septal defect of large size. Pulmonary blood flow increases rapidly at birth in normal infants. In the presence of a ventricular septal defect, pulmonary blood flow increases further as pulmonary vascular resistance falls. Pulmonary arterial pressure normally falls rapidly after birth; the fall is delayed at high altitude, and pressure remains slightly elevated. Pulmonary arterial pressure does not fall when a large ventricular septal defect is present, and it increases as systemic arterial pressure rises. The muscle in the pulmonary arteries does not regress as rapidly as normal in infants at high altitudes. In infants with ventricular septal defect, the muscle does not regress normally and soon after birth increases in amount. (From Rudolph, A. M.: The changes in the circulation after birth; their importance in congenital heart disease, Circulation **41:**343, 1970. By permission of the American Heart Association, Inc.)

adequately (as in the respiratory distress syndrome) and Po_2 remains low, the pulmonary vascular resistance and pressure may remain high and there may be prolonged patency of the ductus and persistent right-to-left shunting of blood (Strang and MacLeish, 1961).

Under normal postnatal conditions, the systemic and pulmonary vascular beds are connected in series to form a continuous circuit. While the systemic circulation has a high vascular resistance with a large pressure gradient between the arteries and veins, the pulmonary circulation presents a low resistance to flow.

Both hypoxemia and hypercapnia constrict the pulmonary vascular bed and increase resistance to flow. Chronic hypoxemia at high altitude or in diseases such as severe cystic fibrosis with emphysema is associated with a pulmonary hypertension that returns to or toward normal when hypoxemia is corrected (Goldring and others, 1964). Pulmonary hypertension that persists for months or, more frequently, for years results in cor pulmonale, which then further complicates the existing pulmonary insufficiency.

Under normal circumstances the arterial blood from the left ventricle contains up to 5% unsaturated blood (venous admixture). This comes mainly from the bronchial circulation but also partly from blood in the pulmonary circulation bypassing the alveoli and from blood flowing through the thebesian veins. It results in a depression of the arterial Po_2 from approximately 102 to 97 torr. In certain conditions, such as ventilation-perfusion imbalance (including decreased diffusing capacity), the amount of the venous admixture through the lungs increases sufficiently to cause significant arterial hypoxemia. Venous admixture also occurs because of intrapulmonary shunting as the result of atelectasis, pulmonary arteriovenous fistula, pulmonary hemangiomas, and increased collateral (bronchial) circulation as in bronchiectasis. In addition, shunting may occur at the cardiac level when there is congenital heart disease with right-to-left shunts.

Pulmonary hemodynamics vary significantly during the respiratory cycle. Small vessels and capillaries in the alveolar wall are apparently exposed to the pressure in the alveoli. These vessels may therefore be compressed or even collapsed during positive pressure breathing, particularly when the patient is hypovolemic. In contrast, pressure surrounding larger vessels outside of alveoli would reflect the pleural pressure and tend to distend these vessels during inflation (West and others, 1964).

VENTILATION-PERFUSION RELATIONSHIPS

To achieve normal gas exchange in the lung, the regional distribution of ventilation and perfusion must be balanced. Without this balance, pulmonary gas exchange would be impaired even though the overall levels of ventilation and perfusion might be adequate. The normal value for the ventilation-perfusion ($\dot{V}_A/\dot{Q}$) ratio is about 0.8.

Studies with radioactive gases have shown that the elastic and resistive properties of various parts of the lung as well as the pulmonary blood flow are influenced by gravity. Thus, both components of the $\dot{V}_A/\dot{Q}$ ratio are affected by changes in the position of the patient (West, 1965).

In the upright position, blood flow and ventilation are both less in the apex than in the base of the lungs. Since the difference in blood flow between apex and base is relatively greater than that for ventilation, the $\dot{V}_A/\dot{Q}$ ratio increases from the bottom to the top of the lungs, as shown in Fig. 3-18. Thus, the apical regions (high $\dot{V}_A/\dot{Q}$) have higher alveolar Po_2 and lower Pco_2 and P_{N_2}, whereas the basal areas (low $\dot{V}_A/\dot{Q}$) have lower Po_2 and higher Pco_2 and P_{N_2}. Gravity has a greater effect on the $\dot{V}_A/\dot{Q}$ ratio in hypotensive and hypovolemic patients and may be exaggerated with positive pressure breathing. In the supine position, similar differences exist between the anterior and posterior parts of the lung but are of smaller magnitude. During exercise, pulmonary arterial pressure and blood flow as well as ventilation are in-

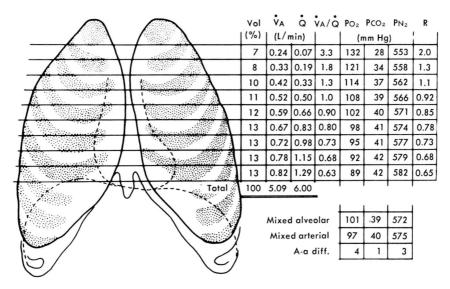

Vol (%)	$\dot{V}_A$ (L/min)	$\dot{Q}$	$\dot{V}_A/\dot{Q}$	PO_2 (mm Hg)	PCO_2	PN_2	R
7	0.24	0.07	3.3	132	28	553	2.0
8	0.33	0.19	1.8	121	34	558	1.3
10	0.42	0.33	1.3	114	37	562	1.1
11	0.52	0.50	1.0	108	39	566	0.92
12	0.59	0.66	0.90	102	40	571	0.85
13	0.67	0.83	0.80	98	41	574	0.78
13	0.72	0.98	0.73	95	41	577	0.73
13	0.78	1.15	0.68	92	42	579	0.68
13	0.82	1.29	0.63	89	42	582	0.65
Total 100	5.09	6.00					

	PO_2	PCO_2	PN_2
Mixed alveolar	101	.39	572
Mixed arterial	97	40	575
A-a diff.	4	1	3

Fig. 3-18. Effect of distribution of ventilation and perfusion on regional gas tensions in erect man. The lung is divided into nine horizontal slices, and the position of each slice is shown by its anterior rib markings. *Vol %*, relative lung volume; $\dot{V}_A$, regional alveolar ventilation; $\dot{Q}$, regional perfusion; $\dot{V}_A/\dot{Q}$, ventilation-perfusion ratio; *R*, respiratory exchange ratio. (From West, J. B.: J. Appl. Physiol. **17**:893, 1962.)

creased and are distributed more evenly. In infants and children, the distribution of pulmonary blood flow is more uniform, since the pulmonary arterial pressure is relatively high and the gravity effect in the lungs is less.

In diseased lungs, changes in the $\dot{V}_A/\dot{Q}$ ratio occur as the result of uneven ventilation and/or perfusion; e.g., compression or occlusion of pulmonary vessels, reduced pulmonary vascular bed, or intrapulmonary anatomic right-to-left shunt may contribute to nonuniform perfusion. In congenital heart conditions with increased pulmonary blood flow due to left-to-right shunting, the $\dot{V}_A/\dot{Q}$ ratio is decreased, but it is increased when perfusion is diminished, as in cases of tricuspid atresia or pulmonic stenosis.

There may be an intrinsic regulatory mechanism in the lung that, to a limited extent, functions to preserve a normal $\dot{V}_A/\dot{Q}$ ratio. In areas in which $\dot{V}_A/\dot{Q}$ ratios are high, a low PCO_2 tends to constrict airways and dilate pulmonary vessels, and the opposite occurs in areas in which regional $\dot{V}_A/\dot{Q}$

ratios are low. In the latter case, low PO_2 also contributes to the vascular constriction. Administration of isoproterenol abolishes this regulatory mechanism, resulting in an increase in intrapulmonary shunting (Goldzimer and others, 1974).

Several methods are available to assess ventilation-perfusion relationships. Uneven $\dot{V}_A/\dot{Q}$ ratios in various parts of the lungs cause an increase in gradient between gas tensions of mixed alveolar air and arterial or, more specifically, mixed pulmonary venous blood. However, an increased A-a PO_2 gradient (A-aDO_2) may also be the result of alterations in diffusion and/or direct venous admixture. Differential diagnosis of these factors can be made by changing the inspired PO_2 (Rahn and Fahri, 1964). If the A-aDO_2 is relatively unchanged by changes in inspired PO_2, the most likely cause of the increased gradient is $\dot{V}_A/\dot{Q}$ imbalance. When the A-aDO_2 increases with low inspired oxygen tensions (PO_2 <50 mm Hg), an impairment of diffusing capacity is the most probable cause. If, on the other hand, the A-aDO$_2$ increases with high inspired oxygen tensions, the underlying pathology is most likely to be due to right-to-left shunting (Fig. 3-19). Nelson and associates (1963) reported a higher A-aDO$_2$ in newborns than in adults and attributed their findings to increased right-to-left shunting rather than to uneven $\dot{V}_A/\dot{Q}$ ratios.

Ventilation-perfusion imbalance, particularly the presence of high $\dot{V}_A/\dot{Q}$ areas, increases the a-A gradient of PCO$_2$ (a-ADcO$_2$). Increased a-ADcO$_2$ is most apparent in cases of pulmonary hypoperfusion such as peripheral pulmonic stenosis, pulmonary artery ligation as the result of the superior vena cava–right pulmonary artery shunt procedure, and massive pulmonary embolism. An a-ADcO$_2$ as high as 20 torr may be seen in these cases.

Nonuniform $\dot{V}_A/\dot{Q}$ ratios throughout the lungs, particularly the presence of low $\dot{V}_A/\dot{Q}$ areas, will also cause an increased a-A gradient of PN$_2$. Utilization of the PN$_2$ gradient has definite advantages over PO$_2$, since the former is only slightly affected by

diffusion and is not influenced by venous admixture. Since nitrogen is inert and PN$_2$ during the steady state is essentially the same in the body fluids PN$_2$ in the urine may be used as an index of arterial PN$_2$. The normal value for a-ADN$_2$ thus obtained is below 10 mm Hg (mean, 3 to 5). The a-ADN$_2$ during the first 24 hours of life is significantly elevated (ΔPN$_2$ >20 mm Hg) (Fahri, 1964). This indicates that the pulmonary ventilation is not properly matched with increased pulmonary perfusion (a low $\dot{V}_A/\dot{Q}$ ratio) during the neonatal period. The a-ADN$_2$ decreases rapidly toward normal values within a few days of life (Fig. 3-3). In severe $\dot{V}_A/\dot{Q}$ imbalance, such as occurs in severe cystic fibrosis, PN$_2$ gradients may be significantly increased. Fig. 3-19 summarizes the physiologic diagnosis based on arterial blood gases and A-a gas tension differences (Nelson, 1976).

The difference between physiologic and anatomic dead space may also be used as an index of uneven perfusion, since this difference (alveolar dead space) would increase

Defect		Air-breathe		Increase in A-aDO$_2$			Increase in a-ADcO$_2$	Increase in a-ADN$_2$
		Pa$_{O_2}$	Pa$_{CO_2}$	On air (21% O$_2$)	100% O$_2$	14% O$_2$		
Hypoventilation		Low	High	None	None	None	None	None
Venous admixture (shunt)		Low	NI	Moderate	Large	Slight	Un-measurable	None
Diffusion limitation		Low	NI to low	Slight	Un-measurable	Mod-erate	Un-measurable	None
Uneven $\dot{V}_A/\dot{Q}_c$	High $\dot{V}_A/\dot{Q}_c$	NI to high	NI to low	Moderate	Slight	Slight	Large	Slight
	Low $\dot{V}_A/\dot{Q}_c$	Low	NI to high	Moderate	Slight	Slight	Slight	Large

Fig. 3-19. Classification of respiratory disturbances: physiologic diagnosis is based on arterial blood gases and alveolar-arterial gas pressure differences while breathing air, as well as on their behavior during the breathing of hyperoxic and hypoxic gas mixtures. (From Nelson, N. M.: Respiration and circulation after birth. In Smith, C. A., and Nelson, N. M., editors: The physiology of the newborn infant, ed. 4, Springfield, Ill., 1976, Charles C Thomas, Publisher, p. 227.)

when ventilated areas are not well perfused (Severinghaus and Stupfel, 1957). By using xenon with a gamma camera and an appropriately programmed computer it is possible to get both pictorial and numerical information on ventilation and perfusion (Treves and others, 1974).

OXYGEN TRANSPORT

Oxygen must be supplied continuously to all body tissues to maintain normal metabolism. Changes in oxygen demand are met by the integrated response of three major functional components of the oxygen transport system: pulmonary ventilation, cardiac output, and blood hemoglobin concentrations and characteristics. In acute oxygen demand such as severe exercise, high fever, or acute hypoxemia (Pa_{O_2} <60 torr), oxygen transport is increased mainly by the increase in cardiac output while the alveolar ventilation is increased to maintain proper levels of alveolar P_{O_2} and P_{CO_2}. Chronic hypoxemia increases erythropoietin production and results in increased erythrocyte production from a normal daily rate or approximately 1% of circulating red cell mass to about 2%. Thus, increase in red cell mass in response

to chronic hypoxemia is a slow process (Finch and Lenfant, 1972). Increased hemoglobin concentrations above normal levels (15 g/dl) raise viscosity and increase blood flow resistance until the plasma volume also is increased (Thorling and Erslev, 1968).

The amount of oxygen carried by the plasma depends on its solubility and is small (approximately 0.3 ml/dl/100 torr). The majority of oxygen molecules in blood are combined reversibly with hemoglobin to form oxyhemoglobin. Each molecule of hemoglobin combines with four molecules of oxygen; 1 g of oxyhemoglobin is combined with 1.34 ml of oxygen.

The oxygen-hemoglobin dissociation curve reflects the affinity of hemoglobin for oxygen (Fig. 3-20). As blood circulates through the normal lungs, oxygen tension increases from the mixed venous level of near 40 torr to approximately 100 torr, and hemoglobin is saturated about 97% in arterial blood. The shape of the dissociation curve is such that further increases in P_{O_2} result in a very small increase in oxygen saturation (S_{O_2}) of hemoglobin.

As blood circulates through the capillaries, oxygen is taken up by the tissues, and P_{O_2}

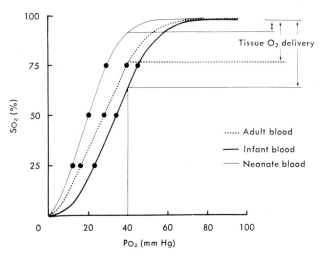

Fig. 3-20. Schematic representation of oxygen-hemoglobin dissociation curves with different oxygen affinities. In infants above 3 months of age with high P_{50} (30 torr vs 27 in adults), tissue oxygen delivery per gram of hemoglobin is increased. In neonates with a lower P_{50} (20 torr) and a higher oxygen affinity, tissue oxygen unloading at the same tissue P_{O_2} is reduced.

as well as So_2 fall. In the normal adult, blood So_2 decreases to 50% when Po_2 falls to about 27 torr at 37° C and pH of 7.4. The P_{50}, which is Po_2 of whole blood at 50% So_2, indicates the affinity of hemoglobin for oxygen. It is known that the affinity of hemoglobin for oxygen increases when the blood pH increases (Bohr effect). A decrease in temperature also increases the oxygen affinity and shifts the oxygen-hemoglobin dissociation curve to the left; a decrease in pH or an increase in temperature has the opposite effect (Comroe, 1974).

Benesch and Benesch (1967) and Chanutin and Curnish (1967) demonstrated that the oxygen affinity of hemoglobin solution can be decreased by the addition of organic phosphate, in particular 2,3-DPG and ATP, which bind to deoxyhemoglobin but not to oxyhemoglobin. Human erythrocytes contain an extremely high concentration of 2,3-DPG, averaging about 4.5 μmole/ml, as compared with ATP (1.0 μmole/ml) and other organic phosphates (Oski and Delivo-

ria-Papadopoulos, 1970). Thus, an increase in red cell 2,3-DPG decreases the oxygen affinity of hemoglobin, increases P_{50} (shift to the right of the dissociation curve), and increases the unloading of oxygen at the tissue levels. Such an increase in 2,3-DPG and P_{50} has been found in chronic hypoxemia.

In the newborn, blood oxygen affinity is extremely high and P_{50} is low (approximately 19 torr) because fetal hemoglobin reacts poorly with 2,3-DPG. Postnatally, P_{50} increases rapidly (Oski and Deliveria-Papadopoulos, 1970); it exceeds the normal adult value by 3 months of age and remains high during the first decade of life (Motoyama and others, 1974). This high P_{50} is associated with increased levels of ATP and 2,3-DPG (Fig. 3-21), probably related to the process of general growth and development and high plasma levels of inorganic phosphate (Card and Brain, 1973). These observations provided Card and Brain with a hypothesis to explain why the hemoglobin levels in infants

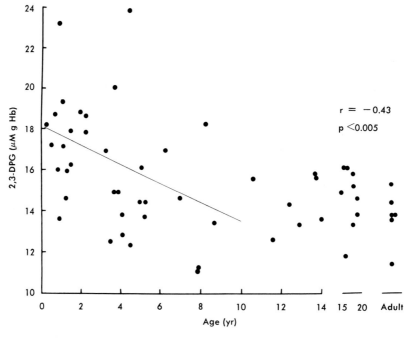

Fig. 3-21. Blood 2,3-DPG level vs the age of healthy infants and children. The 2,3-DPG level is high in infants and decreases toward the adult level by age 10. This increase in 2,3-DPG is associated with higher levels of P_{50}. (From Motoyama, E. K., Zigas, C. J., and Troll, G.: Am. Soc. Anesth. Abstract, 1974, pp. 283-284.)

and children are lower than in adults ("anemia" of childhood). Since infants and children have a lower oxygen affinity for hemoglobin, oxygen unloading at the tissue levels is increased. A lower level of hemoglobin in infants and children would therefore be just as efficient, in terms of tissue oxygen delivery, as a higher hemoglobin level in the adults. Table 3-5 shows the theoretical equivalent of hemoglobin concentrations in terms of tissue oxygen unloading.

These findings have important clinical implications for anesthesiologists. Infants and children with a hemoglobin level less than 10 g/dl are often the cause of controversy as to whether they are acceptable for general anesthesia and surgery. Such a level of hemoglobin has been used arbitrarily without the knowledge of different oxygen affinity and tissue oxygen unloading. It appears from Table 3-5 that if a hemoglobin level of 10 g/dl is acceptable for an adult with a P_{50} of 27 torr, 8.2 g/dl should theoretically be adequate for an infant more than 3 months old with an average P_{50} of 30 torr (without considering the high level of metabolism and oxygen consumption). In contrast,

for a 2-month-old premature infant with a P_{50} of 24 torr, a hemoglobin level of 10 g/dl is only equivalent to 6.8 g/dl in adults, and this may be inadequate to provide adequate tissue oxygenation.

It is interesting to note that the presence of cyclopropane in blood significantly decreases oxygen affinity and increases P_{50} by 3 torr, whereas 2,3-DPG level is unaffected. Halothane, on the other hand, has little effect on the P_{50} of adult blood (Table 3-6). Apparently this effect of cyclopropane is the direct physical interaction with hemoglobin since the incubation of red blood cells with cyclopropane has no effect on P_{50} (Orzalesi and others, 1971). From the viewpoint of tissue oxygen delivery, cyclopropane appears to be an excellent agent for surgery involving massive blood losses and shock.

SURFACE ACTIVITY AND LUNG FUNCTION

The alveolar surfaces of the human lungs are lined with surface-active materials with unique properties that are responsible for the stability of air spaces. These materials, which contain specific phospholipids and

Table 3-5. Hemoglobin requirement for equivalent tissue O_2 delivery

	P_{50} (torr)	Hb for equivalent O_2 delivery (g/dl)						
Adult	27	7	8	9	10	11	12	13
Infant >3 mo	30	5.7	6.5	7.3	8.2	9.0	9.8	10.6
Neonate <2 mo	24	10.3	11.7	13.2	14.7	16.1	17.6	19.1

Calculated from data of Motoyama, E. K., Zigas, C. J., and Troll, G.: Functional basis of childhood anemia, Am. Soc. Anesth. Abstract, 1974, pp. 283-284.

Table 3-6. Effect of presence of anesthetics on blood P_{50} and 2,3-DPG content

	Control	Anesthetics	ΔA-C	p
Halothane 3% (N = 6)				
P_{50} **(torr)**	26.1 ± 0.2	26.6 ± 0.3	0.5 ± 0.1	<0.05
2,3-DPG (μM/L RBC)	3.67 ± 0.24	3.94 ± 0.32	0.27 ± 0.31	ns*
Cyclopropane 25% (N = 6)				
P_{50} **(torr)**	26.4 ± 0.4	29.2 ± 0.4	2.8 ± 0.2	<0.001
2,3-DPG (μM/ml RBC)	4.45 ± 0.33	4.20 ± 0.34	−0.25 ± 0.13	ns

Data from Orzalesi, M. M., Cowan, M. J., and Motoyama, E. K.: The invitro effect of cyclopropane and halothane on the oxygen affinity of human blood, Am. Soc. Anesth. Abstract, 1971, pp. 187-188.
*ns, not significant.

proteins (discussed later), are collectively called pulmonary surfactant.

The relation between pressure (P), surface tension (T), and radius (r) of a sphere, such as a soap bubble, is expressed by the Laplace equation:

$$P = \frac{2T}{r}$$

It can be seen from this equation that if surface tension were constant, when a number of spheres are connected, the smallest sphere would have the highest pressure. Thus, the spheres with the smaller radii would empty their gas contents into the larger ones. If lung units are substituted for

spheres in this concept, the lungs would be unstable, with collapse of most of the units into several large ones, as in cases of the respiratory distress syndrome. This instability does not take place in normal lungs. As Clements and associates (1958) first demonstrated with a modified Wilhelmy balance, saline extract of normal lungs exhibits an extremely low level of surface tension (0 to 5 dynes/cm) during dynamic compression of the surface area while the tension increases (30 to 50 dynes/cm) during expansion of surface area (Fig. 3-22). Their findings indicate that, in normal lungs, as the alveolar radius decreases so does the surface tension, and thus the stability of the air spaces is main-

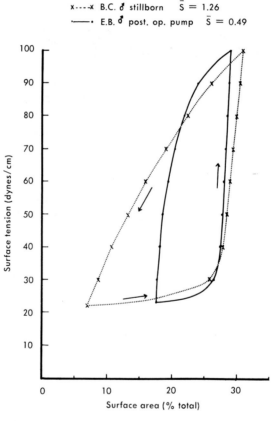

Fig. 3-22. Surface area–surface tension relations for two lung extracts measured on the Wilhelmy balance. $\bar{S}$ (stability index) equals (the maximum surface tension minus the minimum surface tension) times 2 divided by (the maximum surface tension plus the minimum surface tension). $\bar{S}$ above approximately 0.85 is normal and below is abnormal. Minimum surface tension below 15 dynes/cm is normal and above is abnormal. The lung extract of a stillborn infant had normal surface activity, whereas that of a patient dying following cardiac surgery with a bypass pump did not.

tained regardless of the size of each lung unit (Fig. 3-23).

The alveolar lining layer obtained from lung lavage contains approximately 10% lipoprotein and 90% phospholipid of which dipalmitoyl phosphatidylcholine (lecithin) is the major fraction responsible for the unique surface activity and stability of the lungs (King, 1974). These substances are apparently produced by the type II alveolar epithelial cells (granular pneumocytes), stored in the osmiophilic lamellar inclusions within these cells, and excreted into the air space to form surface-active alveolar lining layers (Kikkawa and others, 1965) (Figs. 3-24 and 3-25).

Not only are the surface-active properties of the alveolar lining important in normal pulmonary function whether they provide the basis for lung stability, but inadequacy or deficiency of the surfactant system has been shown to be important in several clinical conditions. Avery and Mead (1959) showed that the minimum surface tension of lung extracts from infants dying of the respiratory distress syndrome (hyaline membrane disease) was unusually high when measured on the Wilhelmy balance. Surface-active lecithins are markedly decreased or even absent in the alveolar linings in these lungs (Boughton and others, 1970). These findings explain, at least in part, the atelectasis and low compliance of lungs from infants with this syndrome.

A second condition with decreased surface activity of the lungs is the so-called wet lung or shock lung syndrome seen in some patients that is associated with a variety of clinical conditions, such as open heart surgery with prolonged cardiopulmonary bypass, shock, pancreatitis, near-drowning, smoke inhalation, and head trauma (see Chapter 27). Under these circumstances there is increased venous admixture, decreased pulmonary compliance, atelectasis, and decreased surface activity of the lung extract. A similar condition occurs after prolonged inhalation of high concentrations of oxygen (Caldwell and others, 1965; Northway and others, 1967). The pulmonary pathology includes thickening of alveolar membranes, interstitial and intra-alveolar edema, capillary congestion, and atelectasis. Surface activity is also decreased. Whether the decrease in surface activity of the lung is a primary or secondary factor in the pathogenesis of these conditions remains to be elucidated.

CILIARY ACTIVITY

The cilia in the respiratory tract play an important role in the removal of mucosal secretions and harmful material. In animals (and presumably in humans), these cilia move in a synchronous, whiplike fashion at the rate of about 600 to 1300 times per minute and are able to move particles toward the upper part of the respiratory tract at the rate of around 1.5 cm/min. The ciliary function is influenced by a number of factors, such as the viscosity of the surrounding mucus and the thickness of the mucous layer. In addition, inspired air with a high concentration of oxygen or a relative humidity below 50%, certain air pollutants, cig-

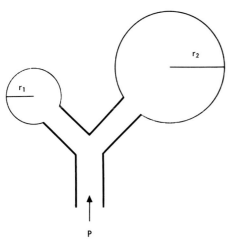

$$r_1 = 20\ \mu \qquad\qquad r_2 = 120\ \mu$$

$$T_1 = 5\ \text{dynes/cm} \qquad\qquad T_2 = 30\ \text{dynes/cm}$$

$$P = \frac{2\,T_1}{r_1} = \frac{2\,T_2}{r_2} = 5\ \text{cm } H_2O$$

Fig. 3-23. Schematic drawing of stable alveoli of different sizes.

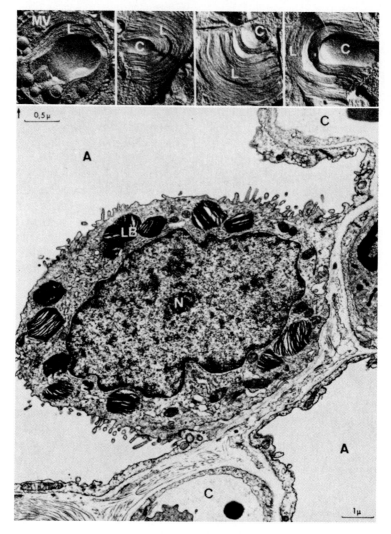

Fig. 3-24. Granular pneumocyte (type II). Cytoplasm around the nucleus *(N)* contains many organelles, particularly osmiophilic lamellar bodies *(LB)*. *A,* alveolar space; *C,* capillary space. Insets show lamellar bodies in freeze-etched preparation revealing form and existence of central core *(C)* around which lamellae *(L)* are stacked. (×22,400.) (From Weibel, E. R.: Physiol. Rev. **53**:419, 1973.)

arette smoke, and some anesthetic gases are among the factors reducing the function of the respiratory cilia. Electrolytes, particularly hydrogen and potassium ions, are also known to have a profound effect on ciliary activity, and cocaine produces paralysis. In tissue culture some viral infections reduce ciliary motion by as much as 50%, and repeated infections in vivo can destroy the cilia entirely (Kilburn and Salzano, 1966).

It has been shown by Spock and associates (1967) that serum from homozygotes with cystic fibrosis as well as from heterozygotes inhibits the normal ciliary beating pattern of rabbit tracheal explants. Similar findings were also reported with oyster gill cilia (Bowman and others, 1969). Conover and associates (1974) believe that they have possibly identified a factor biochemically, but these findings have been difficult for other investigators to reproduce. The relation of this serum dyskinesia factor to the clinical status of patients with cystic fibrosis remains to be established, since mucociliary clear-

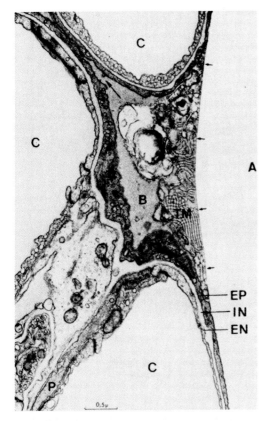

Fig. 3-25. Perfusion-fixed rat lung showing three capillaries *(C)* and the extracellular lining layer toward the alveolus *(A)* composed of a base layer *(B)* and an osmiophilic lining layer *(short arrows)*. Base layer contains tubular myelin figures *(TM)* and extends into a cleft between capillaries closely opposed because of septal folding *(long arrow)*. *EP,* alveolar epithelial cell (type I); *EN,* capillary endothelial cell; *IN,* interstitium; *P,* pericyte. (×23,000.) (From Weibel, E. R.: Physiol. Rev. **53:**419, 1973.)

ance of these patients has been reported to be unaffected (Sanchis and others, 1973). It is clear, however, that further knowledge about the cilia of the respiratory tract should help in the management of airway secretions in various respiratory diseases as well as during and after general anesthesia.

PRENATAL DEVELOPMENT OF THE LUNGS

The most dramatic and crucial adaptation that occurs at the time of birth involves the introduction of air into the previously fluid-filled lungs and a rapid transfer within seconds from placental to pulmonary gas exchange. This adjustment requires an effective neuronal drive of ventilation that in turn depends on the adequate morphologic and biochemical maturation of the lung tissues. It is worthwhile, therefore, to review briefly the process of prenatal development of human lungs and respiration.

The fetal lungs begin to form within the first several weeks of the embryonic period when the fetus is only 3 mm long. A groove appears in the ventral aspect of the foregut, creating a small pouch. The outgrowth of the endodermal cavity with a mass of surrounding mesenchymal tissue projects into the pleuroperitoneal cavity and forms lung buds. The future alveolar membranes and mucous glands are derived from the endoderm, whereas the cartilage, muscle, elastic tissue, and lymph vessels originate from the mesenchymal elements surrounding the lung buds (Emery, 1969). During the pseudoglandular period, which extends until the seventeenth week of gestation, the budding of the bronchi and lung growth take place rapidly into a loose mass of connective tissue. Morphologic development of the human lung is illustrated in Fig. 3-26.

By 16 weeks' gestation, all preacinar branching of the airways (down to the terminal bronchioli) is complete (Reid, 1967). Disturbance of the free expansion of the developing lung in this stage, as in the case of diaphragmatic hernia, results in hypoplasia of the airways as well as lung tissue (Areechon and Reid, 1963).

The canalicular period occupies the middle part of gestation when the future respiratory bronchioli develop as the relative amount of connective tissue diminishes. There is growth of capillaries adjacent to the respiratory bronchioli, and the whole lung becomes more vascular (Emery, 1969). At about 24 weeks' gestation the lung enters the terminal-sac (alveolar) period, which is characterized by the appearance of clusters of terminal air sacs, termed saccules, with flattened epithelium (Hislop and Reid, 1974). These

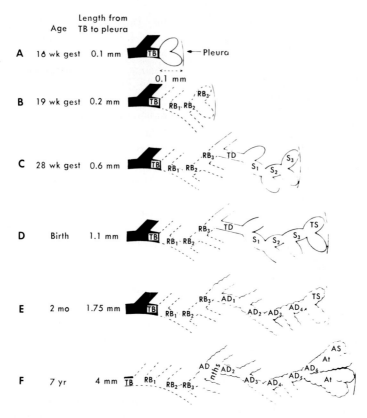

Fig. 3-26. Development of the acinus in human lungs at various ages. *TB,* terminal bronchiole; *RB,* respiratory bronchiole; *TD,* transitional duct; *S,* saccule; *TS,* terminal saccule; *AD,* alveolar duct; *At,* atrium; *AS,* alveolar sac. (From Hislop, A., and Reid, L.: Thorax **29**:90, 1974.)

saccules are large and irregular in comparison with the adult alveoli (Boyden, 1969). At about 26 to 28 weeks' gestation, proliferation of the capillary network surrounding the terminal air spaces becomes sufficient for pulmonary gas exchange (Potter, 1961). These morphologic developments may occasionally occur earlier, since infants born at 24 to 25 weeks' gestation have been known to survive. From 28 weeks' gestation to term there is further lengthening of saccules with possible growth of additional generations of air spaces. In some species, such as the rat, there are no mature alveoli at birth (Burri, 1974). Whether the proliferation of alveoli in humans starts prenatally or postnatally is debatable, but it is generally agreed that most of the alveolar formation takes place during the first decade of postnatal life (Thurlbeck, 1975).

More recently, much interest and investigation have been focused on the ultrastructural and biochemical maturation of the fetal lung. Of particular interest have been the type II alveolar epithelial cells (granular pneumocytes) that appear at about 24 to 26 weeks' gestation but occasionally as early as 20 weeks (Spear and others, 1969; Lauweryns, 1970).

It appears that the type II cells produce the surface-active material (pulmonary surfactant) that forms the alveolar lining layer and accounts for much of the stability of the lungs (Kikkawa and others, 1965). Since the most common cause of maladaptation of the newborn, the respiratory distress syndrome, is largely the result of incomplete maturation of the surfactant-producing system and hence is almost invariably associated with prematurity, factors that influence the metabolism of pulmonary surfactant are currently being intensively studied. In addition, there is some evidence that intrauterine distress in fetuses with borderline maturity of the lungs and surfactant system can result in a clinically apparent deficiency at or shortly after birth (Reynolds and others, 1965).

On the other hand, there is definite experimental evidence from work with animals that certain pharmacologic agents such as cortisol (deLemos and others, 1970; Motoyama and others, 1971), thyroxine (Wu and others, 1973), and heroin (Tauesch and others, 1973) administered to the maternal organism or directly to the fetus will accelerate the maturation of the lungs, with early appearance of the type II pneumocytes and surfactant.

Since these substances are potentially toxic to other organs of the fetus, the encouraging preliminary results indicating that corticosteroids accelerate maturation of the human fetal lung (Liggins and Howie, 1972) should be evaluated cautiously; routine clinical use of such drugs must await proof that they are reasonably safe as well as effective. In any case, none of these drugs have proved effective in preventing or ameliorating respiratory distress syndrome when used postnatally in high-risk infants (Baden and others, 1972).

For many years it has been believed that respiratory movements do not occur in utero, but Boddy and Dawes (1975) and Boddy and Robinson (1971) have established the presence of breathing-type movements in the human fetus by the application of ultrasound techniques. In experimental animals it has been shown (Dawes, 1974) that these movements are easily depressed by sedation, hypoxia, hypoglycemia, and it appears that the human fetus responds in the same way.

The respiratory movements of the fetus result in the inflow and outflow of a small amount of lung fluid; however, the net flow is usually from the lungs to the amniotic fluid, and it is this "excretion" of lung fluid that is the basis for estimating biochemical lung maturity by examination of amniotic fluid for the presence or absence of surface-active phospholipids (Gluck and others, 1971).

Under some circumstances of fetal distress, in utero "gasping" may occur, and amniotic fluid and debris (e.g., meconium or bacteria) can be deposited in the alveolar spaces. Chemical or bacterial (especially streptococcal) pneumonia may then become apparent after the onset of breathing at birth; both of these conditions may lead to serious respiratory insufficiency. Neonatal streptococcal penumonia is usually rapidly progressive and frequently fatal even when recognized or suspected almost immediately and treated specifically (Franciosi and others, 1973).

NEONATAL RESPIRATORY ADAPTATION

As indicated earlier, there seems little doubt that respiratory movements occur in utero for many weeks before birth. These are of both the gasplike and rhythmical varieties. Surely there are also a number of inhibitory mechanisms that limit such movements before birth and are at least partially eliminated or overcome with birth. The mechanisms involved in the onset of respiration at birth have been well reviewed by Purves (1974), and this should be consulted for further details.

The first breath involves the introduction of air into fluid-filled lungs, and therefore large surface forces must be overcome. In the usual situation, 15 to 25 cm H_2O pressure are necessary for the initial breath, but in some normal infants 70 cm H_2O must be exerted (Karlberg and others, 1962) (Fig. 3-27). The fluid is at first rapidly removed via the upper airways, and then more gradually the residual fluid leaves the lungs through the pulmonary capillaries and lymphatics over the first few days of life, and the changes in compliance parallel this time course. These changes are all retarded in the prematurely born infant.

With expansion of the lungs with air, the pulmonary vascular resistance drops dramatically and the pulmonary blood flow markedly increases, thus allowing gas ex-

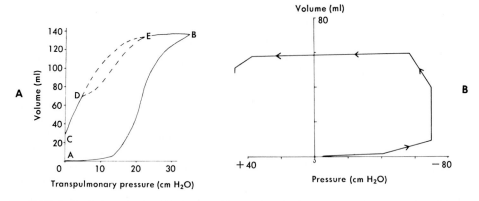

Fig. 3-27. A, Typical pressure-volume curve of expansion of a gas-free lung. A-B represents the initial expansion. In the example, approximately 13 cm H_2O pressure will be necessary to overcome surface forces. C represents deflation to zero pressure with gas trapping. **B,** Pressure-volume relationships during the first breath of a newborn weighing 4.3 kg. Here, 60 to 70 cm H_2O pressure were necessary to overcome the surface forces. (From Karlberg, P., Cherry, R. B., Escardó, F. E., and Köch, G.: Acta Paediatr. Scand. **51:**121, 1962.)

change to occur (Fig. 3-17). It appears that changes in Po_2, Pco_2, and pH are largely responsible for this decrease in pulmonary vascular resistance (Cook and others, 1963). With these adjustments, the cardiopulmonary system approaches adult levels of $\dot{V}_A/\dot{Q}$ balance within a few days (Nelson and others, 1962, 1963). It should be remembered that these changes are delayed in the immature organism.

The process of expansion of the lungs during the first few hours of life is greatly influenced by the presence or absence of adequate amounts of pulmonary surfactant. In the mature newborn, surfactant is present in sufficient amounts and forms an alveolar lining layer that is the major factor in the stability of the lungs, i.e., in the prevention of serious atelectasis.

This brief review of neonatal respiratory adaptation should indicate the necessity of adequate maturation of the lungs as preparation for alveolar gas exchange and the multiple changes that must occur in the lungs and their circulation with the onset of air breathing if the organism is to survive separation from the functioning placenta. In spite of the fact that the lungs in utero have had no contributory function in gas exchange, the adjustments to extrauterine

existence must occur within a few moments after birth (Fig. 3-28). Failure to adjust may be the result of immaturity, depression of the respiratory center (drugs, asphyxia, or trauma), or peripheral cardiopulmonary disease or anomalies.

Once birth has occurred, it is useful to realize that the minimal energy requirement exists at the neutral temperature of the infant (usually about 36.5° to 37.5° C) (Brück and others, 1962). Above and below this temperature, energy expenditure increases.

POSTNATAL DEVELOPMENT OF THE LUNGS

The human lung is not fully mature at birth but continues to develop during the first decade of life. It is conceivable, therefore, that lung function in healthy infants and young children may be quite different from that of older children and young adults. Such a difference may account for the high incidence of lower airway disease in infants (Glezen and Denny, 1973).

Considerable amounts of morphologic data have been accumulated in recent years on the postnatal development and growth of the human lung and have been compiled by Emery (1969) and Thurlbeck (1975). Although the development of the pulmonary

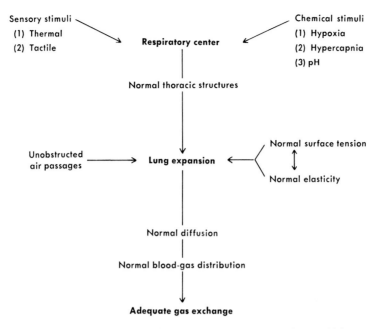

Sensory stimuli
(1) Thermal
(2) Tactile

Respiratory center

Chemical stimuli
(1) Hypoxia
(2) Hypercapnia
(3) pH

Normal thoracic structures

Unobstructed air passages → Lung expansion ← Normal surface tension / Normal elasticity

Normal diffusion

Normal blood-gas distribution

Adequate gas exchange

Fig. 3-28. Schematic representation of the onset of breathing at birth.

airway system down to terminal bronchioli (approximately sixteenth generation) are completed as early as 16 weeks' gestation, most if not all pulmonary alveolar formation takes place postnatally (Reid, 1967). There is a rapid increase in the number of alveoli during the first few years of life, approaching the adult level at about 6 years of age (Dunnill, 1962; Hogg and others, 1970), but the lung maturation and alveolar formation may continue throughout childhood and adolescence (Emery and Wilcock, 1966; Thurlbeck and Angus, 1975). The latter findings are of particular interest, since the functional maturation of the lung also appears to continue until 15 to 18 years of age.

Static recoil pressure of the lungs (see Mechanics of breathing, p. 51) is relatively high (lung compliance is relatively low) in healthy young adults and decreases gradually with age, presumably because of the loss of elastic fibers from aging or air pollution (Turner and others, 1968). Such changes are associated with a progressive increase in lung compliance, closing capacity, and air trapping (Anthonisen and others, 1969).

In the newborn, the static recoil pressure

of the lung is low (lung compliance is high), somewhat resembling that of emphysematous lungs in the aged (Gribetz and others, 1959; Fagan, 1969). Recent studies have indicated that static recoil pressure steadily increases (compliance, normalized for lung size, decreases) throughout infancy and childhood toward the normal values for young adults (Motoyama, 1977; Zapletal, Misur, and Sammanek, 1971). Such a low elastic recoil or unusually high distensibility of the lungs in infants and children tends to collapse small airways and increase the closing capacity (Mansell and others, 1972).

Information on airway dynamics in the developing lungs is still limited and controversial. It appears, however, that the flow resistance of the total airways (as well as the lower airways), when normalized for lung volumes, is disproportionately lower, rather than higher, in infants than in older individuals (Polgar, 1967; Motoyama, 1977). These findings do not necessarily contradict clinical evidence that infants are prone to severe obstruction of small airways. Since the absolute (not relative) airway diameters in infants are much smaller than those in

Table 3-7. Characteristics of lung mechanics in infants

Function	Clinical manifestation
Static	
High lung compliance (low Pstl)	Instability of small airways, increased closing capacity
High thoracic compliance (low Pstw)	Prone to lower airway disease (bronchiolitis, status asthmaticus)
Dynamic	
Upper airway resistance	
High in absolute terms	Upper airway obstruction (croup)
Low for lung size	Protective against obstruction?
Lower airway resistance	
High in absolute terms	Prone to lower airway disease
Very low for lung size	Probably protective against small airway disease

older individuals, relatively mild bronchiolar inflammation, secretions, or peribronchiolar edema would lead to far greater degrees of obstruction in this age group.

Based on the above information, the characteristics of respiratory mechanics in infants and young children may be summarized as follows: (1) Compliance of the lung is high; it tends to cause premature closure of small airways. (2) Compliance of the thorax is also high in infants; it tends to decrease FRC to a lower level and accentuate the airway closure. (3) The upper airway resistance is high in absolute terms, although it appears lower in infants than in older children when normalized for lung volumes. Severe upper airway obstruction seen in infants (croup, epiglottitis) is related to the small absolute caliber. (4) The lower airway resistance, when the lung size is taken into account, appears relatively lower in infants than in older individuals. However, since the caliber of the lower airways in absolute terms is smaller in this age group, a relatively mild disease process would result in disproportionately severe obstructions; hence, there is a higher incidence of lower airway disease in infants (Table 3-7).

MEASUREMENT OF PULMONARY FUNCTION IN CHILDREN

Ventilatory function tests provide qualitative and quantitative evaluation of the lung function, although they usually do not help in making a specific diagnosis. However, the measurement of pulmonary function is helpful because it provides an objective assessment of the general type of disability, the extent of the impairment, and the efficacy of various forms of treatment, either medical or surgical. From the practical point of view, most of the simple, clinically applicable tests require the understanding of the patient and his active participation. Therefore, most of the tests cannot be used with children under 5 or 6 years of age.

The standard spirometry, including the helium (or nitrogen) dilution technique, will provide information on VC, TLC, FRC, RV, and their ratios (Fig. 3-5). During the forced vital capacity (FVC) maneuver, spirometry also provides forced expiratory volume at 0.5, 1.0, and 3.0 seconds (FEV_t) and maximum midexpiratory flow rate (MMFR), or the mean flow rate during the middle half (by volume) of expiration. For further details of various techniques for pulmonary function studies, publications by Polgar and Promadhat (1971) and by Bates and associates (1971) should be consulted.

The most frequent types of pulmonary disability may be classified under the general headings of (1) restrictive diseases and (2) obstructive diseases, although there is considerable overlap between the two groups. Restrictive disorders, whether intrapulmonary or extrapulmonary in origin, result in a reduction of the patient's lung volumes.

R.K., 17 yr, hemosiderosis

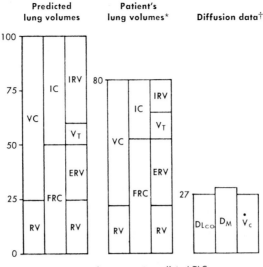

Fig. 3-29. Pulmonary function changes in a disease (idiopathic pulmonary hemosiderosis) characterized by pulmonary fibrosis. The changes in lung volumes are moderate except for decreases in inspiratory capacity (IC) and inspiratory reserve volume (IRV). The decreases in total lung diffusing capacity
(DL_{CO}), diffusing capacity of the membrane (D_M), and pulmonary capillary blood volume ($\dot{V}_c$) are striking. These are all approximately 27% of the predicted values. (From Bucci, G., Cook, C. D., and Barrie,
H.: J. Pediatr. **58:**820, 1961.)

Relatively common restrictive disorders in
the pediatric age group from the anesthesiologist's point of view include respiratory distress syndrome and diaphragmatic hernia in
the newborn period, congestive heart failure (also obstructive), pulmonary fibrosis,
kyphoscoliosis, abdominal distension, and a
partial paralysis due to muscle relaxants.
Fig. 3-29 shows an example of pulmonary
function in a patient with pulmonary fibrosis.

In postoperative patients, especially those
who have been given muscle relaxants, VC
will be a practical guide to muscle strength.
VC of at least 30 ml/kg of body weight (normal range, 60 to 70 ml/kg) appears to be
necessary for the maintenance of adequate
spontaneous ventilation. The measurement
of occlusion airway pressure (inspiratory
and expiratory) at FRC will provide additional information (see Chapter 27).

Obstructive pulmonary disorders may
be subdivided into upper and lower airway
diseases. Most of the severe upper airway

diseases, such as acute epiglottitis and subglottic croup, occur in infancy and early
childhood. Occasionally, however, upper airway obstruction can be seen in children with
chronic hypertrophic tonsillitis, vascular
ring, and subglottic stenosis associated with
prolonged intubation or tracheostomy. Congenital heart diseases with large left-to-right
shunts, such as atrial or ventricular septal
defects, sometimes are complicated by the
obstruction of major bronchi by the enlarged
left heart or pulmonary arteries.

The lower airway disorders commonly
seen among children include cystic fibrosis,
bronchial asthma, and heart disease with
left-sided obstruction (mitral and aortic
valvular diseases) with pulmonary venous
hypertension. Generally, in lower airway diseases such as cystic fibrosis, VC is decreased;
TLC, FRC, and RV as well as FRC/TLC
and RV/TLC ratios are increased because of
air trapping. Peak expiratory flow rate and
airway resistance may be within normal

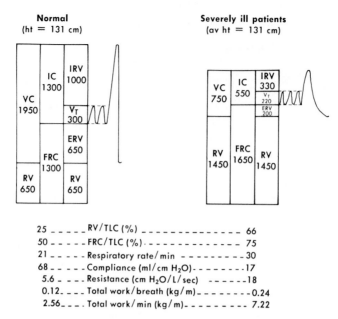

Fig. 3-30. Average values from the respiratory studies of the most severely affected patients with cystic fibrosis of the pancreas compared with predicted values for a normal child of the same height. (From Cook, C. D., Helliesen, P. J., Kulczycki, L., and others: Studies of respiratory physiology in children. II. Lung volumes and mechanics of respiration in 64 patients with cystic fibrosis of the pancreas, Pediatrics **24:**181, 1959. Copyright American Academy of Pediatrics 1959.)

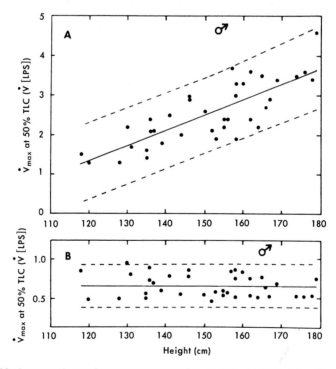

Fig. 3-31. A, Maximum expiratory flow rate at 50% TLC vs standing height in boys. *Drawn line,* regression equation (Table 3-8); *dashed lines,* 95% confidence limits. **B,** Same data with flow rates in TLC/sec. *Drawn and dashed lines,* average and 95% confidence limits.

Table 3-8. Normal values for maximum expiratory flow rate ($\dot{V}_{max}$) at different lung volumes and peak expiratory flow rate (PEFR) (L/sec) in relation to body height (cm)

y		N	a*	b*	130 cm	150 cm	170 cm
$\dot{V}_{max}$ at 25% VC	♂	39	−2.3069	+0.02817	1.36 ± 0.41	1.92 ± 0.40	2.48 ± 0.43
	♀	26	−1.8576	±0.02483	1.35 ± 0.42	1.87 ± 0.40	2.36 ± 0.43
$\dot{V}_{max}$ at 50% VC	♂	39	−4.5848	+0.05430	2.48 ± 0.50	3.35 ± 0.47	4.65 ± 0.53
	♀	26	−3.3655	+0.04470	2.45 ± 0.50	3.35 ± 0.49	4.25 ± 0.53
$\dot{V}_{max}$ at 50% TLC	♂						
	♀						
		37	−3.4163	+0.03946	1.73 ± 0.50	2.50 ± 0.46	3.29 ± 0.50
		24	−2.3030	+0.03162	1.81 ± 0.42	2.44 ± 0.41	3.07 ± 0.44
PEFR	♂						
	♀						
		39	−6.9865	+0.08060	3.49 ± 0.84	5.10 ± 0.82	6.72 ± 0.90
		26	−5.3794	+0.06594	3.19 ± 0.87	4.51 ± 0.84	5.83 ± 0.92

From Zapletal, A., Motoyama, E. K., van de Woestijne, K. P., and others: Maximum expiratory flow-volume curves and airway conductance in children and adolescents, J. Appl. Physiol. **26**:308, 1969.
*a, b = coefficients in regression equations of the type $y = a + bx$, where y is the measurement and x is height in cm. N = number of observations. Data for height 130, 150, and 170 cm are predicted values ± standard error.

limits, especially in mild cases, since they are mostly determined by the upper airway resistance. $FEV_{1.0}$ and MMFR are moderately decreased. Fig. 3-30 shows the pulmonary function of severely ill patients with cystic fibrosis.

As previously mentioned, the measurement of maximum expiratory flow rates ($\dot{V}_{max}$) on the descending limb of MEFV curves (Fig. 3-10) is by far the most sensitive test to detect lower airway obstruction. Besides simplicity (it can be measured during the FVC maneuver), an additional advantage of using MEFV curves in children is that $\dot{V}_{max}$ in low lung volumes is, to a considerable extent, independent of the degree of effort made by the subject. This is in contrast to the conventional tests of ventilatory function, which are heavily influenced by the degree of effort and cooperation of the patient. The normal values of $\dot{V}_{max}$ for children are shown in Fig. 3-31 and Table 3-8. Examples of MEFV curves from normal children and from those with cystic fibrosis and asthma are shown in Fig. 3-32.

Diffusion studies, evaluation of distribution of ventilation, and the assessment of ventilation-perfusion ratios require specialized equipment and personnel. However, a considerable amount of information can be obtained from the careful measurements of arterial blood gases (Fig. 3-19).

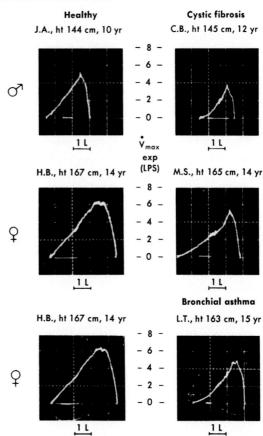

Fig. 3-32. Representative examples of maximum expiratory flow-volume curves in patients with clinically mild cystic fibrosis and asthma, each compared with the curve of a healthy child of the same sex and similar height and age. (From Zapletal, A., Motoyama, E. K., Gibson, L. E., and Bouhuys, A.: Pediatrics **48**:64, 1971. Copyright American Academy of Pediatrics 1971.)

LUNG ASPIRATION AND BIOPSY

Although most conditions involving the lung may be diagnosed by means of an adequate history together with physical and radiologic examinations, pulmonary function tests, suitable cultures, and skin and serologic tests, it may occasionally be necessary to perform a lung aspiration or biopsy for more direct culture or examination of the lung tissue. Tumor masses should, of course, be examined and if possible removed, but in cases of diffuse, unexplained disease, biopsies, if done early in the course of the illness, may be useful for diagnostic (e.g., pulmonary hemosiderosis) or therapeutic (e.g., *Pneumocystis carinii*, fungal infections, cytomegalic inclusion body disease) purposes (Stinger and others, 1968). Microscopic examination as well as cultures may then be obtained and may provide definite answers.

The relative safety of open lung biopsy, even in the extremely ill child, has recently been emphasized by Roback and associates (1973). On the other hand, Hyde and associates (1973) have pointed out that before undertaking the more major procedures, the various alternatives to open biopsy should be considered carefully. These are mediastinoscopy, needle biopsy with a cutting or trephine needle, transbronchial biopsy, percutaneous pleural biopsy, and fiberoptic biopsy. With regard to the last technique, the review by Sackner (1975) should be consulted for further details of the many diagnostic and therapeutic uses now established for bronchofibroscopy.

BIBLIOGRAPHY

Anthonisen, N. R., Danson, J., Robertson, P. C., and Ross, W. R. D.: Airway closure as a function of age, Respir. Physiol. 8:58, 1969.

Areechon, W., and Reid, L.: Hypoplasia of lung with congenital diaphragmatic hernia, Br. Med. J. 1:230, 1963.

Assali, N. S., and Morris, J. A.: Maternal and fetal circulations and their interrelationships, Obstet. Gynecol. Surv. 19:923, 1964.

Avery, M. E., Chernick, V., Dutton, R. E., and Permutt, S.: Ventilatory response to inspired carbon dioxide in infants and adults, J. Appl. Physiol. 18:895, 1963.

Avery, M. E., and Fletcher, B. D.: The lung and its disorders in the newborn infant, ed. 3, Philadelphia, 1974, W. B. Saunders Co., p. 55.

Avery, M. E., and Mead, J.: Surface properties in relation to atelectasis and hyaline membrane disease, Am. J. Dis. Child. 97:517, 1959.

Baden, M., Bauer, C. R., Colle, E., and others: A controlled trial of glucocorticoids in the treatment of respiratory distress syndrome, Pediatrics 50:526, 1972.

Ball, W. C., Stewart, P. B., Newsharn, L. C. S., and Bates, D. V.: Regional pulmonary function studied with xenon-133, J. Clin. Invest. 41:519, 1962.

Barcroft, J.: Researches on prenatal life, vol. 1, Oxford, 1946, Blackwell Scientific Publications Ltd., p. 260.

Bartlett, D., Jr., Jeffery, P., Sant'Ambrogio, G., and Wise, J. C. W.: Location of stretch receptors in the trachea and bronchi of the dog, J. Physiol. 258:409, 1976.

Bates, D. V.: Respiratory disorders associated with impairment of gas diffusion, Annu. Rev. Med. 13:301, 1962.

Bates, D. V., Macklem, P. T., and Christie, R. V.: Respiratory function in disease, ed. 2, Philadelphia, 1971, W. B. Saunders Co.

Benesch, R., and Benesch, R. E.: The effect of organic phosphates from the human erythrocytes on the allosteric properties of hemoglobin, Biochem. Biophys. Res. Commun. 26:162, 1967.

Boddy, K., and Dawes, G. S.: Fetal breathing, Br. Med. Bull. 31:3, 1975.

Boddy, K., and Robinson, J. S.: External method for detection of fetal breathing in utero, Lancet 2:1231, 1971.

Boughton, K., Gandy, G., and Gairdner, D.: Hyaline membrane disease. II. Lung lecithin, Arch. Dis. Child. 45:311, 1970.

Bowman, B. H., Lockhart, L. H., and McCombs, M. L.: Oyster ciliary inhibition by cystic fibrosis factor, Science 164:325, 1969.

Boyden, E. A.: The pattern of the terminal air spaces in a premature infant of 30-32 weeks that lived 19¼ hours, Am. J. Anat. 126:31, 1969.

Bradley, G. W., von Euler, C., Marttila, I., and Roos, B.: A model of the central and reflex inhibition of inspiration in the cat, Biol. Cybern. 19:105, 1975.

Brück, K., Parmelee, H., Jr., and Brück, M.: Neutral temperature range and range of "thermal comfort" in premature infants, Biol. Neonate 4:32, 1962.

Bucci, G., and Cook, C. D.: Studies of respiratory physiology in children. VI. Lung diffusing capacity, diffusing capacity of the pulmonary membrane, and pulmonary capillary blood volume in congenital heart disease, J. Clin. Invest. 40:1431, 1961.

Bucci, G., Cook, C. D., and Barrie, H.: Studies of respiratory physiology in children. V. Total lung diffusion, diffusing capacity of pulmonary membrane, and pulmonary capillary blood volume in normal subjects from 7 to 40 years of age, J. Pediatr. 58:820, 1961.

Bureau, M., and Bouverot, P.: Blood and CSF acid-base

changes and rate of ventilatory acclimatization of awake dogs to 3,500 m, Respir. Physiol. **24:**203, 1975.

Burns, B. D.: The central control of respiratory movements, Br. Med. Bull. **19:**7, 1963.

Burri, P. H.: The postnatal growth of the rat lung. III. Morphology, Anat. Rec. **178:**711, 1974.

Butler, J., and Smith, B. H.: Pressure-volume relationships of the chest in the completely relaxed anaesthetised patient, Clin. Sci. **16:**125, 1957.

Caldwell, P. R. B., Giammona, S. T., Lee, W. L., and Bondurnat, S.: Effect of oxygen breathing at one atmosphere on the surface activity of lung extracts in dogs, Ann. N. Y. Acad. Sci. **121:**823, 1965.

Card, R. T., and Brain, M. C.: The "anemia" of childhood; evidence for a physiologic response to hyperphosphatemia, N. Engl. J. Med. **288:**388, 1973.

Chanutin, A., and Curnish, R. R.: Effect of organic and inorganic phosphates on the oxygen equilibrium of human erythrocytes, Arch. Biochem. **121:**96, 1967.

Chernick, V., Faridy, E. E., and Pagtakhan, R. D.: Role of peripheral and central chemoreceptors in the initiation of fetal respiration, J. Appl. Physiol. **38:**407, 1975.

Clark, F. J., and von Euler, C.: On the regulation of depth and rate of breathing, J. Physiol. (Lond.) **222:** 267, 1972.

Clements, J. A., Brown, E. S., and Johnson, R. P.: Pulmonary surface tension and mucus lining of the lungs; some theoretical considerations, J. Appl. Physiol. **12:** 262, 1958.

Comroe, J. H., Jr.: Physiology of respiration, Chicago, 1974, Year Book Medical Publishers, Inc., pp. 183-196.

Conover, J. H., Conod, E. J., and Hirschhorn, K.: Studies on ciliary dyskinesia factor in cystic fibrosis. IV. Its possible identification as anaphylatoxin (C_{3a})-IgG complex, Life Sci. **14:**253, 1974.

Cook, C., D., Cherry, R. B., O'Brien, D., and others: Studies of respiratory physiology in the newborn infant. I. Observations on the normal premature and full-term infants, J. Clin. Invest. **34:**975, 1955.

Cook, C. D., Drinker, P. A., Jacobson, H. N., and others: Control of pulmonary blood flow in the foetal and newly born lamb, J. Physiol. (Lond.) **169:**10, 1963.

Cook, C. D., and Hamann, J. F.: Relation of lung volumes to height in healthy persons between the ages of 5 and 38 years, J. Pediatr. **59:**710, 1961.

Cook, C. D., Helliesen, P. J., Kulczycki, L., and others: Studies of respiratory physiology in children. II. Lung volumes and mechanics of respiration in 64 patients with cystic fibrosis of the pancreas, Pediatrics **24:**181, 1959.

Cook, C. D., Sutherland, J. M., Segal, S., and others: Studies of respiratory physiology in the newborn infant. III. Measurements of mechanics of respiration, J. Clin. Invest. **36:**440, 1957.

Cross, K. W., Klaus, M., Tooley, W. H., and Weisser, K.: The response of the newborn baby to inflation of the lungs, J. Physiol. (Lond.) **151:**551, 1960.

Cross, K. W., and Oppé, T. E.: The effect of inhalation of high and low concentrations of oxygen in the respiration of premature infants, J. Physiol. **117:**38, 1952.

Dawes, G. S.: Revolutions and cyclical rhythms in prenatal life; fetal respiratory movements rediscovered, Pediatrics **51:**965, 1973.

Dawes, G. S.: Breathing before birth in animals and men, N. Engl. J. Med. **290:**557, 1974.

deLemos, R. A., Shermeta, D. W., Knelson, J. H., and others: Acceleration of appearance of pulmonary surfactant in the fetal lamb by administration of corticosteroids, Am. Rev. Respir. Dis. **102:**459, 1970.

Derenne, J. P., Couture, J., Iscoe, S., and others: Occlusion pressures in men rebreathing CO_2 under methoxyflurane anesthesia, J. Appl. Physiol. **40:**805, 1976.

Dripps, R. D., and Comroe, J. H., Jr.: The effect of the inhalation of high and low oxygen concentrations on respiration, pulse rate, ballistocardiogram and arterial oxygen saturation (oximeter) of normal individuals, Am. J. Physiol. **149:**277, 1947.

Dripps, R. D., and Comroe, J. H., Jr.: The respiratory and circulatory response of normal man to inhalation of 7.6 and 10.4 percent CO_2 with a comparison of the maximal ventilation produced by severe muscular exercise, inhalation of CO_2 and maximal voluntary hyperventilation, Am. J. Physiol. **149:**43, 1947a.

Dunnill, M. S.: Postnatal growth of the lung, Thorax **17:**329, 1962.

Dutton, R. E., Chernick, V., Moses, H., and others: Ventilatory response to intermittent inspired carbon dioxide, J. Appl. Physiol. **19:**931, 1964.

Edelman, N. H., Lahiri, S., Brando, L., and others: The blunted ventilatory response to hypoxia in cyanotic congenital heart disease, N. Engl. J. Med. **282:**405, 1970.

Emery, J. L.: The anatomy of the developing lung, London, 1969, Heinemann Medical Books, Ltd.

Emery, J. L., and Wilcock, P. F.: The postnatal development of the lung, Acta Anat. (Basel) **65:**10, 1966.

Euler, C. von, and Trippenbach, T.: Cyclic excitability changes of the inspiratory "off switch" mechanism, Acta Physiol. Scand. **93:**560, 1975.

Fagan, D. G.: Functional development of the human lung. In Emery, J., editor: The anatomy of the developing lung, London, 1969, Heinemann Medical Books, Ltd., pp. 191-202.

Fahri, L. E.: Atmospheric nitrogen and its role in modern medicine, J.A.M.A. **188:**984, 1964.

Fenner, A., Jansson, E. H., and Avery, M. E.: Enhancement of the ventilatory response to carbon dioxide by tube breathing, Respir. Physiol. **4:**91, 1968.

Finch, C. A., and Lenfant, C.: Oxygen transport in man, N. Engl. J. Med. **286:**407, 1972.

Finley, T. N., Swenson, E. W., and Comroe, J. H., Jr.: The cause of arterial hypoxemia at rest in patients with "alveolar-capillary block syndrome," J. Clin. Invest. **41:**618, 1962.

Forster, R. E.: Exchange of gases between alveolar air

and pulmonary capillary blood; pulmonary diffusing capacity, Physiol. Rev. 37:391, 1957.

Foster, H. V., Dempsey, J. A., and Chosy, L. W.: Incomplete compensation of CSF(H$^+$) in man during acclimatization to high altitude (4,300 m), J. Appl. Physiol. 38:1067, 1975.

Franciosi, R. A., Knostman, J. D., and Zimmerman, R. A.: Group B streptococci neonatal and infant infections, J. Pediatr. 82:707, 1973.

Freund, F., Roos, A., and Dodd, R. B.: Expiratory activity of the abdominal muscles in man during general anesthesia, J. Appl. Physiol. 19:693, 1964.

Gautier, H., and Bertrand, F.: Respiratory effects of pneumotaxic center lesions and subsequent vagotomy in chronic cats, Respir. Physiol. 23:71, 1975.

Glenn, W. W. L., Holcomb, W. G., Hogan, J., and others: Diaphragm pacing by radiofrequency transmission in the treatment of chronic ventilatory insufficiency, J. Thorac. Cardiovasc. Surg. 66:505, 1973.

Glezen, W. P., and Denny, F. W.: Epidemiology of acute lower respiratory disease in children, N. Engl. J. Med. 288:498, 1973.

Gluck, L., Kulovich, M. V., Borer, R. C., and others: Diagnosis of the respiratory distress syndrome by amniocentesis, Am. J. Obstet. Gynecol. 109:440, 1971.

Goldring, R. M., Fishman, A. P., Turino, G. M., and others: Pulmonary hypertension and cor pulmonale in cystic fibrosis of the pancreas, J. Pediatr. 65:501, 1964.

Goldzimer, E. L., Konopka, R. G., and Moser, K. M.: Reversal of the perfusion defect in experimental canine lobar pneumococcal pneumonia, J. Appl. Physiol. 37:85, 1974.

Goodrich, J. K., Jones, R. H., Coulam, C. M., and Sabiston, D. C., Jr.: Xenon-133 measurement of regional ventilation, Radiology 103:611, 1972.

Gribetz, I., Frank, N. R., and Avery, M. E.: Static volume pressure relations of excised lungs in infants with hyaline membrane disease; newborn and stillborn infants, J. Clin. Invest. 38:2168, 1959.

Guz, A., Noble, M. I. M., Eisele, J. H., and Trenchard, D.: The role of vagal inflation reflexes in man and other animals. In Porter, R., editor: Breathing; Hering-Breuer centenary symposium, London, 1970, Churchill, pp. 17-40.

Harned, H. S., and Ferreiro, J.: Initiation of breathing by cold stimulation; effects of changes in ambient temperature on respiratory activity of the full term fetal lamb, J. Pediatr. 83:663, 1973.

Hart, M. C., Orzalesi, M. M., and Cook, C. D.: Relation between anatomic respiratory dead space and body size and lung volume, J. Appl. Physiol. 18:519, 1963.

Hislop, A., and Reid, L.: Development of the acinus in the human lung, Thorax 29:90, 1974.

Hogg, J. C., Williams, J., Richardson, J. B., and others: Age as a factor in the distribution of lower-airway conductance and in the pathologic anatomy of ob-structive lung disease, N. Engl. J. Med. 282:1283, 1970.

Hughes, J. M. B., Rosenzweig, D. Y., and Kivitz, P. B.: Site of airway closure in excised dog lung; histologic demonstration, J. Appl. Physiol. 29:340, 1970.

Hukuhara, T.: Functional organization of brain stem respiratory neurons and rhythmogenesis, In Umbach, W., and Koepchen, H. P., editors: Central rhythmic and regulation, Stuttgart, 1974, Hippokrates-Verlag GmbH, pp. 35-49.

Hyatt, R. E., Okeson, G. C., and Rodarte, J. R.: Influence of expiratory flow limitation on the pattern of lung emptying in normal man, J. Appl. Physiol. 35:411, 1973.

Hyde, R. W., Hall, C. B., and Hall, W. J.: New pulmonary diagnostic procedures; are they practical alternatives to open lung biopsy? Am. J. Dis. Child. 126:292, 1973.

Karlberg, P., Cherry, R. B., Escardó, F. E., and Köch, G.: Respiratory studies in newborn infants. II. Pulmonary ventilation and mechanics of breathing in the first minutes of life, including the onset of respiration, Acta Paediatr. Scand. 51:121, 1962.

Kikkawa, Y., Motoyama, E. K., and Cook, C. D.: Ultrastructure of lungs of lambs; the relation of osmiophilic inclusions and alveolar lining layer to fetal maturation and experimentally produced respiratory distress, Am. J. Pathol. 47:877, 1965.

Kilburn, K. H., and Salzano, J. V., editors: Symposium on structure, function and measurement of respiratory cilia, Am. Rev. Respir. Dis. 93:1, 1966.

King, R. J.: The surfactant system of the lung, Fed. Proc. 11:2238, 1974.

Lahiri, S., Brody, J. A., Velasquez, T., and others: Relative role of environmental and genetic factors in respiratory adaptation to high altitude, Nature 261:133, 1976.

Lauweryns, J. M.: "Hyaline membrane disease" in newborn infants; macroscopic, radiographic and light and electron microscopic studies, Hum. Pathol. 1:175, 1970.

Leusen, I.: Regulation of cerebrospinal fluid composition with reference to breathing, Physiol. Rev. 52:1, 1972.

Liggins, G. C., and Howie, R. N.: A controlled trial of antepartum glucocorticoid treatment for prevention of the respiratory distress syndrome in premature infants, Pediatrics 50:515, 1972.

Macklem, P. T., and Mead, J.: Resistance of central and peripheral airways measured by a retrograde catheter, J. Appl. Physiol. 22:395, 1967.

Mansell, A., Bryan, C., and Levison, H.: Airway closure in children, J. Appl. Physiol. 33:711, 1972.

McIlroy, M. B., Marshall, R., and Christie, R. V.: The work of breathing in normal subjects, Clin. Sci. 13:127, 1954.

Mead, J.: Control of respiratory frequency, J. Appl. Physiol. 15:325, 1960.

Mead, J.: The lung's "quiet zone," N. Engl. J. Med. 282:1318, 1970.

Mead, J., and Collier, C.: Relation of volume history of lungs to respiratory mechanics in anesthetized dogs, J. Appl. Physiol. 14:668, 1959.

Mead, J., Turner, J. M., Macklem, P. T., and Little, J. B.: Significance of the relationship between lung recoil and maximum expiratory flow, J. Appl. Physiol. 22:95, 1967.

Milic-Emili, J.: Recent advances in the evaluation of respiratory drive, Int. Anesthesiol. Clin. 15:39, 1977.

Milic-Emili, J., and Grunstein, M. M.: Drive and timing components of ventilation, Chest 70:131, 1976.

Miller, H. C., and Behrle, F. C.: The effects of hypoxia on the respiration of newborn infants, Pediatrics 14:93, 1954.

Mills, J. E., Sellick, H., and Widdicombe, J. G.: Epithelial irritant receptors in the lungs. In Porter, R., editor: Breathing; Hering-Breuer centenary symposium, London, 1970, Churchill, pp. 77-92.

Mitchell, R. A.: Cerebrospinal fluid and the regulation of respiration. In Caro, C. G., editor: Advances in respiratory physiology, Baltimore, 1966, The Williams & Wilkins Co., pp. 1-47.

Mitchell, R. A., and Burger, A. L.: Neural regulation of respiration, Am. Rev. Respir. Dis. 111:206, 1975.

Mitchell, R. A., Carman, C. T., Severinghaus, J. W., and others: Stability of cerebrospinal fluid pH in chronic acid-base disturbances in blood, J. Appl. Physiol. 20:443, 1965.

Mitchell, R. A., and Herbert, D. A.: Synchronized high frequency synaptic potentials in medullary respiratory neurons, Brain Res. 75:350, 1974.

Motoyama, E. K.: Pulmonary mechanics during early postnatal years, Pediatr. Res. 11:220, 1977.

Motoyama, E. K., and Cook, C. D.: Unpublished observations.

Motoyama, E. K., Orzalesi, M. M., Kikkawa, Y., and others: Effect of cortisol on the development of fetal rabbit lungs, Pediatrics 48:547, 1971.

Motoyama, E. K., Zigas, C. J., and Troll, G.: Functional basis of childhood anemia, Am. Soc. Anesth. Abstract, 1974, pp. 283-284.

Munson, E. S., Larson, C. P., Jr., Babad, A. A., and others: The effects of halothane, fluroxene and cyclopropane on ventilation; a comparative study in man, Anesthesiology 27:716, 1966.

Nelson, N. M., Prod'hom, L. S., Cherry, R. B., and others: Pulmonary function in the newborn infant. II. Perfusion-estimation by analysis of the arterial-alveolar carbon dioxide differences, Pediatrics 30:975, 1962.

Nelson, N. M., Prod'hom, L. S., Cherry, R. B., and others: Pulmonary function in the newborn infant; the alveolar-arterial oxygen gradient, J. Appl. Physiol. 18:534, 1963.

Nielsen, M., and Smith, H.: Studies on the regulation of respiration in acute hypoxia, Acta Physiol. Scand. 24:293, 1951.

Noble, M. I. M., Eisele, J. H., Trenchard, D., and Guz, A.: Effect of selective peripheral nerve blocks on respiratory sensations. In Porter, R., editor: Breath-

ing; Hering-Breuer centenary symposium, London, 1970, Churchill, pp. 233-246.

Northway, W. H., Jr., Rosan, R. C., and Porter, D. Y.: Pulmonary disease following respiratory therapy of hyaline-membrane disease, N. Engl. J. Med. 276:357, 1967.

Olinski, A., Bryan, M. H., and Bryan, A. C.: Influence of lung inflation on respiratory control in neonates, J. Appl. Physiol. 36:426, 1974.

Orzalesi, M. M., Cowan, M. J., and Motoyama, E. K.: The in vitro effect of cyclopropane and halothane on the oxygen affinity of human blood, Am. Soc. Anesth. Abstract, 1971, pp. 187-188.

Oski, F. A., and Delivoria-Papadopoulos, M.: The red cell, 2,3-diphosphoglycerate, and tissue oxygen release, J. Pediatr. 77:941, 1970.

Paintal, A. S.: Vagal sensory receptors and their reflex effects, Physiol. Rev. 53:159, 1973.

Pappenheimer, J. R., Fenci, V., Heisey, S. R., and Held, D.: Role of cerebral fluids in control of respiration as studied in unanesthetized goats, Am. J. Physiol. 208:436, 1965.

Perlstein, P. H., Edwards, N. K., and Sutherland, J. M.: Apnea in premature infants and incubator-air-temperature changes, N. Engl. J. Med. 282:461, 1970.

Pitts, R. F.: Organization of the respiratory center, Physiol. Rev. 26:609, 1946.

Polgar, G.: Opposing forces to breathing in newborn infants, Biol. Neonate 11:1, 1967.

Polgar, G., and Promadhat, V.: Pulmonary function testing in children; techniques and standards, Philadelphia, 1971, W. B. Saunders Co.

Potter, E. L.: Pathology of the fetus and infant, Chicago, 1961, Year Book Medical Publishers, Inc.

Purves, M. J.: Onset of respiration at birth, Arch. Dis. Child. 49:333, 1974.

Radford, E. P., Jr., Ferris, B. J., Jr., and Kriet, B. C.: Clinical use of nomogram to estimate proper ventilation during artificial respiration, N. Engl. J. Med. 251:877, 1954.

Rahn, H., and Fahri, I. E.: Ventilation, perfusion and gas exchange; the $\dot{V}_A/\dot{Q}$ concept. In Fenn, W. O., and Rahn, H., editors: Handbook of physiology, vol. 1, section 3: Respiration, Washington, D.C., 1964, American Physiological Society, pp. 735-766.

Reid, L.: The embryology of the lung. In DeReuck, A. V. S., and Porter, R., editors: Development of the lung, Ciba Foundation Symposium, London, 1967, Churchill, pp. 109-130.

Reynolds, E. O. R., Jacobson, H. N., Motoyama, E. K., and others: The effect of immaturity and prenatal asphyxia on the lungs and pulmonary function of newborn lambs; the experimental production of respiratory distress, Pediatrics 35:382, 1965.

Rigatto, H., and Brady, J. P.: Periodic breathing and apnea in preterm infants. I. Evidence for hypoventilation possibly due to central respiratory depression, Pediatrics 50:202, 1972.

Rigatto, H., Brady, J. P., and Verduzco, R. T.: Chemoreceptor reflexes in preterm infants. I. The effect of gestational and postnatal age on the ventilatory response to inhalation of 100% and 15% oxygen, Pediatrics **55:**604, 1975.

Roback, S. A., Weintraub, W. H., Nesbit, M., and others: Diagnostic open lung biopsy in the critically ill child, Pediatrics **52:**605, 1973.

Rohrer, F.: Der Strömungswiderstand in den menschlichen Atemwegen und der Einfluss der unregelmässigen Verzweigung des Bronchialsystems auf den Atmungsverlauf in verschiedenen Lungenbezirken, Pflügers Arch. **162:**225, 1915.

Rudolph, A. M.: The changes in the circulation after birth; their importance in congenital heart disease, Circulation **41:**343, 1970.

Sackner, M. A.: Bronchofiberscopy, Am. Rev. Respir. Dis. **111:**62, 1975.

Sanchis, J., Dolovich, M., Rossman, C., and others: Pulmonary mucociliary clearance in cystic fibrosis, N. Engl. J. Med. **288:**651, 1973.

Sellick, H., and Widdicombe, J. G.: Vagal deflation and inflation reflexes mediated by lung irritant receptors, J. Exp. Physiol. **55:**153, 1970.

Severinghaus, J. W.: Hypoxic respiratory drive and its loss during chronic hypoxia, Clin. Physiol. **2:**57, 1972.

Severinghaus, J. W., and Mitchell, R. A.: "Ondine's curse"; failure of respiratory center automacity while awake, Clin. Res. **10:**122, 1962.

Severinghaus, J. W., Mitchell, R. A., Richardson, B. W., and Singer, M. M.: Respiratory control at high altitude suggesting active transport regulation of CSF pH, J. Appl. Physiol. **18:**1155, 1963.

Severinghaus, J. W., and Stupfel, M.: Alveolar dead space as an index of distribution of blood flow in pulmonary capillaries, J. Appl. Physiol. **10:**335, 1957.

Sørensen, S. C., and Severinghaus, J. W.: Irreversible respiratory insensitivity to acute hypoxia in man born at high altitude, J. Appl. Physiol. **25:**217, 1968.

Spear, G. S., Vaeusorn, O., Avery, M. E., and others: Inclusions in terminal air spaces of fetal and neonatal human lung, Biol. Neonate **14:**344, 1969.

Spock, A., Heick, H. M. C., Cress, H., and Logan, W. S.: Abnormal serum factor in patients with cystic fibrosis of the pancreas, Pediatr. Res. **1:**173, 1967.

Stahlman, M. T., and Meece, N. J.: Pulmonary ventilation and diffusion in the human newborn infant, J. Clin. Invest. **36:**1081, 1957.

Steinschneider, A.: Prolonged apnea and the sudden infant death syndrome; clinical and laboratory observations, Pediatrics **50:**646, 1972.

Stinger, R. J., Stiles, Q. R., Lindesmith, G. G., and others: Use of lung biopsy in diagnosis of pulmonary lesions in children, Ann. Surg. **34:**810, 1968.

Strang, L. B., and MacLeish, M. H.: Ventilatory failure and right-to-left shunt in newborn infants with respiratory distress, Pediatrics **28:**17, 1961.

Tauesch, H. W., Jr., Carson, S. H., Wang, N. S., and Avery, M. E.: Heroin induction of lung maturation and growth retardation in fetal rabbits, J. Pediatr. **82:**869, 1973.

Thorling, E. B., and Erslev, A. J.: The "tissue" tension of oxygen and its relation to hematocrit and erythropoiesis, Blood **31:**332, 1968.

Thurlbeck, W. M.: Postnatal growth and development of the lung, Am. Rev. Respir. Dis. **111:**803, 1975.

Thurlbeck, W. M., and Angus, G. E.: Growth and aging of the normal human lung, Chest **67:**35, 1975.

Treves, S., Ahnberg, D. S., Laguarda, R., and Streider, D. J.: Radionuclide evaluation of regional lung function in children, J. Nucl. Med. **15:**582, 1974.

Wade, J. G., Larson, C. P., Jr., Hickey, R. F., and others: Effect of carotid endarterectomy on carotid chemoreceptor and baroreceptor function in man, N. Engl. J. Med. **282:**823, 1970.

Weibel, E. R.: Morphometry of the human lung, New York, 1963, Academic Press, Inc.

Weibel, E. R.: Morphometric estimation of pulmonary diffusion capacity. V. Comparative morphometry of alveolar lungs, Respir. Physiol. **14:**26, 1972.

Weibel, E. R.: Morphological basis of alveolar-capillary gas exchange, Physiol. Rev. **53:**419, 1973.

West, J. B.: Topographical distribution of blood flow in the lung. In Fenn, W. O., and Rahn, H., editors: Handbook of physiology, vol. 2, section 3: Respiration, Washington, D.C., 1965, American Physiological Society, pp. 1437-1451.

West, J. B., Dollery, C. T., and Naimark, A.: Distribution of blood flow in isolated lung; relation to vascular and alveolar pressures, J. Appl. Physiol. **19:**713, 1964.

Westbrook, P. R., Stubbs, S. E., Sessler, A. D., and others: Effect of anesthesia and muscle paralysis on respiratory mechanics in normal man, J. Appl. Physiol. **34:**81, 1973.

Whitelaw, W. A., Derenne, J. P., and Milic-Emili, J.: Occlusion pressure as a measure of respiratory center output in conscious man, Respir. Physiol. **23:**181, 1975.

Widdicombe, J. G.: Reflex control of breathing. In Widdicombe, J. G., editor: Respiratory physiology, MTP international review of science, series 1, vol. 2, Borough Green, Kent, 1974, Butterworth & Co., Publishers, Ltd., pp. 273-302.

Woolcock, A. J., Vincent, N. J., and Macklem, P. T.: Frequency dependence of compliance as a test for obstruction in small airways, J. Clin. Invest. **48:**1097, 1969.

Wu, B., Kikkawa, Y., Orzalesi, M. M., and others: The effect of thyroxine on the maturation of fetal rabbit lungs, Biol. Neonate **22:**161, 1973.

Zapletal, A., Misur, M., and Sammanek, M.: Static recoil pressure of the lungs in children, Bull. Physiopath. Respir. (Nancy), **7:**139, 1971.

Zapletal, A., Motoyama, E. K., Gibson, L. E., and Bouhuys, A.: Pulmonary mechanics in asthma and cystic fibrosis, Pediatrics **48:**64, 1971.

Zapletal, A., Motoyama, E. K., van de Woestijne, K. P., and others: Maximum expiratory flow-volume curves and airway conductance in children and adolescents, J. Appl. Physiol. **26:**308, 1969.

CHAPTER 4

Preparing children for operation

PHYSICAL AND EMOTIONAL FACTORS

Preparation of any child for anesthesia and operation demands attention to all details of his *physical condition*, which generally is accorded, plus concern for his *emotional condition*, which can be of even greater importance (Potts, 1956) but frequently is inadequately carried out.

Part of the explanation for this difference is because standards of evaluation and treatment have been established for most physical qualities but are vague or entirely lacking in psychic and emotional areas, leaving us with much theory but few rules or tools with which to work. Since emotional preparation may be started prior to hospital admission, this will be considered first.

For years, psychiatrists and other physicians have emphasized the emotional stress experienced by hospitalized children and the danger of lasting aftereffects (Levy, 1945; Wallgren, 1955; Gofman and others, 1957; Bowlby, 1953; Vernon, 1965).

Most discussions on this subject have concerned normal children of fond parents, scheduled for tonsillectomy or herniorrhaphy (Lipton, 1963; Kennell and Gergen, 1966;

Rosen and Brueton, 1970). While this situation may involve problems enough, a huge variety of situations exist that complicate the problem considerably. Consider, for example, the different emotional involvement in the following situations: (1) normal children facing single uncomplicated elective procedures, (2) various abnormal situations, including neurotic children (and parents), children facing repeated operations (over 100 for one child recently encountered), and chronically ill, crippled, retarded, maltreated, burned, and traumatically injured children, and (3) that group of unfortunate young patients facing, and often expecting, fatal outcome from cystic fibrosis, leukemia, or other diseases (Smith, 1973; Bird, 1973).

Management of each individual must vary greatly, but in general *the phases of emotional conditioning include home and preadmission preparation, admission to the hospital, preoperative care, and anesthetic induction, followed by postoperative assurance,* with the possible repetition of the whole procedure in mind (Eckenhoff, 1953; Eckenhoff and Helrich, 1958; Davenport and Werry, 1970).

HOME AND PREADMISSION PREPARATION

The first upsetting incident in the child's operative experience may be in learning that he is to have an operation. Under most circumstances this happens at the doctor's office, and the manner in which it is broached will depend on the insight of the physician involved.

Should one have a choice, there are advantages to telling the child about the operation

4 to 6 days before the date of admission. This gives the child time to get used to the idea but not long enough to dwell on it or to pick up unpleasant ideas from friends or chance television programs. Certainly, there are no fixed rules in this matter.

From the beginning it is essential to consider the special needs of each child. If a child is apt to be badly upset by the prospect of an operation, more time may be necessary to work with him or to obtain assistance from others, including his pediatrician or surgeon, a psychiatrist, or even occasionally a visit with another child who has had the same operation and who will be visible evidence that survival is possible.

Although the preadmission preparation of children must be individualized, there are several essentials that pertain to all, and even though they are familiar, they bear repeating.

The child must always be dealt with honestly. Parents frequently mislead children badly, even though their motives may be excellent. Shielding the child from the truth or distorting it to save tears or, in some cases, to avoid being the bearer of bad tidings is no kindness, for the truth will be doubly bitter when it is finally revealed.

It is questionable how deeply one needs to go into details (Francis and Cutler, 1957), for children can be frightened by hearing too much, but some warning of the coming events is definitely in order.

It is important to *emphasize the pleasant, positive aspects* of hospital life, such as television and toys, as well as to mention the less enjoyable finger-sticking and ear, nose, throat, and rectal examinations. To many children the hospital stay can be an interesting experience—no school, continuous television, attention from all sides, lots of children, lots of toys and presents from parents, cards from friends, and a chance to be a hero afterwards. Even repeated hospitalization may have its compensations. One 8-year-old boy who barely survived an 80% burn gradually learned so much about the hospital that he "took over" on each return and proudly supervised the other children in his area.

The fact that hospital life can be a series of horrible experiences for other children does not need to be mentioned.

A parent should try to find out *what particular fears or questions* bother a child and deal with them directly. Young children who are afraid that their parents will leave them should be reassured that the parents can stay with them much of the time and will always be close at hand. Those about to enter the hospital for the first time may have vague, exaggerated fears, many of which can be corrected quite easily. Children who have had a previous operation should be questioned both about features they liked and about those they disliked, and they should be reassured that efforts will be made to act on this information. Sometimes it is some simple but unsuspected item that has been most upsetting, such as hospital scrambled eggs, a certain overzealous nurse, or rectal thermometers, which can be readily avoided once identified.

Hospital preadmission programs

In many children's hospitals an attempt is made to ease the shock of admission by organizing preadmission parties for preschool-aged children and hospital visits for older children. These can serve several purposes. The first trip to the hospital will be a happy one, yet while the cookies are being devoured the children will see uniforms, hospital beds, and children on crutches. They will also see play areas, television sets, and speedy go-carts being used by obviously happy children, all of which are much more reassuring than promises made by parents who are not quite sure themselves.

Preadmission examination

It also may help to bring the children to the hospital before admission for preoperative checkup and routine laboratory work. If these are performed in advance, the child can get this part over with and go home again, thus deleting one of the more objectionable items usually crowded into the day of admission. At this time it is helpful if the anesthesiologist can have a few minutes with the child, so that they can be on more friend-ly terms on the night before operation.

Explaining the reason for hospitalization

Parents should be aware of several strange misunderstandings that are quite common among children. One of these is the child's belief that he is being sent to the hospital as a punishment and that the entire illness is some form of retribution. Although this could be based on parental threats, this is rarely the case, and parents should make a point of eradicating such beliefs, whether they are voiced or not (Haller, 1967).

One of the best ways to present the child's need for hospitalization is to suggest that the child must go to get something fixed, just the way a car must be taken to the repair shop to get fixed. If the lesion is a visible lump or a crooked toe, little more need be said. When the problem is more abstruse, or if there is an ominous note, it may be more difficult to choose the right words or to know how much to say. After the child is told the main facts, it is usually best to confine oneself to answer-ing the child's questions. Here again, ex-planations need not be too explicit unless the child insists on knowing all the details.

Parents can gain considerable help from articles on the care of hospitalized children as well as from books written for children, among which are such well-known ones as *Johnny Goes to the Hospital* (Sever, 1953), and *Elizabeth Gets Well* (Weber, 1970).

HOSPITAL ADMISSION

A child should be admitted to the hospital in sufficient time to provide for the necessary workup without requiring an exhaustive pro-cession of tests, examinations, and consulta-tions. In many cases, 3 to 5 days will be needed to allow for adequate medical evalua-tion and a chance for the child to become ad-justed to hospital surroundings.

Much depends on the organization of ad-mission. It is essential to keep parent and child together as much as possible, to actual-ly treat them as one. They have prepared for this together and to separate them at the doorstep would be a great injustice to both (Mayer, 1964).

A history taken at admission details many of the child's emotional responses to every-day items and provides insight into the child's behavior pattern. This may be used to good advantage by the anesthesiologist, since it usually includes many pet likes and dis-likes. It has proved very helpful to show groups of children around the ward together, to have them visit the playrooms, and to have a routine introduction for different age groups and those facing different operations. This has been especially important for chil-dren scheduled for cardiac operations, spinal fusion, and other extensive procedures where recovery will involve unfamiliar pro-cedures.

During the process of admission, the child may find himself being "taken over" by the professionals who carry the traditional belief that they know more about children than their parents do. Parents are naturally un-willing to relinquish their role of protector and thus contest the takeover. The resultant stress may become obvious, with the child the ultimate loser (Bird, 1973).

There have been great strides in hospital-parent-child relationships, and parents now are allowed to stay with their child through-out much of the hospital stay, some presently showing much determination to be with the infant or child during both the induction and recovery phases of anesthesia. At present there is considerable disagreement as to how far this should be allowed to go. Both Mellish (1969) and Koop (1973) stated that overpro-tective parents who follow their child to the operating room may add to the emotional tension and confusion, and Lee and Greene (1969, 1970) added that too much may have been done to promote parental participation in the care of hospitalized children. Yet, when reasonable parents who are aware of the postoperative behavior problems ask to stay with their child, we are hardly justified in denying them unless we can guarantee complete elimination of emotional stress, which, as yet, we have been unable to do (Linde, 1968).

PREANESTHETIC VISIT

The anesthesiologist's preoperative visit is especially important when the patient is a child (Egbert and others, 1965; Downes and Nicodemus, 1969). Because of the varied nature of their problems and the great difference in their sizes and emotional attitudes, children can be evaluated properly only by firsthand inspection.

The chart

Before speaking to the patient or his parents, the anesthesiologist should learn as much as possible from the hospital chart. This will enable him to analyze the problem, know what to look for in the child, and avoid repetition of unnecessary questions or examination.

From the chart one should get the *child's first name*, for this will promote friendly personal relations. His *age* and *weight* are noted, because both must be considered in planning anesthetic management and fluid therapy. The *history* provides essential information concerning *symptoms*, *diagnosis*, and *intended operation* in addition to a number of lesser details. *Birth history* is reviewed to see if the child had a normal delivery, whether there was any delay in crying, or if there was cyanosis or any other sign suggestive of birth injury, congenital disease, or hypoxia. Subsequent *growth* and *development* are noted, for retarded growth may accompany serious organic diseases. Special attention must be paid to warnings concerning *sensitivity* to penicillin or other drugs the child may have received. History of *severe* or *recurrent infection* is important and may suggest decreased resistance from such causes as anemia or agammaglobulinemia or the existence of complicating lesions such as otitis, rheumatic fever, or low-grade renal infections.

Regardless of the child's age, one should look for history of *previous operations*. A 1-month-old infant may already have undergone several major procedures. The anesthesiologist should know the reason for previous operations, the type of anesthesia used, and the child's emotional and physical reaction to the experience. It is especially important to recognize any danger signals.

If the child had a *high fever following* use of halogenated agents, this should be considered in choosing subsequent anesthetics. Unless associated with upper abdominal pain, jaundice, or elevated enzyme levels, fever does not necessarily contraindicate repeated use of halothane.

History of *high fever during* the operative period in the patient or any relatives suggests a tendency toward malignant hyperpyrexia, and both halothane and succinylcholine should be avoided (Britt and others, 1973; Denborough and others, 1973). Similarly, a *hyperirritable* or *neurotic* child must be accorded special preparation in order to avoid protracted psychic disturbances, and ketamine should be avoided.

The *system history* should not be overlooked. Briefly, the following may be of special significance:

1. **Central nervous system.** History of hydrocephalus, mental retardation, or convulsions should be noted. The etiology of convulsions should be investigated, since they may be due to epilepsy, infection, trauma, or other causes. When children have been receiving anticonvulsant therapy, this should *not* be discontinued prior to operation. Additional preoperative medication usually should be reduced, however, to prevent excessive depression.
2. **Cardiovascular system.** Cyanosis, fainting, poor physical development, clubbed fingers, weakness, or history of murmur should be noted. Reduced exercise tolerance is most significant.
3. **Respiratory system.** Recurrent infections, stridor, cough, respiratory obstruction, croup, and cyanosis are important. Children are more frequently subject to asthma and tracheitis than are older patients. History of previous tracheostomy or any laryngotracheal irritation, especially if recent, will be a deterrent to endotracheal intubation.
4. **Gastrointestinal system.** Recurrent vomiting associated with the presenting lesion will suggest dehydration and electrolyte depletion. History of poor nutritional habits may also be of significance.

A number of medical diseases are now treated with *therapeutic agents* that complicate anesthesia. Children receive *cortisone* for a variety of conditions, including poison ivy, asthma, rheumatic fever, and thrombocytopenic purpura. Whatever the reason for its use, one of its effects is depression of adrenal cortical activity. To avoid hypotensive complications, some believe that patients who have received corticoids during the 6 months before operation should receive cortisone supplementation, advising for adults 100 mg of hydrocortisone (IM or IV) on the day before, the day of, and the day after surgery. Although such hypotension has been reported several times (Lewis and others, 1953; Alper and others, 1963; Vandam, 1962), routine use of cortisone is not advised unless it has been administered recently or in relatively high dosage. The anesthesiologist should certainly know if patients have received such drugs in order to evaluate various intraoperative or postoperative reactions.

Although less frequently encountered, other therapeutic agents offer individual problems. Chlorpromazine, also used for a variety of conditions including malignancy, prolonged vomiting, hiccoughs, and fever, can potentiate the depressant effect of anesthetics (Bourgeois-Gavardin and others, 1955). Antihypertensive drugs, such as rauwolfia serpentina or reserpine (Serpasil), were also believed to be dangerous unless discontinued 1 or 2 days before operation (Coakley and others, 1956), but they are now considered to involve less danger if maintained under careful observation.

The antineoplastic agent doxorubicin hydrochloride (Adriamycin) is a potent cardiotoxic drug (Rinehart and others, 1974). If total dosage exceeds 350 mg/m^2, a complete cardiac evaluation should be performed prior to anesthesia.

L-Dopa, currently used in neuromuscular disorders, is another drug that may induce vasomotor instability. Goldberg and Whitsett (1971) and Beven and Burn (1973) advised its discontinuation 2 to 7 days before operation, but increasing experience has led many to believe it reasonable to maintain its use during the entire operative period.

Reviewing the findings of the physical examination as listed on the chart is important. Although the anesthesiologist should evaluate the child's general physical condition

himself and perform essential details of the physical examination, he can learn much from the chart and save the child from unnecessary poking and prodding. In the report of the physical examination one can gain valuable assistance if detailed examination of the nervous system, muscle strength, or cardiac lesions has been performed. Reports from special studies such as pneumoencephalograms, cardiac catheterization, and respiratory function tests are invaluable in assessing patients with specific disorders. Any reports of consultations should be read carefully, since these usually contain the essentials of the patient's problem presented in the chief resident's most concise and carefully worded terms. The consultant's reply, if legible, may be of further assistance.

Laboratory reports are examined next. Hemoglobin or hematocrit determination, red cell count, and urinalysis are required in all children prior to general anesthesia. It is now general policy to test all blacks for sickle cell abnormality prior to anesthesia (Gilchrist, 1973).

A question that constantly arises is whether one should set minimal acceptable preoperative levels for hematocrit and hemoglobin in children, and, if so, what they should be (Herbert and Hammond, 1963; Rackow and Salanitre, 1969). With adults, whose average hemoglobin is 15 g/dl, a minimum acceptable level of 10 g/dl has been traditional. Because of so-called anemia of childhood, during which a child's average hemoglobin is approximately 11 g/dl, many argue that the acceptable level should be lowered to 9 g/dl.

This is truly a dilemma of increasing proportions. Several factors make a slight or moderate anemia appear less crucial than formerly believed. In impoverished areas, innumerable children and adults have survived anesthesia and operation with hemoglobin levels of 6 to 8 g/dl, and at The Children's Hospital Medical Center we have had similar experience with children suffering from chronic renal failure. Elevation of 2,3-DPG level (Oski, 1973) and other responses have been found to compensate for reduced hemoglobin levels (p. 19). On the other hand, there are recurring reports of complications involving questionable hypoxic episodes followed by seizures, retarded development, or death.

If a 1-month-old infant who is scheduled for inguinal herniorrhaphy is found to have a hemoglobin level of 9 g/dl one of three choices may be made: (1) one may cancel the operation and send the infant home for a 2- or 3-week trial of iron therapy (with questionable effect), (2) one may transfuse the child, or (3) one may operate without transfusion. If the first choice is made, the hernia could become strangulated during the interim—an infrequent occurrence, but worth considering if the family lives far from the hospital. If the child is transfused there is the ever present risk of various reactions; the risk is variable but usually would be greater than the risk of operating in the presence of borderline anemia. If one does go ahead without transfusion, there is the specter of the child who suffers temporary hypoxia due to glottic spasm and never fully recovers. Should this happen to a child who had substandard hemoglobin concentration, one might be in for a hard time if the case were taken to court, for exaggerated importance is frequently attributed to any minor discrepancy of this nature.

As Gillies (1974) pointed out in his excellent review, there are many variables to be considered, and while the minimum level of hemoglobin is admittedly elastic, one is still not justified in taking risks that are not necessary.

It has been our practice to set no strict rule but to consult with the surgeon in every situation where the child's hemoglobin level is near or below 10 g/dl. The relative advantages and disadvantages are considered in an attempt to find the most reasonable decision. If the operation is postponed, simple anemias may be corrected by administration of 1 teaspoon of ferrous sulfate two or three times daily in an elixir containing 7½ grains (370 mg) per teaspoon. If it is decided to go ahead in the presence of a reduced hemoglobin level, this is noted on the child's chart with due

explanation. It is also explained to the child's parents.

Whether it is decided to proceed, transfuse, or delay, it is obviously of paramount importance to take immediate steps to find the cause of the anemia and institute the suitable form of therapy (Gilchrist, 1973).

It is of interest to note that a record has been kept at our hospital during the past 5 years of all anesthetized children who had a hemoglobin level of less than 10 g/dl. To date there has been no increase in operative or postoperative complications in these children.

An effort should be made to avoid routine testing and extensive laboratory studies that involve discomfort, expense, and sometimes significant blood loss. Greater reliance on clinical signs should be encouraged in the care of small patients.

Differential blood smears are examined for abnormal types or numbers of red and white cells.

Bleeding and clotting times are not routinely tested, but if there is any history suggestive of increased bleeding or if patients are undergoing extensive procedures, template bleeding time, prothrombin time (PT), and partial thromboplastin time (PTT) usually are ordered, and recent ingestion of aspirin is investigated.

Serum electrolytes are frequently important, especially in the presence of acid-base imbalance and gastrointestinal disorders. Chest x-rays may be indicated for children with varied specific problems, but neither chest x-rays nor electrocardiograms are standard requirements.

The chart may be checked further to note the child's temperature over a period of several days prior to operation, for it may be found that a child whose temperature is normal immediately before operation previously had been running a spiking fever.

The nurse's bedside notes may also prove valuable, since one may find details not noted elsewhere. Frequently the nurse will observe coughing, hoarseness, or vomiting that the doctor has either missed or regarded as unimportant. The fluid intake and output are of special significance in small children who may be upset by hospitalization and become dehydrated quite rapidly, even when facing nothing more extensive than a herniorrhaphy.

In conditions in which roentgen-ray films give significant information, as in pulmonary or cardiac lesions, the anesthesiologist will profit by viewing these. If there is still uncertainty concerning the diagnosis, the anesthesiologist should make his own attempt to analyze the situation and be able to add his opinion to those of other physicians.

In most instances, reviewing the patient's chart and other data need not take more than a few minutes. However, if the patient is seriously ill or if the situation is a complicated one, the anesthesiologist is obligated to spend considerable time in pursuing all the evidence and, if necessary, to request any additional information that he believes essential.

Meeting the child

Once satisfied that he has the pertinent facts, the anesthesiologist is ready to see the patient and his parents. It should be emphasized that this is not only a responsibility of the anesthesiologist but also an important opportunity for him, since by personal contact he can learn much that he would miss if he confined himself to the operating room. In addition, he has a chance to win the confidence of the patient and the gratitude of the parents, if they are present.

Sincere interest in patients before and after their trip to the operating room will be rewarded not only by greater clinical success with the patients but also by increased respect on the part of one's professional associates. Lack of interest may naturally lead in the opposite direction.

The actual interview with the child may have its problems. Rather than being in his own bed, the patient is more likely to be three rooms down the hall watching a neighbor's television program. This may put the anesthesiologist at a disadvantage; however, it is essential that he see the child alone for a few minutes.

Before making any statements about the operation, the anesthesiologist must find out if the child knows there is to be one. If not, the unexpected announcement of an operation can throw both patient and parents into turmoil. Probably the safest way to bring up the business at hand is to ask the child why he is in the hospital. If the answer shows some comprehension of the situation and the parents remain calm, it will be safe to go ahead. However, if a child is old enough to understand, but obviously has no idea of the coming operation, and the parents suddenly start to interrupt, it is evident that the child has not been told.

It is usually best to take the parents aside and convince them that the child should know of the operation. Sometimes the parents are obdurate in their refusal. To comply with their wishes is unfair to the child and is also unsafe, for it invites the increased risk that sudden fear and excitement impose on the hazards of induction.

For most children, *fear of needles* predominates before, during, and after the operative period. This seems a reasonable dislike that we should treat with more concern and relieve by honestly promising to use other methods whenever possible. Children who have been anesthetized previously may have developed a strong aversion to the standard *anesthesia mask*, another feature that needs improvement. Many vague fears may be expressed before operation. Some children ask if they will ever wake up; others are afraid they will awaken during operation. Some want to know how they will be cut open. The sight of other children emerging from the operating room undoubtedly chills some, but others seem strangely unaffected ("Gee, look at Jimmy bleed," etc.).

Moderately concerned children, more often adolescents, can be helped immeasurably if the parent or surgeon alerts the anesthesiologist several days before operation, thus allowing him extra time to fortify the child's morale and, when indicated, to establish accurate preliminary sedative control.

While sedation can do much to obtund preoperative anxiety, it must be borne in mind that the child who awakens with a painful tube pulling at his chest, casts on his legs, or both eyes covered by bandages will be badly shocked if his only warning was that he was going to the hospital "to have his picture taken" (Fig. 4-1).

It is always advisable to explain to the parents that the anesthesia will not entail any force or mishandling. Parents' fears are often carried over from unpleasant memories of their own early experiences.

Solicitous parents often want someone else to break the news to the child. Children frequently accept the truth more calmly than the parents had anticipated, and all are relieved after the feeling of uncertainty is cleared.

It may be best to avoid mentioning the time of the operation, because this could invite an unpleasant night of anticipation. Certain terms should also be omitted. To tell a child you are going to put him to sleep will not sound pleasant if his pet has recently been "put to sleep."

After the child understands that he is going to go to sleep and have something fixed, the need for further discussion of the operation depends mainly on the child. If he has been happily engrossed in a television program, comic books, or his parents, it seems unwise to describe all the details of the operating room. It is possible that with moderate seda-

tion he will doze through his trip to the operating room and remember little of it. It seems far better to get the child's attention back to his interests and not to upset him.

On the other hand, if a child of reasoning age is crying or evidently upset, if he has been given false impressions about the hospital, or if he remembers previous difficulty, it may be necessary to devote considerable time and skill to getting this child into a more optimistic frame of mind.

Many children withhold their fears from all but their most trusted associates. Thus, a ward aide or a fellow patient may know more about a child than one can learn directly in a single visit. I have rarely had a child admit fear of castration, but nurses report this to be fairly common. Death is mentioned occasionally, but not in the form of the "death wish" occasionally encountered in adults. A child may scream "you're killing me" in frantic excitement but usually does not mean it. Some know, and say nothing. A 13-year-old girl with severe cystic fibrosis who was told about her scheduled tracheostomy simply said, "I know, my three sisters had it."

Excessive fear may be suggested by tears and wild remonstrance or by boisterous overactivity. More frequently it is seen in the quiet child who stares ahead mutely and refuses to eat (Bothe and Galdston, 1972).

The use of continued sedation for many of

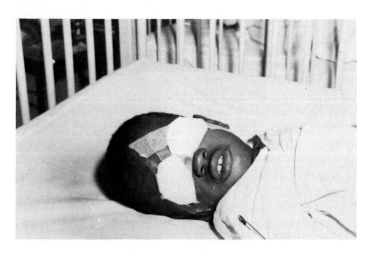

Fig. 4-1. A child who is to awaken with painful dressings or bandaged eyes should be allowed some previous word of preparation.

these worried children seems a natural expedient, and it was expected that one of the many tranquilizing agents would answer this need. Although diazepam and hydroxyzine have been of some help, neither has been entirely satisfactory.

For children who are truly neurotic or are faced with the unsurmountable emotional stress of a major amputation or a potentially terminal procedure, a psychiatrist who is specially experienced in this field can be of tremendous assistance (Smith, 1964; Wolff, 1969; Petrillo and Sanger, 1972).

Morale building. One of the best ways to build a child's morale is to focus attention on *who he is* and *what he can do*. As soon as a child can communicate, he willingly accepts praise for any accomplishment. An older child likes to talk about his pets and projects. By discussing them with him, one gets into the "inner circle" of his confidence.

Establishing the patient as a special individual and *gaining his acceptance of the anesthesiologist as a confidante* are both important achievements, for they provide great solace to the child and are invaluable to the anesthesiologist at the time of induction. For children who return for repeated operations, such a relationship becomes increasingly helpful.

Physical examination. The extent of the physical examination that the anesthesiologist performs will depend on the circumstances. If a small infant scheduled for a minor operation has been crying all afternoon and has finally dropped off to sleep, it would seem wiser not to awaken him. One can observe from the bedside the child's general nutritional state, skin color, character of respiration, and presence of nasal discharge. The surgeon's notes may be relied on for the rest of the examination, and these may be rechecked in the morning prior to operation.

With an older child, the anesthesiologist should evaluate his general state of health while talking with him and his parents and then perform any procedure indicated. It seems desirable for the anesthesiologist to examine the heart, lungs, nose, mouth, and throat of all patients he is to anesthetize.

In the examination of a child one should look for somewhat different signs than in an adult. Between the age of 4 and 8 years, children must be examined for loose teeth. Finding an empty socket after operation is less alarming if one knew that the child lost the tooth before admission. There is always the danger of rapid onset of an upper respiratory tract infection with cough, runny nose, and red throat. Children must be checked for this repeatedly. If an infant has a runny nose, it may be hard to tell whether it is due to an infection or is simply the result of crying. Enlarged cervical nodes and otitis also occur rather frequently with respiratory tract infection. Infants develop fever and rashes rapidly, and their temperatures must be observed closely. Dehydration, as evidenced by sunken fontanels, loose, dry skin, and acidotic breath, may also appear unexpectedly.

Respiratory obstruction of all types is common in children and may be due to infection, anatomic anomalies, or tumors. Exact diagnosis should be made before anesthesia is started. Bear in mind that unilateral nasal discharge is unusual and suggests a foreign body (or rarely choanal atresia).

When a child is scheduled for procedures such as repair of lacerations, removal of a tumor, or excision of a nevus, the anesthesiologist should see for himself where the lesion is and how large it is (Fig. 4-2). A tumor may be the size of a pea or a pumpkin, whereas a nevus may be a spot on a child's elbow or may cover half his head. The anesthesia cannot be planned intelligently without knowledge of these points.

Summary of patient evaluation

After completing the interview, the anesthesiologist writes a preoperative note on the chart, recording the chief complaint, relevant findings, history of previous operations, anesthetic experience, drugs taken during the past 6 months, allergies and sensitivities, family history of intraoperative fever, or other potential complications. The operative lesion is examined and described if possible, with the size and location of mass, degree of

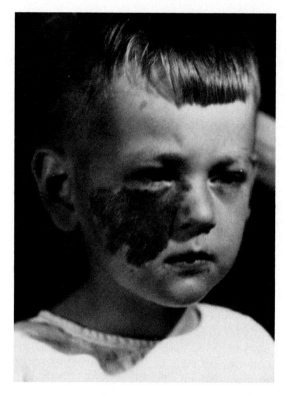

Fig. 4-2. Operation was scheduled as "excision of nevus." Only by firsthand inspection can the anesthesiologist evaluate problems.

curvature of the spine, and similar specific findings noted. A record is made of any laceration, bruise, or loose or missing teeth so that these cannot be ascribed to events during the trip to the operating room. It is also of value to assess the child's anxiety level on a scale from 0 through 3 (p. 104).

The diagnosis is listed, and complications are noted. The anesthesiologist states whether he accepts the patient as scheduled, requests a delay for consultation or more information, or advises cancellation. If accepted, the plan of anesthetic management is noted.

Cancellation of operation

Request for delay of operation seldom causes serious problems, but advice to cancel is apt to be upsetting, especially if it comes on the morning of operation. If the anesthesiologist decides that the operation should not be done, he should notify the surgeon as promptly as possible and hear the surgeon's opinion before taking final action. While many so-called contraindications would justify abandonment of an elective operation on a poor-risk patient, the same conditions might be disregarded completely if the operation involved the saving or prolongation of a life. One may also find that a surgeon will appear relieved when strongly advised to cancel an operation that involved major problems.

PREANESTHETIC ORDERS AND SEDATION

Preoperative orders may be written by the surgeon or anesthesiologist in part or in toto, but both should know what was ordered and why as well as know something of the effect of the prescribed therapy.

Minimal general orders concerning restriction of diet, activity, and routine laboratory work can be written by any physician. Those related to the special surgical procedure may reasonably be left to the surgeon, while the anesthesiologist would be expected to rule on sedation. Since preoperative sedation is an important and extensive topic, it will be given proportional consideration.

General orders: restriction of oral intake

Whereas it is extremely important that a child's stomach be free of solids prior to anesthesia, it is also important that his fluid intake be interrupted no longer than necessary. Consequently, small infants are given sugar and water feedings until 4 hours before operation and are listed for an early place in the day's operating schedule.

The following regimen is suggested:

1. **From birth to 6 months of age.** No solids or milk after midnight; clear fluids until 4 hours before operation.
2. **From 6 months to 3 years of age.** No solids or milk after midnight; clear fluids after 2:00 AM.
3. **Three years of age or older.** Nothing by mouth after midnight.
4. **Children to be operated on in the afternoon.** Sweetened, clear fluids until 4 hours before operation; grape juice, apple juice, and cola drinks offer fluid and calories; milk and orange juice are not permitted (Woodbridge, 1943).

Enema

Although the soapsuds enema was traditional for many years, it is tiring and upsetting to most patients, and its value is questionable. It may be indicated occasionally, but it is a routine procedure only when surgery on the lower bowel is planned.

Laboratory studies

A *complete blood count* (CBC), *hemoglobin* or *hematocrit*, and *urinalysis* are standard preoperative requirements in most hospitals. Unless individual conditions alter the situation, these tests may be performed as early as 10 days before operation. There is seldom difficulty in obtaining blood samples, but it may be difficult to obtain urine specimens from small children, especially before emergency operations. It is considered reasonable to proceed without the urinalysis at such times.

As noted previously, it has been our practice at The Children's Hospital Medical Center to regard the *sickle cell test* as routine for all blacks but not to insist that it be performed prior to emergency procedures unless the surgeons expect to use a tourniquet to reduce bleeding. In such cases the test must be performed. At the present time, no tourniquet is used on any patient who has the disease, but tourniquets are allowed on patients who have only the trait.

Crossmatch for transfusion should be obtained. If blood transfusion is probable during an operation, the blood should be ordered and prepared the day before (unless fresh blood is indicated).

Other tests, x-rays, and medication are ordered according to individual indications.

PREANESTHETIC SEDATIVES FOR ANXIETY

Efforts to control children's voiced reactions, as well as their silent autonomic responses to the emotional stress of the operative period, have been concentrated chiefly on administration of sedative and vagolytic drugs (Shearer, 1960, 1961). Toward this end, Waters (1938) wrote a classic paper on preanesthetic medication of children in which he prescribed morphine and scopolamine in a 20:1 ratio given according to the child's age and/or weight.

It is not to our credit that efforts have continued to be limited to a search for new and better sedatives and that the results are little better than those of Waters. To make pediatric patients more receptive to general anesthesia and better operative subjects, anesthesiologists have certainly exhausted the pharmacopeia, and the literature on pediatric premedication, though of slight value, greatly exceeds that on any other phase of this specialty. Other methods of controlling the fears of hospitalized children will be described, but first it seems reasonable to review some of the sedatives that have been advocated.

Out of the confusing variety of drugs and dosages, three general approaches have predominated: (1) *basal anesthesia,* in which a sound sleep is induced, (2) *moderate seda-tion*, aimed at producing "sedation without depression," and (3) *no medication*, with reliance on diverting the child by pleasant, relaxed surroundings until time for operation.

Basal anesthesia

Rectal administration of thiopental sodium (Pentothal) in doses of 20 to 30 mg/kg and methohexital sodium (Brevital), 10 to 15 mg/kg, has the great advantage of inducing sleep without mask or needle.* The chief disadvantage is the time required to administer the agent plus a minimal 10-minute wait for effect. Since this is actually induction of anesthesia, it should be performed by the anesthesiologist rather than a ward nurse and should be carried out in the operating room area. Other disadvantages include the variable effect of the drug and the fact that since its use is delayed until a few minutes before operation, the child is denied the usual early morning sedative that reduces preoperative hunger, thirst, and apprehension. Delayed awakening is another disadvantage of this form of sedation.

Ketamine also induces basal anesthesia but is given by injection and thus lacks the advantage of painless administration. Its use is more suitable for highly resistant children who refuse a suppository.

Tribromoethanol (Avertin), once popular for basal anesthesia, is no longer marketed.

Moderate sedation

The standard approach to premedication during the past 30 years has been to use a belladonna agent to reduce vagal responses and salivation plus one or more sedative agents to control fear and restlessness (Table 4-1). The aim here is not necessarily a sleeping child but a state of sedation without depression (Fig. 4-3).

Barbiturates and narcotics have been employed most frequently for sedation, but

tranquilizers of all types have been tried. The accepted method has been to use each agent in a single inaccurate dose estimated by weight and injected shortly before the child is taken from his bed and shuttled off to the operating room.

Innumerable combinations of sedatives thus administered give similarly imperfect results. At best about 75% of the children are satisfactorily sedated; most of the others are still apprehensive and unhappy about their recent "shots" and dry tongues, while a few lie oversedated and depressed.

Anticholinergics. For many years the use of an anticholinergic agent was considered to be mandatory. Atropine was generally favored for pediatric premedication because of its superior vagolytic action (Eger, 1962), but some have preferred scopolamine for its greater drying effect and additional sedative effect that is quite devoid of respiratory depression (Stephen and others, 1956; Wyant and Dobkin, 1957).

During recent years the picture has undergone considerable change. Without ether, a drying agent is no longer a necessity in all cases. Ketamine and neostigminelike drugs are the only remaining agents used in anesthesia that stimulate excessive secretions. A vagal blocking agent is important in pediatric anesthesia to prevent bradycardia due to mechanical stimulation or increased concentrations of halothane and especially following succinylcholine administration, but these indications are by no means universal. Furthermore, the hypodermic injection and the prolonged unpleasantness of a dry, sticky mouth are sufficient reason to delay administration until the patient has been put to sleep.

When atropine is used for premedication, a relatively heavy dosage is recommended for children. Our preference is to start the neonate with 0.15 mg, increasing by 0.05 to 0.10 mg up to a maximum of 0.6 mg in full-grown patients. A formula to fit our dosage scale would be approximately:

$$0.15 \text{ mg} + 0.01 \text{ mg/kg}$$

It has been customary to give this hypoder-

*Details of the preparation and administration of drugs are described in Chapter 7.

Table 4-1. The Children's Hospital Medical Center preanesthesia medication schedule

Age	Average weight (kg)	Pentobarbital (Nembutal) (mg)	Morphine (mg)	Atropine (mg)
Newborn	3.3	—	—	0.15
6 mo	8.1	30 PR	—	0.2
1 yr	10.6	45 PR	1.0	0.2
2 yr	14.0	60 PR	1.5	0.3
3 yr	15.0	60 PR	2.0	0.3
4 yr	17.1	90 PR	3.0	0.3
5 yr	19.4	90 PR	3.0	0.3
6 yr	22.0	90 PR	4.0	0.4
7 yr	24.7	90 PR	5.0	0.4
8 yr	27.9	100 PO	5.0	0.4
9 yr	31.4	100 PO	5.0	0.4
10 yr	35.2	100 PO	6.0	0.4
11 yr	39.6	100 PO	6.0	0.4
12 yr	44.4	100 PO	6.0	0.4
13 yr	49.1	100 PO	8.0	0.4
14 yr	54.4	100 PO	8.0	0.4
15 yr	58.8	100 PO	8.0	0.4
16 yr	61.9	100 PO	8.0	0.4

1. This table is a guide to be followed for average, well-developed patients. Increases or reductions in medication must be made for patients who do not fall in this category, i.e., hyperactive, obese, or poor-risk patients.
2. Pentobarbital (Nembutal) should be given at least 90 minutes before surgery.
3. Morphine should be given 30 to 45 minutes (IM or SC) before surgery.
4. Suggested guide for pentobarbital when followed by morphine is 4.0 mg/kg for rectal use (maximum 120 mg) and 3.0 mg/kg for oral use (maximum 100 mg).
5. Suggested guide for morphine is 0.75 mg/yr of age.

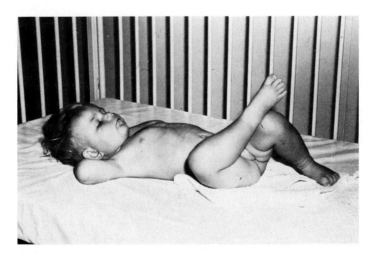

Fig. 4-3. Sedation without depression. Such evident relaxation decreases the risk of major operation. This little boy was about to undergo repair of ventricular septal defect.

mically, with morphine, 45 minutes to 1 hour before operation.

The most potent argument against preoperative administration of atropine lies in the fact that it has usually passed the most effective period of action by the time its protection is needed and must be repeated for reliable effect.

Several anticholinergic drugs have enjoyed brief popularity, but until recently none has threatened to displace atropine or scopolamine. One of the newer agents is the quaternary ammonium compound glycopyrrolate. According to Young and Sun (1962), Franko and associates (1962), Wyant and Kao (1974), and Salem and associates (1976), this agent is safe and effective, and a dose half that of atropine produces equal or better anticholinergic effect over a longer period. Emphasis has been placed by Salem and associates on the reduced volume and acidity of gastric secretions associated with glycopyrrolate as compared with those following the use of atropine. A final advantage noted by Gillick (1974) is that the drug does not pass the blood-brain barrier in sufficient amount to cause danger of central nervous system irritation or depression.

If the practice of routine preoperative administration of an anticholinergic still existed, the adoption of glycopyrrolate might be a popular move. In view of the present trend to use atropine for specific indications only, there appears to be more reluctance to substitute a new and more expensive drug for one as well known and as effective as atropine.

Hypnotics and narcotics. For healthy, normal children, a sedative such as pentobarbital sodium (Nembutal) may be added at 6 months of age to control restlessness without inducing respiratory depression. Morphine may be added at 1 year to increase the tranquilizing effect without inducing the excitement occasionally encountered when larger doses of barbiturate alone are relied on. Most satisfactory results using this method are obtained by giving pentobarbital at least 90 minutes before operation and morphine 30 to 40 minutes before operation. Since dosage is grossly inaccurate, nothing is gained by intramuscular injection of pentobarbital. Rectal administration of pentobarbital is preferable in most children under 8 years of age and the oral route thereafter. The dosage of all drugs *must* be individualized, but a suggested guide for pentobarbital, when followed by morphine, is 4.0 mg/kg for rectal use (maximum 120 mg) and 3.0 mg/kg for oral administration (maximum 100 mg).

When children are not to be operated on until well into the day's schedule, pentobarbital is given at 8:30 AM to reduce anxiety during the waiting period. Morphine is administered on call, approximately 30 minutes before operation.

Even with this standard method there are *numerous variations*. Barbiturates and narcotics are reduced or eliminated in critically ill children. During excessive environmental heat or when children have fever, atropine dosage is reduced, delayed until after anesthetic induction, or omitted entirely.

While the combination of atropine, morphine, and pentobarbital has probably been the most widely used approach, there are innumerable alternatives. Chloral hydrate is relatively safe and effective, though bitter. Stetson and Jessup (1962) recommended its use in a syrup, approximately 5 mg/kg. Boyd and Manford (1973) studied a similar drug, trichloroethanol (triclofos), which they gave by mouth in a dosage of 71 mg/kg; they reported it to be superior to diazepam and trimeprazine tartrate (see below).

Most of the highly vaunted nonbarbiturate tranquilizers have been disappointing, being unreliable as sedatives as well as expensive, toxic, unpalatable, or prepared in pills or capsules too large for children to swallow. Among those that have been tried and found wanting are meprobamate, glutethimide, hydroxyzine, and perphenazine (Smith and Miller, 1961).

Droperidol, the long-acting cycloplegic component of Innovar, has been tested alone as a premedicant. Werry and Davenport (1965) reported postoperative motor disturbances, and Bush (1972) found it so unsuitable that he abandoned it during preliminary trials; however, Stiles (1975), using 1 mg/20 lb (0.1 mg/kg) for children over 1 year old, finds it highly reliable, even for the severely crippled.

It is interesting to note current practices in established pediatric strongholds. For children over 1 year, C. R. Stephen in St. Louis (1970) and Downes in Philadelphia (1976) both favored the standard combination of pentobarbital, morphine and atropine, which has also been most heavily used at our institution. In Chicago, Levin at Children's Memorial Hospital reported use of intramuscular pentazocine lactate (Talwin), 1.2 mg/kg, and atropine (1973). At Los Angeles Children's Hospital a move has been under way to abandon sedatives in all children under 10 years of age, a practice already established at The Hospital for Sick Children in Toronto. In Liverpool, Rees has preferred trimeprazine, 1.5 mg/kg, given orally 4 hours before operation, while others have used diazepam (Valium), 0.2 to 0.4 mg/kg, perphenazine (Trilafon), 0.2 mg/kg, and promethazine (Phenergan), 1 mg/kg.

In 1948 Poe and Karp advocated one of the most accurate methods of sedation, in which the agent is given in small repeated doses, thus enabling one to titrate the child to the desired end point.

It is gratifying to see more attempts made to use oral medication. Root and Loveland (1973) found that oral administration of diazepam (0.3 mg/kg) and scopolamine (0.025 to 0.5 mg/kg) gave the best results, 58.7% being moderately to deeply hypnotized. Boyd and Manford (1973), comparing triclofos (71 mg/kg) with oral diazepam (0.2 mg/kg), found triclofos satisfactory in 88% and diazepam in 77% of trials. Table 4-2 shows several types of sedatives that are suitable for oral use in children.

Although many reports have been loosely assembled, several careful attempts to eval-

Table 4-2. Sedatives for oral use

Sedative	Form	Concentration	Total dose (70-kg adult)	Dose (mg/kg) Anxiety level				Time to act
				0	1	2	3	
Chloral hydrate	Syrup Elixir Capsule	50, 100 mg/ml 50, 100 mg/ml 250, 500 mg	500 mg	0	6	8	10	30 minutes
Diazepam (Valium)	Ampule Tablet	2, 5, 10 mg/ml 2, 5, 10 mg	10-20 mg	0	0.1	0.2	0.3	30 minutes
Flurazepam (Dalmane)	Capsule	15 mg	10-30 mg	0	0.1	0.2	0.3	30 minutes
Hydroxyzine pamoate (Vistaril)	Syrup Vial Tablet	2 mg/ml 25, 50 mg/ml 10, 25, 50, 100 mg	100 mg	0	1	2	3	30 minutes
Meperidine	Tablet	50 mg	100 mg	0	1	1.5	2	30-45 minutes
Pentobarbital (Nembutal)	Capsule	30, 50, 100 mg	100-150 mg	0	4.0	5.0	6.0	30 minutes
Promethazine (Phenergan)	Syrup Vial Tablet	1.25 mg/ml 50 mg/ml 12.5, 25, 50 mg	25 mg	0	0.5	1.0	1.5	30 minutes
Triclofos	Liquid		1500 mg	0	50	70	90	15-30 minutes
Trimeprazine (Temaril)	Syrup Capsule Tablet	0.5 mg/ml 5 mg 2.5 mg	100 mg	0	1.0	1.5	2.0	4 hours

uate comparable sedative action have been made, including those by Freeman and Bachman (1959), Cope and Glover (1959), Doughty (1962), Rackow and Salanitre (1962), Root and Loveland (1973), Smith and Jeffries (1959), Keller and associates (1968), and Barker and Nisbet (1973). Thus far, the more accurate the report, the more positive the finding that most sedative drugs presently known, given as a *single dose based on age and weight, produce quite variable and unsatisfactory results.*

No medication

There has been a definite trend toward reduction of use of preoperative sedatives over the past 20 years. Beginning with a few individuals who had the interest, talent, and time, it was found that many children fared better without sedatives and the attendant needles and side effects. The concept has been fostered, and a "no medication" policy has been adopted in several pediatric anesthesia departments around the country.

An important factor in the increasing success of this policy has been the changing attitude of the hospital organization as a whole. The current tendency to play down formality and promote more homelike surroundings fits nicely into the scheme. Children find it easier to relax in play areas that are supervised by girls in sports clothes rather than nurses in starched uniforms.

The usual procedure in the no medication approach is for the anesthesiologist to visit the child on the eve of the operation, and in the morning the child is brought to a play area in the operating suite. There he will be attended by suitably trained personnel who will ply him with toys, games, and things to do. In talking to the children, these young attendants often can detect some of the fears and anxieties that the children have not voiced to physicians or nurses.

How much the parent should participate in this preoperative approach is difficult to say, as evidenced by the different policies currently in force; some do not allow parents to be with the child at all on the morning of operation, others allow them to go to the preoperative area and stay until the child is taken away, and a few arrange it so that the parents can be with the child throughout induction of anesthesia.

By far the most distressing event of the preoperative period is the moment of parting between a small frightened child and his equally upset parents. To witness a 2-year-old being taken from the arms of her parents screaming "Mummy, Daddy—don't leave me," as she is taken off for an operation of dubious outcome, is particularly soul-wrenching.

To avoid this, one can either have the parent leave the child the evening before operation and not return or give the child enough sedation to prevent it. If sedation is not given, the parting is going to be difficult wherever it occurs, and the process is apt to be a howling failure unless the parents are allowed to stay through the induction. Thus, for children under 4 years of age, the no medication approach seems advisable chiefly for children undergoing less extensive operations and in cases where parents can be allowed to stay through induction.

When these provisions can be observed, the no medication policy has been applauded by parents, psychiatrists, and other observers. Movies of this method showing parent participation have been especially popular, and those produced under Epstein at Children's Hospital of Washington, D.C. have enjoyed wide circulation.

One should make it clear that it cannot be used for all children. Even in the institutions where it is most popular there are many exceptions. Children who are facing cardiac or other extensive procedures and those who, because of mental retardation, language problems, or hyperexcitability, cannot be made to understand or cooperate are usually given adequate sedation (basal or moderate) before leaving their beds.

REVIEW OF FAULTS

There are many faults in the present methods of preoperative management of children. Most are recognized, and efforts have been made to correct them, but since the situation is still quite unsatisfactory, it seems reasonable to point out some of the more apparent weaknesses.

1. There is a lack of evidence as to the basic cause of anxiety in children, and it is not possible even to tell how much of the anxiety is related to the operative experience.
2. The traditional dosage of sedative drugs is based on the weight and height of a child, when it is their emotional condition that is being treated.
3. No measure of stress or anxiety in children of the same age has been established.
4. We quite irrationally expect reliable results from a single dose of a guessed amount of sedative.
5. The comparison of different sedatives has often been made without a previous attempt to determine the most effective dose of the agents used.
6. Evaluation of sedatives has often been based on whether a child was quiet or excited after medication without regard to whether he had been quiet or excited before medication.
7. Ordering atropine for every child, with resultant thirst and cracked lips, is illogical and unkind if the effect of the drug wears off before the operation has started.
8. Perhaps the greatest failure to date has been the lack of individualization in preoperative management of children. Although efforts have been made to improve methods, the tendency has been to adopt a single method and attempt to use it for all, whether it is basal, moderate, or no medication.

PROPOSED CHANGES IN THE MANAGEMENT OF HOSPITALIZED CHILDREN

After 35 years it has become obvious that we cannot improve on Waters' approach simply by juggling the types and dosages of sedative agents or by omitting them. There are indications that several changes should be made, both in general approach and in the use of sedatives.

First, we must accept the fact that the management of emotional stress has become a matter of far greater concern than it was 35 years ago. This has been due in part to the introduction of many more distressing forms of treatment involved in the excessive

procedures now undertaken (e.g., prolonged endotracheal intubation) and in part to the greater awareness of the public, and parents in particular, of the fact that psychic trauma can have a lasting effect, that it often can be avoided, and that in many situations the emotional stress involved in an operation far outweighs the hazards of the surgery. This is evident in the growing number of parents who bring their children to the hospital openly admitting that the possibility of emotional trauma is their chief concern.

Evidence should be obtained to determine what part the operative experience plays in the child's response to hospitalization. Until we can define the particular factors that cause lasting disturbances, it is wrong to concentrate entirely on the preoperative phase. With less distasteful methods of induction and more unpleasant postoperative experiences, anesthesia may no longer be the most upsetting event. In a study by Visintainer and Wolfer (1975), anesthetic induction was not included among the six leading causes of stress in hospitalized children. Similar findings were reported by Meyers and Muravchick (1976), who compared the behavior of hospitalized children following anesthesia with that of children who had not had anesthesia. The lack of significant difference seemed a highly significant finding.

In some areas, better relationships between parents and professionals must be worked out. Intercommunication between physician, hospital, parent, and child should be developed to prevent misunderstanding and insecurity. Parents should be allowed to participate in the care of the hospitalized child to a definite degree without interfering with his welfare; otherwise the dissatisfaction and insecurity of the parents will be transferred to the child. The interplay between all of the participants is highly involved (Fig. 4-4).

In regard to sedation, the concept must be accepted that each child is different and has different fears and a different anxiety level. We must try to find both the type and degree of the child's anxiety. Most of all, we

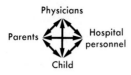

Fig. 4-4. Important interrelationships in contending with child's anxieties.

should be on the lookout for the hyperanxious child so that he may be accorded special treatment that will prevent excessive psychic shock.

It is clear that we can improve the present situation by discontinuation of known fallacies, but better methods have yet to be established. Efforts should be made in the following directions:

1. Elimination of needles for sedation.
2. Use of atropine only as indicated, and then given by preexisting infusion or after anesthetic induction has rendered the child analgesic.
3. Establishment of a system of evaluation of the level of anxiety to be used as a guide to dosage of sedative agents.
4. Development of special management technics for children suspected of having increased risk of emotional trauma.
5. Greater attempts to uncover the fears and anxieties of individual children and their parents, and methods of controlling them.
6. Continuation of the search for a drug or combination of drugs that will provide reliable sedation without depression or other side effects.

During the preoperative examination, it would be advantageous for the anesthesiologist to estimate the child's level of anxiety and record it on a scale of 0 through 3 as outlined in the guide below. Such an estimate may be made by first considering the predisposing factors and then by talking directly to the child.

GUIDE TO CLASSIFICATION OF ANXIETY LEVELS

Anxiety level 0

Sleeps soundly.
When awake is relaxed, responsive.
Occupies himself with toys, things to do.
Plays pleasantly with others.
Eats well.
Submits to treatments.

Anxiety level 1

Awakens easily, slightly restless.
Whines when alone, needs help, satisfied when entertained.
Cries when parents leave.
Eats slowly.
Communicates, responds.
Will apply himself when encouraged to draw, etc.

Anxiety level 2

Sleeps fitfully, quite restless.
Unhappy, unpleasant, whiney.
Avoids attendants, resists examination and treatment.
Difficult to pacify, but will respond in time.
Older child either withdrawn or hyperactive.
Has many fears, demands, dislikes.
May have had previous anesthetic misfortune.

Anxiety level 3

Cries and screams much of the time.
Sick, spoiled, psychotic.
Completely uncooperative, withdrawn, combative.
Unable to speak English or to be understood.
Fights off all approach.
Intensely worried by real or imagined plight.

As noted by Smith, and associates (1976), there are several factors that predispose children to high anxiety states. These include the following:

1. Age 1 to 4 years.
2. Inability to communicate.
3. Emotional or neurotic parents.
4. Previous traumatic hospital experience.
5. Fear of expected operation—amputation, cardiac surgery, or other extensive procedure.

Inability to communicate is one of the most distressing of the factors, whether it is because of foreign tongue, mental retardation, cerebral palsy, or simply not being old enough to talk.

By talking to the child one can gather more evidence by which to classify him according to anxiety levels. The guide above shows some of the significant signs that help evaluate infants and children. Among these signs, one is most apt to miss the significance of the very quiet child and the one who is hyperactive, both of whom might appear relatively normal while actually under appreciable strain (Wolff, 1969). In addition, by eliciting some of the major likes and dislikes of the child one also gains considerable insight into his emotional status (Korsch, 1975).

After the child is evaluated on a scale of variable need there should be a variable method of treatment that can be adjusted accordingly. Wherever possible, a child's emotional needs should be answered by personal attention, reassurance, diversion, and communication, with sedation used as a supplementary agent. However, the use of sedation will reasonably increase with more severe and complicated forms of emotional problems. Sedatives will also be relied on more heavily when personnel have less time, less interest, and less ability to deal directly with these unhappy patients.

As a general guide, the following steps are suggested.

Management of children in level 0. Mostly 7 to 12 years old. Talk to the child or play with him long enough to have him become accustomed to your appearance and the sound of your voice. Find out an older child's interests, something he likes to talk or think about or something he does well, so that the topic can be resumed before the operation. Find something to praise or compliment him about. Reevaluate at least an hour before operation in the morning, renew acquaintance, and strengthen relationship between parent, child, and yourself.

Sedation may be added if necessary, using minimal dose by oral or rectal route (pentobarbital, 3 mg/kg; diazepam, 0.1 mg/kg; etc.).

Management of children in level 1. Increase attempt to build friendship and confidence of the child and parents. Emphasize good things around the child while trying to find out what might be disturbing him. Some of the quieter 1- to 4-year olds will be in this group. If the parents are nearby, keep them around as much as possible but try to prevent an emotional parting just before the operation. Most of the normal, older children should be found in this group and should be relatively easy to deal with using encouragement, honest attention to their questions, reassurance, and establishment of some common topic of interest, such as a TV program, Little League baseball, or collecting bottle tops.

Light sedation on the morning of the operation will be helpful; use pentobarbital, 4 mg/kg PR or 3 mg/kg PO, or similar agent at least 90 minutes before operation.

Management of children in level 2. These moderately excited children will need additional attention, with supplemental help from parents and attendants in the form of encouragement and understanding. There may be a definite problem of misunderstanding, a reasonable fear, or history of a sensitizing event that needs airing but requires time to discover. Sickness and discomfort may be added factors. Moderate amounts of sedation may be used but only after an honest attempt has been made to find out if there is some unrecognized factor that can be corrected by communication rather than by medication.

A small dose of sedative at bedtime followed by a moderate amount of sedation well before the hour of operation should give reasonably good results. It will be especially helpful to visit any Level 2 or Level 3 child on the morning of operation early enough to check the general emotional response and add a word of reassurance as well as an additional half dose of sedative and a request for those around the child to tread lightly.

Management of children in level 3. For these children, an all-out attempt must be made to avoid adding further trauma to patients who may already be sensitized. Parents should be interviewed, and help may be sought from nurses and wardmates as to the reasons for the child's distress. An attending psychiatrist may be of much help, especially if he has been in contact with the child. It should be noted that this discussion pertains to the types of seriously ill, deformed, and discouraged children seen more frequently in pediatric centers specializing in kidney transplants, cardiac malformation, mental retardation, and other relatively unusual situations.

Sedation should be administered with greater generosity but not to excess. It is wise to try the intended sedative a day or two prior to operation to test the child's reaction to it and to establish a mild degree of desensitization with hydroxyzine or phenobarbital (enzyme induction may be a consideration).

Dosage of pentobarbital should not exceed 6 mg/kg PR or 5 mg/kg PO. Significantly greater response to the morning sedation will be obtained if a moderate dose of the agent has been given at bedtime. Again, much attention should be devoted to markedly distressed children on the morning of operation, and supplemental medication should be ordered if necessary. When the situation is acute and prompt control is necessary, one may induce anesthesia by intravenous administration of thiopental, but one should not force a mask on an upset child (see Chapter 7).

Sedation for children in unusual circumstances. There are situations where more precision is needed in controlling children prior to operation, one example being the child with fracture of cervical vertebrae who must not be allowed to move quickly at any time. In these cases, personal attention will be of much value, but neither this nor any one-shot pharmaceutical approach will provide sufficient reliability. A more profound state of sedation will probably be required, such as that produced by droperidol or by a slow intravenous infusion to which morphine and diazepam may be added in small divided doses, in order to titrate the patient to the desired level of quiescence.

The above suggestions are offered for trial by those interested in narrowing the gap between the present high level of care of anesthetized children and the unsatisfactory state of our control of children while awake.

The traditional method of barbiturate, morphine, and atropine is still widely employed and may be preferable for many patients who require major procedures and who are not in danger of experiencing severe emotional trauma.

SUMMARY

The importance of both physical and emotional preparation of children must be recognized. Physical preparation has become satisfactorily standardized, but attempts to prepare children for the emotional stresses of hospitalization have been unsatisfactory, with the chief reliance being on the use of sedatives.

Anesthesiologists have failed to recognize the fact that emotional distress often causes greater suffering than such familiar anesthetic complications as nausea and headache. A child who cries for weeks after leaving the hospital and who will not leave his mother's side is certainly suffering from an equally severe insult.

Emotional complications can be reduced by greater reliance on personal communication between hospital personnel, physicians, parents, and patients and by the application of sedatives in appropriate supportive roles.

BIBLIOGRAPHY

Ainsworth, M. D., and Boston, M.: Psychodiagnostic assessments of a child after prolonged separation in early childhood, Br. J. Med. Psychol. **25:**169, 1952.

Alper, M. H., Flacke, W., and Krayer, O.: Pharmacology of reserpine and its implications for anesthesia, Anesthesiology **24:**524, 1963.

Barker, R. A., and Nisbet, H. I. A.: The objective measurement of sedation in children; a modified scoring system, Can. Anaesth. Soc. J. **20:**599, 1973.

Beven, J. C., and Burn, M. D.: Acid-base changes and anesthesia, the influence of preoperative starvation and feeding in paediatric surgical patients, Anaesthesia **28:**415, 1973.

Bird, B.: Talking with patients, ed. 2, Philadelphia, 1973, J. B. Lippincott Co.

Bothe, A., and Galdston, R.: The child's loss of consciousness; a psychiatric view of pediatric anesthesia, Pediatrics **50:**252, 1972.

Bourgeois-Gavardin, M., Nowill, W. K., Margolis, G., and Stephen, C. R.: Chlorpromazine; a laboratory and clinical investigation, Anesthesiology **16:**829, 1955.

Bowlby, J.: Some pathological processes engendered by early mother-child separation. In Senn, M. F. E., editor: Infancy and childhood, transaction of Seventh Conference of Josiah Macy, Jr., Foundation, New York, March 23-24, 1953.

Boyd, J. D., and Manford, M. L.: Premedication in children; a controlled clinical trial of oral triclofos and diazepam, Br. J. Anaesth. **45:**501, 1973.

Britt, B., Kalow, W., Gordon, A., Humphrey, J. G., and Newcastle, N. B.: Malignant hyperthermia; an investigation of five patients, Can. Anaesth. Soc. J. **20:**431, 1973.

Bush, G. H.: Evaluation of droperidol as premedicant, personal communication, 1972.

Coakley, C. S., Alpert, S., and Boling, J.: Circulatory responses during anesthesia of patients on rauwolfia therapy, J.A.M.A. **161:**1143, 1956.

Cope, R. W., and Glover, W. J.: Trimeprazine tartrate for premedication in children, Lancet **1:**858, 1959.

Davenport, H. T., and Werry, J. S.: Effect of general anesthesia, surgery and hospitalization upon the behavior of children, Am. J. Orthopsychiatry **40:**806, 1970.

Denborough, M. A., Dennett, X., and Anderson, R. M.: Central-core disease and malignant hyperpyrexia, Br. Med. J. **1:**272, 1973.

Diggs, L. W.: Sickle cell crises, Am. J. Clin. Pathol. **44:**1, 1965.

Doughty, A.: Oral premedication in children; a controlled clinical trial of pecazine, trimeprazine and methylpentynol, Br. J. Anaesth. **34:**80, 1962.

Downes, J. J.: Personal communication, 1976.

Downes, J. J., and Nicodemus, H.: Preparation for and recovery from anesthesia, Pediatr. Clin. North Am. **16:**601, 1969.

Eckenhoff, J. E.: Relationship of anesthesia to postoperative personality changes in children, Am. J. Dis. Child. **86:**587, 1953.

Eckenhoff, J. E., and Helrich, M. H.: Study of narcotics and sedatives for use in preanesthetic medication, J.A.M.A. **167:**415, 1958.

Egbert, L. D., Lamdin, S. J., and Hacket, T. P.: Psychological problems of surgical patients. In Eckenhoff, J. E.: Science and practice in anesthesia, Philadelphia, 1965, J. B. Lippincott Co.

Eger, E. I.: Atropine, scopolamine, and related compounds, Anesthesiology **23:**365, 1962.

Francis, L., and Cutler, R. P.: Psychological preparation and premedication for pediatric anesthesia, Anesthesiology **18:**106, 1957.

Franko, B. V., Alphin, R. S., Ward, J. W., and others: Pharmacodynamic evaluation of glycopyrrolate in animals, Ann. N.Y. Acad. Sci. **99:**174, 1962.

Freeman, A., and Bachman, L.: Pediatric anesthesia; an evaluation of preoperative medication, Anesth. Analg. (Cleve.) **38:**429, 1959.

Gilchrist, G. S.: Preoperative hematologic evaluation and management. In Gans, S. L., editor: Surgical pediatrics, New York, 1973, Grune & Stratton, Inc.

Gillick, J. S.: Atropine toxicity in a neonate, Br. J. Anaesth. **46:**793, 1974.

Gillies, I. D. S.: Anaemia and anaesthesia, Br. J. Anaesth. **46:**589, 1974.

Gofman, H., Buckman, W., and Schade, G. H.: The child's emotional response to hospitalization, Am. J. Dis. Child. **93:**157, 1957.

Goldberg, L. I., and Whitsett, T. L.: Cardiovascular effects of levodopa, Clin. Pharmacol. Ther. **12:**376, 1971.

Haller, G. A., editor: The hospitalized child and his family, Baltimore, 1967, The Johns Hopkins University Press.

Herbert, W., and Hammond, D.: Preoperative evaluation of the anemic child, Am. Surg. **29:**660, 1963.

Jackson, K.: Psychological preparation as a method of reducing emotional trauma of anesthesia in children, Anesthesiology **12:**293, 1951.

Joos, H. A.: Atropine intoxication in infancy, Am. J. Dis. Child. **79:**855, 1950.

Keller, M. L., Sussman, S., and Rochberg, S.: Comparative evaluation of combined preoperative medications for pediatric surgery, Anesth. Analg. (Cleve.) **47:**199, 1968.

Kennell, J. H., and Gergen, M. E.: Early childhood separations, Pediatrics **37:**291, 1966.

Koop, E. C.: Preparing the patient and his family for hospital and surgery. In Gans, S. L., editor: Surgical pediatrics, New York, 1973, Grune & Stratton, Inc.

Korsch, B. M.: The child and the operating room, Anesthesiology **43:**251, 1975.

Lee, J. S., and Greene, N.: Parental presence and emotional state of children prior to surgery, Clin. Pediatr. (Phila.) **8:**126, 1969.

Lee, J. S., and Greene, N.: Anxiety in children, Anesthesiology **33:**652, 1970.

Levin, R. M.: Pediatric anesthesia handbook, Flushing, N.Y., 1973, Medical Examination Publishing Co., Inc.

Levy, D. M.: Psychic trauma of operation in children, Am. J. Dis. Child. **69:**75, 1945.

Lewis, L., Robinson, R. F., Yee, J., and others: Fatal adrenal cortical insufficiency precipitated by surgery during prolonged continuous cortisone treatment, Ann. Intern. Med. **39:**116, 1953.

Linde, S. M.: When children need their parents most; rooming-in with hospitalized children, Today's Health **46:**26, 1968.

Lipton, B.: Current concepts in the management of pediatric anesthesia, Pediatr. Digest **5:**13, 1963.

Love, H. D.: Your child goes to the hospital; a book for parents, Springfield, Ill., 1972, Charles C Thomas, Publisher.

Mayer, J.: Reactions of children during hospital admission; three diaries, Ment. Hyg. **48:**576, 1964.

McKenzie, A. L., and Pigott, J. F. G.: Atropine overdosage in three children, Br. J. Anaesth. **43:**1088, 1971.

Mellish, R. W. P.: Preparation of a child for hospitalization and surgery, Pediatr. Clin. North Am. **16:**543, 1969.

Meyers, E. R., and Muravchick, S.: Anesthesia induction techniques in pediatric patients; a controlled study of behavioral consequences, paper presented at Midwest Anesthesia Residents' Conference, Iowa, 1976, Anesth. Analg. (Cleve.) **56:**538, 1977.

Morse, M., Cassels, D. E., and Holder, M.: The position of the oxygen dissociation curve of the blood in normal children and adults, J. Clin. Invest. **29:**1091, 1950.

Morton, H. G.: Atropine intoxication; its manifestations in infants and children, J. Pediatr. **14:**755, 1939.

Oski, F. A.: Hemoglobin and hematocrit values; what is normal? J. Pediatr. **82:**543, 1973.

Oski, F. A., and Norman, J. L.: Hematologic problems in the newborn, Philadelphia, 1966, W. B. Saunders Co.

Petrillo, M., and Sanger, S.: Emotional care of hospitalized children, Philadelphia, 1972, J. B. Lippincott Co.

Poe, M. F., and Karp, M.: Seconal as a basal anesthetic for children, Anesth. Analg. (Cleve.) **27:**88, 1948.

Potts, W. J.: The heart of a child, J.A.M.A. **161:**487, 1956.

Rackow, H., and Salanitre, E.: A dose-effect study of preoperative medication in children, Anesthesiology **23:**747, 1962.

Rackow, H., and Salanitre, E.: Modern concepts in pediatric anesthesiology, review, Anesthesiology **30:**208, 1969.

Rinehart, J. J., Lewis, R. P., and Balcerzak, S. P.: Adriamycin cardiotoxicity in man, Ann. Intern. Med. **81:**475, 1974.

Root, B.: Problems of evaluating effects of premedication in children; presentation of a key-sort card, Anesth. Analg. (Cleve.) **41:**180, 1962.

Root, B., and Loveland, J. P.: Pediatric premedicaiton

with diazepam hydroxyzine; oral vs intramuscular route, Anesth. Analg. (Cleve.) **52:**717, 1973.

Rosen, M., and Brueton, M.: Emotional disturbances in children having tonsillectomy and adenoidectomy aged 5-6 years, Excerpta Medica Foundation 686, 1970.

Salem, M. P., Wong, A. Y., Maui, M., and others: Premedicant drugs and gastric juice pH volume in pediatric patients, Anesthesiology **44:**216, 1976.

Sargarminiga, J., and Wygands, J. E.: Atropine and the electrical activity of the heart during induction of anesthesia in children, Can. Anaesth. Soc. J. **10:** 328, 1963.

Sever, J.: Johnny goes to the hospital, Boston, 1953, Houghton Mifflin Co.

Shearer, W. M.: The evolution of premedication, Br. J. Anaesth. part I **32:**554, 1960; part II **33:**219, 1961.

Smith, M. J., and Miller, M. M.: Severe extrapyramidal reaction to perphenazine treated with diphenhydramine, N. Engl. J. Med. **264:**396, 1961.

Smith, R. M.: Children, hospitals and parents, Anesthesiology **25:**461, 1964.

Smith, R. M.: The responsibilities of the anesthesiologist in pre- and postoperative care. In Gans, S. L., editor: Surgical pediatrics, New York, 1973, Grune & Stratton, Inc.

Smith, R. M., Fox, D., and Anderson, S.: Preoperative anxiety factors in children, paper presented to American Society of Anesthesiologists, San Francisco, October 11, 1976.

Smith, R. M., and Jeffries, M.: The evaluation of sedative agents for preoperative use in children, Anesth. Analg. (Cleve.) **38:**166, 1959.

Stephen, C. R., Ahlgren, E. W., and Bennett, E. J.: Elements of pediatric anesthesia, Springfield, Ill., 1970, Charles C Thomas, Publisher.

Stephen, C. R., Bowers, M. A., Nowill, W. K., and Martin, R. C.: Anticholinergic drugs in preanesthetic medication, Anesthesiology **17:**303, 1956.

Stetson, J. G., and Jessup, B. V. S.: Use of chloral hydrate mixtures for pediatric premedication, Anesth. Analg. (Cleve.) **41:**203, 1962.

Stiles, C. M.: personal communication, 1975.

Vandam, L. D.: Effects of prior drug therapy on the course of anesthesia. In Eckenhoff, J. E., editor: Science and practice of anesthesia, Philadelphia, 1962, J. B. Lippincott Co.

Vernon, D. A.: The psychological responses of children to hospitalization and illness, Springfield, Ill., 1965, Charles C Thomas, Publisher.

Visintainer, M. A., and Wolfer, J. A.: Psychological preparation for surgical pediatric patients, Pediatrics **56:**187, 1975.

Wallgren, A. J.: Children in hospitals, J. Pediatr. **46:** 458, 1955.

Waters, R. M.: Pain relief for children, Am. J. Surg. **39:**470, 1938.

Weber, A.: Elizabeth gets well, New York, 1970, Thomas Y. Crowell Co., Inc.

Werry, J. S., Davenport, H. T., and Nissenbaum, R.: The psychological effects of premedication for paediatric anaesthesia; a pilot study, New Zeal. Med. J. **64:**641, 1965.

Wolff, S.: Children under stress, London, 1969, Penguin Publishing Co., Ltd.

Woodbridge, P. D.: Preanesthetic breakfast, Anesthesiology **4:**81, 1943.

Wyant, G. M., and Dobkin, A. B.: Antisialagogue drugs in man, Anaesthesia **12:**203, 1957.

Wyant, G. M., and Kao, E.: Glycopyrrolate methobromide. I. Effect on salivary secretion, Can. Anaesth. Soc. J. **21:**230, 1974.

Young, R., and Sun, D. C. H.: Effects of glycopyrrolate on antral motility, gastric emptying and intestinal transit, Ann. N.Y. Acad. Sci. **99:**131, 1962.

CHAPTER 5

Choice of inhalation agents

GENERAL CONSIDERATIONS

This entire chapter could be written by some authorities in one sentence: "All pediatric operations can be very nicely managed under endotracheal intubation using nitrous oxide, oxygen, and relaxants."

The entire chapter could also be written by other experts with equal brevity but different wording: "Halothane is especially useful for children and may be used for practically all types of operations."

Both statements are reasonable, but the situation is not that simple. I for one do not want to start every anesthesia with a needle, or intubate all patients, or use relaxants for children with airway obstruction. Nor do I want to put every child to sleep or have to force a mask on a resisting child. Though we are getting closer, we still do not have one technic that can be suited to all patients.

In a changing situation in which new agents are continually being introduced and new surgical procedures are being attempted on sicker patients, the choice of anesthetic agent must be under continual scrutiny and be subject to alteration in step with increasing information and developing conditions.

Several important changes have already occurred in relation to choice of agents for pediatric anesthesia. One no longer may claim that any one anesthetic approach is best for a particular surgical procedure, since excellent results are now recorded for practically any operation using a number of methods.

The basis on which evaluation is made also has changed. For many years, the fact that ether stimulates respiration outweighed the disadvantages of its flammability. Now flammability outlaws any anesthetic, while the effect on respiration is a relatively minor consideration.

Choice has widened because of introduction of new drugs and lack of any single all-purpose agent, so that the final decision in complicated situations, especially those with legal overtones, actually is rendered more difficult. Thus, for an infant with biliary atresia, the logical choice based on scientific evidence could be halothane, but the possibility of unsound, yet time-consuming, litigation could influence one to use another approach, such as a relaxant technic.

The decision concerning agents and methods often appears to be made without a moment's consideration. When situations have been repeated innumerable times this can occur, but the decision usually represents much forethought, experience, and judgment.

Under other conditions, the correct choice is difficult and demands the weighing of several important considerations, often with no perfect answer, e.g., the child who comes to the hospital with a lacerated eyeball and a full stomach.

Fortunately, one change for the better is that we have discarded that outworn maxim "the right agent is the one the anesthesiolo-

109

gist knows best."* Although there are times when this does apply, it could also serve as an excuse for great ignorance. An anesthesiologist might use open-drop ether for the child with the lacerated eyeball. Because he has failed to learn newer methods, that would be the approach he knows best, but obviously it would not be acceptable under any circumstances.

To set up a system that will be continuously useful in choosing agents and methods, it is advisable first to postulate *what is needed*, or the *ideal method* (it may not be an agent), next to consider *what is available*, and finally to decide *how to make the choice.*

WHAT IS NEEDED

The ideal method must enable one to provide hypnosis, analgesia, control of reflexes, and relaxation (Woodbridge, 1957) as well as immobilization (Snow, 1858). The above elements must be individually controllable, rapidly effective, potent, and promptly reversible.

The method must be safe, without danger of explosion, toxicity, undesirable side effects, or alteration of bodily functions and should maintain airway protection.

It should be practical, available, inexpensive, and universally acceptable to patients without the discomfort of needles or the disturbance of masks.

Obviously nothing of the kind exists, but a multichanneled electronic device that is controlled via stick-on skin tabs could be imagined, perhaps as some outgrowth of acupuncture.

WHAT IS AVAILABLE

Examination of what is actually available promptly brings us back to reality. The principal agents include the following:

1. Local anesthetics: procaine, tetracaine, lidocaine, carbocaine, bupivacaine, and others.
2. General anesthetics: nitrous oxide, halothane, enflurane, fluroxene, methoxyflurane, ether, cyclopropane.

---

*This maxim also condemned by Greene, N. M.: Anesthesiology **44:**101, 1976.

3. Sedatives, hypnotics, tranquilizers, dissociative agents, and narcotics given by intravenous, intramuscular, oral, or rectal route.
4. Muscle relaxants: succinylcholine, *d*-tubocurarine, gallamine, pancuronium, metocurine.
5. Hypnosis.
6. Electronarcosis.
7. Acupuncture.

HOW TO CHOOSE

When a 4-year-old black child known to have diabetes is brought to the hospital comatose with head injury and ruptured liver, how do we manage anesthesia?

With a complicated problem, an attempt is made to arrange all pertinent data in order of importance, one's brain working as a computer, organizing, matching, sorting, eliminating, and coming up with an answer. Choice is determined, often without our realization, by a three-stage process; first meeting *basic anesthetic requirements*, then fitting them to the *specific situation*, and finally altering the technic to *suit personal preference.*

Basic anesthetic requirements are those of safety (freedom from explosion, toxicity, and depression) as well as those of practicality. These are similar in all age groups, with minor exceptions.

Factors related to the *specific situation* that must be considered in choosing the anesthetic agent are the child's age, his physical and emotional state, his previous experiences and expressed dislikes, the operation planned, and the special needs of the surgeon. As always, the child's greater tendency to airway obstruction and lack of temperature control are borne in mind.

Personal preference of the anesthesiologist often appears in the choice between methods of induction, use of circle or T-tube system, or relaxant as opposed to inhalation technic.

In the case of the black comatose diabetic child with head injury and ruptured liver, there is actually little room for choice, since treatment of the ruptured liver demands priority, and other than supportive measures, the only anesthetic management needed for a comatose patient would be endotracheal intubation and oxygen.

Choice of anesthetics for the child with the lacerated eyeball and full stomach is far more difficult.

Basic anesthetic requirements of adequate oxygenation and safety would allow almost any agent except ether and cyclopropane. The requirements of the specific situation are control of intraocular pressure and prevention of aspiration. To meet these requirements one must eliminate excitement and straining (often caused by needles and mask induction) and drugs that raise intraocular pressure, i.e., ketamine and probably succinylcholine. It seems questionable that preliminary d-tubocurarine would be adequate protection for the use of succinylcholine. Although some prefer "crash" induction and intubation with intravenous agents for full stomach, it would seem doubly dangerous here.

My choice of the least upsetting method would be thiopental (Pentothal) by rectum without preliminary needles, then nitrous oxide–halothane induction, establishment of an infusion, and administration of atropine, followed by endotracheal intubation without a muscle relaxant.

Another important decision that would be required concerns the proper time to extubate this child. While early extubation would increase the danger of aspiration of vomitus, the intense straining often associated with delayed extubation might endanger the eye. Ophthalmologists state that the repair of a recently torn eyeball cannot be expected to withstand high tensions. It is our belief, consequently, that if the stomach of such a patient is washed out reasonably well during the operation, a suitably equipped anesthesiologist probably could prevent aspiration of vomitus encountered with early extubation but would have difficulty in averting serious damage caused by increased intraocular pressure under late extubation. Our choice, therefore, is to extubate before the return of coughing and gagging.

Choice of agent depends on thorough knowledge of those available. Rather than listing further personal preferences that might become outdated, a brief summary of currently used agents is presented below with attention directed toward their pediatric application.

INHALATION AGENTS
Nitrous oxide (N_2O)

A musty-smelling nonexplosive gas compressed to a liquid in cylinders at 750 lb/sq in, N_2O is the most widely used anesthetic in both the pediatric and adult fields. Its popularity as an induction agent and supplemental anesthetic is because of its inoffensive odor, low solubility (Table 5-1), hypnotic and analgesic effect, compatibility with all other drugs, and freedom from depressant effect. The use of N_2O reduces the requirement of other agents that carry greater risk or more prolonged effect.

Although no absolute contraindications exist for N_2O, there are several situations where its use demands special consideration. Nitrous oxide often proves *ineffective for induction of infants under 1 month of age*, unless excessive concentrations are used. Because small infants accept halothane quite readily, this agent is used to initiate induction. Of greater importance is the problem of *accumulation of N_2O during procedures involving gas-containing spaces*. Eger and Saidman (1965) noted that N_2O was more soluble than nitrogen in blood and therefore would distend any air-containing space to which it was carried. Stomach, bowel, cerebral ventricles, and eustachian tubes are thus exposed during procedures for diaphragmatic hernia, bowel obstruction, pneumoencephalography, or tympanoplasty, respectively.

In *situations where maximum oxygenation is essential*, as in bronchoscopy, major burns, shock, or marked debility, the use of N_2O in effective concentrations (50% or more) would be open to question.

Once believed to be entirely nontoxic, N_2O has aroused increasing suspicion on several counts. Lymphocyte depression, reported by Eastwood and associates (1963), was viewed with more interest than alarm; however, subsequent reports of increased in-

Table 5-1. Pharmacology of halogenated anesthetics

	Enflurane (compound 347)	Isoflurane (compound 469)	Methoxyflurane	Halothane
Trade name	Ethrane	Forane	Penthrane	Fluothane
Formula	F F F / H–C–C–O–C–H / F Cl F	F H F / F–C–C–O–C–H / F Cl F	Cl F H / H–C–C–O–C–H / Cl F H	F Br / F–C–C–Cl / F H
Boiling point	56.5	48.5	104.6	50.2
Molecular weight	184.5	184.5	165.0	197.4
Vapor pressure at 20° C	180	250	22.5	243
Solubility or partition coefficients				
Oil/gas	98.5	99.0	825.0	236
Blood/gas	1.91	1.4	13.0	2.3
Odor	Mild	Mildly pungent	Mild	Mild
MAC				
Infant, 0-3 yr	2.0	1.7		1.08
Child, 3-10 yr	2.5	1.4		0.9
Adult	1.7	1.15	0.16	0.76
Induction	Rapid	Less rapid due to odor	Slow	Rapid
Recovery	Rapid	Very rapid	Slow	Rapid
Metabolism	2.5%	Nil or minimal	High (40%)	18-20%
Flammability	No	No	7.0% in air 5.4% in O$_2$	No
Chemical stabilizer	Not necessary	Not necessary	Required	Required

Adapted from Lowe, H. J.: Dose-regulated Penthrane (methoxyflurane) anesthesia, North Chicago, Ill., 1972, Abbott Laboratories.

cidence of miscarriage (Whitcher and others, 1971; Bruce, 1973; Cohen and others, 1971), testicular damage (Kripke and others, 1976), cancer (Corbett and others, 1973; Cohen, 1976), teratogenicity (Smith and others, 1965), and other responses to prolonged exposure to N_2O (Fink and Cullen, 1976), while not yet definitive, have convinced us that operating room personnel are in greater danger than patients, and we can no longer use N_2O with our previous abandon. Methods of reducing its accumulation in operating rooms are described in Chapter 6.

Nitrous oxide shows significant alteration of potency with barometric pressure, becoming less effective at high altitudes (e.g., Denver, Colo.) and more effective at or below sea level and in hyperbaric devices (Smith, 1965).

Trichloroethylene (C_2HCl_3)

Trichloroethylene is a relatively weak, nonexplosive agent that was used for many years for outpatient procedures and neurosurgical operations, but tachypnea, cardiac irregularities, occasionally hepatotoxicity, and incompatibility with soda lime combine to prevent it from being of major value either alone or as a supplementary agent.

Cyclopropane (C_3H_6)

A sweet, almost sickish smelling explosive gas compressed to a liquid in (orange) cylinders at 75 lb/sq in, cyclopropane affords rapid induction, full hypnosis, analgesia, and relaxation, adequate reflex control, and minimal toxicity. Although cyclopropane is incompatible with epinephrine, and arrhythmias occur frequently, it causes peripheral vasoconstriction and has been considered the agent of choice for patients having hypovolemia. With the additional advantage of preserving body heat and moisture, cyclopropane enjoyed considerable popularity as an induction agent and for maintenance in infants and children with cardiac defects and other poor-risk patients. In spite of these advantages, the introduction of nonexplosive agents that are equally effective has rendered cyclopropane obsolete.

Diethyl ether ($C_2H_5OC_2H_5$)

Ether has much in its favor, including the fact that it is effective for almost any procedure, has excellent signs of depth and controllability, offers cardiorespiratory support and full relaxation, and is neither toxic nor epinephrine-sensitive. In addition, it can be administered by open drop, insufflation, nonrebreathing, or closed methods. Its disadvantages include an unforgettable, choking odor and respiratory and gastrointestinal irritation. Small infants are especially difficult to anesthetize regardless of the method and easily develop breath-holding spells with resultant cyanosis and bradycardia. In spite of the prolonged dominance of ether in pediatric anesthesia, its explosive quality has rendered it virtually obsolete in many parts of the world, its continued use being limited chiefly to areas where expense bars the use of nonflammable agents.

Fluroxene ($C_4H_5OF_3$)

An unsaturated halogenated hydrocarbon, fluroxene (Fluoromar) was synthesized by Krantz in 1953, well before halothane, and was tried and marketed. It is sweet, relatively inoffensive, and nonirritating and is believed to cause little myocardial depression. It was also believed to be nonhepatotoxic. These features earned it some use among elderly patients, but lack of potency limited its value for healthy younger subjects, and high incidence of nausea and vomiting prevented its general acceptance. More recently, two reports of fatal hepatotoxicity (Reynolds and others, 1972; Tucker and others, 1973) and evidence that fluroxene undergoes enzyme induction when used in conjunction with several other drugs (Harrison and Smith, 1973) have fairly effectively obliterated any remaining enthusiasm for its use.

Halothane ($C_2HClBrF_3$)

Halothane (Fluothane) is presently the most widely used primary agent in pediatric anesthesia and may retain its lead in spite of any competing anesthetics now in sight. Because of its extensive use, it deserves detailed consideration. Since most of our knowledge of the agent is derived from work with adults, this is discussed first.

Halothane was developed by Raventos (1956) and Suckling (1957), and the initial clinical trial was made in 1956 by Michael Johnstone of Manchester, England. The structural formula is that of a saturated aliphatic two-carbon molecule (Table 5-1). Evidence that halothane was neither flammable nor explosive in oxygen within clinically employed limits gave it an immediate advantage over existing agents, but its multiple-halogenated structure aroused fear of hepatotoxicity. Abajian and associates (1959) did much to overcome the doubts of Americans and establish the drug in adult use in this country, and Stephen (1957) was one of the first proponents of its use in children.

Halothane is prepared as a clear fluid, having a sweet, fruity, nonirritating odor. It decomposes very slowly and is stabilized by storage in amber bottles. Its blood/gas solubility coefficient of 2.3 gives it the potential of relatively rapid action.

As an anesthetic agent for adults, halothane has been moderately successful, but widespread popularity has been limited by several minor disadvantages, the existence of numerous alternative methods (intravenous, relaxant, regional) and the continuing uncertainty about hepatic necrosis and other toxic effects.

In adult use, halothane fulfills the prime requisites of an anesthetic agent reasonably well. It provides reliable hypnosis and satisfactory analgesia (excellent with supplemental nitrous oxide), and reflexes are adequately controlled, leaving relaxation the one factor that is inadequate for many procedures in large patients. In elderly patients, hypotension limits its value.

Ease of administration, unapproached by any other drug, is an outstanding advantage. The initial danger of overdosage was largely overcome by the introduction of finely calibrated, out-of-circuit vaporizers.

Freedom from airway irritation is an outstanding characteristic of halothane and makes it the drug of choice in the presence of airway pathology. Pharyngeal reflexes are also obtunded sufficiently to allow use of an artificial airway relatively early in induction.

During the stimulation of operation, spontaneous respiration often is adequate. In general, however, respiration is depressed at relatively light levels of anesthesia and usually requires assistance, especially if narcotics have been administered before or during operation.

Halothane depresses cardiovascular activity, the mean arterial blood pressure falling in proportion to the depth of anesthesia (Eger and others, 1971). Skovsted and associates (1969) have shown that central nervous system receptors and baroreceptors have little to do with this response, which is the result of direct negative inotropic action on myocardium (Goldberg, 1968), cardiac slowing due to action on the sinoatrial node, and reduction of peripheral resistance (Eger and others, 1970). While the depression of arterial blood pressure may be excessive in debilitated patients or when halothane is the sole agent, with average patients the customary addition of nitrous oxide so reduces the required concentration of halothane that hypotension rarely affects anesthesia at moderate depth.

It has also been observed that the initial hypotensive action of halothane is not progressive but with prolonged anesthesia (5 hours) shows some reversal due, presumably, to stimulation of the sympathetic nervous system (Eger and others, 1971).

The release of catecholamines is reduced under halothane, and consequently ventricles are less irritable, but arrhythmias do occur in the ventricles, atrioventricular node, and atria.

The untoward effect of halothane is also seen in its sensitization of the myocardium to epinephrine, which, according to Katz and Epstein (1968), if used at all in the presence of halothane, should be strictly limited (see dosage guide below). In comparison, enflurane shows significantly less myocardial sensitization than halothane, and isoflurane shows hardly any at all (Joas and Stevens, 1971).

ADULT ALLOWANCE OF EPINEPHRINE DURING HALOTHANE ANESTHESIA*

100 μg (10 ml) 1:100,000 in 10 minutes
100 μg (20 ml) 1:200,000 in 10 minutes
300 μg (30 ml) 1:100,000 in 30 minutes
300 μg (60 ml) 1:200,000 in 30 minutes

Significant circulatory effects of halothane include decreased peripheral resistance and increased right-to-left shunting (Price, 1969) as well as marked hepatic vasoconstriction (Berger and others, 1975).

Halothane has been shown to cause appreciable elevation of CSF pressure, an action shared by most inhalation agents with the exception of enflurane (Smith and Wollman, 1972; Shapiro, 1975). Initial reports of the effect of halothane on spinal fluid pressure aroused brief efforts to outlaw its use for neurosurgery, but it continues to be one of the more popular agents in that field.

The relationship of halothane to *changes in body temperature* is one of the most important aspects of the agent. Under normal conditions, halothane causes peripheral vasodilation and increased peripheral circulation with resultant loss of body heat. This cooling is especially significant in small infants and of itself causes respiratory depression, delayed awakening, and other undesirable responses. Because halothane, like other anesthetic gases, becomes more soluble as the blood cools, the same inspired concentration of halothane will produce a deeper plane of anesthesia and even greater depression.

The role of halothane in relation to the development of hyperthermia has been less clear, but as reported by Strobel (1971), Britt and associates (1976), Gronert and Theye (1976), and others, there is increasing evidence that halothane may trigger the onset of malignant hyperthermia by its effect on the myoplasmic calcium content of muscular tissue. This is discussed in Chapter 26.

An important finding was that of Eger (1974), who showed that if a patient's temperature rose above 39° C, his MAC for halothane would fall sharply. Although the mech-

anism could hardly be related to that associated with the cooling mentioned above, the result would be similar in that the level of anesthesia would become deeper while the patient was breathing the same concentration of halothane. In hyperthermic patients, however, whether one is dealing with malignant hyperthermia or not, there would be more acute danger than in moderate hypothermia.

Problems of toxicity and metabolism. Obviously the chief limiting factor in the use of halothane has been the question of its toxicity. At the time of introduction of halothane, the presence of five halogen atoms in each halothane molecule caused reasonable concern. However, when tests by Duncan and Raventos (1959) failed to show evidence of metabolic breakdown, much of the fear was allayed. The tests, considered to be reliable at the time, involved postanesthetic examination of the urine of two dogs for trichloroacetic acid, urinalysis for halide and bromide in several rats, and examination of the blood of three rats for halothane metabolites.

The reports of fatal hepatic necrosis that followed shortly after the release of halothane (Virtue and Payne, 1958; Brody and Sweet, 1963; Bunker and Blumenfeld, 1963) brought little surprise to the original doubters. Halothane was immediately implicated, and innumerable and widely varied restrictions were suggested for its use.

Attempts to prove that "halothane hepatitis" was a specific entity were unsuccessful. Pathologic lesions in the liver were indistinguishable from those found in infectious and serum hepatitis. Furthermore, since the response did not appear to be either dose-related or reproducible, halothane could not be termed toxic in the exact sense of the word.

Failure to place the onus on toxicity led to the concept that the hepatitis was caused by a sensitization response to the drug. Popper (1960), Trey and associates (1969), Klatskin and Kimberg (1969), and others constructed a convincing argument that patients developed an immune reaction, evidenced by eosinophilia, lymphocyte response, and fever. Although there have been many incon-

*Adapted from Katz, R. L., and Epstein, R. A.: The interactions of anesthetic agents and adrenergic drugs to produce arrhythmias, Anesthesiology **29**:763, 1968.

sistencies in the concept, it still appears possible that metabolites of halothane react with proteins or lipids to produce irreversible binding, "thereby providing the basis for possible allergic mechanisms of halothane necrosis" (Uehelke and others, 1973). Evidence for and against the theory of sensitization response is found in articles by Cohen and associates (1971), Morley (1974), Mathieu and associates (1974), and others. The importance accorded this theory seems considerably reduced at present, greater interest now being directed toward biotransformation and enzyme induction (Brown, 1974; Rehder and Sessler, 1974; Cohen and others, 1975).

Both Stier (1964) and Van Dyke and associates (1965) reported evidence of metabolism of halothane. Since nontoxic trifluoroacetic acid, bromide, and chloride were believed to be the only by-products, this was not regarded with great concern. Following the demonstration of the biotransformation of methoxyflurane (Holaday and others, 1970; Mazze and Cousins, 1973; Dobkin and Levy, 1973) and the release of fluoride, a definite toxic end product, it was shown that from 10% to 23% of halothane administered to humans might undergo metabolism

(Rehder and others, 1967; Cascorbi and others, 1970) and that at least three metabolic pathways were possible. Cohen's discovery of N-trifluoro-acetyl-2-aminoethanol and N-acetyl-S-(2-bromo-2-chloro-1,1-difluoroethyl) cysteine in human urine in addition to trifluoroacetic acid showed that many potentially toxic metabolites might be formed, depending on the route of metabolism (Fig. 5-1). The usual path involves oxidative action by mixed-function microsomal enzymes, reduced nicotinamide adenine dinucleotide phosphate (NADPH), and molecular oxygen (Brown, 1974), the most important factor in the enzyme system being the cytochrome P450 (Van Dyke and Wood, 1973). It has been shown that variations in the amount and route of metabolism may be caused by enzyme induction, enzyme inhibition, hypoxia, and other factors. The evidence produced by Widger and associates (1976) that anaerobic metabolism of halothane may produce appreciable amounts of fluoride suggests an important clue to the etiology of halothane hepatitis.

Because of the inconsistency of the appearance of hepatotoxicity, one suspects that it may be due to a chance interaction of several factors. Dykes (1970) has named 12 possible

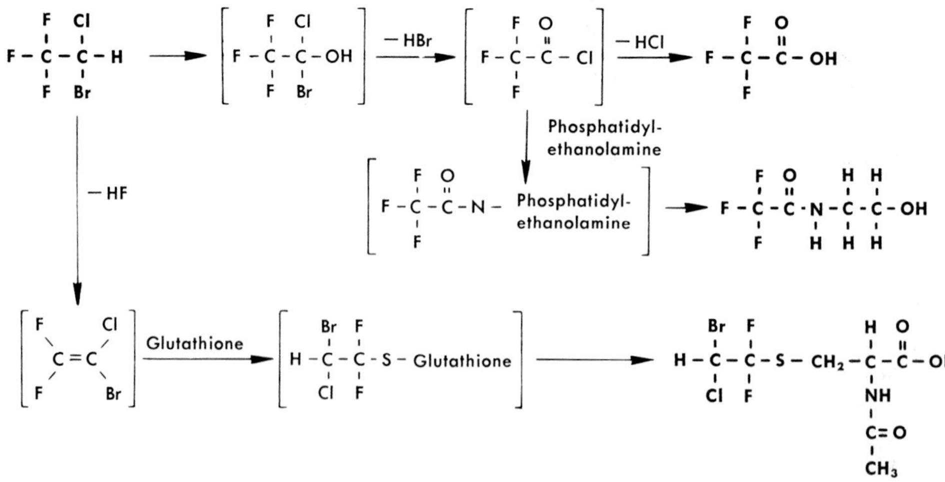

Fig. 5-1. Scheme for metabolic route for the production of three major urinary metabolites of halothane: trifluoroacetic acid, phosphatidylethanolamine, and 2-bromo-2-chloro-1,1-difluoroethylene. (From Cohen, E. N., Trudell, J. R., Edmunds, H. N., and Watson, E.: Anesthesiology **43**:392, 1975.)

contributing causes, including anaphylaxis, diet, genetic factors, and repeated anesthesia.

More recently, greater attention has been directed toward problems of chronic toxicity involving depression of organ systems of operating room personnel who are exposed to waste metabolites over prolonged periods. The possibility of increased toxicity of halothane when used in the presence of x-ray was brought out by Chambers and associates (1964) and by Hughes and Powell (1970). The report of Karis and associates (1976) that ultraviolet light increased the toxicity of halothane caused some alarm and led our institution, the Children's Hospital Medical Center, to attempt to repeat Karis's investigation. A medical engineering firm engaged for the study* was unable to find any evidence of increased toxicity.

Pediatric use of halothane. The initial trials of halothane in pediatric anesthesia aroused some anxiety. Junkin and associates (1957) warned that the agent was potent and should be administered drop by drop, not poured on the mask. Others found it hard to regulate even with a bubble-through ether vaporizer. With increasing sophistication, however, halothane became the preferred agent not only for tonsillectomy and herniorrhaphy but for most abdominal and cardiac surgery, and within 10 years it was the undisputed favorite for pediatric anesthesia throughout most of the Western world.

It was clear that halothane was far more valuable in its application to children than when used for older patients. Its advantages were more distinct, its disadvantages less evident. One could almost believe that the first all-purpose pediatric anesthetic had been found.

The principal factors responsible for the greater value of halothane in pediatric anesthesia are (1) the increased importance of an inoffensive agent, (2) the higher incidence of airway problems that require a nonirritant agent, (3) more satisfactory relaxation obtained, and (4) the decreased incidence of complications, especially hepatotoxicity.

The acceptability of halothane is more important with children, because adults will endure unpleasant jabs or odors that would completely disrupt the induction of a frightened child. In adult anesthesia it is *desirable* that an anesthetic be inoffensive—for pediatric patients it is *mandatory*.

The avoidance of airway irritation is of increased importance because of the presence of a large tongue and narrow air passages in the child as well as the high incidence of inflammatory lesions, tumors, and congenital defects. In any form of airway pathology, whether caused by enlarged tonsils, cystic fibrosis, or aspirated safety pins, halothane is still the choice. As noted by Reynolds (1962), the ease with which the airway may be controlled under halothane markedly reduces the need for endotracheal intubation. This is especially advantageous in smaller children who have greater incidence of postintubation croup (Koka and others, 1977).

While relaxation under halothane is inadequate for many operations on adults, it is sufficient in children for all but the most demanding operations, such as dissection of retroperitoneal nodes or liver transplantation.

To compare the complications and side effects of halothane in infants and adults, one should have more data than are now available. The more rapid uptake of halothane reported by Salanitre and Rackow (1961) and by Eger (1974) and the increased blood concentration required for anesthesia (Gregory and others, 1969) are characteristic of the responses of younger patients to all anesthetics, as noted in Chapter 2.

The depression of respiration was immediately evident when halothane was used for small children. Podlesch and associates (1966) provided definite data showing a rise in end-tidal CO_2 and stated that respiration should be assisted or controlled during anesthesia with this agent. The study of Graff and associates on acid-base balance under halothane (1964) showed that infants and children could maintain a normal Pa_{CO_2} at

---

*Technology in Medicine, Inc., 3 New England Park, Burlington, Mass.

light planes but required increased work at deeper planes and soon developed acidosis if not assisted.

The effect of halothane on the cardiovascular system of young infants has caused reasonable concern. Leigh and Belton (1960) warned of the sudden depression of cardiac function during surgery under halothane. Reliable studies of cardiac response to halothane were made in normal children by McGregor and associates (1958) and in children undergoing cardiac surgery by Taylor and Stoelting (1961). Both teams found that very light concentrations of halothane must be maintained (0.25% and 0.8%, respectively, with 50% nitrous oxide) to prevent cardiac depression, which became severe with halothane concentrations of 2% or 3%. These workers, as well as Reynolds (1962) and Stephen and associates (1970), have emphasized the importance of using atropine when giving halothane to young children, in order to pre-

vent vagal activity, bradycardia, and decreased output. Without atropine, 1% to 1.5% halothane may produce reduction in blood pressure and limit the use of halothane. With 0.02 to 0.03 mg of atropine per kg, however, one usually can administer 2% to 3% halothane before encountering the same degree of hypotension.

Clinical observations have been confirmed by the work of Barash and associates (1978). Using noninvasive echocardiographic technic to measure cardiac function in 13 children between the ages of 19 months and 12 years, they found that with 2% halothane, systolic blood pressure, pulse rate, and cardiac output decreased to 82%, 94%, and 72% of control values, respectively. After intravenous administration of 0.02 mg of atropine per kg, pulse rate increased by 49% and cardiac output increased by 47% over control values (Fig. 5-2).

Cardiac arrhythmias are encountered dur-

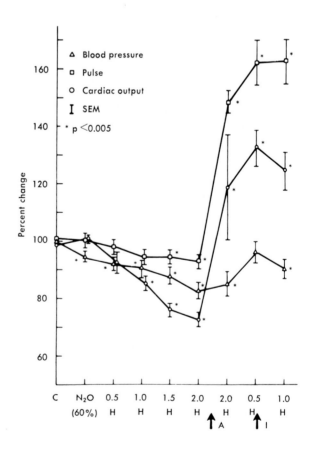

Fig. 5-2. Changes in blood pressure *(triangle)*, pulse *(square)*, and cardiac output *(circle)* with increasing concentration of halothane. *A,* atropine, *I,* intubation. (From Barash, P. G., Glanz, S., Katz, J. D., and others: Anesthesiology **49**:79, 1978.)

ing halothane anesthesia in children, especially during operations on the face, eyes, or abdomen where either deeper anesthesia or greater irritability may be a factor. Reporting on halothane sensitization of the myocardium in the presence of epinephrine, Melgrave (1970) voiced his conviction that children tolerate epinephrine better than adults. As yet there does not seem to be sufficient evidence to disregard the potential danger. While the use of epinephrine with halothane may not be entirely contraindicated, restrictions similar to those for adults are recommended (see dosage guide on p. 115).

The effect of halothane on body temperature has particular importance in young patients. Rapid loss of body heat, easily explained by peripheral vasodilation and relatively large body surface area, was promptly reported by Bull and associates (1958), Harrison and associates (1960), Hackett and Crosby (1960), and others, while the role of halothane in hyperthermic states was noted somewhat later by Stephen and associates (1970) and Berman and associates (1970).

Hepatotoxicity in children. An important influence on the broad use of halothane in children has been the general belief that children rarely if ever contract the hepatitis that has been such a problem in adults. Instead of just one question here, however, we are faced with two: are children actually less susceptible, and if so, why?

There have been few documented accounts of fatal posthalothane hepatic necrosis in pediatric patients, and only one report attempts to sum up known cases. Carney and Van Dyke (1972) described 11 children between the ages of 5 months and 12 years who had signs of liver toxicity following halothane anesthesia. The oldest and youngest of these children died. While the death of the 12-year-old was typical of "halothane hepatitis," hemolytic anemia and other complications confused the infant's diagnosis. The role of halothane was considered significant in only three of the survivors.

In an effort to gather more evidence on which to evaluate the safety of halothane in children, a review of the literature for pub-

lished cases was coupled with information gained from a survey to collect unpublished cases in patients under 21 years of age. As of January 1977, seven published cases and nine unpublished cases of fatal hepatic toxicity following halothane (plus many more reports of children who had developed jaundice and recovered) had been assembled. Of the total, six patients were under 10 years old, ten were 10 years or over, and eight were believed to be prepubertal. Of the 16, only three appeared to be simple cases that did not have such contributing factors as multiple operations, chronic illness, shock, or open-heart operations. Details of these cases will be found in Chapter 26.

While it is impossible to draw statistical meaning from such incomplete material, it is known that the figures represent at least 1 million halothane anesthetics in patients under 21 years of age. It is also possible to state with greater assurance that while children cannot be assumed to be immune to acute postoperative hepatic necrosis, the incidence is extremely low.

Several theories for the low incidence of this complication have been suggested. Carney and Van Dyke (1972) believe that it is simply due to an aging process, the liver becoming more and more easily irritated throughout life. The possibility that it is related to an immune, or sensitization, response has been upheld by those who state that children are less subject to sensitization responses, a view that seems difficult to defend. Brown (1974) stated that it is decided by a decreased rate of metabolism of the drug in young children, enzymal activity being markedly increased at puberty by the surge of androgenic activity.

It appears increasingly probable that any difference discovered will be found to be in the amount of halothane metabolized and the pathway involved. The simplest metabolic route, producing trifluoroacetic acid, bromide, and chloride and requiring the least complicated enzymatic participation, is thought to be the normal route during childhood, while alternate routes, producing more irritant metabolites, are believed to be followed only because of injury or depression of hepatic cells.

The last 10 years have seen little change in the uncertainties of "halothane hepatitis." However, a more definite case has been established to show the danger of toxicity arising from chronic exposure of operating room personnel to spillage of waste nitrous oxide and halothane (Bruce, 1973; Cohen and others, 1971; Sawyer and others, 1971). Because of the popular use of T-systems for infants and small children, this hazard tends to be magnified in the pediatric age group. Efforts to overcome this depend on economy in the use of agents and more efficient scavenging of excess gases (see Chapter 6).

Current view of halothane for children. At the present time, the belief that children are more tolerant than adults to halothane is widespread but not universal. Benson (1975) has informally stated that halothane is safe for anyone under 15 years old, while Richards (1976) has formulated a more conservative policy, and Melman (1976) has imposed the same restrictions as those used on adults. Theories followed at our hospital are briefly summarized as follows:

The danger of halothane hepatitis in prepubertal children is slight but cannot be completely disregarded.

Young children may receive halothane without limit as to total number of exposures or the interval between exposures. (Solosko and associates [1972] and several others have reported children who have received halothane over 100 times. The fact that most of these exposures were relatively brief probably reduced their hazard.)

Postoperative fever is not a contraindication to subsequent halothane unless associated with other symptoms such as abdominal pain, jaundice, eosinophilia, or elevated enzyme levels.

The presence of cholestatic jaundice, as in biliary atresia, does not contraindicate halothane anesthesia in infants. However, to use halothane in any case where liver dysfunction is present or probable tends to invite unwarranted litigation.

Following the onset of puberty, young people respond to halothane as do adults and should be subject to the restrictions applied to adults.

Although halothane is excellent for approximately 90% of pediatric procedures, the following situations would suggest alternative agents.

Relative contraindications

1. For induction of a child with an infusion running on arrival in the operating room.
2. For induction of a child who voices preference for intravenous or other methods over mask induction.
3. Situations requiring extreme degrees of relaxation (e.g., excision of large abdominal tumor).
4. Facial deformities, burns, and other obstacles to the use of an anesthesia mask.
5. Extremely poor-risk cardiac patients with cardiac enlargement.
6. History of numerous operations, the presence of severe trauma or debilitating disease, or the probability of encountering massive blood loss or generalized infection that might alter hepatic function.
7. Exceptionally small premature infants, who require only supportive care plus local infiltration or incision.
8. The occasional outpatient with a full stomach or recent coma and other candidates for local or regional anesthesia.
9. Patients who show unexpected hypotension or dangerous arrhythmias during anesthesia.
10. Operations of more than 4 hours' duration for which nonhalogenated agents could serve as well.

Definite contraindications

1. History of liver failure.
2. History of hyperthermic reaction of patient or relative during previous anesthesia.

Methoxyflurane ($C_3H_4OCl_2F_2$)

Methoxyflurane (Penthrane), a halogenated ether, was introduced by Artusio and Van Poznak (1960) after clinical trials had shown it to cause less cardiac irritability than teflurane and halopropane and to offer more relaxation than halothane. Because methoxyflurane is characterized by low vapor pressure and high blood solubility (Table 5-1), users immediately encountered prolonged induction and recovery time, which they learned to overcome by employing intravenous induction agents and/or special vaporizers (Pentec) and by discontinuing administration well before the end of the operation. With high concentration, muscle relaxation is good and respiration less depressed than with halothane, making it especially popular for bronchography.

In 1964 Davenport and Quan recommended methoxyflurane for children, and Topkins (1967) and Volpitto (1968) also advocated it for pediatric plastic and bronchoscopic work.

Disadvantages of the agent, in addition to the unpleasant smell and difficulties of administration, first appeared in marked skin pallor (Dobkin and others, 1966), which had been interpreted by Hudon (1961) as being due to peripheral vasoconstriction in compensation for cardiac depression. Our own early use of the drug was marked by prolonged recovery and excessive nausea and vomiting, possibly related to use in high dosages without endotracheal intubation (Lewis and Smith, 1965). Hart and associates (1964) stated that because of delayed awakening, methoxyflurane was contraindicated in cardiac surgery in children.

In 1964 Paddock and associates reported renal impairment following methoxyflurane anesthesia. Subsequently, the fatalities reported by Crandell and associates (1966), Pezzi and associates (1966), Panner and associates (1970), and others involving high-output urinary failure, hypernatremia, elevated blood urea nitrogen level, and renal oxalate deposition aroused great alarm. Holaday and associates (1970) described the biodegradation of methoxyflurane by microsomal liver enzymes that starts almost immediately after administration is begun and may continue for 9 to 12 days afterwards. It involves the release of inorganic fluoride, dichloroacetic acid, methoxyfluoro-acid, and oxalic acid. The renal toxicity has been related to body type, obesity, preexisting renal disease, and tetracycline therapy (Kuzucu, 1970), and age has not appeared to be a protective factor.

The repeated warnings of Mazze (1973, 1976) concerning the predictable toxicity of methoxyflurane are difficult to overlook.

In defense of the drug, there is good evidence that renal damage is definitely associated with depth of anesthesia or with concentration and duration of serum drug levels. Dobkin and Levy (1973) showed release of inorganic fluoride ion to be within safe levels under light anesthesia, and Lowe and Hagler (1971) have developed a highly systematized method that predetermines methoxyflurane dosage by MAC, body weight, and expected duration of the operation. Using this approach, they believe toxic renal complications can be avoided.

Although opinion remains divided, the potential for serious problems, the complicated methods required to avoid them, and the lack of definite clinical advantages seem to leave few, if any, indications for the use of methoxyflurane in pediatric anesthesia.

Enflurane ($C_3H_2OClF_5$) and isoflurane

Enflurane (Ethrane) and isoflurane (Forane) are two fluorinated anesthetic agents that were discovered by Terrell in 1963 and 1965 in an endeavor to avoid the problem of hepatic toxicity. The first of these, enflurane, was tested for anesthetic effect in animals by Krantz in 1953 and in humans by Virtue and associates in 1966 and was released in 1972. The drug resembles methoxyflurane in its three carbon–ether molecular structure (Table 5-1), but the placement of halogen ions suggests greater stability, and its biodegradation is only 2.6% as compared with 25% in halothane (Cascorbi and others, 1970).

In clinical use, enflurane is basically similar to halothane, but with an MAC of 1.3, higher concentrations are required, induction concentration approaching 5% and maintenance concentration of 2% to 3%. The odor is sweet, but the agent causes somewhat more respiratory irritation (Dobkin and Byles, 1969; Horne and Ahlgren, 1973) and increased postoperative nausea.

With enflurane, greater muscular relaxation is achieved without respiratory depression (Linde and others, 1970), and myocardial depression is said to be less than that caused by halothane, but the difference does not appear to be clinically significant (Shimosato and others, 1969). One disadvantage of enflurane is the appearance of epileptiform seizure activity at moderate depth that is clinically manifested at deeper levels (Julien and others, 1972; Rosen and Soderberg, 1975). The tendency is increased by hyperventilation and hypocarbia and after discontinuation of the drug. Although postictal complications have not been reported, this defect reduces the probability of lasting popularity of the agent if confronted by a less fitful competitor.

The second fluorinated agent discovered by Terrell, isoflurane, is an isomer of enflurane and thus a saturated ether (Table 5-1). From the outset, its structural arrangement promised great resistance to metabolic breakdown and consequently maximal freedom from hepatorenal toxicity. This has been confirmed by several investigators, who have found halothane and methoxyflurane to undergo considerable biodegradation, enflurane little, and isoflurane least of all (Halsey and others, 1971; Byles and others, 1971).

Initially it appeared that isoflurane was nonflammable, stable, potent, and free from any damaging side effects. Shortly before expected release of the drug, evidence of possible carcinogenic properties was reported (Corbett and others, 1973). Approval of the drug was delayed, and intensive study was undertaken to determine the extent of the danger involved. Investigation of the clinical properties and metabolic processes of isoflurane continue to reveal information that should be of considerable value after official clearance of the agent.

Isoflurane is prepared as a colorless liquid, requires no stabilizing agent, and may be stored in clear glass bottles. Its odor is considerably more pungent than that of halothane and may cause airway irritation and coughing on induction.

Since the blood/gas solubility coefficient of isoflurane is lower than that of halothane, more rapid induction and excretion would be expected were it not for the irritant effect. Excretion and recovery follow predicted faster rates.

MAC for isoflurane in adults is 1.38, that for children 1.5, and that for neonates 1.7; thus, it is rated as having half the potency of halothane in spite of the fact that it produces greater relaxation at anesthetic concentration.

Greater repiratory depression occurs with isoflurane than with any commonly used inhalation anesthetic (Fourcade and others, 1971).

With increasing depth of anesthesia, isoflurane shows no increase in respiratory rate to compensate for reduced tidal volume. The resultant rise in Pa_{CO_2}, decrease in inspiratory/expiratory ratio (I/E), and decrease in response to CO_2 make controlled ventilation mandatory.

Isoflurane has a direct negative inotropic effect on myocardium and causes marked reduction of peripheral resistance. It is considered to have a less depressant effect than halothane on the cardiovascular system, however, since cardiac output is more adequately sustained during hypotension by compensatory increase in heart rate. In normal adults, both drugs cause reduction in blood pressure with increasing depth of agent when used without supplementation, the hypotension with halothane being greater.

With prolonged use, isoflurane does not produce the cardiovascular stimulation seen with halothane and other agents. Stevens and associates (1973) showed that after 5 hours halothane causes increasing cardiac output, stroke volume, heart rate, oxygen consumption, and cardiac index and decreasing total peripheral resistance and right atrial pressure, none of which are seen with isoflurane. They consider this an advantage of isoflurane in that changes due to hypovolemia or other clinical abnormalities would be more easily recognized.

In the management of poor-risk patients, Kemmotsu and associates (1973) showed that in the presence of congestive heart failure, isoflurane has a significantly greater negative inotropic effect than halothane, and thus the advantage held by isoflurane in normal patients would be lost in those at increased risk.

Of less importance is the effect of increased peripheral flow on temperature control, the increased heat loss working toward the advantage or disadvantage of individual patients.

As previously noted, isoflurane has a con-

Table 5-2. Comparison of halothane, enflurane, and isoflurane in children

	Halothane (%)	Enflurane (%)	Isoflurane (%)
Induction excitement—minimal	19	46	37
Induction excitement—moderate	6	11	16
Induction excitement—severe	0	3	0
Induction breath-holding	7	10	16
Induction cough	5	16	27
Induction hiccough	1	8	0
Induction laryngospasm	1	5	12
Clonic movement	0	4	0
Recovery delirium	8	37	19
Recovery nausea	5	5	6
Recovery vomiting	5	3	4

From Horne, J., and Ahlgren, E. W.: Halothane, enflurane, and isoflurane for outpatient surgery; a pediatric case series, presented before American Society of Anesthesiologists, San Francisco, October 1973.

siderable advantage over halothane in relation to myocardial sensitization by epinephrine (Joas and Stevens, 1971). With deeper anesthesia the advantage is increased, since sensitivity under isoflurane decreases, while that under halothane remains practically the same.

It is obviously important as well as interesting that isoflurane shows no clinical or electroencephalographic evidence of the seizure activity noted in its isomer enflurane (Clark and others, 1973).

The fact that isoflurane causes three times more potentiation of d-tubocurarine than does halothane is definitely important and could easily cause complications.

The report of Horne and Ahlgren (1973) comparing the use of halothane, enflurane, and isoflurane is most interesting. As shown in Table 5-2, the incidence of side effects with enflurane and isoflurane is appreciable and includes a variety of respiratory, neuromuscular, emotional, and gastrointestinal complications. These findings appear to be representative of the experience of others and promise little to those who change from halothane to the newer agents.

BIBLIOGRAPHY

Abajian, J., Jr., Brazell, E. H., Dente, G. A., and Mills, E. L.: Experience with halothane (Fluothane) in more than five thousand cases, J.A.M.A. **171:**535, 1959.

Artusio, J. F., and Van Poznak, A.: Clinical evaluation of methoxyflurane in man, Fed. Proc. **19:**273, 1960.

Artusio, J. F., Van Poznak, A., Hunt, R. E., and others: A clinical evaluation in man, Anesthesiology **21:**512, 1960.

Barash, P. G., Glanz, S., Katz, J. D., and others: Ventricular function in children during halothane anesthesia; an echocardiographic evaluation, Anesthesiology **49:**79, 1978.

Benson, D. W.: Personal communication, 1975.

Berger, P. E., Culham, J. A. G., Fitz, C. R., and Harwood-Nash, D. C.: Slowing of hepatic blood flow by halothane; angiographic manifestations, Radiology **118:**303, 1975.

Berman, M. C., Harrison, G. G., Bull, A. B., and Kench, J. E.: Changes underlying halothane-induced malignant hyperpyrexia in Landrace pigs, Nature **225:**653, 1970.

Bertram, H.: Halothane in pediatric anesthesia, Zentralbl. Chir. **87:**291, 1962.

Britt, B. A., Endrenyi, L., Cadman, D. L., and others: Porcine malignant hyperthermia; effects of halothane on mitochondrial respiration and calcium accumulation, Anesthesiology **42:**292, 1976.

Brody, G. L., and Sweet, R. B.: Halothane anesthesia as a possible cause of massive hepatic necrosis, Anesthesiology **24:**29, 1963.

Brown, B. R., Jr.: Enzymatic activity and biotransformation of anesthetics, Int. Anesthesiol. Clin. **12:**25, 1974.

Bruce, D. L.: Acute and chronic anaesthetic action on leukocytes, Can. Anaesth. Soc. J. **20:**55, 1973.

Bull, A. B., Du Plessis, C. G. G., and Pretorius, J. A.: Fluothane anaesthesia in infants and children, S. Afr. Med. J. **32:**130, 1958.

Bunker, J. B., and Blumenfeld, C. M.: Liver necrosis after halothane anesthesia; cause or coincidence? N. Engl. J. Med. **268:**531, 1963.

Byles, P. H., Dobkin, A. B., Ferguson, J. H., and Levy, A. A.: Forane (compound 469); crossover comparison with enflurane (Ethrane), halothane and methoxyflurane in dogs, Can. Anaesth. Soc. J. **18:**376, 1971.

Carney, F. M. T., and Van Dyke, R.: Halothane hepatitis; a critical review, Anesth. Analg. (Cleve.) **51**:135, 1972.

Cascorbi, H. F.: Factors causing differences in halothane biotransformation, Int. Anesthesiol. Clin. **12**: 63, 1974.

Cascorbi, H. F., Blake, D. A., and Helrich, M.: Differences in the biotransformation of halothane in man, Anesthesiology **32**:119, 1970.

Chambers, J. S. W., Sewell, P. F. J., and Young, H. B.: Jaundice after halothane and radiotherapy, Br. Med. J. **1**:562, 1964.

Chase, R. E.: Biotransformation of Ethrane in man, Anesthesiology **35**:262, 1971.

Clark, D. L., Hosick, E. C., Adams, N., and others: Neural effects of isoflurane (Forane) in man, Anesthesiology **39**:261, 1973.

Cohen, E. N.: Editorial views; anesthetics and cancer, Anesthesiology **44**:459, 1976.

Cohen, E. N., Bellville, J. W., and Brown, B. W.: Anesthesia, miscarriage and pregnancy; a study of operating room nurses and anesthetists, Anesthesiology **35**: 343, 1971.

Cohen, E. N., and Hood, N.: Application of low-temperature autoradiography to studies of the uptake and metabolism of volatile anesthetics in the mouse, Anesthesiology **30**:306, 1969.

Cohen, E. N., Trudell, J. R., Edmunds, H. N., and Watson, E.: Urinary metabolites of halothane in man, Anesthesiology **43**:392, 1975.

Cohen, R. D., and Simpson, R.: Lactate metabolism, Anesthesiology **43**:661, 1975.

Corbett, T. H., Cornell, R. G., Leiding, K., and others: Incidence of cancer among Michigan nurse anesthetists, Anesthesiology **38**:260, 1973.

Crandell, W. B., Pappas, S. G., and MacDonald, A.: Nephrotoxicity associated with methoxyflurane anesthesia, Anesthesiology **27**:591, 1966.

Davenport, H. T., and Quan, P.: Methoxyflurane anesthesia in pediatrics; a clinical report, Can. Med. Assoc. J. **91**:1291, 1964.

Dobkin, A. B., and Byles, P. H.: New inhalation anesthetics, Clin. Anesth. **3**:295, 1969.

Dobkin, A. B., Byles, P. H., and Neville, J. F., Jr.: Neuroendocrine and metabolic effects of general anesthesia with graded hemorrhage, Can. Anaesth. Soc. J. **13**:453, 1966.

Dobkin, A. B., and Levy, A. A.: Blood serum fluoride levels with methoxyflurane anaesthesia, Can. Anaesth. Soc. J. **20**:81, 1973.

Duncan, W. A. M., and Raventos, J.: The pharmacokinetics of halothane (Fluothane) anesthesia, Br. J. Anaesth. **31**:302, 1959.

Dykes, M. H. M.: Additional possible contributing factors, Int. Anesthesiol. Clin. **8**:407, 1970.

Dykes, M. H. M.: Anesthesia and the liver; history and epidemiology, Can. Anaesth. Soc. J. **20**:34, 1973.

Eastwood, D. W., Green, C. D., Lambdin, M. A., and Gardner, R.: Effect of nitrous oxide on the white-cell count in leukemia, N. Engl. J. Med. **268**:297, 1963.

Eger, E. I. II: Anesthetic uptake and action, Baltimore, 1974, The Williams & Wilkins Co.

Eger, E. I. II, and Saidman, L. J.: Hazards of nitrous oxide anesthesia in bowel obstruction and pneumothorax, Anesthesiology **26**:61, 1965.

Eger, E. I. II, Smith, N. T., Cullen, D. J., and others: A comparison of cardiovascular effects of halothane, fluroxene, ether and cyclopropane in man; a resumé, Anesthesiology **34**:25, 1971.

Eger, E. I. II, Smith, N. T., Stoelting, R. K., and others: Cardiovascular effects of halothane in man, Anesthesiology **32**:396, 1970.

Fink, B. R., and Cullen, B. F.: Anesthetic pollution; what is happening to us? Anesthesiology **45**:79, 1976.

Fourcade, H. E., Stevens, W. C., Larson, C. P., and others: The ventilatory effects of Forane, a new inhaled anesthetic, Anesthesiology **35**:26, 1971.

Gion, H., and Saidman, L. J.: The minimum alveolar concentration of enflurane in man, Anesthesiology **35**: 361, 1971.

Goldberg, A. H.: Effects of halothane on force-velocity, length-tension, and stress-strain curves of isolated heart muscle, Anesthesiology **29**:192, 1968.

Goldberg, A. H., and Phear, W. P. C.: Alterations in mechanical properties of heart muscle produced by halothane, J. Pharmacol. Exp. Ther. **162**:101, 1968.

Graff, T. D., Sewall, K., Lim, T. S., and others: Acid-base balance in infants during halothane anesthesia with use of an adult circle absorption system, Anesth. Analg. (Cleve.) **43**:583, 1964.

Greene, N. M.: Editorial views; familiarity as a basis for the practice of anesthesiology, Anesthesiology **44**:101, 1976.

Gregory, G. A., Eger, E. I. II, and Munson, E. W.: The relationship between age and halothane requirement in man, Anesthesiology **30**:488, 1969.

Gronert, G. A., and Theye, R. A.: Halothane-induced porcine malignant hyperthermia; metabolic and hemodynamic changes, Anesthesiology **44**:36, 1976.

Hackett, P. R., and Crosby, R. N.: Some effects of inadvertent hypothermia in infant neurosurgery, Anesthesiology **21**:356, 1970.

Halsey, M. J., Sawyer, D. C., Eger, E. I. II, and others: Hepatic metabolism of halothane, methoxyflurane, cyclopropane, Ethrane and Forane in miniature swine, Anesthesiology **35**:43, 1971.

Harrison, G. G., Bull, A. B., and Schmidt, H. J.: Temperature changes in children during general anesthesia, Br. J. Anaesth. **32**:60, 1960.

Harrison, G. G., and Smith, J. S.: Massive lethal hepatic necrosis in rats anesthetized with fluroxene, after microsomal enzyme induction, Anesthesiology **39**: 619, 1973.

Hart, S. M., Sloan, I. A., and Conn, A. W.: Pediatric cardiac surgery with methoxyflurane, Can. Anaesth. Soc. J. **11**:42, 1964.

Holaday, D. A., Rudofsky, S., and Treuhaft, D. S.: The metabolic degradation of methoxyflurane in man, Anesthesiology **33**:579, 1970.

Horne, J., and Ahlgren, E. W.: Halothane, enflurane,

and isoflurane for outpatient surgery; a pediatric case series, presented before American Society of Anesthesiologists, San Francisco, October 1973.

Hudon, F.: Methoxyflurane, Can. Anaesth. Soc. J. **8:** 544, 1961.

Hughes, M., and Powell, L. W.: Recurrent hepatitis in patients receiving multiple halothane anaesthetics for radium treatment of carcinoma of the cervix, Gastroenterology **58:**790, 1970.

Joas, T. A., and Stevens, W. C.: Comparison of the arrhythmic doses of epinephrine during Forane, halothane and fluroxene anesthesia in dogs, Anesthesiology **35:**48, 1971.

Johnstone, M.: Human cardiovascular response to fluothane anesthesia, Br. J. Anaesth. **28:**392, 1956.

Joseph, S. I.: Hepatic function and halothane, Anesthesiology **25:**103, 1964.

Julien, R. M., Kavan, E. M., and Elliott, H. W.: Effects of volatile anaesthetic agents on EEG activity recorded in limbic and sensory systems, Can. Anaesth. Soc. J. **19:**263, 1972.

Junkin, C. L., Smith, C., and Conn, A. W.: Fluothane for paediatric anaesthesia, Can. Anaesth. Soc. J. **4:** 259, 1957.

Karis, J. H., Menzel, D. B., Aboudonia, M. B., and Bennett, P. B.: Increase of halothane toxicity by ultraviolet irradiation, presented before American Society of Anesthesiologists, San Francisco, 1976.

Karlin, J. M., and Kutt, H.: Acute diphenylhydantoin intoxication following halothane anesthesia, J. Pediatr. **76:**941, 1970.

Katz, R. L., and Epstein, R. A.: The interactions of anesthetic agents and adrenergic drugs to produce arrhythmias, Anesthesiology **29:**763, 1968.

Kemmotsu, O., Hashimoto, Y., and Shimosato, S.: Inotropic effects of isoflurane on mechanics of contraction in isolated cat papillary muscles from normal and failing hearts, Anesthesiology **39:**470, 1973.

Klatskin, G., and Kimberg, D. V.: Recurrent hepatitis attributable to halothane sensitization in an anesthetist, N. Engl. J. Med. **280:**515, 1969.

Koka, B., Jeon, I. S., Andre, J. M., and others: Postintubation croup in children, Anesth. Analg. (Cleve.) **56:**501, 1977.

Krantz, J. C., Jr., Carr, C. J., Lu, G., and Bell, F. K.: Anesthesia; anesthetic action of trifluoroethyl vinyl ether, J. Pharmacol. Exp. Ther. **108:**488, 1953.

Kripke, B. J., Kelman, A. D., Shah, N. K., and others: Testicular reaction to prolonged exposure to nitrous oxide, Anesthesiology **44:**104, 1976.

Kuzucu, E. Y.: Methoxyflurane, tetracycline and renal failure, J.A.M.A. **211:**1162, 1970.

Leigh, M. D., and Belton, M. K.: Pediatric anesthesiology, ed. 2, New York, 1960, Macmillan, Inc.

Lewis, A. A., and Smith, R. M.: The use of methoxyflurane in children, Anesth. Analg. (Cleve.) **44:**347, 1965.

Linde, H. W., Lamb, V. E., Quimby, C. W., Jr., and others: The search for better anesthetic agents; clinical investigation of Ethrane, Anesthesiology **32:**555, 1970.

Lomaz, J. G.: Halothane and jaundice in paediatric anaesthesia, Anaesthesia **20:**70, 1965.

Lowe, H. J.: Dose-regulated Penthrane (methoxyflurane) anesthesia, North Chicago, Ill., 1972, Abbott Laboratories.

Lowe, H. J., and Hagler, K.: Clinical and laboratory evaluation of an expired anesthetic gas monitor (Narko-Test), Anesthesiology **34:**378, 1971.

Marechal, J.: Halothane in pediatric practice, Acta Anaesth. Belg. **18:**35, 1967.

Mathieu, A., and Di Padua, D.: Hypersensitivity reactions to volatile anesthetics and their metabolites, In Mathieu, A., and Kahan, B. D., editors: Immunologic aspects of anesthetic and surgical practice, New York, 1975, Grune & Stratton, Inc.

Mathieu, A., Di Padua, D., Mills, J., and others: Experimental immunity to metabolites of halothane and fluroxene, Anesthesiology **40:**385, 1974.

Mazze, R. I., and Cousins, M. J.: Renal toxicity of anaesthetics; with specific reference to the nephrotoxicity of methoxyflurane, Can. Anaesth. Soc. J. **20:** 64, 1973.

Mazze, R. I., and Hitt, B. A.: Editorial views; methoxyflurane metabolism, Anesthesiology **44:**369, 1976.

McGregor, M., Davenport, H. T., Jegier, W., and others: The cardiovascular effects of halothane in normal children, Br. J. Anaesth. **30:**398, 1958.

Melgrave, A. P.: The use of epinephrine in the presence of halothane in children, Can. Anaesth. Soc. J. **17:**256, 1970.

Melman, E.: Personal communication, 1976.

Moffitt, E. A., Tarhan, S., and McGoon, D. C.: Whole-body metabolism during and after open-heart surgery, Can. Anaesth. Soc. J. **20:**607, 1973.

Morley, T. S.: Halothane; clinical considerations, Int. Anesthesiol. Clin. **12:**72, 1974.

Nicodemus, H. F., Nassiri-Rahimi, C., Bachman, L., and Smith, T. C.: Median effective doses (ED_{50}) of halothane in adults and children, Anesthesiology **31:** 347, 1969.

Paddock, R. B., Parker, J. W., and Guadagni, N. P.: The effects of methoxyflurane on renal function, Anesthesiology **25:**707, 1964.

Panner, B. J., Freeman, R. B., Roth-Mayo, L. A., and others: Toxicity following methoxyflurane anesthesia, J.A.M.A. **214:**86, 1970.

Paronetto, F., and Popper, H.: Lymphocyte stimulation induced by halothane in patients with hepatitis following exposure to halothane, N. Engl. J. Med. **283:**277, 1970.

Pezzi, P. J., Frobese, A. S., and Greenberg, S. R.: Methoxyflurane and renal toxicity, Lancet **1:**823, 1966.

Podlesch, I., Dudziak, R., and Zinganell, K.: Inspiratory and expiratory carbon dioxide concentrations during halothane anesthesia in infants, Anesthesiology **27:** 823, 1966.

Popper, H.: Symposium on toxic hepatic injury, Gastroenterology **38:**786, 1960.

Price, H. L., Cooperman, L. H., Warden, J. C., and

125

others: Pulmonary hemodynamics during general anesthesia in man, Anesthesiology **30:**629, 1969.

Raventos, J.: Action of Fluothane; a new volatile anesthetic, Br. J. Pharmacol. **11:**394, 1956.

Rehder, K., Forbes, J., Alter, H., and others: Halothane biotransformation in man; a quantitative study, Anesthesiology **28:**711, 1967.

Rehder, K., and Sessler, A. D.: Biotransformation of halothane, Int. Anesthesiol. Clin. **12:**41, 1974.

Reynolds, E. S., Brown, B. R., Jr., and Vandam, L. D.: Massive hepatic necrosis after fluroxene anesthesia; a case of drug interaction? N. Engl. J. Med. **286:**530, 1972.

Reynolds, R. N.: Halothane in pediatric anesthesia, Int. Anesthesiol. Clin. **1:**209, 1962.

Richards, C. C.: Personal communication, 1976.

Rosen, I., and Soderberg, M.: Electroencephalographic activity in children under enflurane anesthesia, Acta Anaesth. Scand. **19:**361, 1975.

Saidman, L. J., and Eger, E. I. II: Effect of nitrous oxide and narcotic premedication on the alveolar concentration of halothane required for anesthesia, Anesthesiology **25:**302, 1964.

Salanitre, E., and Rackow, H.: Respiratory complications associated with the use of muscle relaxants in young infants, Anesthesiology **22:**194, 1961.

Sawyer, D. C., Eger, E. I. II, Bahlman, S. H., and others: Concentration dependence of hepatic halothane metabolism, Anesthesiology **34:**230, 1971.

Shapiro, H. M.: Review article; intracranial hypertension, Anesthesiology **43:**445, 1975.

Shimosato, S., Suigai, N., Iwatsuki, N., and others: The effect of Ethrane on cardiac muscle mechanics, Anesthesiology **30:**514, 1969.

Skovsted, P., Price, M. L., and Price, H. L.: The effects of halothane on arterial pressure, preganglionic sympathetic activity and barostatic reflexes, Anesthesiology **31:**507, 1969.

Smith, A. L.: The mechanism of cerebral vasodilation by halothane, Anesthesiology **39:**581, 1973.

Smith, A. L., and Wollman, H.: Cerebral blood flow and metabolism; effects of anesthetic drugs and technics, Anesthesiology **36:**378, 1972.

Smith, B. E., Gaub, M. L., and Moya, F.: Investigations into the teratogenetic effects of anesthetic agents; the fluorinated agents, Anesthesiology **26:**260, 1965.

Smith, R. M.: Anesthesia during hyperbaric oxygenation, Ann. N.Y. Acad. Sci. **117:**768, 1965.

Snow, J.: On chloroform and other anaesthetics; their action and administration, London, 1858, Churchill.

Solosko, D., Frissell, M., and Smith, R. B.: 111 halothane anesthesias in a pediatric patient; a case report, Anesth. Analg. (Cleve.) **51:**706, 1972.

Stefanini, M., Herland, A., and Kosyak, E.: Fatal massive necrosis of the liver after repeated exposure to methoxyflurane, Anesthesiology **32:**374, 1970.

Stephen, C. R., Ahlgren, E. W., and Bennett, E. J.: Elements of pediatric anesthesia, Springfield, Ill., 1970, Charles C Thomas, Publisher.

Stephen, C. R., Grosskreutz, D. C., Lawrence, J. H. A., and others: Evaluation of Fluothane for clinical anaesthesia, Can. Anesth. Soc. J. **4:**246, 1957.

Stevens, W. C., Eger, E. I. II, Joas, T. A., and others: Comparative toxicity of isoflurane, halothane, fluroxene, and diethyl ether in human volunteers, Can. Anaesth. Soc. J. **20:**357, 1973.

Stier, A.: Zur frage der stabilitat von halothan (2brom-2-chlor-1,1,1-tri-fluorathan) im stoffwechsel, Naturwissenschaften **51:**65, 1964.

Stoelting, R. K.: Halothane anesthesia following methoxyflurane-induced nephrotoxicity, Anesthesiology **33:**464, 1970.

Strobel, G. E.: Treatment of anesthetic-induced malignant hyperpyrexia, Lancet **1:**40, 1971.

Strunin, L., and Simpson, B. R.: Halothane in Britain today, Br. J. Anaesth. **44:**919, 1972.

Suckling, C. W.: Some chemical and physical factors in the development of Fluothane, Br. J. Anaesth. **29:**466, 1957.

Taylor, C., and Stoelting, V. K.: Halothane anaesthesia for paediatric cardiac surgery, Can. Anaesth. Soc. J. **8:**247, 1961.

Topkins, M.: The use of methoxyflurane in plastic surgery, monograph no. 8, North Chicago, Ill., 1967, Abbott Laboratories.

Trey, C., Davidson, C. S., and Lipworth, L.: The clinical syndrome of halothane hepatitis, Anesth. Analg. (Cleve.) **48:**814, 1969.

Tucker, W. K., Munson, E. S., Holaday, D. A., and others: Hepatorenal toxicity following fluroxene anesthesia, Anesthesiology **39:**104, 1973.

Uehelke, H., Hellmer, K. H., and Taberelli-Poplawski, S.: Metabolic activation of halothane and its covalent binding to liver endoplasmic proteins in vitro, Arch. Pharmacol. **279:**39, 1973.

Van Dyke, R. A., Chenoweth, M. B., and Van Poznak, A.: Metabolism of volatile anesthetics. I. Conversion in vivo of several anesthetics to $^{14}CO_2$ and chloride, Biochem. Pharmacol. **13:**1239, 1965.

Van Dyke, R. A., and Wood, C. L.: Metabolism of methoxyflurane; release of inorganic fluoride in human and rat hepatic enzymes, Anesthesiology **39:**613, 1973.

Virtue, R. W., Lund, L. O., Phelps, M., Jr., and others: Difluoromethyl 1,1,2-trifluoro-2-chlorethyl ether as an anesthetic agent; results with dogs and a preliminary note on observations with man, Can. Anaesth. Soc. J. **13:**233, 1966.

Virtue, R. W., and Payne, K. W.: Postoperative death after Fluothane, Anesthesiology **19:**562, 1958.

Vitcha, J. F.: A history of Forane, Anesthesiology **35:**4, 1971.

Volpitto, P. P.: Methoxyflurane anesthesia for bronchography in infants and children, monograph no. 14, North Chicago, Ill., 1968, Abbott Laboratories.

Walton, B., Hamblin, A., Dumonde, D. C., and Simpson, R.: Absence of cellular hypersensitivity in patients with unexplained hepatitis following halothane, Anesthesiology **44:**391, 1976.

Whitcher, C. E., Cohen, E. N., and Trudell, J. R.: Chronic exposure to anesthetic gases in the operating room, Anesthesiology 35:348, 1971.

Widger, L. A., Grandolfi, A. J., and Van Dyke, R. A.: Hypoxia and halothane metabolism in vivo; release of inorganic fluoride and halothane metabolite binding to cellular constituents, Anesthesiology 44:197, 1976.

Wilson, L. A., and Harrison, G. A.: Pulmonary ventilation in children during halothane anesthesia, Anesthesiology 25:613, 1964.

Woodbridge, P. D.: Changing concepts concerning depth of anesthesia, Anesthesiology 19:536, 1957.

CHAPTER 6

Design and function of pediatric anesthesia systems

Unassisted ventilation: open systems
Assisted and controlled ventilation
Humidification
Scavenging systems
Summary

A great deal of effort has been expended in the development and analysis of pediatric breathing systems and has left us with a confusion of theories, papers, and discarded equipment. It may be helpful to retrace some of the steps that led to this situation.

UNASSISTED VENTILATION: OPEN SYSTEMS

Prior to 1930, diethyl ether was the standard pediatric anesthetic, with occasional recourse to chloroform, ethyl chloride, and divinyl ether. All of these agents could be dropped onto a gauze-covered mask, poured into a towel-wrapped "cone," or vaporized with the aid of an electric pump and blown into the patient's mouth or pharynx by a metal "ether hook" or other device. Surgery was comparatively simple, ventilation was spontaneous, and unassisted respiratory technics usually were sufficient.

This approach was believed to be adequate. Anesthetic deaths occurred, however, primarily due to overdosage, aspiration of vomitus, or hyperpyrexia.

Advantages that can still make open administration of ether practical in exotic situations are the simplicity of the equipment required and the degree of analgesia and relaxation that can be provided without cardiorespiratory depression.

Several factors limit the use of open-drop ether. Because of a vapor pressure of 442 mm Hg and a boiling point of 34.6° C, its volatility is markedly reduced in a humid environment or when the liquid ether is cooled. Thus, with rapid administration a gauze-covered mask may become both saturated and cold, markedly reducing vaporization of ether and at the same time contributing to heat loss in the child. Covering the mask to achieve greater anesthetic concentration obviously increases rebreathing. To correct this, metal nipples have been placed on masks to facilitate addition of oxygen.

Obvious disadvantages of open methods include the dead space under the mask or cone, the gross inaccuracy of control, and the danger of irritating skin or eyes by contact with raw ether or saturated masks. The danger of fatal explosion was not great when ether was used freely in room air. Cautery, x-ray, electric vaporizer (or in one case the anesthetist's cigar) might cause a loud pop or brief flame, but these events seldom did any harm.

Following the introduction of absorption technics, ignition of ether in enclosed systems with high concentrations of oxygen caused much more destructive explosions and consequently brought more stringent regulations.

The greatest disadvantage of open technics, the inability to assist respiration, became evident with the introduction of anesthetic agents that did not support respiration and with the pediatric surgeon's entry into the chest.

ASSISTED AND CONTROLLED VENTILATION

The common factor of all current pediatric breathing systems is some method of assisting or controlling respiration. The numerous variations that have been developed fall into two basic categories of CO_2 control. One is structured on the use of CO_2 absorption and includes both to-and-fro and circle absorption systems. The other technic is based on controlling CO_2 either by nonrebreathing valves that eliminate all expired air or by accurately matching the flow of fresh gases with the volume of expired air. Obviously the latter includes all of the variations on the Ayre system. A general comparison can be made between the advantages of the two basic technics:

Absorption systems	Nonrebreathing systems
1. Conserve heat 2. Retain moisture 3. Reduce pollution 4. Save anesthetic agents 5. Reduce explosive hazard	1. More accurate control of anesthetic concentrations 2. More mobile 3. Apparatus simpler, less expensive 4. Valves may be eliminated 5. Easily cleaned 6. No carbon dioxide absorption needed 7. Lightweight

Absorption systems are definitely *safer for administration of explosive agents* and *more economical*. Their retention of respiratory moisture is usually a desirable feature. The retention of body warmth is advantageous in infants but can be dangerous in older children. The evidence that exposure to anesthetic agents can be harmful to operating room personnel (Cohen and others, 1971) is an added point in favor of absorption technics.

The original aim of nonrebreathing systems was to provide a *simple, lightweight, mobile* technic that could easily be adapted to small patients in a variety of positions. This has been achieved to a great extent. The

large canisters and heavy breathing tubes have been effectively eliminated. As will be seen, however, continuing modification of the technic has resulted in loss of the original simplicity. The principal remaining advantage of nonrebreathing systems, and a most important one, is *accuracy of control of anesthetic concentration*. This has become of increasing value as more potent agents have been introduced.

Although use of nonrebreathing technic results in greater expenditure for anesthetic consumed, the apparatus itself is considerably cheaper than those designed for closed systems and carbon dioxide absorption technics.

Carbon dioxide absorption

To-and-fro systems. The advantage of cyclopropane for neonatal surgery led to the use of miniaturized to-and-fro apparatus in the early 1930s. Abdominal procedures, then tracheoesophageal fistula repair, and the first cardiac procedure (ligation of patent ductus arteriosus by Gross in 1938) were performed under to-and-fro cyclopropane using mask and headstrap (Lank, 1953). The design of the to-and-fro apparatus was similar to that introduced by Waters in 1924 (see Waters and Mapleson, 1961) in which the avoidance of valves and passage of expired gases through the absorber on both expiration and inspiration were considered important assets.

Cannisters of 90-, 120-, and 250-ml capacity were initially made of metal but subsequently of Plexiglas. Breathing bags of 150, 250, 350, and 500 ml were fitted to one end of the canister, and wide-bore, curved adapters holding from 10 to 20 ml of dead space were interposed between canister and mask or endotracheal tube (Fig. 6-1). An airtight system was achieved by mask with headstrap or by endotracheal tube; cyclopropane or ether could be used at economic flows with nitrous oxide and oxygen, and ventilatory assistance or control could be provided. Excellent and even excessive heat retention occurred, the canister often becoming considerably overheated when used with larger

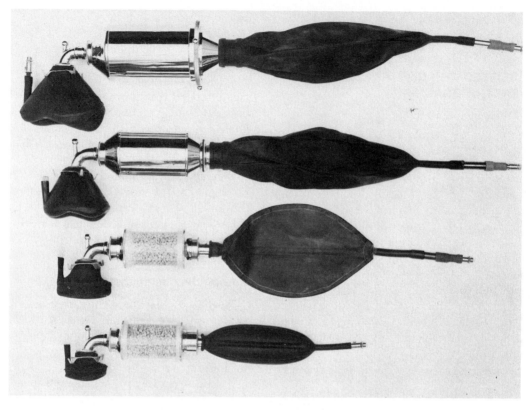

Fig. 6-1. To-and-fro carbon dioxide absorption apparatus.

children. Moisture was conserved, and the explosive hazard of escaping dry gas was reduced, but not eliminated, as evidenced by several explosions (including two of our own). Three chief disadvantages of this system led to its demise: (1) dead space was excessive at the start of each use and increased with exhaustion of soda lime, (2) the apparatus was clumsy and difficult to handle, and (3) the soda lime crumbled, and powder was blown into the patient's face and airway.

Circle absorption systems. Circle absorption systems were first used in 1887, and modifications have been appearing ever since, many of them for pediatric use. In the adaptation of the circle system to small patients, it was originally assumed that all components of the apparatus should be reduced in proportion to the patient's size in order to prevent dead space and resistance. Numer-

ous attempts to achieve a satisfactory combination were made without complete success. Among the last to appear were the Ohio and Bloomquist models. Both offered advantages provided by to-and-fro apparatus, i.e., provision of ventilatory assistance, economy of gas, and heat and moisture conservation. In addition, dead space was reduced, and inhalation of soda lime dust was eliminated. However, all infant circle systems have involved a considerable nuisance factor in requiring complete change-over from adult systems and have been even more difficult to maneuver than to-and-fro systems. Of greater importance, the addition of valves was a disadvantage. The assumption that smaller valves would cause less resistance proved to be in error.

As shown in the formula

$$R = \frac{4 \times W}{d^2}$$

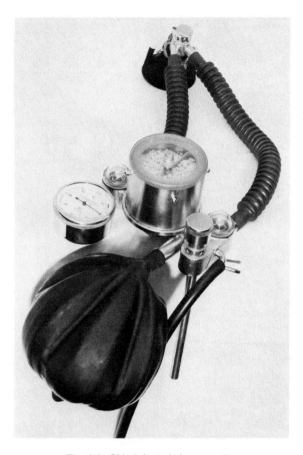

Fig. 6-2. Ohio infant circle apparatus.

where W is the weight of the valve and d the diameter, resistance is inversely proportional to diameter of the valve (Hunt, 1955). The smaller valve did not reduce resistance but with a small amount of moisture became considerably more resistant than the larger valves.

The Ohio infant circle system (Fig. 6-2) consists of a 250-ml upright cylindrical canister held by a support that can be mounted on the side of the operating table. Two corrugated rubber breathing tubes (2 cm internal diameter and 26 cm long) are joined by a light metal Y piece. The dead space, usually 4 cm in such Y pieces, is reduced by a dividing segment that extends to the rim of the fitting. Horizontally placed valves, 2.5 cm in diameter and fixed to the stand, and a 500-ml bag complete the apparatus. In use, its

adaptability is seriously limited by its required fixation to the operating table and the shortened breathing tubes.

The infant circle apparatus devised by Bloomquist (1957) is swung on a mobile supporting arm that is attached to the anesthesia machine (Fig. 6-3). It consists of a 350-ml plastic canister set vertically into a 5 × 5 inch baseplate, with two corrugated breathing tubes originally joined by a Sierra valve. This device, with two rubber valves 2 cm in diameter positioned close to the child's face, contains an appreciable amount of dead space, and the original valves used became wet and resistant frequently. A later modification of this apparatus replaced the Sierra valve with two horizontally seated valves set into the baseplate, with greatly improved action. The 500-ml breathing bag is similar

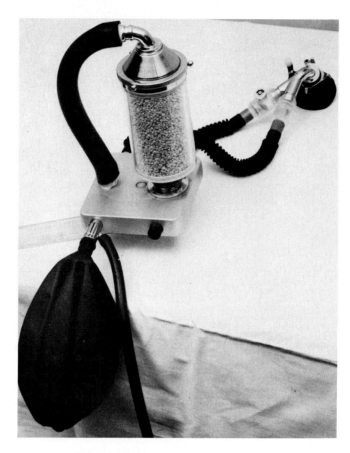

Fig. 6-3. Bloomquist infant circle apparatus.

to that of the Ohio circle. In both systems, the fitting of the bag to the rest of the apparatus is poorly arranged.

Modifications of adult circle absorption system. Several attempts have been made to adapt circle technics to infants and children. Adriani and Griggs (1953) incorporated a rubber squeeze bulb into the circle system that was intended to help circulate gases in the system. Revell (1959) and Roffey and associates (1961) introduced a small turbine pump powered by suction or oxygen to create a constant flow of gases and eliminate both dead space and resistance (Fig. 6-4).

Neff and associates (1968), with a similar goal in view, designed a double-barrelled Venturi injection system that they inserted in the inspiratory limb of the circle absorber.

These modifications were designed to overcome resistance, dead space, and work

and even to enable one to remove the valves from the circle apparatus. Clinical trial and analysis have thrown some doubt on the value of the adaptations. Each of the devices involves some additional expense, preparation, and attention. Furthermore, unless the system is airtight, any of these circulating devices will blow anesthetic gases out of the system and entrain room air, thereby greatly diluting the anesthetic. Thus, induction is best started with regular valves in place and use of the circulating devices withheld until the system can be closed effectively. In their study of the Neff circulator, Jones and Prosser (1973) found that resistance and work of breathing were reduced but improved ventilation did not occur, probably because of CO_2 washout.

Considerable misspent energy can be attributed to the ingrained assumption that

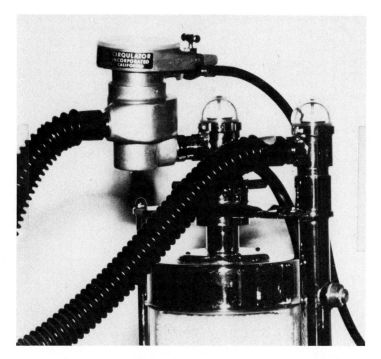

Fig. 6-4. Revell circulator.

smaller patients need smaller breathing apparatus. Graff and associates (1964) brought many traditional misconceptions to light by measuring the ventilatory response of infants to adult circle apparatus. They showed that under light endotracheal halothane–nitrous oxide anesthesia, infants tolerate adult circle apparatus as well as the Ayre T-piece system. Breathing spontaneously, infants are able to overcome the resistance and dead space of either apparatus by expenditure of additional work for an appreciable time without showing hypercarbia or respiratory acidosis. Under deeper anesthesia this response becomes depressed.

Convictions about the superiority of different types of pediatric apparatus have largely dissolved with the abandonment of spontaneous respiration once possible with ether. The advisability of assisted or controlled respiration is generally accepted and has been documented by Reynolds (1966), Podlesch and associates (1966), Freeman and associates (1964), and others.

A most valuable modification of the adult circle system has been the elimination of the heavy rubber breathing tubes and masks and the metal Y-adapters. The substitution of lightweight plastic breathing tubes and masks has reduced the bulk and drag of the equipment greatly (Fig. 6-5). Plastic Y-adapters with a central dividing septum to reduce dead space have produced further refinement.

It now appears that an adult circle system with standard canisters and valves, lighter breathing tubes, and modified Y-adapter is acceptable for all ages if used with assisted or controlled respiration.

Nonrebreathing systems

It should be noted at the outset that the term *nonrebreathing system* used in Canada and the United States and the term *rebreathing system* used in England both refer to the same type of apparatus, i.e., that by which the accumulation of CO_2 is limited by washout rather than by absorption. Since the technic, when applied to T-systems, is designed with the intention of retaining a nor-

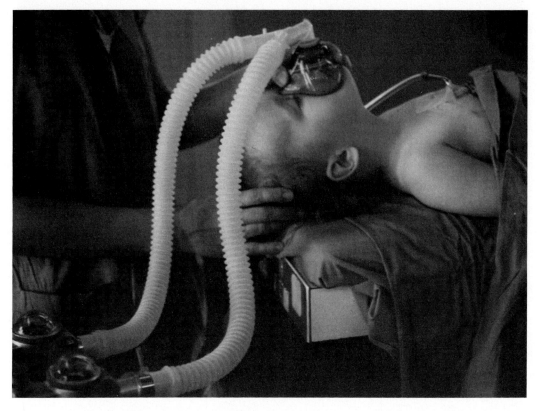

Fig. 6-5. Adult circle system with short plastic breathing tubes, adapter, and mask.

mal amount of CO_2, the British term is the more accurate. For the sake of consistency, however, the term *nonrebreathing* will be used here to include both the T-piece systems and nonrebreathing valves.

Nonrebreathing technics have been the most extensively used methods for small children during recent years. Although Ayre is justly credited with establishing the basic T-piece system for children (1937, 1937a, 1937b), the fundamental concept had been introduced, along with modern endotracheal anesthesia, by Sir Ivan Magill during World War I. His apparatus consisted of a single, long breathing tube with an expiratory valve close to the patient's face and a reservoir bag next to the anesthesia machine, often 6 feet from the patient. This was used for administration of ether to adults under spontaneous respiration, with fresh gas flow (FGF) equal to the patient's minute volume (MV). The system was effective and continued

in popular use whenever spontaneous respiration was retained. It remains one of the basic variations of the Ayre T-system today.

Ayre was fully mindful of Magill's contributions when he first described his classic T-technic. Intended for use during harelip correction and neurosurgical procedures in neonates, it was designed to eliminate airway obstruction and anoxemia, provide adjustable rebreathing, and reduce vascular congestion. Simplicity was one of Ayre's principal goals. His apparatus consisted of a metal T-piece with rubber connectors for the endotracheal tube, the inlet hose, and the expiratory limb (Fig. 6-6). Ayre specified that the internal diameter must nowhere be less than 1 cm. His diagram showed the tip of the inlet hose to be directed toward the patient, although this detail does not appear to have been a fixed item. He suggested the use of an expiratory limb, chiefly for monitoring res-

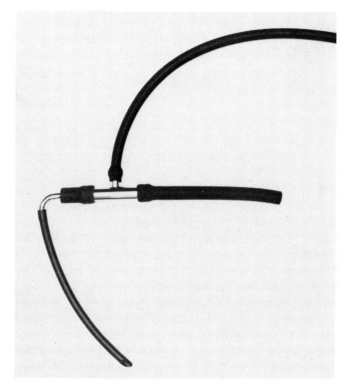

Fig. 6-6. Original Ayre T-tube nonrebreathing system.

piration when the child was covered by drapes.

The innumerable modifications and complicated evaluations of T-system technics that have appeared subsequently have made this one of the most confusing areas of pediatric anesthesia. In actuality, however, one can reduce the essential components of all T-systems to the basic T-tube with expiratory limb, as described by Ayre, followed by addition of a reservoir bag and then an expiratory valve (or valves), thus reestablishing the original Magill combination. Many other variations have appeared in the position and type of valves, the length of the rebreathing tube, and the angle of the T-tube. Each elaboration reduces the advantage of simplicity. Recent attempts to provide heat and moisture and to siphon off excess gases so compound the system that the device can become hopelessly complicated.

Several workers have analyzed the nonrebreathing method from different viewpoints. The required FGF has been extensively investigated. Magill originally calculated that since inspiration consumed one third of the respiratory cycle, an FGF of 3 MV should suffice. The algebraic confirmation of this simple logic was worked out by Onchi and associates (1947), with the aid of the following formula:

$$S_{t_1}^{t_2} \frac{\pi T}{C} \sin \frac{2\pi}{C} \, tdt - S_{t_1}^{t_2} \, adt =$$
$$T_{cos} \sin^{-1} \frac{ac}{T\pi} + \frac{ac}{\pi} \sin^{-1} \frac{ac}{T\pi} - \frac{ac}{2}$$

This is presented more for interest than for information. Their conclusion was that the FGF should be 3.14 MV (a remarkable relationship to π). Comparable figures were reached by Inkster (1956) and Harrison (1964) using models and by Nightingale and associates (1965) using clinical measurement.

Harrison (1964) assessed the effects of varying lengths of the expiratory limb and compared systems with no expiratory limb, those with an expiratory limb volume less than tidal volume, and those with an expiratory limb volume greater than tidal volume. As noted in subsequent pages, investigation following the introduction of the Bain system altered many previous concepts of required FGF and MV for maintenance of proper Pa_{O_2} and Pa_{CO_2}.

The simplest and most foolproof of all non-rebreathing systems is the T-piece without any expiratory limb. (A metal Y or even a straight metal or rubber tube with side vent [Lewis and Spoerel, 1961] may be substituted for the T.) The metal Y was used extensively for ether, where assisted respiration rarely was necessary. There is no valve, no bag, no resistance, no dead space, and an inexhaustible supply of room air. During spontaneous respiration, an FGF of 3 to 5 MV is required to prevent air dilution, but rebreathing cannot occur. Reduction of FGF simply means greater inhalation of room air. Respiration can be controlled, if necessary, by intermittent occlusion, or "thumbing," of the expiratory spout. Then there will be no air dilution, and FGF may be regulated to the patient's normal MV.

The advantage of an expiratory limb, in addition to Ayre's use for observing respiration, is that it reduces air dilution and thereby allows delivery of greater concentrations of oxygen and anesthetic. With a limb holding less than tidal volume, the FGF required to prevent air dilution varies with the volume of the tube. When the tube volume exceeds tidal volume, no air dilution is possible during spontaneous ventilation, while 2.5 or 3 MV may be required during controlled respiration to prevent dilution (in valveless systems).

The disadvantages of an expiratory tube are the possibility of rebreathing and the danger of kinking the elongated tube, with resultant distension of the lungs by oxygen at tank pressure.

The addition of a reservoir bag to T-tube and expiratory limb constitutes the *Rees modification of Ayre's technic* (Rees, 1960). The bag greatly facilitates ventilatory assistance or control and was a natural result of the changeover to a relaxant technic.

The Rees apparatus features a smooth-bore expiratory tube with a volume greater than the patient's tidal volume and a 500-ml open-end bag. Ventilation is assisted by manually closing the vent and compressing the bag. Variations on this theme have included using corrugated tubing for easier flexion, different sizes of bags, and different types of mask and endotracheal tube adapters. In the United States, the corrugated expiratory tube with the Keats elbow has been widely used and has been our preference at The Children's Hospital Medical Center (Fig. 6-7).

Rees and others continued without the addition of valves, which probably is the safest as well as the simplest method but requires FGFs of 2 to 3 MV, making it impractical for children weighing more than about 20 kg. By incorporation of a valve (to make a Mapleson A or D), the FGF may be reduced by 50% or more, enabling one to apply the nonrebreathing system to considerably larger patients without incurring excessive expense.

Valves may be of several types. A clamp partially closing the open end of the bag may serve as a valve, while Davenport (1973) has incorporated a valve into the body of the reservoir bag. Metal valves fitted to the T-piece are most commonly employed. Their position in the system is of fundamental importance.

The major variations of the Ayre system, as classified by Mapleson (1954, 1958) fall into five groups (Fig. 6-8). The patterns of gas flow in each have been nicely described by Sykes (1968). In the *Mapleson A* circuit (the original Magill system), the valve is proximal to the patient, the bag is distal, and fresh gases enter in the vicinity of the bag. With spontaneous respiration, for which the system is designed, on end-inspiration the whole circuit is filled with fresh gas, the reservoir bag deflated, and the valve closed. With beginning expiration, dead-space gas

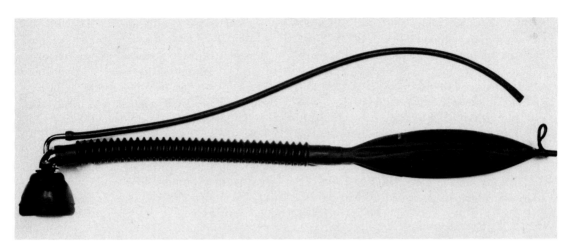

Fig. 6-7. Rees-type modification of Ayre T-system using Keats elbow adapter.

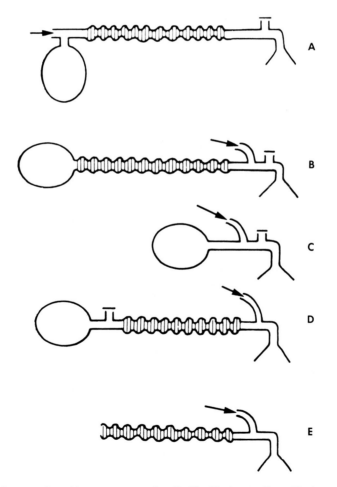

Fig. 6-8. The five nonrebreathing systems as classified by Mapleson. (From Mapleson, W. W.: Br. J. Anaesth. **20:**323, 1954.)

passes the valve, filling the reservoir limb and causing incoming FGF to refill the bag. Pressure builds up, opening the valve early in the cycle, and dumps remaining tidal air, which consists of the alveolar portion. At the end of expiration the valve is open (Fig. 6-9) and the reservoir bag and tube contain fresh gas and reusable dead-space gas but no alveolar air, which extends only as far as the valve. Thus, inspiration will start by rebreathing the alveolar air remaining between patient and valve, then the retained dead-space air, and finally FGF. Varying FGF will alter the rebreathing, but FGFs as low as 0.7 MV have been found sufficient to prevent excess CO_2 accumulation (Eger, 1974).

If controlled ventilation is used with this system (Fig. 6-9), the valve must be more resistant to prevent excess spillage on inflation. On expiration the resistant valve allows greater retention of exhaled gas in the system, and the FGF necessary to clear it out is increased to 3 MV (Norman and others, 1968; Sykes, 1968).

The *Mapleson B and C* have both FGF inlet and valves proximal to the patient, C having an expiratory limb volume less than tidal volume. The bag is a closed limb and contains mixed gases. Both types require FGFs in excess of MV to avoid rebreathing.

The *Mapleson D* system, the most widely used valved circuit, is the most efficient for

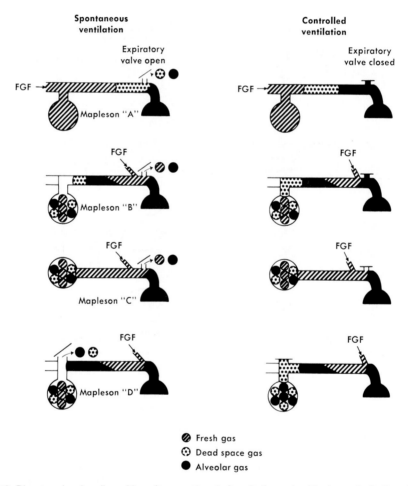

Fig. 6-9. Diagram showing disposition of gases at end of expiration using Mapleson A, B, C, and D circuits in spontaneous ventilation *(left column)* and controlled ventilation *(right column)*.

controlled respiration. The tighter valve opens only during expiration. The FGF inlet is close to the patient, the valve distant. FGF need not exceed MV provided that the expiratory tube volume equals tidal volume. In the Mapleson D during controlled respiration (Fig. 6-9), inspiration begins with inhalation of alveolar air proximal to the FGF inlet, then gas from the FGF inlet, followed by the contents of the reservoir tube and bag. The valve remains closed. Expiration begins with release of pressure on the bag, which refills with a mixture of dead space and alveolar air; then the valve opens and continuing FGF fills the tube, washing expired air toward the valve, which closes toward the end of expiration.

For intelligent use one should know this material thoroughly. For practical application, however, the simplified rules shown in Table 6-1 are suggested.

Variations on the basic T-system appear in endless succession. Early modifications consisted of Y-shaped tubes that were substituted for T-tubes, the FGF being directed toward the patient at either an obtuse or an acute angle. Onchi and associates (1947) demonstrated that resistance was greater in both of these technics than when the FGF enters the system at a right angle.

More recently, Baraka (1969) designed a system consisting of a T-piece, 60-ml expiratory tube and closed bag, and two vents, one proximal and one distal to the patient. For spontaneous ventilation, FGF is brought in through the distal opening and vented proximally, as in Mapleson A. Gases escape through unoccupied vents, which are without valves.

Carden and Nelson (1972) devised a modification of the Mapleson D that reduces the required FGF by 30%. However, they added a second length of corrugated rubber tubing and additional fixtures that detract from the ease of application.

Another arrangement of nonrebreathing apparatus was brought out by Bain and Spoerel, also in 1972. Although this was simply a revision of the standard Mapleson D circuit, it attracted a great deal of interest and stimulated a fresh outburst of investigation of nonrebreathing systems of all types.

The Bain circuit, as introduced in 1972, consists of a fresh-gas inflow tube that is enclosed inside an overlong (6 foot) but lightweight plastic expiratory tube (Fig. 6-10). This arrangement was intended chiefly for easier handling, but it also was believed that the inflow gases might pick up some heat, since the inflow tube was jacketed by warmer expired air. The whole device was actually a slight variation on the coaxial apparatus used by Macintosh and Pask in World War II (Gwilt and others, 1978).

Table 6-1. Basic gas flows for T-systems

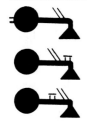

The *Rees system* can be used with FGF twice the child's MV, if the expiratory limb exceeds tidal volume.

Mapleson A is preferable for spontaneous respiration; FGF equal to MV is adequate.

Mapleson D is preferable for controlled ventilation, using:
  a. FGF = 1.5 MV, *or*
  b. Nightingale's formula:
    Under 30 lb, FGF = 3 L/min
    30-80 lb, FGF = 100 ml/lb/min
    Over 80 lb, FGF = 8 L/min

Dead space = 1 ml/lb
Tidal volume (ml) = wt (lb) $\times$ 3, or 3 $\times$ dead space
MV = tidal volume $\times$ respiratory rate

VARIABLES DETERMINING Pa$_{CO_2}$ DURING CONTROLLED VENTILATION WITH A T-PIECE SYSTEM*

1. FGF (fresh gas flow)
2. $\dot{V}_E$ (minute volume)
3. V_D/V_T (the ratio of apparatus and physiologic dead space to tidal volume)
4. Waveform delivered by the ventilator
5. $\dot{V}_{CO_2}$ (carbon dioxide production)
6. a-ADco$_2$ (arterial to alveolar carbon dioxide gradient)

The foregoing dissection and dismemberment of the "simple" Ayre system may appear excessive. In actuality, it is a greatly abbreviated summary of dozens of articles on the subject. Students of pediatric anesthesia should at least be aware of the work that has gone into the development of nonrebreathing systems. For practical daily use, however, when one is dealing with normal children during relatively uncomplicated procedures, it does not seem necessary to use the more complicated formulas. In our work over the past several years we have employed the simple guides shown in Table 6-1 and use both the Bain apparatus and the valveless Rees system with bag-tail scavenger, with assisted or controlled ventilation. I was pleased to find that the same guides and management are used at the Children's Hospital of Philadelphia, except that the Bain apparatus is used for all cases. All agree that when one is dealing with poor-risk patients or those undergoing extensive procedures, blood gases are the most reliable guides to regulation of flow rates and other variables. It is definitely in order to state that the desired maintenance figures include Pa$_{O_2}$ of 50 to 60 torr in neonates and 80 to 100 torr in older infants and children, Pa$_{CO_2}$ of 35 to 45 torr, arterial pH of 7.30 to 7.45, serum potassium level of 3.5 to 5.5 mEq/L, and ionized calcium level of 1.7 to 2.2 mEq/L.

The original Bain system lacks any humidifying device, the proponents of the system having contended that incoming gas is warmed (and moisture preserved) by reason of its passage inside the expiratory tube. In his investigation of this aspect, Weeks (1976) found that while there was enough moisture to prevent injury to tracheal cilia, there was not enough to prevent loss of body temperature. In testing humidifying apparatus, Weeks found that the Garthur Vapor Condenser (HME) was effective but that the 17-ml dead space would be excessive for small infants, while the Cascade humidifier was effective but caused excessive deposition of fluid in the infant airways.

Finally, in respect to the sterilization of the Bain apparatus, Enright and associates (1976) reported that glutaraldehyde was inadequate, but that ethylene oxide was both effective and practical.

Nonrebreathing valves

Leigh introduced the first nonrebreathing valve, which actually consisted of two metal unidirectional valves fed by a reservoir bag (Fig. 6-12). Stephen and Slater (1948), Fink (1954), Lewis and Leigh (1956), Frumin and associates (1959), and others modified the valve, and Stephen devised a mask with an expiratory valve. The original valves were relatively simple, but subsequently the Fink valve and others became more complicated (Loehning and others, 1964). All require high gas flows, and are subject to sticking and therefore somewhat unreliable performance. Their use, even in the United States and Canada, never kept pace with the T-piece, and presently they are in danger of extinction.

HUMIDIFICATION

Humidification is another problem that concerns the pediatric anesthesiologist. Anesthetic gases are dehydrated (moisture content reduced from 22 mg/L to 3 mg/L) to facilitate passage through valves and gauges. The use of these dry gases has aroused greater concern in pediatric anesthesia because of (1) the widespread use of nonrebreathing systems, (2) the increased lability of fluid and temperature balance in smaller patients, and (3) the greater susceptibility of pediatric patients to tracheitis and croup.

---

*From Rose, D. K., and Froese, A. B.: The regulation of Pa$_{CO_2}$ during controlled ventilation of children with a T-piece, Can. Anaesth. Soc. J. **26:**104, 1979.

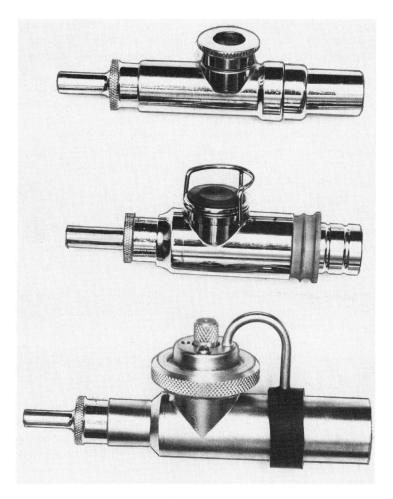

Fig. 6-12. Leigh, Stephen-Slater, and Fink nonrebreathing valves.

The adoption of standard humidification procedures has not occurred, however, and for good reason. Thus far, evidence of gross damage by dry gases is lacking, but under the guise of preventive therapy, humidifying attempts have produced considerable destruction. We are faced with two simple questions: Should humidification be added? And if so, how should it be accomplished?

Effects and defects of humidification

Grounds for humidification of anesthetic gases lie in prevention of both local and general effects of drying. Local effects, maximal when the upper airway is bypassed by endotracheal tube or tracheostomy, include hy-peremia, drying of secretions, crusting, and reduction of ciliary activity (Farmati and others, 1967). Although these reactions are seldom recognizable following operations of moderate duration, they are frequently observed in patients receiving prolonged ventilatory support. With special technics, such as that of Chalon and associates (1972), cytologic damage of ciliated epithelium can be evaluated by cell count after only 1 hour of anesthesia. As yet, however, there have been no follow-up studies on the subsequent course of these patients. An attempt to correlate humidity with the incidence of postoperative airway problems has been made at our hospital with equivocal findings.

With dogs as subjects, Rashad and associates (1967) have shown that inhalation of dry gases may increase pulmonary shunting and reduce compliance.

The local effect of "dry gas" anesthesia most obvious to the anesthesiologist has been drying of secretions inside the endotracheal tube, which can produce complete airway obstruction in the course of a 2- or 3-hour operation.

The generalized effects of dry gas inhalation—loss of body heat and fluid—are frequently emphasized. With the exception of studies by Graff and associates (1964), Rashad and Benson (1967), and Graff and Benson (1969), however, these losses are rarely described in concrete terms. To determine the need for humidification, one should know what is at stake.

The measurement of respiratory fluid loss is complicated because of the changing water content of gases at different temperatures. A liter of air containing 20 mg of water at 23° C is 100% saturated but at 30° C is 66% saturated and at 37° C is 46% saturated.

The respiratory moisture loss of adults is 250 to 300 grams of water in 24 hours under normal conditions* (Déry, 1973a). Hyperventilation in cold, dry air would give maximum respiratory water loss. Respiratory water loss may be determined by several methods. Otis (1964) gives the standard figure of 6 $g/m^2/hr$, while Welsh has developed the formula:

$$L = \frac{A \times RH \times F \times 60}{100,000}$$

where

    L = water loss in grams/hour
    A = milligrams of water per liter of air at ambient temperature under normal conditions
  RH = relative humidity
    F = rate of respirations per minute

The essential calculation, once figures have been determined, is to multiply minute

*Normal conditions: temperature, 70° F; relative humidity, 50%.

ventilation by the gradient between the moisture content of inspiratory and expiratory air, expiratory moisture content usually being constant at 34 mg/L (34 g/m^3).

The respiratory moisture losses of children are comparable to those of adults on the basis of body surface area and may be determined by application of Otis' formula or by direct data. Thus, in a 1-year-old child (weight 20 lb) breathing humidified air:

Respiratory rate = 30/min
MV = 20 × 3 × 30 ÷ 1800 ml = 1.8 L/min
Moisture content expired air = 34 mg/L
Moisture content inspired air = 22 mg/L
Moisture loss = 1.8 × (34 − 22) × 60 = 1.3 g/hr

In the same child during anesthesia with a nonrebreathing system (unhumidified):

Moisture content expired air = 34 mg/L
Moisture content inspired air = 3 mg/L
Moisture loss = 1.8 × (34 − 3) × 60 = 3.3 g/hr

During an operation of conceivable duration, such as 3 hours, the child would lose 167 mg of fluid by the respiratory tract alone. This rate of fluid loss, even when extended over several hours, does not seem impressive and would be easily replaced by infusion.

Heat loss determination

Respiratory loss of body heat is more easily detected and more easily determined than fluid loss, but it is more difficult to control and more dangerous.

For each milligram of water that is lost through vaporization, the body expends 580 small calories. Thus, the heat loss of the 20-lb child if breathing humidified air would have been 2.16 × 580 = 1252.8 calories/hr, but if breathing unhumidified air would have been 5.58 × 580 = 3236.4 calories/hr. The resultant threefold rate of heat loss is evident in the clinical management of small children and infants.

Methods of humidification

There is growing acceptance of the advisability of adding moisture to nonrebreathing systems, although many fail to carry it out. The methods involved vary greatly (Young and Crocker, 1976).

Suggesting simpler technics, Chase and associates (1962a) showed that by wetting the inner surfaces of breathing tubes and bags, the moisture content of inspired gas could be raised from tank level (3 mg/L) to 22 mg/L, which is within the acceptable range (22 to 26 mg/L). Comparable methods have included filling the ether vaporizer with water and passing the gases through this, preferably with a warming jacket around the vaporizer. Déry (1971) and others believe that dry gases intended for nonrebreathing apparatus will be adequately humidified if first passed through a large canister of soda lime. Anhydrous gas (moisture content 4 mg/L) would undoubtedly gain a valuable increment of moisture on passage through soda lime at room temperature, but the resultant moisture content would not approach that of a gas warmed to 32° or 34° C by a heated humidifier.

Devices specially constructed for adding moisture include humidifiers (with or without a heating mechanism), nebulizers (erroneously called vaporizers) that produce droplets or fog, and ultrasonic nebulizers that produce larger volumes of fog. The ingenious "artificial nose" introduced by Toremalm (1961) is designed to capture heat and moisture in exhaled air. Both this and the similar Garthur humidifier are excellent for tracheostomized patients, but increased resistance to ventilation has been reported when used with endotracheal tubes (Steward, 1976).

Choice of apparatus is confused by inadequacies or flaws in each system (Geevarghese and others, 1976). The heavy deposition of water by ultrasonic devices introduces the danger of rapid water overload, especially in small infants (Avery and others, 1967). This form of therapy has little application during anesthesia but has value in delivering aerosolized materials into lower bronchioles during inhalation therapy (Herzog and others, 1964; Stevens and Albregt, 1966). Other nebulizers carry similar danger of excessive wetting of airways. Thus, droplet formation

of any kind is less desirable than saturated air at body temperature, unless specific therapy is intended (Allan, 1966; Modell and others, 1966).

Heated humidifiers are designed to deliver warm saturated gases and thus avoid water fallout. However, any apparatus that can deliver saturated gases at temperatures above 37° C can unload water into the patient and contribute to overhydration. Heated devices also carry the danger of burning patients.

As noted by Steward (1976), many different humidifiers have been produced for use in anesthesia, several of which have been carefully evaluated (Chamney, 1969; Boys and Howells, 1972). The first Bennett Cascade humidifier,* described by Weeks and Broman (1970), was widely used though quite imperfect. It was awkward and shared a common fault of many heated humidifiers in having a long delivery tube that allowed gases to cool and rain out water unless more equipment was added (Garg, 1973), and it had to be otherwise altered to prevent it from blowing its lid. The newer Cascade II* (Fig. 6-13) shows several improvements, including a thermometer at the patient end of the delivery tube and an alarm signal, but it may have to share its popularity with the Conchatherm† (Fig. 6-14) and other competitors. Baker and associates (1977) reviewed the subject, recommended the Fisher-Paykel Heated Humidifier,‡ and included a good list of references. Our experience in current models (1979) is limited to use of the Cascade II and the Conchatherm, both of which fulfill clinical needs.

Contamination by humidifying apparatus is a definite danger but quite controllable (Moffet and Williams, 1967). Disposable humidifiers, such as the high-output humidifier (MacKuanying and Chalon, 1974), eliminate this at a cost, while Cascade and similar humidifiers can be protected simply by add-

---

*Bennett Respiration Products, Inc., 1639 Eleventh Street, Santa Monica, Calif.
†Respiratory Care, Inc., 900 West University Avenue, Arlington Heights, Ill.
‡Fisher-Paykel, New Zealand.

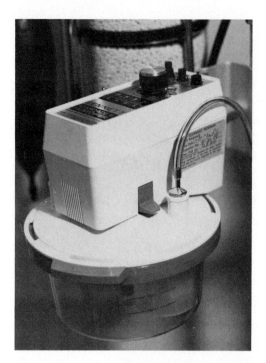

Fig. 6-13. Bennett Cascade II heater-humidifier.

Fig. 6-14. Concha-therm heater-humidifier.

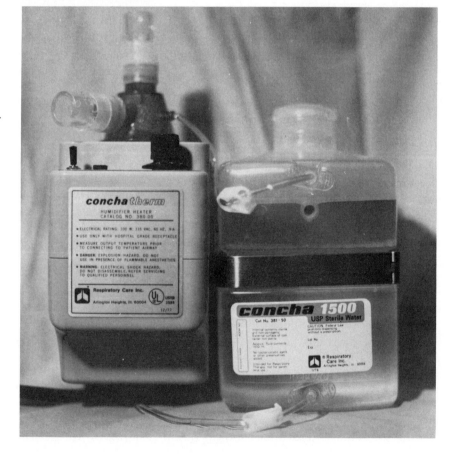

ing 1 drop of 1% silver nitrate to the fluid reservoir. The Emerson humidifier, used by Graff and associates (1964), effectively cleans gases by passing them through a column of copper shavings.

Based on experience and a study of patients anesthetized with and without humidity, we believe that humidification is effective chiefly in maintaining the warmth of small infants. We have found no clinical evidence of increased tracheal irritation when humidifying apparatus was not used.

SCAVENGING SYSTEMS

The growing concern over exposure to waste anesthetic gases is especially pertinent to pediatric anesthesia because of the popular method of blowing large volumes of gases over a child's face during induction and the continued use of high flows with both circle and nonrebreathing technics.

To reduce ambient levels toward the goals of 3 to 30 ppm of nitrous oxide and 0.05 to 5 ppm of halothane suggested by Whitcher and associates (1975), several practices must be modified. With more accurate flowmeters, one may reduce the excessive flow rates currently used in circle absorption rather than nonrebreathing circuits. In addition, the gases escaping from the pop-off valves must be collected and vented through a system independent of the central suction.

The wastage that occurs during pediatric induction can easily amount to 40 or 50 liters. If induction is followed by a long operation, there should be ample time to reestablish acceptable trace concentrations. When there is a succession of short operations, however, as in an outpatient schedule, the buildup can be obvious to all, and the need to alter the situation will be undeniable. To reduce the wastage of induction to a minimum, one may abandon the pleasant practice of "stealing" sleeping children and use intravenous induction for all, or one may compromise and attempt more economical methods of inhalation induction.

At present the reduction of spillage during maintenance of anesthesia under nonrebreathing systems is a considerable nuisance.

As previously noted, the Bain system offers easy adaptation to scavenging and presents little difficulty. The apparatus manufactured by Boehringer* has proved especially reliable. Other systems with exposed valves offer little opportunity for collecting excess gases. The valveless Rees system, which vents through the tail of the breathing bag, can be fitted with a variety of adaptations that make it acceptable though definitely more unwieldy. A device produced commercially under the name Ped-Evac Gas Evacuator† consists of a valve made into the breathing bag that is manipulated by thumb compression.

At The Children's Hospital Medical Center, we presently use the circle absorption system for children weighing more than 15 kg and control waste gases by a Boehringer valve (Fig. 6-15), through which they pass into an independent evacuation system. For smaller children, we use the Bain system in ambulatory surgery, without additional humidification. In the main operating room we use the Rees system with either a Dupaco (Fig. 6-16) or a Boehringer bag-tail adapter to lead waste gases into the evacuation system. Inflow gases are humidified and warmed by means of either a Cascade or a Conchapak heater-humidifier in selected cases, including long procedures, those involving airway pathology or instrumentation, and operations on neonates and poor-risk patients. Since both humidifiers may produce excessive moisture, it is important to mount them at a level below the patient, so that excess water will fall back into the humidifier.

SUMMARY

The principal advantages of the absorption systems are retention of heat and moisture, economy of gases, and easy reduction of pollution. With adaptations required for nonrebreathing systems, their chief remaining advantages are the exact control of anesthetic concentrations and greater mobility.

*Boehringer Labs, Inc., P.O. Box 337, Wynnwood, Pa. 19096
†Ped-Evac Co., P.O. Box 752, Port Angeles, Wash. 98362

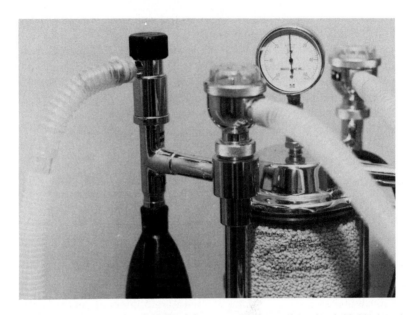

Fig. 6-15. Adult circle system with Boehringer scavenging outlet valve (with black top).

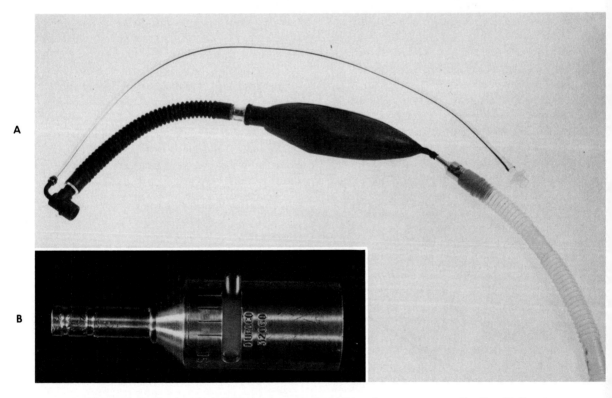

Fig. 6-16. A, Rees system with Dupaco scavenging valve and scavenge evacuation line. **B,** Dupaco scavenging valve.

Generally accepted technics for pediatric use are:

Children under 15 kg

Nonrebreathing systems (with humidity if over 1 hour duration) or modified adult circle

Children 15 kg and over

Standard adult circle system

Type of ventilation

Assisted or controlled
Rate = 30 to 50 respirations/min
Pressure = 15 to 20 cm H_2O
Inspiratory/expiratory duration = 1 to 2

BIBLIOGRAPHY

Adriani, J., and Griggs, T.: Rebreathing in pediatric anesthesia; recommendations and descriptions of improvements in apparatus, Anesthesiology 14:337, 1953.

Allan, D.: Recent advances in pediatric inhalation therapy, Surg. Clin. North Am. 46:1611, 1966.

Avery, M. E., Galina, M., and Nachman, R.: Mist therapy, Pediatrics 39:160, 1967.

Ayre, P.: Anaesthesia for harelip and cleft palate in babies, Br. J. Surg. 25:131, 1937.

Ayre, P.: Anaesthesia for intracranial operations; a new technique, Lancet 1:520, 1937a.

Ayre, P.: Endotracheal anesthesia for babies; with special reference to harelip and cleft palate operations, Anesth. Analg. (Cleve.) 16:330, 1937b.

Bain, J. A., and Spoerel, W. E.: A streamlined anaesthetic system, Can. Anaesth. Soc. J. 19:426, 1972.

Bain, J. A., and Spoerel, W. E.: Flow requirements for a modified Mapleson D system during controlled ventilation, Can. Anaesth. Soc. J. 20:629, 1973.

Bain, J. A., and Spoerel, W. E.: Carbon dioxide output in anaesthesia, Can. Anaesth. Soc. J. 23:153, 1976.

Bain, J. A., and Spoerel, W. E.: Carbon dioxide output and elimination in children under anaesthesia, Can. Anaesth. Soc. J. 24:533, 1977.

Baker, J. D. III, Wallace, C. T., and Brown, C. S.: Maintenance of body temperature in infants during surgery; experience with a new heated humidifier, Anesthesiol. Rev. 4:21, 1977.

Baraka, A.: Rebreathing in a double T-piece system, Br. J. Anaesth. 41:47, 1969.

Berry, F. A., and Hughes-Davies, D. I.: Methods of increasing the humidity and temperature of inspired gases in the infant circle system, Anesthesiology 37:456, 1972.

Best, D. W. S.: A simple inexpensive system for the removal of excess anaesthetic vapors, Can. Anaesth. Soc. J. 18:333, 1971.

Bloomquist, E. R.: Pediatric circle absorber, Anesthesiology 18:787, 1957.

Boys, J. E., and Howells, T. H.: Humidification in anaesthesia; a review of the present situation, Br. J. Anaesth. 44:879, 1972.

Brooks, W., Stuart, D., and Gabel, P.: The T-piece in anesthesia; an examination of its fundamental principle, Anesth. Analg. (Cleve.) 37:191, 1958.

Bruce, D. L., Eide, K. A., Linde, H. W., and Eckenhoff, S. E.: Causes of death among anesthesiologists; a 20 year study, Anesthesiology 29:565, 1968.

Carden, E., and Nelson, D.: A new and highly efficient circuit for paediatric anaesthesia, Can. Anaesth. Soc. J. 19:572, 1972.

Chalon, J., Day, L., and Malebranche, J.: Effects of dry anesthetic gases on tracheobronchial ciliated epithelium, Anesthesiology 37:338, 1972.

Chamney, A. R.: Humidification requirements and techniques, including a review of the performance of equipment in current use, Anaesthesia 24:602, 1969.

Chase, H. F., Kilmore, M. A., and Trotta, R.: Respiratory water loss via anesthesia systems; mask breathing, Anesthesiology 22:205, 1962.

Chase, H. F., Trotta, R., and Kilmore, M. A.: Simple methods for humidifying non-rebreathing anesthesia gas systems, Anesth. Analg. (Cleve.) 41:249, 1962a.

Chu, Y. K., Kang, H. R., and Boyan, C. P.: Is the Bain breathing circuit the future anesthesia system? An evaluation, Anesth. Analg. (Cleve.) 56:84, 1977.

Cohen, E. N., Belleville, J. W., and Brown, B. W.: Anesthesia, miscarriage and pregnancy; a study of operating nurses and anesthetists, Anesthesiology 35:343, 1971.

Davenport, H. T.: Paediatric anaesthesia, ed. 2, Philadelphia, 1973, Lea & Febiger.

Déry, R.: Humidity in anaesthesiology. IV. Determination of the alveolar humidity and temperature in the dog, Can. Anaesth. Soc. J. 18:145, 1971.

Déry, R.: The evolution of heat and moisture in the respiratory tract during anaesthesia with a non-rebreathing system, Can. Anaesth. Soc. J. 20:296, 1973.

Déry, R.: Water balance of the respiratory tract during ventilation with a gas mixture saturated at body temperature, Can. Anaesth. Soc. J. 20:719, 1973a.

Dorsch, J. A., and Dorsch, S. E.: Understanding anaesthetic equipment, Baltimore, 1975, The Williams & Wilkins Co.

Eger, E. I. II: Anesthetic uptake and action, Baltimore, 1974, The Williams & Wilkins Co.

Enright, A. C., Moore, R. L., and Parney, F. L.: Contamination and re-sterilization of the Bain circuit, Can. Anaesth. Soc. J. 23:548, 1976.

Farmati, O., Quinn, J. R., and Fennell, R. M.: Exfoliative cytology of the intubated larynx in children, Can. Anaesth. Soc. J. 14:321, 1967.

Fink, B. R.: A nonrebreathing valve of new design, Anesthesiology 15:471, 1954.

Freeman, A., St. Pierre, M., and Bachman, L.: Comparison of spontaneous and controlled breathing during cyclopropane anesthesia in infants, Anesthesiology 25:597, 1964.

Frumin, M. J., Lee, A. S. J., and Papper, E. M.: New

valve for nonrebreathing systems, Anesthesiology 20: 383, 1959.

Garg, G.: Humidification of the Rees-Ayre T-piece system for neonates, Anesth. Analg. (Cleve.) 52:207, 1973.

Geevarghese, K. P., Aldrete, J. A., and Patel, T. C.: Inspired temperature with immersion heater humidifiers, Anesth. Analg. (Cleve.) 55:331, 1976.

Graff, T. D., and Benson, D. W.: Systemic and pulmonary changes with inhaled humid atmospheres; clinical application, Anesthesiology 30:199, 1969.

Graff, T. D., Holzman, R. S., and Benson, D. W.: Acid-base balance in infants during halothane anesthesia with the use of an adult circle absorption system, Anesth. Analg. (Cleve.) 43:583, 1964.

Graff, T. D., Sewall, K., Lim, T. S., and others: The ventilatory response of infants to airway resistance, Anesthesiology 27:168, 1966.

Gwilt, D. J., Goat, V. A., and Maynard, P.: The Bain system; gas flows in small subjects, Br. J. Anaesth. 50: 127, 1978.

Hanallah, R., and Rosales, J. K.: A hazard connected with re-use of the Bain circuit, case report, Can. Anaesth. Soc. J. 21:511, 1974.

Harrison, G. A.: Ayre's T-piece; a review of its modifications, Br. J. Anaesth. 36:115, 1964.

Harrison, G. A.: The effect of the respiratory flow pattern on rebreathing in the T-piece system, Br. J. Anaesth. 36:206, 1964a.

Hawkins, T. J.: Atmospheric pollution in operating theatres; a review and report on the use of reusable activated charcoal canisters, Anaesthesia 28:490, 1973.

Herzog, P., Norlander, O. P., and Engstrom, C. G.: Ultrasonic generation of aerosol for the humidification of inspired gas during volume-controlled ventilation, Acta Anaesth. Scand. 8:79, 1964.

Hunt, K. H. L.: Resistance in respiratory valves and canisters, Anesthesiology 16:190, 1955.

Inkster, J. W.: The T-piece technique in anaesthesia, Br. J. Anaesth. 28:512, 1956.

Jones, P. L., and Prosser, J.: An assessment of the Neff circulator, Can. Anaesth. Soc. J. 20:659, 1973.

Kain, M. L., and Nunn, J. F.: Fresh gas economics of the Magill circuit, Anesthesiology 29:964, 1968.

Lank, B.: Anesthesia for premature babies, J. Am. Assoc. Nurse Anesth. 21:238, 1953.

Leigh, M. D., and Belton, M. K.: Pediatric anesthesia, ed. 2, New York, 1960, Macmillan, Inc.

Lewis, A., and Spoerel, W. E.: A modification of Ayre's technique, Can. Anaesth. Soc. J. 8:501, 1961.

Lewis, G. B., and Leigh, M. D.: Lewis-Leigh nonrebreathing valve, Anesthesiology 17:618, 1956.

Loehning, R. W., Davis, G., and Safar, P.: Rebreathing with "nonrebreathing" valves, Anesthesiology 25:854, 1964.

MacKuanying, N., and Chalon, J.: Humidification of anesthetic gases for children, Anesth. Analg. (Cleve.) 53:387, 1974.

Magill, I.: Endotracheal anaesthesia, Proc. R. Soc. Med. 22:83, 1928.

Magill, I.: Discussion. In Kain, M. L., and Nunn, J. F.: Fresh gas flow and rebreathing in the Magill circuit with spontaneous respiration, Proc. R. Soc. Med. 60: 749, 1967.

Mansell, W. H.: Bain circuit; "the hazard of the hidden tube," Can. Anaesth. Soc. J. 23:227, 1976.

Mansell, W. H.: Spontaneous breathing with the Bain circuit at low flow rates; a case report, Can. Anaesth. Soc. J. 23:432, 1976a.

Mapleson, W. W.: The elimination of rebreathing in various semi-closed anesthesia systems, Br. J. Anaesth. 20:323, 1954.

Mapleson, W. W.: Theoretical considerations of the effects of rebreathing in two semi-closed anaesthetic systems, Br. Med. Bull. 14:64, 1958.

Mapleson, W. W.: Gas exchange characteristics of anaesthetic systems. In Gray, T. C., and Nunn, J. F., editors: General anaesthesia, Borough Green, Kent, 1972, Butterworth & Co., Publishers, Ltd.

Marrese, R. A.: A safe method for discharging anesthetic gases, Anesthesiology 31:371, 1969.

Modell, J. H., Giammona, S. T., and Alvarez, L. A.: Effect of ultrasonic nebulized suspensions on pulmonary surfactant, Dis. Chest 50:627, 1966.

Moffet, H. L., and Williams, T.: Bacteria recovered from distilled water and mist therapy equipment, Am. J. Dis. Child. 114:7, 1967.

Neff, W. B., Burke, S. F., and Thompson, R.: A Venturi circulator for anesthetic systems, Anesthesiology 29: 839, 1968.

Nightingale, D. A., and Lambert, T. F.: Carbon dioxide output in anaesthetised children, Anaesthesia 33:594, 1978.

Nightingale, D. A., Richards, C. R., and Glass, A.: An evaluation of rebreathing in a modified T-piece system during controlled ventilation of anaesthetized children, Br. J. Anaesth. 37:762, 1965.

Norman, J., Adams, A. P., and Sykes, M. K.: Rebreathing with the Magill attachment, Anaesthesia 23:75, 1968.

Onchi, Y., Hayashi, T., and Veyama, H.: Studies on the Ayre T-piece technique, Far East J. Anesth. 1:30, 1947.

Otis, A. B.: Quantitative relationship in steady-state gas exchange. In Handbook of physiology, respiration, Washington, D.C., 1964, American Physiological Society.

Podlesch, I., Dudziak, R., and Zinganell, K.: Inspiratory and expiratory CO_2 concentration during halothane anesthesia in infants, Anesthesiology 27:823, 1966.

Rackow, H.: Pediatric anesthesia. In Mark, L. C., and Ngai, S. H., editors: Highlights of clinical anesthesiology, New York, 1974, Harper & Row, Publishers, Inc.

Rashad, K. F., and Benson, D. W.: Role of humidity in the prevention of hypothermia in infants and children, Anesth. Analg. (Cleve.) 46:712, 1967.

Rashad, K. F., Wilson, K., Hurt, H. H., Jr., and others: Effect of humidification of anesthetic gases on static compliance, Anesth. Analg. (Cleve.) **46:**127, 1967.

Rayburn, R. L., and Graves, S. A.: A new concept in controlled ventilation of children with Bain anesthetic circuit, Anesthesiology **48:**250, 1978.

Rees, G. J.: Pediatric anaesthesia, Br. J. Anaesth. **32:** 132, 1960.

Revell, D. G.: Circulator to eliminate mechanical dead space in circle absorption systems, Can. Anaesth. Soc. J. **6:**98, 1959.

Reynolds, T. N.: Acid-base equilibrium during C_3H_6 anesthesia and surgery in infants, Anesthesiology **27:** 127, 1966.

Roffey, P. J., Revell, D. G., and Morris, L. E.: An assessment of the Revell circulator, Anesthesiology **22:** 583, 1961.

Rose, D. K., and Froese, A. B.: The regulation of Pa_{CO_2} during controlled ventilation of children with a T-piece, Can. Anaesth. Soc. J. **26:**104, 1979.

Ruben, H.: A new nonrebreathing valve, Anesthesiology **16:**643, 1955.

Seeley, H. F., Barnes, P. K., and Conway, C. M.: Controlled ventilation with the Mapleson D system; a theoretical and experimental study, Br. J. Anaesth. **49:**107, 1977.

Soliman, M. G., and Laberge, R.: The use of the Bain circuit in spontaneously breathing pediatric patients, Can. Anaesth. Soc. J. **25:**276, 1978.

Stephen, C. R., and Slater, H. M.: Nonresisting, nonrebreathing valve, Anesthesiology **9:**550, 1948.

Stevens, H. R., and Albregt, H. B.: Assessment of ultrasonic nebulization, Anesthesiology **27:**648, 1966.

Steward, D. J.: A disposable condenser humidifier for use during anaesthesia, Can. Anaesth. Soc. J. **23:**191, 1976.

Sykes, M. K.: Rebreathing circuits; a review, Br. J. Anaesth. **40:**666, 1968.

Toremalm, N. G.: Air-flow patterns and ciliary activity in the trachea after tracheotomy, Acta Otolaryngol. Scand. **53:**442, 1961.

Ver Steeg, J., and Stevens, W. C.: A comparison of respiratory effect of infants anesthetized with several adult and pediatric systems, Anesthesiology **27:**229, 1966.

Waltemath, C. L., Erbquth, P. H., and Sunderland, W. A.: Increased respiratory resistance after ultrasonic humidification of anesthesia gas; clinical workshop, Anesthesiology **39:**547, 1973.

Waters, D. J., and Mapleson, W. W.: Rebreathing during controlled respiration with various semiclosed anaesthetic systems, Br. J. Anaesth. **33:**374, 1961.

Waters, R. M.: Clinical scope and utilization of carbon dioxide filtration in inhalation anesthesia, Anesth. Analg. (Cleve.) **3:**20, 1924.

Weeks, D. B.: Provision of endogenous and exogenous humidity for the Bain breathing circuit, Can. Anaesth. Soc. J. **23:**185, 1976.

Weeks, D. B., and Broman, K. E.: A method of quantitating humidity in the anesthesia circuit by temperature control; semiclosed circle, Anesth. Analg. (Cleve.) **49:**292, 1970.

Welsh, B., Blackwood, M. J. A., and Conn, A. W.: Evaluation of a laboratory means of estimating respiratory water loss using the T-piece system, Anesth. Analg. (Cleve.) **50:**103, 1971.

Whitcher, C., and others: Developments and evaluation of methods for the elimination of waste anesthetic gases and vapors in hospitals, Publ. No. (N10SH) 75-137, Washington, D.C., 1975, U.S. Department of Health, Education, and Welfare.

Winchell, S. W., and Davis, G.: Sterilization and care of equipment. In Safar, P., editor: Respiratory therapy, Philadelphia, 1965, F. A. Davis Co.

Young, J. A., and Crocker, D.: Principles and practice of respiratory therapy, ed. 2, Chicago, 1976, Year Book Medical Publishers, Inc.

Technics for the induction of anesthesia

The induction of anesthesia can be a crucial event in both the physical and emotional development of a child. It is often handled carelessly, with too little consideration for the anxiety the child is suffering and with inadequate respect for the physiologic stress involved.

No matter how healthy the child or how insignificant the operation, the experience of being placed on an operating table and forcefully put to sleep can be a terrifying and never-to-be forgotten horror. Children who must return for repeated operations may reasonably become emotionally disturbed (Dombro, 1970).

The poor-risk child faces greater emotional strain and additional hazards of cardiorespiratory and neurogenic instability. Since the character of induction may play an appreciable part in the success of the entire operation, considerable attention to details is justified.

The induction of general anesthesia in small infants presents a special set of problems. We assume that preoperative sedative drugs are both unnecessary and unsafe and prefer the infants to be active and responsive. Although they may be less subject to anxiety, infants obviously are disturbed by loud noises, rough handling, needles, cold, and irritant anesthetics. However, gentle handling and reassuring voices have a soothing effect long before words can be understood. Additional support by pacifiers, toys, and music boxes is often helpful. Actual technics of induction of small infants are described in Chapter 15.

Induction of general anesthesia in children old enough to have specific fears calls for further consideration. Several approaches are needed, each of which has individual advantages.

BASAL ANESTHESIA*

Probably the least disturbing method of inducing anesthesia in anxious children is via the rectum, since this involves neither painful injection nor swallowing of suspicious-looking potions. With few exceptions, children under 6 or 8 years of age prefer induction by this technic and often request it on repeat visits. (In the rare exception where the child senses this as some kind of an assault, one naturally desists at once.)

For many years, rectal administration of tribromoethanol (Avertin) was regarded as an ideal method for pediatric induction. Tribromoethanol regularly produced deep sleep in approximately 7 minutes and was particularly

---

* Basal anesthesia is mentioned in Chapter 4 as a method of sedating children. Since it is usually given to children previously unsedated, it serves for both sedation and induction; however, its greater value is for induction of anesthesia.

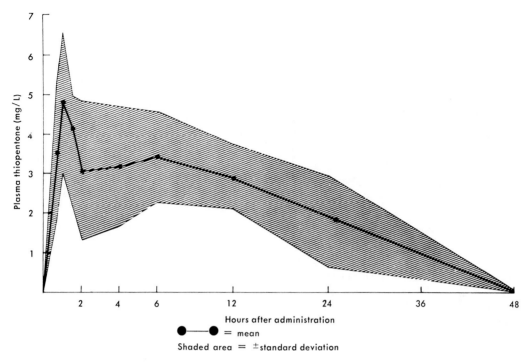

Fig. 7-1. Plasma levels of thiopental in children after administration by rectal suppositories. (From Lindsay, W. A., and Shepherd, J.: Br. J. Anaesth. **41:**977, 1969.)

valuable in that it depressed laryngeal reflexes and caused bronchodilation. It was abandoned largely because it required concoction prior to each administration and often caused rectal stimulation and evacuation.

Thiopental sodium (Pentothal) and methohexital sodium (Brevital) currently are popular for rectal administration. Both agents are rapidly effective and, because they are barbiturates, are more stable than tribromoethanol, but they stimulate rather than depress airway responses.

Thiopental was first prepared for rectal use in aqueous solution (Weinstein, 1939) and subsequently in suppository (Albert and others, 1956) and suspension form (Albert and others, 1959). Dosage and response with different preparations are similar, and for practical purposes the standard 2.0% or 2.5% intravenous solution often is most convenient. The usual dose for children who have not had other sedation is 30 mg/kg (Kaufman, 1973). If given as a supplement to previous but inadequate sedation, 20 mg/kg is advised.

The uptake and distribution of intravenous barbiturates were investigated by Brodie (1952) and others. Albert and associates (1956), Buchmann (1966), and Lindsay and Shepherd (1969) have studied the effects of thiopental following rectal administration. Using thiopental in suppository form, they reported that children with plasma levels of 2.8 mg/L or more were either asleep or adequately sedated and that excretion required 24 to 48 hours (Fig. 7-1).

Methohexital forms a clear solution and lacks the odor and taste of sulfur that is characteristic of thiopental. It is reputed to produce more rapid action and recovery than thiopental, but this is of little clinical significance since any advantage in speed is reduced by greater airway irritability and hiccoughing (during intravenous use).

Methohexital is rated as being two or three times as potent as thiopental (Miller and others, 1973). For rectal use it may be mixed in 1% to 10% solutions, and dosages of 20 mg/kg for unsedated or 15 mg/kg for inadequately sedated children should provide results comparable to those with thiopental.*

With either drug, patients usually fall asleep within 7 to 10 minutes, but this is variable. Following a short general anesthesia, awakening is calm, and children often may be ambulatory in 45 to 60 minutes; however, awakening from thiopental, especially if used as a supplement to other sedatives, may be prolonged.

Induction by rectal medication has special advantages in being suited for administration in the child's bed or when parents wish to be present. It is excellent for resistant children, especially those who are mentally retarded or who, for any reason, comprehend poorly. Because of the rapid onset and profound sedation of basal anesthesia, an anesthesiologist should remain with the child from the time of its administration until the end of the operation. This adds considerably to total anesthesia time and is a major deterrent to its widespread use.

Rectal barbiturates are contraindicated in the presence of airway pathology, since they can cause ventilatory depression and stimulation of laryngeal reflexes. The less pronounced myocardial depression restricts the use of this technic in children with cardiac disease but does not contraindicate it.

INDUCTION BY INTRAMUSCULAR ROUTE

In rare situations, intramuscular injection of *ketamine* is used for infants with difficult veins and for the occasional child who resists all other approaches (Wilson and others, 1967; Page and others, 1972).

This is definitely more rapid and more predictable than rectal induction and is practical for an infant or child who is already on the operating table. The needle is unpleasant, and the amount of solution is excessive, but within 2 or 3 minutes the eyes become fixed and the child can be considered asleep. Although 10 mg/kg is recommended, 6 mg/kg may be sufficient. With either dose, the child usually remains unrelaxed and may

*Goresky and Steward (1979) prefer 25 mg/kg.

move with stimulation but is totally analgesic (Wyant, 1971).

The supportive cardiovascular action of ketamine is especially advantageous for poor-risk patients (Nettles and others, 1973). For this reason, intramuscular ketamine is often used in infants with congenital cardiac defects for preoperative cannulation of vessels but only if they are to have postoperative ventilatory support (see Chapter 16).

INDUCTION BY INTRAVENOUS ROUTE

With children, as with adults, induction by intravenous agents has the advantage of speed plus elimination of the mask, its odors, and the unpleasant sensations of gradual loss of consciousness. The disadvantages are the needle, for which children have a natural dislike (amounting often to terror), and the difficulty of venipuncture, as well as the usual hazards of intravenous agents.

Since venipuncture often must be preceded by reassurance in order to avoid a struggle, it is advisable to make sure that the child does have a promising vein before trying to persuade him that this is the best way. Unless there is a vein that one can be relatively sure of entering on the first try, intravenous induction loses much of its beauty.

Dorsum of the hand, radial vein, and saphenous and other veins of the foot are examined in that order. The volar aspect of the wrist has small visible veins that are inviting, but danger of extravasation and tissue necrosis discourages their use. At The Children's Hospital Medical Center we rarely employ them for induction, never for continued infusion. The scalp occasionally may be used when good veins are not found elsewhere.

At times when it is difficult to find a vein large enough for expected blood replacement, one may use a 25-gauge needle in the antecubital space for induction and place the larger cannulae after anesthetics have caused vasodilation. Metal needles must be removed from the antecubital space immediately after induction (see Chapter 25).

To avoid frightening a child, one should hold the needle out of sight, avoid using the word "needle," and divert attention. Actual insertion, however, is never made without warning. Saying "here comes a little scratch" will help prepare the child and keep him from suspecting that he has been tricked. It is possible to anesthetize the skin by cooling it with ice or ethyl chloride. One should always allow alcohol skin preparation to dry before inserting the needle. The *smallest possible needle* is used, and the least sensitive (dorsal rather than ventral) areas are chosen.

Actual induction with thiopental usually requires 4 to 6 mg/kg. Rather than inducing deep sleep rapidly in apprehensive patients and having the last thing they remember a sharp jab, one can induce gradually and give a posthypnotic suggestion that they are safe and nothing hurts and that this is a good way to go to sleep and when they wake up they are going to feel much better.

Induction is calm, as with adults, but airway obstruction may occur. To prevent this, the patient is asked to lift his chin "way up" as the drug is administered. One should allow 1 or 2 minutes for induction and avoid attempts to hasten the process for fear of causing hypotension.

When a patient is brought to the operating room with an infusion already in place, it offers a rare opportunity that should never be overlooked—that of inducing anesthesia without disturbing the child in any way. This advantage is immediately destroyed if a mask is applied for preoxygenation. On request, however, the child who would resent a mask will be proud to take several deep breaths, which would probably be just as beneficial.

Ketamine may be chosen for intravenous induction in specified situations, especially when analgesia is desired without relaxation or when spontaneous respiration without endotracheal intubation is preferable. One should try to maintain the airway by careful positioning of the head rather than insertion of an airway. With a dose of 2 mg/kg a child usually assumes a catatonic condition and is "asleep" within 1 or 2 minutes (see Chapter 12).

INDUCTION BY INHALATION METHODS

At present, inhalation induction technics appear to be more popular than other methods. The reasons for this vary greatly. They include (1) the child's exaggerated fear of needles based on painful intramuscular inoculations, (2) the anesthesiologist's occasional lack of time or ability to use other methods, and (3) the fact that if a child is already dozing quietly, the inhalation method is the least upsetting.

Since inhalation of a nonirritant anesthetic is fundamentally painless and a needle is not, persistence in the attempt to perfect inhalation induction does seem entirely logical.

Two very important components of inhalation induction are (1) the maintenance of patient morale and (2) the administration of the anesthetic, or the mechanics of induction.

Patient morale

A tremendous advance was made by the elimination of ether, making induction much more pleasant for the child and much easier for the anesthesiologist. Other improvements are imminent. Many children still object, however, and though less skill is required to handle the anesthetic, much skill still may be needed to handle the child.

The anesthesiologist must vary his method to suit the individual. If a child has dozed off while waiting his turn for operation, he can be "stolen" by blowing induction agents over his face before he is moved from stretcher to operating table.

A child who is drowsy and quiet needs only gentle handling and a few words so that he will not be startled as he is readied for induction.

The real test is presented by the child who is still awake, sensitive to all that is going on around him, and as ready to cooperate if things please him as he is to tear the place apart if he is upset. The greatest help in this case is the advantage of having seen the child beforehand, so that both anesthesiologist and child know something about each other. If a line of communication has been found through a child's toys or an older patient's interests or hobby, a pet, or a favorite TV program, focussing his attention on this may help him forget his immediate problem. A sense of gentle unhurried efficiency, obviously expecting the child to cooperate, usually shows better results than an oversympathetic attitude.

Because of the hazard of moving anesthetized patients, most children are now put to sleep on the operating table.

The short trip from waiting area to operating room can be important. The child is moved onto a stretcher and wheeled to the operating room, taking his security blanket and best-loved toys with him. If he proves actively resistant at this stage, he is returned to the waiting area and given additional sedation, preferably with rectal thiopental but occasionally with intravenous or intramuscular agents. One is rarely justified in bringing a screaming child into an operating room (see Suggested do's and don'ts in anesthesia induction below). The average child is cooperative but may be frightened by noisy personnel and strange sights. An assistant should help position him on the operating table and stand by, but it is usually best if the anesthesiologist does the talking.

Do's	Don'ts
Check medication effect 30 minutes before anesthesia time.	Don't allow parents to follow child to operating room door.
Reassure parents and ask them to allow child to go to sleep.	Don't take screaming child into operating room.
If child has an infusion already running, use it for induction.	Don't start induction unless you have a working suction apparatus and a catheter to go *inside* endotracheal tube.
If child is asleep before induction, do a "steal" induction.	
If child is awake, keep his attention away from his operation.	Don't induce a patient with distension. A large stomach tube must be passed to relieve pressure.
Attach blood pressure cuff first—they like it.	
Warm the stethoscope before touching it to the chest.	Don't force a child to lie down.
Let child hold his own mask.	Don't use mask induction on a frightened child.

Do's	Don'ts
Let the anesthesiologist be the only one talking to the child during induction.	Don't use a black rubber mask for induction of a nervous child.
Allow extra time to be sure child is asleep before starting surgical preparation.	Don't put mask on child's face abruptly.
	After two venipuncture failures, don't persist in IV induction.
	Don't start induction without attendant standing by.
	Don't pry child's eyes open to see if he is going to sleep.

As nicely stated by Szasz (1974), "dignity is one of the values that men and women—and children, too—cherish, and that often conflicts with the pursuit of health at any cost." Whether adult or child, having one's clothes removed and being wheeled into a room under glaring lights and surrounded by hooded strangers reduces one to a nonentity. It is fundamental to reestablish the patient as an individual, to let all present know that this unclad body is not just an "appendix" or a "cystic" but that he has a name, which should be used, and in addition that he is a Little League pitcher, or has six sisters, or is a ham radio operator, or is the owner of a red whistle, but in any case that he is someone *special* and therefore important. This gives the patient confidence and a little courage as he goes to sleep.

The progress of the procedure should be smooth and continuous, and unbroken by last minute preparation of equipment.

Immediately before the induction is started, a final check is performed to assure the presence of working suction and suitable suction catheters, an airtight breathing apparatus, and a chart that is properly made out with dose and time of administration of premedicant drugs. To this one will add the time of beginning anesthesia and initial heart rate and blood pressure before turning on the gas flows.

Each step in induction is explained in turn. The child enjoys the blood pressure cuff, so

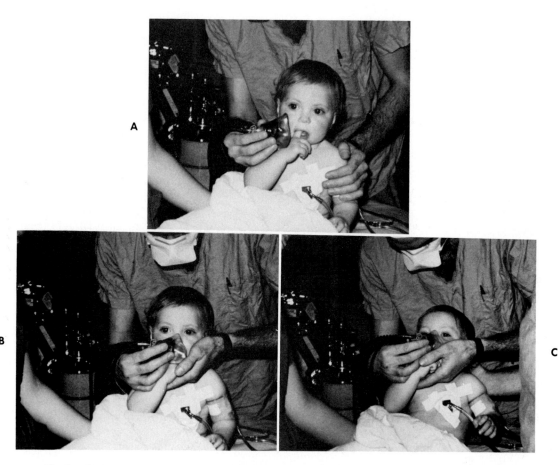

Fig. 7-2. Children who are afraid to lie down on the operating table often have little objection to a "sitting up" induction.

this is applied first and he is encouraged to pump it up and play with it. The stethoscope is less acceptable, especially if cold. It helps to rub it on the child's arm a little, to warn him and to warm the stethoscope, before it is placed on his chest.

At this point it often becomes obvious that a small child has no intention of lying down on the operating table. He may be happy to sit up and play, but nothing will persuade him to lie down. In such cases, it is much better to proceed with induction with him sitting on the table or in someone's lap (Fig. 7-2).

The *mask* is frequently a major problem and must be handled with care, if used at all. To many children it is immediately abhorrent, and they object strenuously to both the sight and smell, even before gases are

started. Because of these emotional reactions, varied approaches may be used. One should never begin by putting a mask on a patient's face abruptly and without warning. The mask should be held away from the patient and shown to him, even if he has seen it previously. Sometimes it helps if the anesthesiologist demonstrates it on himself. By playing that he is "taking turns," he can persuade a suspicious child to take a few breaths at a time and gradually let him have all the turns. One should be sure to tell the child to *breathe through his mouth*, since this reduces the smell. It often helps to start without the mask, simply removing it and blowing the gases over the child's face. This is especially effective if a towel or the child's security blanket is casually draped around the child's face to make a tentlike enclosure, or the hands are cupped over the child's nose and mouth in place of the mask.

Several changes can and should be made in the presently used black masks. They can be decorated with designs and colors, and the smell of rubber (and anesthetics) can be disguised by a drop of perfume or fruit extract placed either on the mask or under the child's nose. With the elimination of explosive anesthetics, conductive (black) masks are no longer mandatory. As emphasized by Stetson (1974), greater use should be made of clear plastic masks (Fig. 7-3), which are much more acceptable to children and also reduce the danger of unrecognized regurgitation. Many children seem delighted to wear surgical masks made out of colored paper, through which one can cut a hole and introduce an effective anesthetic mixture until the child is asleep.

Thermistor and other monitoring devices are usually positioned after the child is unconscious. At the outset, the child may be resistant, apprehensive, alert, responsive, drowsy, or sound asleep, and the treatment must be suited to his mood. The active, resistant child may be taken in by a "super sell"

approach, which captures his attention with rapid jargon while a surreptitious flow of gases reduces him to a more pliant mood. Cyclopropane has been used effectively for rapid inductions (Paymaster and others, 1965) but now is generally outlawed, yielding its place to mixtures of nitrous oxide and halothane.

Lacking the talent of a super-salesman, one does best to rely on the establishment of communication and especially on the building of self-confidence. One can pretend to need a child's help by having him hold the mask on his face all by himself (Fig. 7-4). Have him perform. Ask a 3-year-old to count to 10, or ask a 15-year-old to count backwards by 13s starting at 300. Have a 2-year-old show his strength by squeezing your finger (and be sure to say "ow").

One does not stimulate a quiet child by asking questions and prodding him awake. It is better to discourage activity by suggesting more and more soporific themes and repeating in a mumbled monotone "you're a good boy and you're going to sleep, you're a good boy, you're going to sleep, you're . . . going . . ."

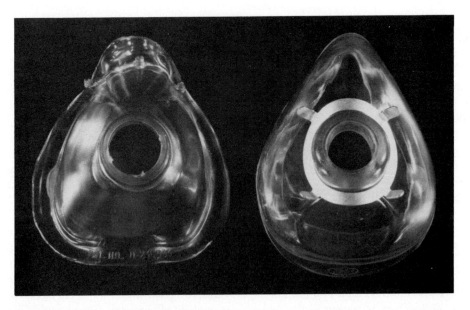

Fig. 7-3. Clear plastic masks are more acceptable and safer than black rubber masks. *Left,* Dryden (Dryden Corporation, 2424 East 55th Place, Indianapolis, Ind. 46220); *right,* Bard Parker (Becton-Dickinson Co., Rutherford, N.J. 07070).

Some degree of hypnosis is involved in almost every inhalation induction. Betcher (1958) has long been an exponent of hypno-induction in children, a favorite ruse being to have the child lose himself in retelling favorite television adventures.

If one is trying to reassure a child, all words with unpleasant connotations should be avoided. These include dizzy, gas, funny smell, cry, hurt, and needles as well as "put you to sleep," for which one can substitute such words as sleep, sweet air, perfume, or sweet smell.

As a patient goes to sleep he may close his eyes and not move, but he may lose consciousness slowly and continue to hear very acutely. Apprehension may increase as he becomes dizzy and disoriented, and he may feel that he is floating off in space, completely helpless and abandoned.

To prevent these sensations, the anesthesiologist must be sure to keep in contact with the patient, continually reminding him by touching him lightly and by telling him that he is all right, everything is fine, and he is going to sleep, going to sleep. . . . The assistant stands quietly beside the patient. Most

children—and many teenagers and adults—appreciate having a hand to hold as they begin to lose control of things.

One must resist the temptation to spring into activity as soon as the child becomes quiet. The anesthesiologist invariably adjusts the head a little, the nurse straightens the hips, and the surgeons have their last joke and then splash cold solutions on the child, who, not being quite asleep, immediately gasps and develops laryngospasm.

It is extremely important to know the signs of early induction and to check them before one disturbs the child. The first sign of early loss of consciousness usually is the appearance of nystagmus, then the eyes close, and the child becomes still. For some time after that he may be only half asleep and will respond to verbal command. One keeps reassuring him and then asks him to take a deep breath. He often obeys, at a point when he appeared to be sound asleep. Until he no longer reacts to one's voice and the lash reflex is gone, one should do nothing to move or stimulate him, unless airway obstruction or similar need arises. Breathing may next become regular and slightly depressed, and

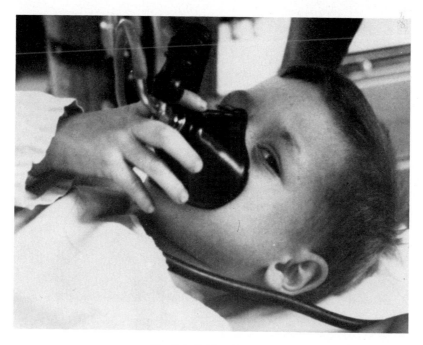

Fig. 7-4. Holding his own.

relaxation gradually increases as the concentration of halothane is advanced to 2.5% or 3.0% in active children. The tongue may fall back, serving as indication for placement of an oral airway. The relaxation of the jaw is noted at this time. With increasing depth, respiration becomes more depressed and should be assisted. Relaxation of the abdominal muscles will become evident, after which the terminal point in inhalation induction comes when the eyes become centered and fixed and the pupils show early constriction. An infusion may be started as soon as the lid reflex is lost, but one should wait for eyeball fixation before attempting intubation or giving the surgeon the word to proceed.

Mechanics of induction

An effective method of induction for healthy children was that of blowing an 8:1 mixture of nitrous oxide and oxygen toward the child's face from a distance of several inches. The fear of accumulating excessive waste gases has made this approach less acceptable, and it is now advisable to reduce the flows to 5 liters of nitrous oxide and 1 liter of oxygen. Trying to accomplish more by persuasion and less by enveloping the child in a cloud of anesthetic, one may use the methods previously described of having the child hold the mask himself, take turns with the anesthesiologist, or count. Another way is to have him take one breath at a time, allowing him to remove the mask in between breaths, while the anesthesiologist carries on an enthusiastic monologue about space men and jet planes.

In this procedure, one must avoid the natural tendency to reduce the nitrous oxide prematurely, before the main anesthetic has reached adequate concentration. Once the stronger agents have been started, halothane, enflurane, or isoflurane may be increased with every two or three breaths as tolerated. Concentrations of 3.5% halothane and 5% enflurane and isoflurane are considered proper limits for induction and should be reduced to approximately 1% and 2% respectively once anesthesia is established.

The widespread use of halothane and

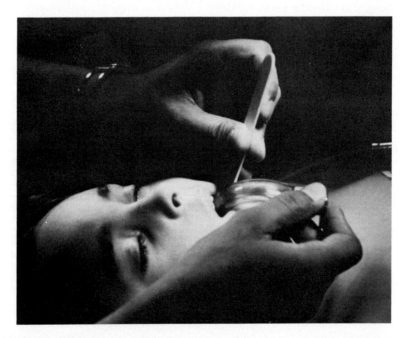

Fig. 7-5. Right way. Pass a tongue depressor (or laryngoscope blade) well in back of the tongue, then press the tongue *forward* and down, and slip the moistened airway over the tongue, with the tip lying free in the hypopharynx.

newer agents has greatly reduced the choking, breath-holding, and vomiting so familiar with ether. Unfortunately enflurane and isoflurane appear to be somewhat more irritating than halothane (Horne and Ahlgren, 1973). Airway obstruction frequently occurs with relaxation of oropharyngeal structures. In addition to elevation of the chin, it is even more important to establish an airtight system with bag and mask and *maintain a moderate but effective pressure (10 to 15 cm H₂O) throughout the entire respiratory cycle* until ventilation becomes unobstructed.

Insertion of an oropharyngeal airway often solves this problem and under halothane is tolerated relatively early in induction; however, it must be inserted correctly. The airway must be large enough to fit behind the tongue and should be inserted with the aid of a tongue depressor to pull the tongue forward (Fig. 7-5). One should avoid the method of inserting the airway upside down to get it past the front teeth and then swinging it around into place (Fig. 7-6). This easily twists out several teeth at once, especially deciduous, decaying, and capped teeth.

If insertion of an airway does not relieve the obstruction, one may continue to apply a moderate amount of manual bag pressure, but if the cords are tightly closed, the use of excessive force simply intensifies the spasm and also may inflate the stomach. If the child is normal, he can tolerate a few moments of spasm. Using 100% oxygen, one can usually squeeze enough through the child's vocal cords to keep him pink and prevent hypoxia. If the child has cardiac disease or if he begins to show bradycardia or cyanosis, one should delay no longer but administer succinylcholine, by vein preferably, and intubate the child as soon as possible.

As compared with airway spasm, vomiting during induction is a rarity. Its prevention and treatment are described in Chapter 26.

The signs of anesthetic depth may be misleading with halogenated anesthetics, since patients often appear to fall asleep rapidly but still have active reflexes. Unless 3 or 4 minutes of induction have passed, one must not attempt endotracheal intubation by such signs. Large, fat individuals and children who have pulmonary disease or shunts, such

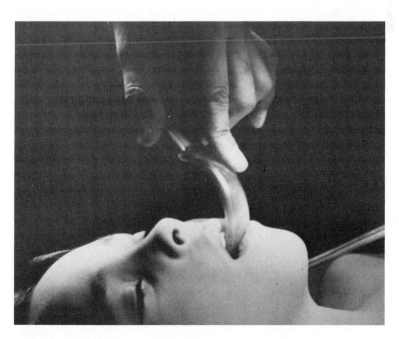

Fig. 7-6. Wrong way. Inserting an inverted airway and rotating it into place looks clever but easily rips out loose or weakened teeth.

as those with cystic fibrosis or tetralogy of Fallot, will take considerably longer to induce than normal children.

Cardiovascular problems during induction may consist of minor arrhythmias and the progressive bradycardia and hypotension denoting excessive concentration of agents.

PARENTAL ATTENDANCE AT INDUCTION

It has been our experience that an intelligent mother can do much to reassure a frightened child. In outpatient areas such a parent is frequently invited to stand beside the child until he has lost consciousness. This proves especially helpful in emergency work, when the child is still upset and often in pain and sedatives have not had time to become effective (Schulman and others, 1967).

There has been increasing pressure from informed parents, often encouraged by psychiatrists, to be allowed to be with their children during induction and recovery phases of major operations (Robertson, 1962; Vernon and others, 1967). Although there has been a traditional sort of resistance to this, it is becoming more obvious that it is not unreasonable and that we might profit considerably by taking a fresh look at the possible advantages to child and parents. One major obstacle at present is the necessity of special areas where induction can be performed outside the operating room, since many modern hospitals have eliminated induction rooms. It is generally agreed that parents (including physicians) should not stay with their children following induction.

THE UNMANAGEABLE CHILD

It has already been suggested that small children may remain resistant and excited in spite of usual medication. For these patients, we prefer to avoid inhalation methods and give rectal thiopental, 20 to 30 mg/kg, allowing 10 minutes for effect prior to moving the child into the operating room. If the child has a readily accessible vein, intravenous induction will save the child from the possibility of delayed awakening.

The most difficult children are those who,

because of mental retardation or severe personality problems, remain entirely unapproachable in spite of all attempts at sedation or persuasion. Although it is often recommended that one should hold the child and "get it over with," forceful mask induction in this situation seems the most brutal method possible. Here the intravenous route becomes the method of choice. Without making the child lie down (or forcibly restraining him), an assistant grasps the child's hand and forearm securely while the anesthesiologist makes the venipuncture. The injection may be felt, but it does not terrorize the child. Induction then may be carried out promptly, to the immediate relief of all; however, it may be preferable to calm the child by partial induction and then try to reduce his fears by reassurance and posthypnotic suggestion.

OTHER INDICATIONS FOR ALTERED INDUCTION TECHNICS

Many pediatric patients require special methods of anesthetic induction. Those with respiratory obstruction at different airway levels, those with a full stomach, "tonsil bleeders," febrile children, others with cardiac or renal disorders, hepatitis, lacerated eyeball, fractured skull, brain tumor, and many other variations all involve special hazards that demand individual consideration. Each of these is discussed in a section devoted to the field involved.

A list of suggested do's and don'ts is offered on p. 156 to summarize important steps and missteps associated with anesthetic induction.

BIBLIOGRAPHY

Albert, S. N., Eccleston, H. N., Boling, J. S., and Albert, C. A.: Basal hypnosis by the administration of a multidose thiobarbiturate suppository, Anesth. Analg. (Cleve.) 35:330, 1956.

Albert, S. N., Henley, E. E., Albert, C. A., and Eccleston, H. N.: Rectal thiopentone in new dosage forms; multidose suppositories or suspension in Abbosert, Anesth. Analg. (Cleve.) 38:56, 1959.

Betcher, A. M.: Hypno-induction techniques in pediatric anesthesia, Anesthesiology 19:279, 1958.

Brodie, B. B.: Physiological disposition and chemical fate of thiobarbiturates in the body, Fed. Proc. 11:632, 1952.

Buchmann, G.: Plasma levels of thiopentone in children after rectal and intravenous administration, Acta Anaesth. Scand. 9:524, 1966.

Dombro, R. H.: The surgically ill child and his family, Surg. Clin. North Am. 50:759, 1970.

Goresky, G. V., and Steward, D. J.: Rectal methohexitone for induction of anaesthesia in children, Can. Anaesth. Soc. J. 26:213, 1979.

Horne, J., and Ahlgren, E. W.: Halothane, enflurane and isoflurane for outpatient surgery; a pediatric case series, report delivered before American Society of Anesthesiology, San Francisco, October 11, 1973.

Kaufman, L.: Anaesthesia for the older child. In Gray, T. C., and Nunn, J. F., editors: General anaesthesia, ed. 3, Borough Green, Kent, 1973, Butterworth & Co., Publishers, Ltd.

Lindsay, W. A., and Shepherd, J.: Plasma levels of thiopentone after pre-medication with rectal suppositories in young children, Br. J. Anaesth. 41:977, 1969.

Miller, J. R., Stoelting, V. K., and Darin, M. W.: A preliminary report on the use of intramuscular methohexital sodium (Brevital) for pediatric anesthesia, Anesth. Analg. (Cleve.) 59:64, 1973.

Nettles, D. C., Herrin, T. J., and Mullen, J. G.: Ketamine induction in poor-risk patients, Anesth. Analg. (Cleve.) 59:64, 1973.

Page, P., Morgan, M., and Loh, L.: Ketamine anaesthesia in paediatric procedures, Acta Anaesth. Scand. 16:155, 1972.

Paymaster, N., Wollman, H., and Bachman, L.: Cyclopropane induction to ether anesthesia in infants and children, Br. J. Anaesth. 37:39, 1965.

Reyber, J.: Hypnosis. In Introduction to psychology; a self selection textbook, Dubuque, Iowa, 1968, William C. Brown, Co., Publishers.

Robertson, J.: Hospitals and children; a parent's eye view, New York, 1962, International Universities Press.

Schulman, J. L., Foley, J. M., Vernon, D. T. A., and Allan, D.: A study of the effect of the mother's presence during anesthesia induction, Pediatrics 39:111, 1967.

Stetson, J. B.: Patient safety; prevention and prompt recognition of regurgitation and aspiration, Anesth. Analg. (Cleve.) 53:142, 1974.

Szasz, T. S.: Illness and indignity, J.A.M.A. 227:543, 1974.

Vernon, D. T. A., Foley, J. M., and Schulman, J. L.: Effect of mother-child separation and birth order on young children's responses to two potentially stressful experiences, J. Pers. Soc. Psychol. 5:162, 1967.

Weinstein, M. L.: Rectal pentothal sodium; new preoperative and basal anesthetic drug in the practice of surgery, Anesth. Analg. (Cleve.) 18:221, 1939.

Wilson, R. D., Nichols, R. J., and McCoy, N. R.: Dissociative anesthesia with CI-581 in burned children, Anesth. Analg. (Cleve.) 46:719, 1967.

Wyant, G. M.: Intramuscular Ketalar (CI-581) in paediatric anaesthesia, Can. Anaesth. Soc. J. 18:72, 1971.

CHAPTER 8

Endotracheal intubation

Advantages
Disadvantages
Indications
Equipment
Technics
Airway and intubation problems

In pediatric anesthesia, the child's airway usually represents the most important and the most insecure factor from the first loss of consciousness throughout the entire operation and well into the recovery period.

Prior to 1940 the use of endotracheal intubation for infants and children was limited to relatively rare occasions, the general belief being that it was too dangerous and traumatic. We are indebted to Deming of Philadelphia and Rees of Liverpool, who, by successful intubation of all their pediatric patients, silenced many critics who had opposed the use of endotracheal tubes in children. At present the majority of pediatric anesthesiologists believe that this procedure, like most, carries inherent hazards and often may be avoided. In representative pediatric centers, the incidence of endotracheal intubation of patients undergoing general anesthesia probably lies between 60% and 75%.

ADVANTAGES

The advantages and disadvantages of intubation of adults are well known. Those related to children differ only slightly. Among the advantages are the following: (1) prevention of aspiration of vomitus (endotracheal intubation is the most reliable means of preventing fatalities in anesthetized patients with full stomach or intestinal obstruction),

(2) prevention of aspiration of blood and tissues from mouth and pharynx, especially in oral, dental, and nasal surgery, (3) control of ventilation in open-chest procedures, apneic states, and resuscitation, (4) ventilatory assistance in the prone position; with children in the face down position, the increased danger of respiratory depression makes endotracheal intubation essential, (5) removal of apparatus from the surgical field (intubation enables the anesthesiologist to relinquish his position and allow the surgeon freedom to work on head, face, or neck), (6) reduction of dead space, and (7) provision for effective clearing of airway by suction.

NOTE: Some may feel that any procedure lasting more than 1 hour calls for intubation. Since a mask is relatively easy to hold on a child's face, and complications as well as anesthetist fatigue increase with added time, intubation for many uncomplicated procedures of 1 to 3 hours would be more advantageous to the anesthetist than to the child.

DISADVANTAGES

The undesirable features of intubation range from minor inconveniences to fatal complications (Flagg, 1951; Gillespie, 1963). They include the following: (1) Narrowing of the airway; the presence of any endotracheal tube significantly reduces the lumen of the child's airway (Orkin and others, 1954; Glauser and others, 1961; Brown and Hustead, 1967). Insertion of the standard adapter inside the tube reduces the lumen even more. (2) At the time of intubation, vocal cord spasm with hypoxia and bradycardia often follows premature attempts at intubation. (3) Loosened and dislodged teeth or lacerations of soft tissues may occur during oral intubation. Nasal intubation adds the danger of hemorrhage from torn mucosal or adenoid tissue (Dingley, 1953). (4) Complications that may occur in intubated patients include passage of the tube beyond the carina with possible collapse of the opposite lung, intubation of the esophagus, obstruction of the tube by kinking, secretions, or biting, and accidental extubation and aspiration of the tube (the only complication not yet personally experienced). (5) Extubation spasm, relatively common after halogenated agents, can be crucial in borderline patients. (6) Postoperative hoarseness, sore throat, tracheal edema, vocal cord ulceration, stricture, and forgotten pharyngeal pack, in that order, should cause increasing concern. A more detailed discussion of the complications is found in Chapter 26.

INDICATIONS

Now that the arguments for and against intubation have been reviewed, situations can be pointed out in which the advantages of intubation outweigh, balance, or are outweighed by the disadvantages, and it can be decided whether intubation is mandatory, preferable, optional, or not indicated (Smith, 1954; Pender, 1954).

Conditions in which endotracheal intubation is mandatory

There are several types of operations in which the advantages of intubation so far outweigh the disadvantages that no patient should be operated on under general anesthesia unless intubation is employed. These include:

1. Operations on patients with full stomach or intestinal obstruction.
2. Intrathoracic procedures.
3. Major operations in the prone position.
4. Intracranial operations.

Conditions in which intubation is definitely preferable

There are operations that are more easily performed with the patient under endotracheal anesthesia but that, under special circumstances, may be managed by nasopharyngeal insufflation or other technics. These include:

1. Operations about the mouth, face, and neck.
2. Operations in the kidney or lateral jackknife position and similar compromising positions.
3. Operations in the upper abdomen.
4. Pneumoencephalogram.
5. If tonsillectomy is performed while the child is sitting up (obsolete Boston technic), intubation is mandatory. If supine, the child should also be intubated, especially if respiratory depressant agents are used. However, it should be noted that some anesthesiologists have insufflated ether for thousands of tonsillectomies without mishap.
6. Infants with pyloric stenosis require special consideration, since they often have 100 ml or more of fluid in their stomachs prior to operation. A sump or Levin tube always must be passed to drain the stomach before anesthesia is started. If the stomach contains only clear, easily removed fluids, an endotracheal tube is not always necessary; however, if barium or milk curds are present, intubation is definitely indicated.

Conditions in which intubation is optional

The following operations are found in this category:

1. Hernia repair in infants and small children.
2. Longer operations on limbs with the patient supine.
3. Minor procedures about the head and neck.
4. Burn dressing and grafting with the patient supine.

Conditions in which intubation is seldom justified

Although experienced personnel may intubate all their patients safely, less skilled individuals, believing this to be the only way, may be led into unnecessary trouble, subjecting children to repeated attempts at intubation with spasm, hypoxia, and tissue damage. Elective procedures that seldom justify intubation include:

1. Short plastic and orthopedic procedures (wire removal, cast change).

2. Perineal operations (circumcision, cystoscopy).
3. Minor surgery on body or limbs.
4. Extraction of three or four milk teeth.
5. Myringotomy.

NOTE: When any of these procedures are performed on an emergency or unscheduled basis, the possible presence of undigested gastric content may automatically make intubation mandatory if general anesthesia is chosen.

EQUIPMENT

Discussion of endotracheal equipment should include consideration of how one should stock the department in which one practices and the care, cleaning, and storage of the equipment, as well as the choice and preparation of the equipment needed for an individual case. Only items of special concern in pediatric patients are discussed.

In an anesthesiology service dealing with a large number of pediatric patients, the wide variety in size of patients, types of pathology, and surgical procedures demands a reasonable assortment of materials. Those that have been found of value in our work at The Children's Hospital Medical Center are listed below.

SUGGESTED ENDOTRACHEAL MATERIALS FOR PEDIATRIC ANESTHESIA SERVICES

Suction devices, permanently fixed in each anesthetizing location, tested daily, metered to minimal 50 cm H_2O suction
Suction catheters, sterile, disposable, vented, sizes 6, 8, 10, 12, and 14
Yankauer tonsil aspirators, plastic or metal
Laryngoscope handles, medium size, lightweight
Laryngoscope blades
  Miller, Nos. 0 (premature), 1 (neonate), 2, and 3
  Macintosh, Nos. 2, 3, and 4
  Wis-Hipple, Nos. 1 and 1½
  Flagg, Nos. 1 and 2
  Kandel, infant
  Phillips, child size
Endotracheal tubes
  Magill, disposable, polyvinylchloride or Silastic, silicone; sizes 2.5 through 7 mm ID, uncuffed; sizes 5 through 8 mm, cuffed
  Cole tubes, sizes 3 through 5 (for diagnostic tracheograms)
  Armored tubes, sizes 3 through 8 mm ID

RAE angled tubes, various types and sizes
Adapters, plastic, straight, for all tubes
Adapters, metal, curved at acute, right, and obtuse angles for operations about the face
Adapter extensions, flexible, metal or rubber
Magill forceps, child and adult sizes
Stylets, Teflon coated, for tube sizes 2.5 to 8.0 mm ID
  Norton, flexible metallic endotracheal tubes, sizes 2.5 through 6 mm ID
  Red rubber Magill endotracheal tubes, sizes 2.5 through 6 mm ID, to be wound with metallic tape for laser surgery of trachea
Lidocaine analgesic lubricant
Fine-spray atomizers
Guedel oropharyngeal airways, sizes 0, 1, 2, and 3
Tongue blades, wooden
Bite blocks

Additional equipment to be immediately available

Bronchoscopic equipment, infant, child, and adult sizes
Anterior commissurescopes
Fiberoptic laryngoscope and bronchoscope
Large-bore needles, short bevel, 12, 14, and 16 gauge
Tracheostomy equipment

The care and cleaning of this material is similar to that used for adults. It is extremely important to keep such essential equipment where it is most easily available in situations in which replacements of supplemental items are needed in a hurry.

Whether one is outfitting a department or preparing equipment for an individual patient, choice of each item will depend on a number of criteria. In the following material an attempt is made to point out some of the more important features by which one may be guided.

Laryngoscopes

More than 100 different laryngoscopes have been advocated during recent years, proving the difficulty involved in designing one that suits all purposes. Handles of standard length are suitable for pediatric use, and although those of smaller diameter may be easier to manipulate, the batteries become exhausted rather quickly. The medium-sized handle is generally more practical, and one of lighter weight now available is especially useful.

In evaluation of laryngoscope blades, the length is of obvious importance, but additional features to note are width and shape of the tip, bore, curvature, and metallic finish.

Inexperienced anesthetists often underestimate the size of a child's face and mouth, using masks, airways, and laryngoscopes that are too small. A laryngoscope blade that is too short or too narrow will not give adequate exposure and will make intubation more difficult and more traumatic. Heavy, wide blades are to be avoided in small children, but it is better to use a long, slender blade such as the No. 2 Miller for a 3-year-old child than the No. 1 Miller, which is intended for a neonate. If one uses a very long blade, such as the No. 3 Miller, on a small child, one has a strong tendency to use it as a lever and pry the mouth open, with resultant pressure on upper teeth, lip, and maxilla. Use of a straight blade requires slightly more relaxa-tion than a curved blade but gives a better exposure in children. The curved tip of the Miller blades makes it possible to retract the epiglottis, as with a Macintosh blade, rather than lift it (Fig. 8-1). With infants, the wider bore of the Wis-Hipple, Flagg, and Kandel blades enables one to see and to pass a tube more easily than with the flattened aperture of the Miller blades. For older children the flatter No. 2 Miller blade becomes more advantageous, since it is less likely to chip large new incisor teeth. The blade designed by Phillips and Duerksen (1973), with a more pronounced terminal curve, has been particularly useful in more difficult situations. For teenage children with stronger jaws and larger mouths, a cuffed endotracheal tube often will be chosen. Then it is usually easier to employ the Macintosh curved blade, which allows more room to pass the bulky cuff. The small curved blade (No. 2 Macintosh) occasionally is useful in special situa-

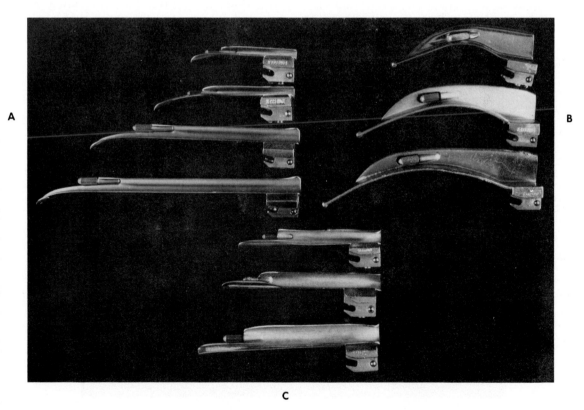

Fig. 8-1. Standard laryngoscope blades employed in pediatric anesthesia: **A,** Miller Nos. 0, 1, 2, and 3. **B,** Macintosh Nos. 2, 3, and 4. **C,** Flagg Nos. 1, 2, and 3.

tions, as in a small child with an ankylosed jaw or in burn contractures of the neck.

The light bulb deserves special attention. For small patients it is important to have the bulb near the tip of the blade. One finds considerable variation in this feature (Fig. 8-2). If the bulb is more than ½ inch from the tip, the soft tissues of the infant's pharynx will close around it and obstruct the light. The larger bulb will carry more light and will be more durable but may obstruct passage of tubes in infants. In some laryngoscopes the bulb is recessed so that it is difficult to change or clean. Conversely, many British blades are built with the bulb on an independent carrier (Fig. 8-3). This is slightly clumsy to use but great for maintenance.

It should be emphasized that when testing a laryngoscope, one should be sure that the light is *white*. One is tempted to accept any bulb that lights, but a yellow or orange light denotes a failing battery or poor connection, and the light obtained may prove quite inadequate. The metal finish of the blade, if shiny, may cause excess reflection; thus, a dull finish is preferable.

It is advisable to have laryngoscopes of several different sizes for pediatric patients because of the wide variation in age, size, and underlying disease. For those who engage in pediatric anesthesia only occasionally, it is suggested that the combination of the Wis-Hipple No. 1 and Miller No. 2 blades will prove the most useful two-blade set (Fig. 8-4). One may start with these and add to them as the occasion arises. When possible, several should be available.

In addition to this equipment, bronchoscopic apparatus should be available at all times for use by the anesthesia service. The anterior commissurescope with slanting leading edge is an excellent instrument for penetrating resistant vocal cords.

Fiberoptic instruments now provide the most effective assistance in difficult intubation (Stiles and others, 1972; Taylor and Towley, 1972; Davis, 1973). Fiberoptic bronchoscopes and laryngoscopes are undergoing

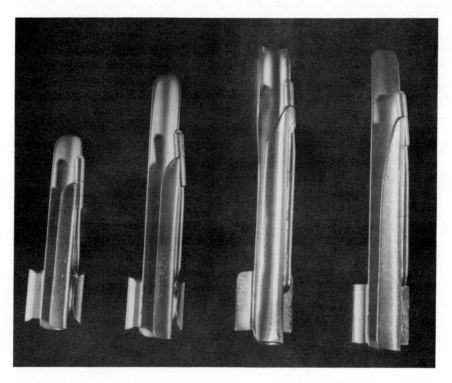

Fig. 8-2. Infant laryngoscope blades *(left to right):* Miller No. 0 (premature), Miller No. 1, Flagg No. 1, Wis-Hipple.

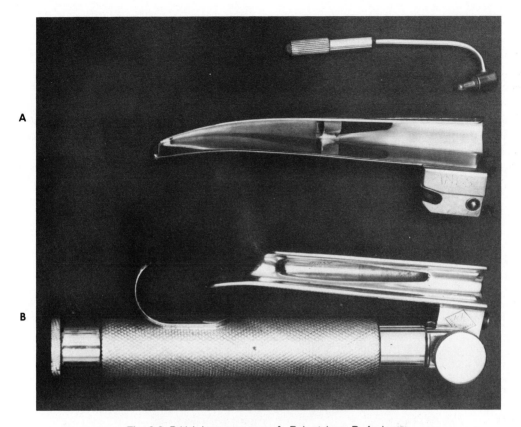

Fig. 8-3. British laryngoscopes: **A,** Robertshaw. **B,** Anderson.

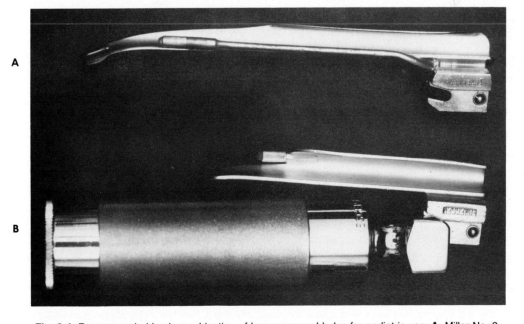

Fig. 8-4. Recommended basic combination of laryngoscope blades for pediatric use: **A,** Miller No. 2. **B,** Wis-Hipple infant blade.

rapid development. At present, as described by Stiles and associates, the bronchoscope is preferable to smaller laryngoscopes because it has a channel intended for passage of a biopsy forceps. The Stiles technic is to advance the bronchoscope until the glottis is visualized and then to pass a cardiac catheter through the channel and down into the trachea. Next, the bronchoscope is withdrawn and a slightly heavier catheter is slipped over the first, to be followed by the endotracheal tube. This method can be used for neonates.

Endotracheal tubes

Any one of several styles of endotracheal tubes may be used for infants and children provided that the individual tube has the proper characteristics. Of the tubes currently favored, the Magill uniform-bore tube is the standard form that can be used for most purposes (Fig. 8-5). It is flexible, easily manipu-

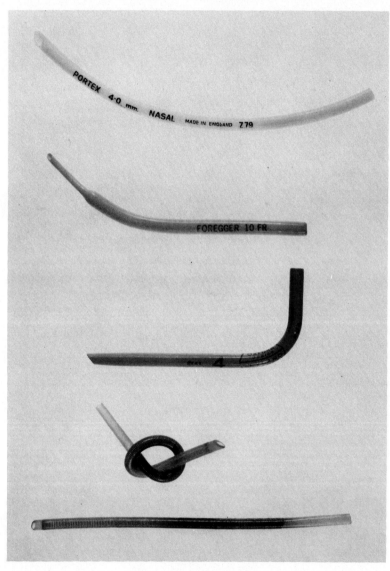

Fig. 8-5. Endotracheal tubes used in pediatric anesthesia *(top to bottom):* Magill, plastic, marked Z-79; Cole, tapered rubber or plastic; Oxford, with right-angle curve; armored tubes, tied in knot and extended.

lated, and may be cut to suit individual needs and preferences. All tubes for pediatric use should have relatively short bevels. An additional hole a short distance from the tip is advantageous.

The reduction of the airway lumen caused by insertion of an adapter of smaller bore formerly was of some significance. The present thin-walled adapters and more expandable tubes have virtually eliminated this problem in all but the smallest sizes.

Disposable endotracheal tubes are now used extensively in the United States and elsewhere and are packaged with a suitable adapter. One should remember to insert the adapter firmly before use and also refrain from resterilizing polyvinylchloride tubes with ethylene oxide (Rendell-Baker and Roberts, 1969).

In 1945 Cole introduced the tapered tube for pediatric use, designed so that only the terminal portion could pass through the vocal cords (Fig. 8-5). The wide remaining portion facilitates air exchange (Glauser and others, 1961) and attachment of an adapter but seriously impedes vision during intubation. Since the shoulder of the tube rides on the vocal cords, use of the tube for prolonged periods, especially for ventilatory therapy, invites cord trauma and is contraindicated (Branstater, 1969). The major problem in the use of Cole tubes has been the tendency of inexperienced persons to choose tubes with tips that are much too narrow and lead to resistance and occlusion. Several infants sent to our hospital with Cole tubes in place have been seriously or fatally affected by this error.

The angulated Oxford endotracheal tube (Fig. 8-5) is believed by some to follow the anatomic lines of the airway more closely. However, intubation is considerably more difficult and requires use of a stylet. Its greatest drawback is the resistance that the angulation offers to passage of suction catheters. In pediatric work, we prefer to avoid curvature of endotracheal tube and adapter whenever possible.

Armored, or anode, endotracheal tubes (Fig. 8-5), consisting of thin latex reinforced by coiled wire, have the advantage of tolerating extreme flexion without kinking. In limited situations they prove valuable, but they have a tendency to become dislodged, the thin latex is easily perforated (Cohen and Dillon, 1972), and there have been reports of many other complications during their use. We prefer Magill tubes for neurosurgical procedures, reserving the anode tubes for exceptional operations about the face.

The Norton metallic endotracheal tube, introduced in 1978 for use during laser surgery of the trachea, is made of coiled metal similar to the sheathing used to cover wire cables. Its application is described in Chapter 21.

Cuffed endotracheal tubes. The addition of an inflatable cuff to the endotracheal tube is especially undesirable in children, since this makes it necessary to use a tube with an internal diameter (ID) at least 1 mm smaller, an important difference in an infant. Fortunately, in children under 6 or 7 years of age the tracheal tissues fit more snugly around the tube, especially at the level of the cricoid cartilage (Colgan and Keats, 1957), and cuffed tubes in sizes less than 5.5 mm ID are seldom needed. In our practice, we use cuffed tubes of 5.5 mm ID or larger.

Stylets. Intubation of normal children rarely calls for use of stylets, and their use is apt to complicate the procedure. Extraction of the stylet after passage of the tube sometimes is difficult, inviting spasm and hypoxia, and the presence of a stiff, pointed object always adds potential trauma. A stylet may help when patients have anatomic abnormalities, however, and should be kept available. Siliconized wire, manufactured for this use, is preferable, but soft copper wire, cut to desired length and with ends turned to avoid injury, is practical and effective.

Criteria for endotracheal tubes. The ideal endotracheal tube should fulfill several requirements. It should (1) have sufficient internal diameter to allow adequate air exchange and passage of a suction catheter, (2) have sufficient strength to prevent collapse or kinking, (3) have sufficient softness to be malleable and prevent laceration of tissues by the pointed edge, (4) be composed of nonirritant material, (5) be clean enough to preclude contamination, and (6) if resterilized, be free of any chemical cleansing agent.

When tracheal intubation was first employed in children, methods were admittedly crude, and surgeons reported numerous instances of gross trauma to mouth, pharynx, and vocal cords. Little attention was paid to cleansing tubes until the hazards of tracheitis were emphasized (Smith, 1953; Zindler and Deming, 1953). Endotracheal tubes initially were made of rubber, often thick and irritant or thin and collapsible.

Concern over airflow resistance and increased work of breathing during spontaneous respiration led to numerous studies of endotracheal tube design (Macon and Bruner, 1950; Orkin and others, 1954; Glauser and others, 1961; Cave and Fletcher, 1968). Emphasis on reduction of airflow resistance hastened the development of better tubes and led to the use of the largest tubes possible. Reduction of airway dead space was also considered a valuable feature in endotracheal intubation. This has become less impressive since routine arterial gas measurements have revealed a tendency to overventilate patients during anesthesia (probably more than is good for them). In like fashion, the increased tendency to assist or control respiration eliminates inspiratory work and the importance of reducing inspiratory airway resistance. Also, fear of increased expiratory resistance is dispelled by reported benefits of positive end-expiratory pressure (PEEP) in many situations.

Real concern over airflow resistance during anesthesia has thus shifted considerably and now centers on elimination of valves that carry increased danger of sticking or malfunction and on elimination of endotracheal tubes that easily become kinked or occluded or cannot be effectively cleared (e.g., Oxford tubes) or any tubes attached to curved adapters. Lesser degrees of resistance imposed by minor reduction of tube lumen have been of importance chiefly during weaning from ventilators if patients must breathe without assistance. This situation has become relatively

uncommon since the introduction of intermittent mandatory ventilation (IMV).

Two important features of endotracheal tubes are the composition of the tube and the method of sterilization. Early endotracheal tubes of red rubber have given way to plastics such as polyvinylchloride. Though plastic materials have a smoother surface, tissue irritation has occurred with many of the tubes and was shown by Guess and Stetson (1968) to be caused in part by organotin compounds used as stabilizing agents in the manufacture of polymers. With prolonged use, the organotin leaches out of the tube, causing inflammatory tissue reaction. Manufacturers have been alerted to this, and tubes should now bear the mark Z-79 or IT (implant tested) to show that they come from a lot that has been tested and proved to be free of irritants. Silicone (Silastic) is the least irritating of all plastics yet tried, and endotracheal and tracheostomy tubes of this material are in great favor. They can be autoclaved, do not deteriorate with time, are soft, and do not stick to tissue.

Several problems have arisen concerning sterilization of endotracheal tubes. Ethylene oxide is effective, but unless the tubes are aired for 72 hours or air-cleaned in a special chamber (Thomas and Levy, 1970), retained ethylene oxide can act as a severe irritant (Winchell and Davis, 1965; Rendell-Baker and Roberts, 1969). Other methods such as boiling, autoclaving, or soaking in sterilizing solutions may shorten the life of most tubes (Bosomworth and Hamelberg, 1965). In the United States, the conversion to sterile disposable endotracheal tubes has largely solved the problem of resterilization. Whether this change will bring appreciable reduction in the incidence of tracheal irritation has not yet become evident.

Preparation of equipment

When intubation of an infant or child is intended, preparation is of increased importance because of the mobility of the child's head, the insecurity of the tube, and the relatively heavy equipment attached to it. After insertion of the tube, the anesthesiologist must not abandon it to tear tape or look for adapters. *All of the necessary equipment should be fully prepared before induction of anesthesia* (see below).

When intubation is not intended, as in herniorraphy or circumcision, suitable laryngoscope, endotracheal tube, and suction catheters should be at hand for emergency use, but additional equipment need not be prepared beforehand.

EQUIPMENT TO BE PREPARED FOR INDIVIDUAL TRACHEAL INTUBATION

All cases

Suction catheters, two that will pass easily through endotracheal tubes of anticipated size (this is the most frequently neglected item)
Suction catheters, two of larger size, for clearing nose, mouth, and pharynx
Laryngoscope
Endotracheal tubes, three sizes—the expected size plus the next size larger and the next size smaller
Lubricant: lidocaine jelly or spray or clean water
Clean syringe, if cuffed tube is to be used
Nasogastric tube
Oropharyngeal airways, expected size and one size larger
Tape, torn and ready for use
Head ring or small pillow

Special indications

Nasotracheal intubation
    Longer endotracheal tubes
    Magill forceps (small size for children under 6 years old)
    4% cocaine solution
Full stomach
    Bite block
    Mouth gag
    Tonsil suction instrument
    Additional large and small suction catheters
    Larger-bore nasogastric tube
Expected difficult intubation
    Several different laryngoscope blades
    Stylet
    Magill forceps
    Endotracheal tubes with different curvatures
    Anterior commissurescope
    Fiberoptic bronchoscope or laryngoscope
    Bronchoscopic equipment and tracheostomy materials immediately available
    Surgical assistance available

The choice of a suitable laryngoscope is seldom difficult. The choice of a proper endotracheal tube is of utmost importance, and mistakes are both common and costly.

The type of tube, whether Magill, Cole, or Oxford, is largely a matter of personal preference, as is the choice between disposable and reusable tubes.

It is the size (diameter) of the endotracheal tube that is the most critical aspect. Although a tube that is too small may demand more respiratory effort, one that is too large may cause the development of laryngotracheal edema. There is little margin for error, but it appears preferable to avoid an oversized tube at all costs.

Various methods have been devised for choice of correct diameter of endotracheal tubes. Some use the lumen of the external naris or the diameter of the little finger (distal joint) as a guide to the size of the glottic chink.

Several formulas to determine the proper tube diameter have been suggested and prove useful but not exact:

Cole's formula (1957):

$$\text{Tube size (Fr)} = \text{Age in years} + 17$$

Penlington's formula (1972):

For children under 6 years old:

$$\text{Tube size (mm ID)} = \frac{\text{Age (yr)}}{3} + 3.5$$

For children 6 years and over:

$$\text{Tube size (mm ID)} = \frac{\text{Age (yr)}}{3} + 4.5$$

The logical basis for choice of endotracheal tube size would seem to be actual anatomic measurement. Considerable data have been obtained by postmortem dissection (Engel, 1962; Butz, 1968) and in living subjects by instrumentation with graduated bougies (Chodoff and Helrich, 1967; Keep and Manford, 1974; Mostafa, 1976) and by roentgenographic studies (Wittenborg and associates, 1967; Donaldson and Thompsett, 1952). Although such measurements demonstrate the dimensional range of the developing trachea, the variation is so great that measurements are not dependable for accurate selection of endotracheal tubes whether related to age, weight, or body length. Table 8-1 from the detailed study of Butz (1968) is informative,

173

Table 8-1. Tracheal length and cross-section areas in children of various ages

Specimen number	Age	Height (in)	Weight (lb)	Trachea length (mm)	Tracheal origin Size (mm)	Tracheal origin Area (mm²)	I	Midtrachea Size (mm)	Midtrachea Area (mm²)	I
213-66	Hours	14.0	1.8	22.0	2.0 × 2.6	4.08	.97	1.3 × 2.8	2.86	.76
221-61	Hours	12.4	3.1	29.0	2.6 × 3.6	7.34	.95	2.1 × 4.0	6.60	.82
112A62	26 days	18.0	4.7	32.0	3.9 × 4.1	12.55	.99	3.1 × 3.2	7.78	.99
102A62	2 days	18.0	5.1	32.0	4.0 × 4.0	12.55	1.00	2.9 × 4.8	10.92	.88
244-61	12 hr	18.4	5.6	29.0	4.0 × 4.4	13.82	.99	2.6 × 4.0	8.16	.91
39A62	8 days	21.2	7.0	34.0	3.9 × 4.0	12.26	1.00	2.8 × 4.0	8.80	.94
139-60	9 days	21.4	7.2	38.0	4.1 × 5.1	16.41	.98	2.4 × 5.2	9.80	.82
11-61	24 hr	19.5	7.4	32.0	3.8 × 3.9	11.65	1.00	2.6 × 4.6	9.40	.86
75A65	3 wk	20.5	7.8	37.0	3.6 × 4.6	13.00	.95	3.6 × 5.4	15.26	.92
13A65	2 mo	21.4	8.3	39.0	4.5 × 4.7	16.60	1.00	3.7 × 4.9	14.24	.96
4A61	4.5 mo	22.5	8.4	41.0	4.7 × 5.0	18.46	1.00	2.9 × 5.5	12.53	.82
31A63	4 mo	21.4	8.8	37.0	4.4 × 4.4	15.20	1.00	3.5 × 4.4	12.10	.97
48A64	4 mo	25.4	14.2	46.0	4.1 × 4.1	13.20	1.00	4.1 × 5.3	17.08	.97
17A65	4 mo	25.5	15.2	46.0	4.4 × 4.5	15.56	1.00	4.3 × 5.5	18.58	.97
77-66	5 mo	28.5	16.1	45.0	4.5 × 5.9	20.86	.96	3.9 × 6.2	19.00	.88
50A65	1 yr	29.0	25	48.0	4.9 × 4.9	18.86	1.00	4.0 × 6.7	21.06	.89
19A66	2 yr	—	32	54.0	5.8 × 6.6	30.10	.99	5.1 × 6.6	26.46	.97
34A63	3 yr	40.6	40	58.0	6.8 × 7.0	37.4	1.00	6.0 × 9.0	42.5	.92
11A66	4 yr	36.5	50	54.0	6.9 × 6.9	37.4	1.00	5.3 × 7.9	32.9	.90
199-66	10 yr	54.5	55	71.0	8.2 × 10.2	65.7	.98	8.0 × 11.2	70.4	.95
150-65	9 yr	53.0	69	66.0	8.4 × 9.4	62.0	.99	8.0 × 12.0	75.4	.92
41A66	10 yr	—	91	69.0	6.9 × 8.0	43.3	.99	7.9 × 8.2	50.9	1.00
123-65	15 yr	61.8	130	74.0	11.6 × 11.8	107.5	1.00	7.3 × 11.1	63.6	.92
68-65	14 yr	56.0	155	76.0	11.1 × 12.1	105.4	1.00	13.6 × 14.1	150.6	1.00

From Butz, R. O., Jr.: Length and cross-section growth patterns in the human trachea, Pediatrics **42:**336, 1968. Copyright American Academy of Pediatrics 1968.

although postmortem shrinkage may have introduced some error.

For choice of tube diameter, our preference has been to use a table similar to that of Slater and associates (1955) based on our own experience and related to age, which not only is the simplest correlate to follow but, as shown by Chodoff and Helrich (1967), is the most accurate. This table (Table 8-2) is posted above the endotracheal storage area. One chooses the tube indicated by the chart and also takes the next larger and next smaller tubes. Of these three, one should be correct. Tube diameters listed here tend to be smaller than in some previous charts, since we aim to have some leak around every tube as evidence that size is not excessive.

Much concern has also been shown in establishing the proper lengths for oral and nasal endotracheal tubes at different ages

(Shellinger, 1964; Fearon and Whalen, 1967; Coldiron, 1968; Mattila and others, 1971). While it is unhealthy for the tube either to extend beyond the carina or to be retracted above the vocal cords, anatomic variations again prove too great to allow reliance on any predetermined reference scale.

The length of tubing that extends out of the mouth is an important safety factor. We prefer to have at least 4 cm extend beyond the lips so that the adhesive tape may be fixed to the tube itself, rather than the adapter. Should tube and adapter become separated, the tube would still be held by the tape and could not pass into the trachea. The added 4 cm is further insurance that the tube will not pass beyond the cords if, by any chance, it should be aspirated (no such aspiration has occurred in our experience).

Rather than estimating the position of

TABLE 8-2

Age or weight	Endotracheal tube size			Suction catheter (French)
	Internal diameter (mm)	External diameter (French)	Length (cm)	
Under 1500 g	**2.5** uncuffed	12	8	6
Newborn-6 mo	**3.0** uncuffed	14	10	6
6-18 mo	**3.5** uncuffed	16	12	8
18 mo-**3** yr	**4.0** uncuffed	18	14	8
3-5 yr	**4.5** uncuffed	20	16	8
5-6 yr	**5.0** uncuffed	22	16	10
6-8 yr	**5.5** cuffed	24	18	10
8-10 yr	**6.0** cuffed	26	18	10
10-12 yr	**6.5** cuffed	28	20	12
12-14 yr	**6.5** cuffed	28	20	12
14-16 yr	♂ **7.0** cuffed	30	22	12
	♀ **6.5** cuffed	28		
16-21 yr	♂ **7.5** cuffed	32	22	12
	♀ **7.0** cuffed	30		

NOTE: Endotracheal tube should fit so as to allow full expansion of both lungs on manual inflation but allow a definite leak with pressure of 20 to 25 cm H_2O.

ENDOTRACHEAL TUBE SIZE

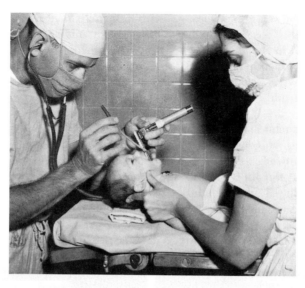

Fig. 8-8. Intubation of the awake infant requires correct positioning of the head. Infant should be held with the head extended and the shoulders down to prevent arching of the back.

keeps it in his right hand until time for insertion. He should not have to grope around for the tube on the table behind him after exposing the glottis. With the infant's head held in the "sniffing" position, the anesthesiologist dips the blade of the laryngoscope into warm water and then inserts the tip over the infant's tongue, gently opening the mouth and sweeping the tongue to the left. Due to the remarkable incidence of nosocomial infections in the newborn, *fingers are not used to pry open the mouth.* The blade is advanced slowly, so that *the baby continues to breathe and cry,* even when the glottis has been exposed. If the baby chokes or stops breathing, the laryngoscope is withdrawn just enough to let him breathe and then advanced again. The blade should not be completely withdrawn from the mouth, for then the entire process must be started all over again.

To overcome the large tongue, one must resist the temptation to pull back on the handle of the laryngoscope and instead lift it forcibly in the direction of the handle, so that the blade does not touch the upper jaw. At this point the glottis should be visualized but may appear too far anterior to allow intubation. The assistant can now depress the larynx down and caudalward to bring the glottis

into position. A much superior method is for the anesthesiologist to do this himself. By holding the laryngoscope near the blade, one can use the little finger of the left hand to position and hold the glottis precisely as needed (Fig. 8-9). This maneuver is also seen in illustrations in the work of Wilton and Wilson (1965) and Gregory (1974).

Four centimeters separate the infant's vocal cords from the carina, so the tip of the tube should be advanced 2 cm beyond the cords (Fig. 8-10). The tube must be held firmly until checked for position by visible motion of the chest and by auscultation; then it is taped in place and the anesthesia apparatus attached.

Intubation under general anesthesia alone

Although intubation of anesthetized or relaxed patients can more nearly approach perfection, all methods involve potential hazards. Picking the right moment for intubation is a ticklish matter, for a premature attempt may induce anoxic spasm, while delay invites cardiac depression.

Under ether anesthesia, signs of regular respiration, general relaxation, and fixed, dilating pupils are easy to read. With cyclo-

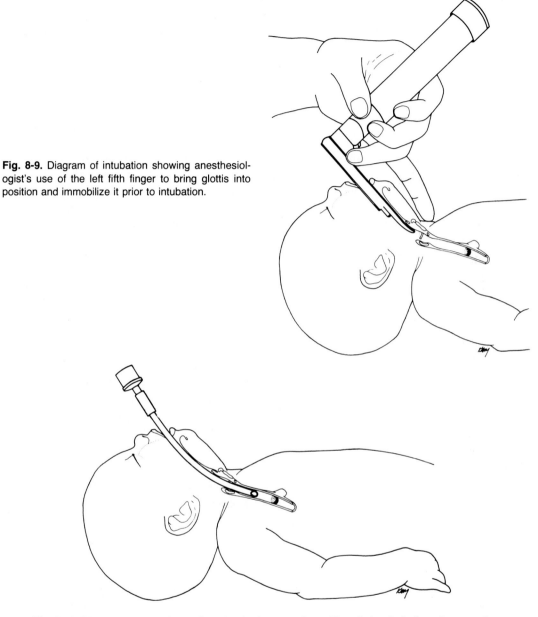

Fig. 8-9. Diagram of intubation showing anesthesiologist's use of the left fifth finger to bring glottis into position and immobilize it prior to intubation.

Fig. 8-10. Diagram showing the endotracheal tube properly positioned, the tip halfway between the vocal cords and carina.

propane and halogenated agents, respiratory depression and muscular relaxation progress rapidly and with less recognizable signs. After an infant has remained motionless and apneic, it is natural to assume that he is ready for intubation, but one is often badly mistaken. When halothane is used, unless there have been 2 or 3 minutes of gradual induction with good ventilatory exchange and 3.0% to 3.5% concentration for at least 1 minute, an attempt at intubation is apt to be met with active responses, often severe laryngospasm. For intubation under halothane one must come dangerously close to overdosage, with sudden bradycardia and hypotension. If attempting this method, one must use full atropinization beforehand and be on strict guard against change in heart rate or blood pressure. This danger is reduced in older children but is sufficient to make the method one to avoid in infants.

When this approach is used in older children, signs of increasing depth and time for intubation are immobility, loss of eyelash and eyelid response, apnea, jaw relaxation, flaccidity of arms and hands, relaxation of abdominal muscles, and centrally fixed eyeballs with beginning pupillary fixation. An infant's eyes should not be pried open for this purpose, but in children more than 6 months old this is the most reliable sign of suitable depth for intubation (after the child has been asleep for several minutes). The child whose eyes are still upturned is not ready for intubation, and to attempt it is a definite mistake. Since respiration becomes depressed as the level of anesthesia deepens, one must first assist and then control ventilation in order to gain adequate concentrations for intubation. If one is not overzealous, this can be done without forcing air into the stomach, since the child usually is ready to intubate before the esophagus loses its natural tone.

Use of relaxant alone

For intubation of the uncomplicated newborn, intramuscular succinylcholine seems definitely superior to all other methods. While many prefer an apneic dose of 2 mg/kg, it is safer to reduce this to 1.0 to 1.5 mg/kg, with the intention to reduce struggling but allow the infant to maintain his own oxygenation. Before intramuscular succinylcholine is given, atropine is advised but is not mandatory. It may be given (0.1 mg) by intravenous route within 30 minutes before anesthesia and is effective within 30 seconds. By intramuscular route, 0.2 mg of atropine may be given from 5 to 45 minutes before anesthesia but should not be given simultaneously with succinylcholine, since the initial vagal slowing of atropine and that of succinylcholine can be dangerous when acting together.

With intramuscular succinylcholine, the technic of intubation is similar to that used in awake intubation but greatly simplified. The stethoscope is applied and oxygen is administered, but topical lidocaine is omitted (it has been shown that relaxants reduce responses and that awake subjects tolerate intubation without discomfort). Ventilation is assisted as the relaxant becomes effective. Biceps tone decreases, and after 90 to 120 seconds the infant is still breathing spontaneously but hyperactivity is gone. The jaw can be opened without resistance and the glottis easily exposed, immobile and open, allowing accurate evaluation of tube size needed and immediate intubation. If the tube is too large, resistance will be sensed as it is introduced, and it can be changed. Anesthesia apparatus is promptly attached, the infant is oxygenated, the aeration of both lungs is checked to confirm tube position, and the tube is taped in place. After intubation there will be less danger of spasm and breath-holding than with inhalation methods.

Intramuscular succinylcholine can also be used for larger children but has less marked advantage. Since intubation is less hazardous and more easily performed and veins are more accessible, the intravenous route is usually chosen.

Use of general anesthesia plus relaxant

The two methods most frequently used for children beyond infancy are general anesthesia with additional intravenous relaxant and conventional intravenous induction with thiopental and relaxant. The management of both methods is much the same for children as for adults. When general anesthesia is used, one starts with nitrous oxide and adds halothane to establish an even, light plane, seldom using more than a 2% concentration and thus avoiding danger of any cardiac depression. The infusion is placed, and atropine is added if none has been given within 45 minutes, followed by succinylcholine (approximately 1.5 mg/kg as described in Chapter 13). Preliminary administration of an antidepolarizing agent has not appeared necessary prior to adolescence.

This method is popular with children who fear needles. It is relatively fast and allows maximal ease of intubation. Since children often have airway obstruction, and hypoxia develops rapidly, it is not to be used for patients in whom intubation may be difficult.

If *d*-tubocurarine is used for intubation of infants, one should be warned that apnea occurs almost immediately after administration.

Use of intravenous anesthetic plus relaxant

For anesthesiologists who prefer an intravenous anesthetic for induction, this is the standard technic. If there is an easily entered vein, it is a quick and effective approach. Administration of atropine, thiopental, and succinylcholine followed by immediate apnea, flaccidity, intubation, fixation of tube, and establishment of controlled ventilation all can be accomplished in less than 2 minutes under most circumstances. In healthy, well-prepared children and adolescents this is a popular and acceptable method. It also carries maximum potential for dangerous complications. While a child's intense aversion to needles and the absence of suitable veins should be considered reasonable contraindications, it is my belief that *any airway problem or gastrointestinal distension should be considered a major contraindication to intravenous anesthetic induction for endotracheal intubation.* In the presence of airway or ventilatory problems, it is inexcusable to induce apnea with relaxants unless one is certain that respiration can be carried on passively. Similarly, in patients with distension, the complete flaccidity that follows intravenous relaxants calls for both speed and dexterity to prevent regurgitation and aspiration. As described in Chapter 22, methods that require neither the headlong haste nor the superior skill of the "crash" induction are more dependable for standard use in critical situations.

Use of morphine, hypnotic, and topical anesthetic

Since the introduction of naloxone (Narcan), morphine has become extremely valuable as a controllable agent for safe, gradual anesthetic induction of patients with severe airway problems or cardiorespiratory disease. Given a child with fracture of cervical vertebrae, retropharyngeal abscess, or cardiac failure, one can administer increments of 0.5 to 1.0 mg of morphine, add enough hydroxyzine or diazepam to produce light sleep, and apply generous topical lidocaine spray. Adequate anesthesia can be obtained for visualization of the glottis and intubation without evident respiratory or cardiac depression and without stimulation of laryngeal responses. Should there be any morphine excess, it can be promptly reversed with naloxone. This relatively unappreciated method is probably the most useful for a variety of difficult situations and offers greater safety, controllability, and patient acceptability than any other, with minimal requirement for expert manipulative ability. It is especially valuable in many situations in which awake intubation had previously been chosen in adults but for which no satisfactory method had been found for children.

Nasal intubation

The nasal route of intubation is indicated for a number of operations about the mouth and face, and we prefer to use it when patients are expected to require postoperative ventilatory assistance, since the tube can be more securely fixed, is less irritating, and cannot be bitten. Nasal intubation is more difficult to perform and can start profuse hemorrhage from the nose or pharynx (Dingley, 1953). Furthermore, pieces of adenoid can be torn away, and these and other scrapings may be carried into the trachea, increasing the danger of pulmonary infection (Davenport and Rosales, 1959; Berry and others, 1973).

Before starting anesthesia one should check the patency of the nares by having the child breathe through his nose while each nostril is blocked off successively (Block and Brechner, 1973). One frequently finds that one nostril is larger than the other and thus a better one to use. If either nostril is not patent, one should look for the cause. (We recently withdrew the metal eraser-end of a pencil from the nostril of an unsuspecting 3-year-old.)

In preadolescent children one may expect to use uncuffed tubes of the same size that would be required for oral intubation. Older patients may require a nasal tube that is a half or full size smaller, with cuff. Nasal tubes should be approximately 20% longer than oral tubes. Special equipment should include topical spray (4% lidocaine) and child- or adult-sized Magill forceps.

Nasal intubation may be expected to take longer, and consequently one needs a well-established plane of anesthesia. Spontaneous respiration lends an extra factor of safety but is not mandatory. In addition to analgesic jelly on the endotracheal tube, use of topical spray to the nostrils, pharynx, and glottis prolongs the period available for manipulation and reduces the chance of inducing laryngeal responses. A nasal decongestant may be useful if the turbinates appear swollen.

When the child is suitably anesthetized, nasal intubation is started by elevating the tip of the nose and inserting the tube *horizontally* along the floor of the nasal cavity (if pointed toward the eyes, as frequently attempted, the tube must gouge its way through the turbinates to reach the nasopharynx). When properly directed, the tube may meet mild resistance, which often may be overcome by gently rotating the tube as it is advanced. Solid obstruction should be taken as a sign to desist.

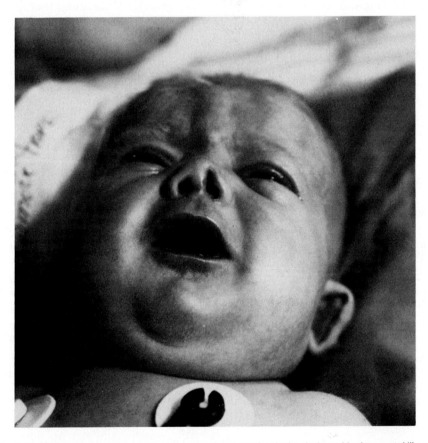

Fig. 8-11. Nasal ulceration caused by pressure of endotracheal tube during critical neonatal illness.

As previously noted, there is distinct danger of shearing off adenoidal tissue in children, with bothersome bleeding and additional danger that pieces of adenoid will either be carried into the trachea or remain as obstructing plugs in the tube. To prevent this, one can insert a suction catheter through the endotracheal tube, its tip projecting slightly beyond the end of the tube and thus acting as a guide and a foil as the tube is advanced.

When the tube has reached the pharynx, the laryngoscope is passed to visualize tube and glottis. It may be possible by elevating the head to maneuver the glottis into position to receive the endotracheal tube; otherwise a Magill forceps will be needed to direct the tube into the glottic chink, with an assistant ready to advance the tube when it is properly positioned. If the tube is the correct size, the main difficulty usually will be related to the curvature of the tube. If the tube is too straight, the head should be extended. If the tube is too sharply curved, the head must be lifted and the neck flexed.

In taping the nasotracheal catheter in place, it is extremely important to avoid pressure of the tube against the edge of the nostril, for this easily produces ulceration followed by nasal scarring and obvious facial distortion (Fig. 8-11). The tube should be taped so that the entire upper rim of the nostril is visible (Fig. 8-12) and may be observed throughout the operation and during postoperative ventilation, should this be necessary.

"Blind" nasal and oral intubation

Nasal-endotracheal intubation without laryngoscopic assistance occasionally may be useful in children, but the narrower passages

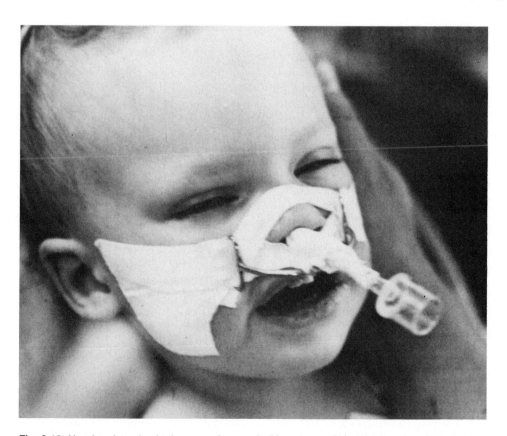

Fig. 8-12. Nasal endotracheal tubes must be taped with care to avoid pressure, ulceration, and unsightly scarring. It is best to leave the upper half of the nostril uncovered by tape. Logan bow is used here for additional long-term support.

and less adaptable tubes make the process more difficult, and the soft tissues and increased adenoidal masses add to the incidence of trauma and hemorrhage. Because of even greater difficulty in infants, the blind nasal approach is hardly ever indicated.

When one is dealing with children, adult technics for nasal intubation are applied as recommended by Magill (1930, 1975), Gillespie (1963), Bennett and associates (1978), and others, and the same preliminary steps are followed as in visual nasal intubation previously described. When the tube has reached the hypopharynx, however, one proceeds under the guidance of breath sounds rather than by visual guidance. Much importance has been given to the necessity for spontaneous ventilation to maintain audible breath sounds. This may involve some reduction of relaxation and return of bothersome reflexes. To prevent this situation, one may apply generous amounts of topical anesthetic to the trachea and glottis. However, we have found it preferable to attain full relaxation with greater depth of general anesthesia, or occasionally by use of relaxants, and then provide the breath sounds by rhythmic compression of the patient's chest. Palpation and simple external visual observation, as described by Bennett and associates (1978), help to direct the tube through the glottis. It should be emphasized that forceful or continued attempts are to be avoided.

The practice of blind oral intubation, once used by obstetricians, may be of value in children and especially in infants. To do this, one stands facing the patient, retracts the tongue with index and middle fingers, the tips reaching nearly to the epiglottis, and passes the tube with the other hand.

Selective bronchial blocking

Removal of infected lung tissue frequently is performed with the patient in a lateral position with the diseased hemithorax uppermost. In 1969 Vale reported successful management of such a case using a Fogarty balloon-tipped catheter to block the infected bronchus, followed by insertion of an endotracheal tube by standard technic. Hogg and Lorhan (1970), Cullum and associates (1973), and Cay and associates (1975) reported comparable experiences.

In similar situations where lobectomy is performed on children with cystic fibrosis, our preference has been to use the Overholt prone position with the head slightly lowered, so that secretions will drain into the pharynx and mouth. This is effective, simply done, and causes minimal interference with respiration.

Position, size, and fixation of endotracheal tubes

Numerous complications are caused by incorrect placement of endotracheal tubes and their dislodgment after intubation. Erroneous intubation of the esophagus is seen occasionally and may be difficult to recognize. Passage of the tip of the tube beyond the carina is a common occurrence.

Following passage of an endotracheal tube, one watches for equal expansion of the chest and pronounced lift of the sternum and upper ribs. Decreased breath sounds on either side call for retraction of the tube until both sides are equal. As shown by Bosman and Foster (1977), flexion and extension of the head can cause considerable movement of the tube. Consequently one should have the patient's head in the intended position when confirming breath sounds and avoid subsequent motion. Bednarek and Kuhns (1975) recommend palpation of the suprasternal notch as a method of positioning the endotracheal tube, and several other methods have been suggested.

For clinical anesthesia, immediate and continued stethoscopic auscultation has served well, provided that extreme caution is taken to avoid dislodgment during any movement of the child's head or body. If the head is moved either laterally or vertically, the anesthesiologist holds both tube and face so that there will be no change in relative position. If the child's body is to be moved, the tube is disconnected from the breathing apparatus until the new position has been established, the tube again being held in place during the movement. When intubation is intended for prolonged ventilatory support, x-ray confirmation of its position is considered essential at the outset and at subsequent intervals as indicated.

At this time one checks the size of the endotracheal tube. Postoperative tracheitis has been found to be caused by excessive tube size more than any other factor (Koka and others, 1977). When the tube has been satisfactorily positioned, the anesthesiologist inflates the patient's chest with a pressure of 20 to 25 cm H_2O, at which pressure there should be an audible gas leak around the endotracheal tube. If there is no leak or if the leak is obviously excessive, the tube should be replaced by one of more suitable size.

For fixation of endotracheal tubes, the common cloth-backed adhesive tape usually serves well. Both tube and face should be clean and dry. Tincture of benzoin may be used on tender skin or before prolonged cases, but it seldom is needed for the average operation. Tape that is ½ inch wide, in strips long enough to circle the tube and extend half way to the ear on each side with one strip below the mouth and another above, will usually suffice. Rather than several pieces of tape being wrapped around the same ½ inch of tube, much better fixation is gained by winding at least one strip of tape over another area on the tube, as is done in the taping of chest tubes. As was noted in reference to nasal tubes, one must be careful to avoid strapping endotracheal tubes so as to cause undue pressure. Oral tubes are apt to be forced too far into the corners of the mouth, with the skin of the face pulled into tight folds.

AIRWAY AND INTUBATION PROBLEMS

There is a rich assortment of airway problems that offer the pediatric anesthesiologist exciting opportunities for heroism or homicide. Although solutions to all are not known, there are several important rules that must be observed if one is to avoid disaster.

As with most dangerous situations, the first essential is to know when to expect trouble (the second, how to avoid it; and the third, if caught, how to get out of it). An organized approach is mandatory (Ament, 1978).

Many know enough to expect difficulties with epiglottitis or Pierre Robin syndrome (Dennison, 1965), but the diagnosis of Hurler's syndrome or Ludwig's angina may not be appreciated until the anesthesiologist finds that he has uncorked a catastrophe. A list of some of the problems is given below. This list, arranged in etiologic categories, is by no means complete. Such references as Warkany (1971) and Gray and Skandalakis (1972) could add dozens of less common anomalies. However, familiarity with the diverse situations represented here should furnish a basic comprehension of the field.

CLINICAL CONDITIONS INVOLVING DIFFICULT INTUBATION

Congenital anomalies
Conjoined twins
Encephalocele
Double harelip
Pierre Robin syndrome, micrognathia
Craniofacial deformity (Crouzon, Apert)
Branchial cleft, Treacher Collins syndrome

Tumors
Cystic hygroma
Hemangioma of tongue, pharynx
Teratoma

Infection
Pharyngeal abscess
Epiglottitis
Tracheobronchitis
Ludwig's angina

Muscular and skeletal problems
Ankylosis of jaw, spine
Wired teeth, jaws
Dislocated cervical vertebrae
Cervical cord tumor
Halo traction apparatus
Hurler's disease

Trauma
Facial fractures, lacerations
Burns of mouth, airway
Foreign body aspiration

The difficulties involved are quite varied, and a better classification might be based on the type of problem, the simplest being merely positional (a child with normal airway and ventilation who must be intubated in prone position) and the most hazardous being

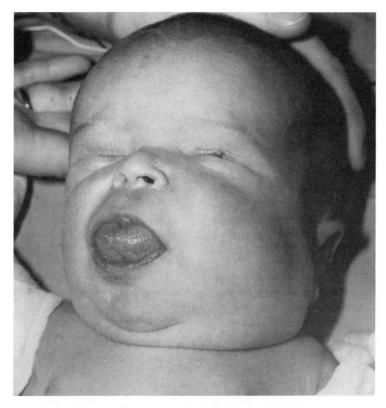

Fig. 8-14. Problems in intubation. Cystic hygromas frequently occur around neck and face. Like this, many are soft and allow awake intubation with only moderate difficulty.

rocessed maxilla and bulging eyes impede mask fit, nares are often stenotic, tongue is large, and cricoid is abnormally narrow (Colgan and Keats, 1957). Topical anesthetic and insertion of nasopharyngeal airway prior to anesthesia may be necessary. Perform halothane-oxygen induction. For Tessier midface advancement, preoperative tracheostomy is often advisable (Tessier, 1971).

Ankylosis of jaw, halo head and neck fixation, dislocated cervical spine. Respiration is neither obstructed nor depressed, but intubation is impeded by abnormal or limited anatomic position. Gain patient cooperation by giving graded increments of sedative and narcotic plus topical anesthesia until apprehension is relieved—then intubate using stylet (Block and Brechner, 1973), retrograde transtracheal guide (Powell and Ozdil, 1967; Nolan, 1969), or fiberoptic bronchoscope (Stiles and others, 1972).

Scar contracture of mouth or neck — no airway obstruction. Ketamine may be used if mouth is not to be stimulated (Patterson, 1972). Incision of

lateral cervical contracture cords may help cervical extension and allow passage of laryngoscope (Epstein and others, 1966).

Hurler's syndrome (gargoylism). Airway is normal at birth, but gradual infiltration of the pharynx and submandibular area by firm lymphoid tissue makes laryngoscopy increasingly difficult by 3 to 4 years of age. Preoperative evaluation is mandatory. Disease is fatal by 8 to 10 years of age. Elective procedures are not indicated if airway is obstructed. Perform preliminary tracheostomy under local anesthesia if operations are necessary during a later stage.

Ludwig's angina or massive submandibular cellulitis. Airway is inaccessible in severe cases, but patient can ventilate spontaneously. Relaxants and ketamine are contraindicated. In 1941 Williams and Marcus advised exposing the trachea through incision under local anesthesia in case of emergency and then proceeding under thiopental and nitrous oxide anesthesia to incise infected area. A rapidly reversible inhalation anesthesia (nitrous oxide–halothane) might be preferable

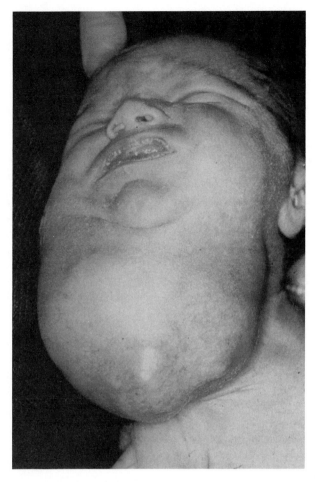

Fig. 8-15. This rock-hard teratoma compressed the trachea. Difficult awake intubation was followed by tracheostomy.

today, preceded by full atropinization (Gross and Nieburg, 1977).

If papillomas or severe swelling make it impossible to find the true glottic passage, forceful compression of the chest or abdomen (Heimlich maneuver) often blows the cords apart, showing the proper route for intubation.

In many of the above situations that threaten acute airway occlusion, one can prevent disaster by emergency tracheostomy through the cricothyroid interspace or by insertion of 12- to 18-gauge needles at the same site. If needles are used, one must blow oxygen through them, for patients are not able to survive by spontaneous ventilation on

room air (Reed and others, 1954; Jacoby and others, 1951).

BIBLIOGRAPHY

Allen, H. L., Metcalf, D. W., and Biering, C.: Anesthetic management for the separation of conjoined twins, Anesth. Analg. (Cleve.) **38:**109, 1959.

Ament, R.: A systemic approach to difficult intubations, Anesthesiol. Rev. **5:**12, 1978.

Aro, L., Takki, S., and Aromaa, U.: Technique for difficult intubations, Br. J. Anaesth. **43:**1081, 1971.

Bednarek, F. J., and Kuhns, L. R.: Endotracheal tube placement in infants determined by suprasternal palpation; a new technique, Pediatrics **56:**224, 1975.

Bennett, E. J., Grundy, E. M., and Patel, K. P.: Visual signs in blind nasal intubations; a new technique, Anesthesiol. Rev. **5:**18, 1978.

Bennett, J. M.: Anesthetic management for drainage of

abscess of submandibular space (Ludwig's angina), Anesthesiology **4:**25, 1943.

Berry, F. A., Jr., Blankenbaker, W. L., and Ball, C. G.: A comparison of bacteremia occurring with nasotracheal and orotracheal intubation, Anesth. Analg. (Cleve.) **52:**873, 1973.

Biller, H. F., Harvey, J. B., Bone, R. C., and Oguira, J. G.: Laryngeal edema; an experimental study, transactions of American Laryngeal Association **91:**68, 1970.

Block, C., and Brechner, K. L.: Unusual problems in airway management. II. Anesth. Analg. (Cleve.) **50:**114, 1973.

Bosman, Y. K., and Foster, P. A.: Endotracheal intubation and head positions in infants, S. Afr. Med. J. **52:**71, 1977.

Bosomworth, P. P., and Hamelberg, W.: Effect of sterilization technics on safety and durability of endotracheal tubes and cuffs, Anesth. Analg. (Cleve.) **44:**576, 1965.

Bougas, T. P., and Smith, R.: Pathologic airway obstruction in children, Anesth. Analg. (Cleve.) **37:**137, 1958.

Boutros, A. R.: Arterial blood oxygenation during and after endotracheal suctioning in the apneic patient, Anesthesiology **32:**114, 1970.

Branstater, B.: Dilatation of the larynx with Cole tubes, Anesthesiology **31:**378, 1969.

Branstater, B., and Muallem, M.: Atelectasis following tracheal suction in infants, Anesthesiology **31:**468, 1969.

Brown, E. S., and Hustead, R. F.: Rebreathing in pediatric anesthesia systems, Anesthesiology **28:**241, 1967.

Butz, R. O., Jr.: Length and cross-section growth patterns in the human trachea, Pediatrics **42:**336, 1968.

Calderwood, H. W., and Ravin, M. B.: The cat as a teaching model for endotracheal intubation, Anesth. Analg. (Cleve.) **51:**258, 1972.

Cave, P., and Fletcher, G.: Resistance of nasotracheal tubes used in infants, Anesthesiology **29:**588, 1968.

Cay, D. L., Csenderits, L. E., Lines, V., and others: Selective bronchial blocking in children, Anaesth. Intensive Care **3:**127, 1975.

Chodoff, P., and Helrich, M.: Factors affecting pediatric endotracheal tube size; a statistical analysis, Anesthesiology **28:**779, 1967.

Cohen, D. D., and Dillon, J. B.: Hazards of armored endotracheal tubes, Anesth. Analg. (Cleve.) **51:**856, 1972.

Coldiron, J. S.: Estimation of nasotracheal tube length in neonates, Pediatrics **41:**823, 1968.

Cole, F.: A new endotracheal tube for infants, Anesthesiology **6:**87, 1945.

Colgan, F. J., and Keats, A. S.: Subglottic stenosis; a cause of difficult intubation, Anesthesia **18:**265, 1957.

Cullum, A. R., English, I. C., and Branthwaite, M. A.: Endobronchial intubation in infancy, Anaesthesia **28:**66, 1973.

Davenport, H. T., and Rosales, J. K.: Endotracheal intubation of infants and children, Can. Anaesth. Soc. J. **6:**65, 1959.

Davis, N. J.: A new fiberoptic laryngoscope for nasal intubation, Anesth. Analg. (Cleve.) **52:**807, 1973.

Dennison, W. M.: The Pierre-Robin syndrome, Pediatrics **36:**336, 1965.

Dingley, A. R.: Nasal intubation; danger and difficulties, Br. Med. J. **1:**693, 1953.

Donaldson, S. W., and Thompsett, A. C., Jr.: Tracheal diameter in the normal newborn infant, Am. J. Roentgenol. Radium Ther. Nucl. Med. **67:**785, 1952.

Eckenhoff, J.: Some anatomic considerations of the infant larynx influencing endotracheal anesthesia, Anesthesiology **12:**401, 1951.

Engel, S.: The child's lung, ed. 2, London, 1962, Edward Arnold, Publishers, Ltd.

Epstein, B. S., Rudman, H. L., Harday, D. L., and Downes, H.: Comparison of orotracheal intubation with tracheostomy for anesthesia in patients with face and neck burns, Anesth. Analg. (Cleve.) **45:**352, 1966.

Fearon, B., and Whalen, J. S.: Tracheal dimensions in the living infant, Ann. Otol. **76:**964, 1967.

Flagg, P. J.: Endotracheal inhalation anesthesia; special reference to postoperative reactions and suggestions for their elimination, Laryngoscope **61:**1, 1951.

Gellis, S. S., and Feingold, M.: Apert's syndrome, Am. J. Dis. Child. **115:**721, 1968.

Gillespie, N. A.: Endotracheal anesthesia, ed. 3, Madison, Wis., 1963, University of Wisconsin Press.

Glauser, E. M., Cook, C. D., and Bougas, R. P.: Pressure flow characteristics and dead spaces of endotracheal tubes used in infants, Anesthesiology **22:**339, 1961.

Gray, E. W., and Skandalakis, J. E.: Embryology for surgeons, Philadelphia, 1972, W. B. Saunders Co.

Gregory, G. A.: In Shnider, S. M., and Moya, F., editors: The anesthesiologist; mother and newborn, Baltimore, 1974, The Williams & Wilkins Co.

Gross, S. J., and Nieburg, P. O.: Ludwig's angina in children, Am. J. Dis. Child. **131:**291, 1977.

Guess, W. L., and Stetson, J. B.: Tissue reactions to organotin stabilized polyvinyl chloride (PVC) catheters, J.A.M.A. **209:**118, 1968.

Hallowell, P.: Endotracheal intubation of infants and children, Int. Anesthesiol. Clin. **1:**135, 1962.

Hedden, M., Smith, R. B. F., and Torpey, D. J.: A complication of metal spiral-imbedded latex endotracheal tubes, Anesth. Analg. (Cleve.) **51:**859, 1972.

Hogg, C. E., and Lorhan, P. H.: Pediatric bronchial blocking, Anesthesiology **33:**560, 1970.

Jacoby, J. J., Reed, J. P., Hamelberg, W., and others: Simple method of artificial respiration, Am. J. Physiol. **167:**798, 1951.

Jordan, W. S., Graves, C. L., and Elwyn, R. A.: New therapy for post-intubation laryngeal edema and tracheitis in children, J.A.M.A. **212:**585, 1970.

Kahn, A., and Fulmer, J.: Acrocephalosyndactylism, N. Engl. J. Med. **252:**379, 1955.

Karis, J. G.: Misadventure during endotracheal anesthesia, J.A.M.A. **226:**676, 1973.

Keep, P. J., and Manford, M. L.: Endotracheal tubes for children, Anaesthesia **29**:181, 1974.

Koka, B. V., Jeon, S., Andre, J. M., and others: Postintubation croup in children, Anesth. Analg., (Cleve.) **56**:501, 1977.

Macon, E. B., and Bruner, H. D.: The scientific aspect of endotracheal tubes, Anesthesiology **11**:313, 1950.

Magill, I. W.: Technique in endotracheal intubation, Br. Med. J. **2**:817, 1930.

Magill, I. W.: Blind nasal intubation, Anaesthesia **30**:476, 1975.

Mattila, M., Heikel, P. E., Suutarinen, T., and Lindfors, E. L.: Estimation of a suitable nasotracheal length for infants and children, Acta Anaesth. Scand. **15**:239, 1971.

Mostafa, S. M.: Variation in subglottis size in children, Proc. R. Soc. Med. **69**:793, 1976.

Nolan, R. T.: Nasal intubation, Anaesthesia **24**:447, 1969.

Norton, M. L., and de Vos, P.: New endotracheal tube for laser surgery of the larynx, Ann. Otol. **87**:554, 1978.

Orkin, L. K., Siegel, M., and Rovenstein, E. A.: I. Resistance to breathing by apparatus used in anesthesia, Anesth. Analg. (Cleve.) **33**:217, 1954.

Pappas, M. T., Katz, J., and Finestone, S. C.: Problems in anesthetic and airway management with Gardner's syndrome; report of a case, Anesth. Analg. (Cleve.) **50**:340, 1971.

Patterson, J. F.: Anesthesia in Vietnam, Anesth. Analg. (Cleve.) **51**:306, 1972.

Pender, J. W.: Endotracheal anesthesia in children; advantages and disadvantages, Anesthesiology **15**:495, 1954.

Penlington, G. N.: Endotracheal tube sizes for children, Br. J. Anaesth. **29**:494, 1974.

Phillips, O., and Duerksen, R. L.: Endotracheal intubation; a new blade for direct laryngoscopy, Anesth. Analg. (Cleve.) **52**:691, 1973.

Powell, W. F., and Ozdil, T.: A translaryngeal guide for tracheal intubation, Anesth. Analg. (Cleve.) **46**:231, 1967.

Reed, J. P., Kemph, J. P., Hamelberg, W., and others: Studies with endotracheal artificial respiration, Anesthesiology **15**:28, 1954.

Rendell-Baker, L., and Roberts, R. B.: Hazards of ethylene oxide sterilization, Anesthesiology **30**:349, 1969.

Robin, P.: La chute de la base de la langue considéré comme une nouvelle cause du gêne dans la respiration naso-pharyngienne, Bull. Acad. Natl. Med. (Paris) **89**:37, 1923.

Salem, M. R., Mathrubhutham, M., and Bennett, E. J.: Difficult intubation, N. Engl. J. Med. **295**:879, 1976.

Shellinger, R. R.: The length of the airway to the bifurcation of the trachea, Anesthesiology **25**:169, 1964.

Slater, H. M., Sheridan, C. A., and Ferguson, R. H.: Endotracheal tube sizes for infants and children, Anesthesiology **16**:950, 1955.

Smith, R. M.: The prevention of tracheitis in children following endotracheal anesthesia, Anesth. Analg. (Cleve.) **32**:102, 1953.

Smith, R. M.: Indications for endotracheal anesthesia in pediatric anesthesia, Anesth. Analg. (Cleve.) **33**:107, 1954.

Stiles, C. M., Stiles, Q. R., and Denson, J. S.: A flexible fiberoptic laryngoscope, J.A.M.A. **221**:1246, 1972.

Tahir, A. H.: Endotracheal tube lost in the trachea, J.A.M.A. **222**:1061, 1972.

Tahir, A. H., and Renegar, O. J.: A stylet for difficult orotracheal intubation, Anesthesiology **39**:337, 1973.

Taylor, P. A., and Towley, R. M.: The broncho-fiberscope as an aid to endotracheal intubation, Br. J. Anaesth. **44**:611, 1972.

Tessier, P.: The definitive plastic surgical treatment of the severe facial deformities of craniofacial dysostosis; Crouzon's and Apert's diseases, Plast. Reconstr. Surg. **48**:419, 1971.

Thomas, E. T., and Levy, A. A.: Dissipation of ethylene oxide from anesthesia equipment; use of a mechanical aerator, Anesthesiology **32**:261, 1970.

Urban, B. J., and Weitzner, S. W.: Avoidance of hypoxemia during endotracheal suction, Anesthesiology **31**:473, 1969.

Vale, R.: Selective bronchial blocking in a small child, Br. J. Anaesth. **41**:453, 1969.

Warkany, J.: Congenital malformations; notes and comments, Chicago, 1971, Year Book Medical Publishers, Inc.

Williams, A. C., and Marcus, P. S.: Choice of anesthesia in Ludwig's angina, Anesth. Analg. (Cleve.) **20**:160, 1941.

Wilton, T. N. P., and Wilson, F.: Neonatal anaesthesia, Philadelphia, 1965, F. A. Davis Co.

Winchell, S. W., and Davis, G.: Sterilization and care of equipment, In Safar, P., editor: Respiratory therapy, Philadelphia, 1965, F. A. Davis Co.

Wittenborg, M. H., Gyepes, M. T., and Crocker, D.: Tracheal dynamics in infants with respiratory distress, stridor, and collapsing trachea, Radiology **88**:653, 1967.

Zindler, M., and Deming, M. V.: Anesthetic management of infants for surgical repair of congenital atresia of esophagus with tracheo-esophageal fistula, Anesth. Analg. (Cleve.) **32**:180, 1953.

CHAPTER 9

Maintenance and monitoring, or signs of life and depth

A 4-year-old boy who has had successful induction with nitrous oxide, oxygen, and halothane is intubated with a 4.5 mm ID endotracheal tube and is well stabilized on a circle absorption system. For the next 4 hours he will undergo a ureteral reimplantation. What problems lie ahead for the anesthesiologist?

The varied tasks involved in anesthetic maintenance can be sorted out in several ways but ultimately may be reduced to *two major (and conflicting) responsibilities:* one is *to provide adequate depth and working conditions for the surgeon;* the other is *to provide maximum supportive care of the child.*

To carry out these major functions requires continued undivided attention to the patient, observation of signs of depth and danger, and ability to interpret and act on the information gained.

SIGNS OF ANESTHETIC DEPTH

Years ago, the dominant thought during anesthesia was to keep the patient asleep. The classic guides to ether anesthesia first described by Snow in 1858 and later developed by Guedel (1937) (Fig. 9-1) were *measures of depression* of respiration, muscle activity, and pupillary responses. Although children react more rapidly than adults to anesthesia, and signs of anesthetic depth, especially in

infants, are more difficult to distinguish, Guedel's signs served for pediatric use of ether, and monitors played a very small role.

Agents now in use have divergent patterns of action, with little resemblance to ether, and we must rely on *evaluation of the individual components of general anesthesia* as suggested by Woodbridge in 1957. These are *hypnosis, analgesia, muscle relaxation,* and *control of reflex responses* (Fig. 9-2). While all four components may be affected equally by some anesthetics, several agents show marked action on one phase and little or none on others (e.g., thiopental causes deep hypnosis with poor relaxation, but *d*-tubocurarine has the exact opposite effect).

Evaluation of proper depth is further affected by altered responses of children of different ages and the changing anesthetic requirements of different operations.

Evaluation of hypnosis is not usually difficult under halothane or other potent general anesthetics. Children often fall asleep rapidly, especially if previously sedated. The 4-year-old patient mentioned above probably would have drifted off in the first 2 minutes of induction, with nystagmus showing early loss of consciousness, followed by closing eyes and loss of eyelash and eyelid responses. Other signs of loss of consciousness are roving, dissociated eyeball movements and airway obstruction caused by relaxation of tongue and jaw. One can be badly mistaken, however, by assuming that a child is unconscious simply because he lies quietly with his eyes closed. He may inhale a low concen-

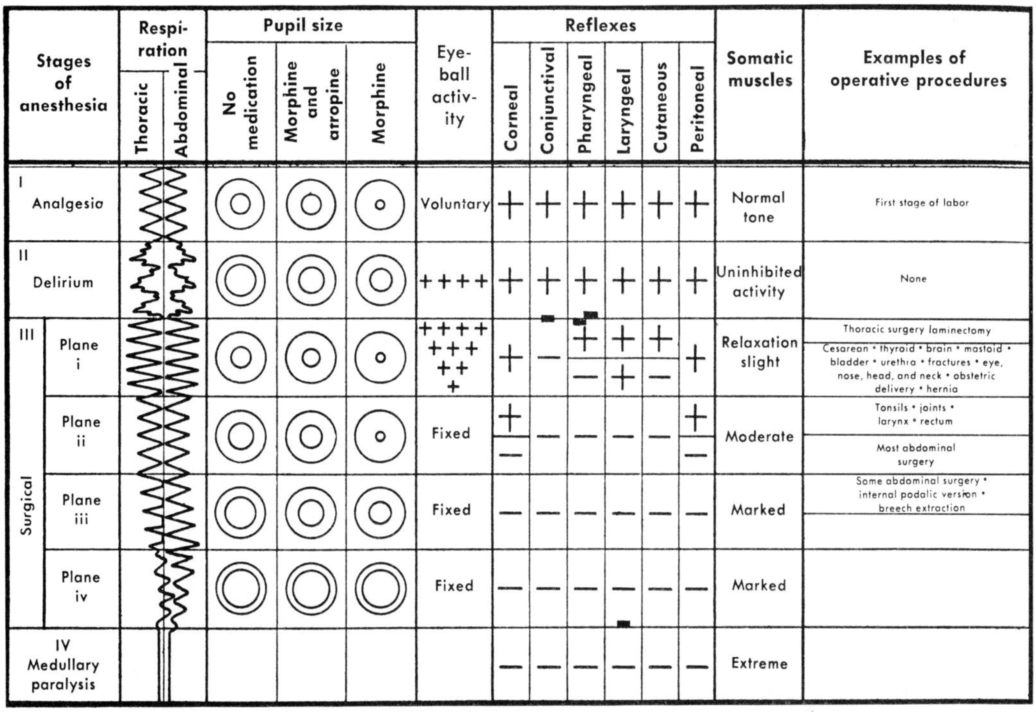

Stages of anesthesia		Respiration		Pupil size			Eye-ball activity	Reflexes						Somatic muscles	Examples of operative procedures
		Thoracic	Abdominal	No medication	Morphine and atropine	Morphine		Corneal	Conjunctival	Pharyngeal	Laryngeal	Cutaneous	Peritoneal		
I Analgesia				◎	◎	○	Voluntary	+	+	+	+	+	+	Normal tone	First stage of labor
II Delirium				◎	◎	◎	++++	+	+	+	+	+	+	Uninhibited activity	None
III Surgical	Plane i			◎	◎	○	++++ +++ ++ +	+	−	+ + −	+ +		+	Relaxation slight	Thoracic surgery laminectomy. Cesarean • thyroid • brain • mastoid • bladder • urethra • fractures • eye, nose, head, and neck • obstetric delivery • hernia
	Plane ii			◎	◎	○	Fixed	+ −	−	−	−	−	+ −	Moderate	Tonsils • joints • larynx • rectum. Most abdominal surgery
	Plane iii			◎	◎	◎	Fixed	−	−	−	−	−	−	Marked	Some abdominal surgery • internal podalic version • breech extraction
	Plane iv			◎	◎	◎	Fixed	−	−	−	−	−	−	Marked	
IV Medullary paralysis								−	−	−	−	−	−	Extreme	

Fig. 9-1. Stages and planes of ether anesthesia. (From Goodman, L. S., and Gilman, A.: The pharmacological basis of therapeutics, ed. 4, New York, 1970, Macmillan, Inc.)

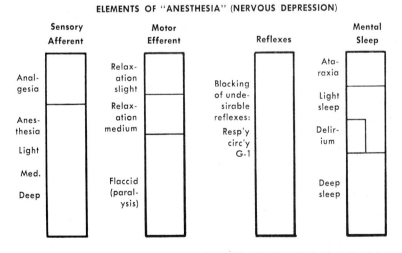

ELEMENTS OF "ANESTHESIA" (NERVOUS DEPRESSION)

Sensory Afferent — Analgesia, Anesthesia, Light, Med., Deep

Motor Efferent — Relaxation slight, Relaxation medium, Flaccid (paralysis)

Reflexes — Blocking of undesirable reflexes: Resp'y circ'y G-1

Mental Sleep — Ataraxia, Light sleep, Delirium, Deep sleep

Fig. 9-2. Four components of general anesthesia. (From Woodbridge, P. D.: Anesthesiology **19:**536, 1957.)

Most signs of anesthetic depth are relatively easy to follow when more soluble agents are used, but potent rapid-acting anesthetics wipe out finer changes in muscle tone and grades of respiratory depression. With halothane and other halogenated agents, heart rate and blood pressure become the primary guides. In addition, the more accurately calibrated vaporizers take on the role of monitors, helping to gauge the level of anesthesia by rate of administration of agent. With the exception of these aids, monitoring devices play a comparatively small part in determination of depth during pediatric anesthesia.

SIGNS OF LIFE

The anesthesiologist's responsibility for providing supportive care to the child involves more diverse and more complicated problems than those related to meeting the needs of the surgeon. To deal with these problems one must adhere to basic principles of patient care and also be proficient in clinical and technical methods of diagnosis and treatment.

The phrase "He that keepeth thee shall not slumber" (Psalm 120) was originally intended as reassurance but serves as well for admonition. Whether punishable by damnation or litigation, to leave an anesthetized patient physically unattended by leaving the room or mentally unattended by reading or sleeping is inexcusable patient neglect.

The general care of an infant or child during operation is slightly different from that of an adult. Personnel must be restrained in their tendency to move a child abruptly, with resultant trauma, hypotension, or displacement of endotracheal tube or intravenous infusion. Care must also be taken to see that the child is not exposed to excessive cooling during preparation nor too deeply buried under drapes and that the surgeons neither lean on his chest nor use it as an instrument table.

Precepts for prescribed positive performance include remaining at the head of the patient, maintaining continuous stethoscopic observation of heart and lungs, and, when possible, retaining accessibility to the patient's head. The anesthetic chart, doubly valued as a clinical monitor and legal document, is initiated before anesthetic induction and maintained with accuracy but without losing contact with the progress of the operation. During prolonged operations, boredom and fatigue must be recognized as major hazards to be overcome by rational methods of prevention (see below).

Specific measures of supportive care are aimed at enabling the child to withstand the combined effect of the illness, the operation, and the anesthetic.

Rather than watching for signs of depression, one must concentrate on *evaluation and regulation of the essential physiologic functions: respiration, circulation, tissue oxygenation and metabolism, and temperature control.* In this, the anesthesiologist should use early signs of aberrant function rather than wait for the appearance of danger signs, just as the motorist should be able to stay on the road without relying on the guard rail.

It requires some knowledge of the variables of pediatric physiology to determine the difference between normal and abnormal in each age level. Thus, if our 4-year-old has a heart rate of 140 per minute, systolic blood pressure of 90 mm Hg, and measured blood loss of 160 ml, are these findings abnormal? Do they represent indication for transfusion?

If the limits of normal function are exceeded and danger signs appear, the anesthesiologist must recognize them promptly and treat them effectively. Failure to recognize signs of mounting danger or to take measures to correct them certainly reflect decreasing levels of competence.

SPECIFIC METHODS OF EVALUATING AND CONTROLLING PATIENT CONDITION
Clinical observation

To evaluate the various factors that determine the child's "condition," the anesthesiologist relies primarily on continuous *clinical observation*, assisted by monitoring devices as needed. In pediatric anesthesia it is mandatory to be fully aware of the progress of the operation at all times; consequently, the anesthesiologist should remain standing, with the whole patient in view, throughout the procedure (Fig. 9-4).

As stressed by Artusio and associates (1973), information picked up by the five senses, instantly interpreted by the brain, is more widely useful than that provided by any instruments or computers yet known. In the management of the anesthetized child its value is obvious. *Normal respiration* is observed in proper rate and depth (see Chapter 2), freedom from obstruction, equal expansion of both sides of the chest, easy compliance (especially when intubated), and normal color of skin and blood. *Abnormal respiration* would be evident in noisy, obstructed, depressed, or irregular respiration, unequal expansion, tracheal tug, hiccough, bucking, glottic spasm, or apnea. *Normal cardiovascu-*

lar function is evident in suitable heart rate, rhythm, pulse volume, vascular tone, capillary refill, and skin color. During intrathoracic procedures one can view the heart directly and watch it contract, fill, dilate, fibrillate, slow, or exsanguinate. One can often diagnose a significant arrhythmia more quickly by direct vision than by electrocardiograph, since the force of contraction is easily visible.

Blood loss can be estimated reasonably well by visual estimation of bleeding, pulse rate, and volume, by color of the conjunctivae, and by counting of blood-soaked sponges.

Temperature is best measured, but heating and cooling of the skin is often sensed manually, especially when associated with flushing, sweating, or cyanosis.

Neuromuscular tone is easily estimated by

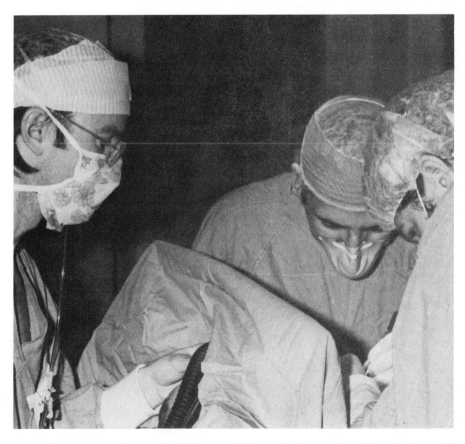

Fig. 9-4. Continuous visual monitoring of the surgical procedure is mandatory for optimal care of the child.

passively extending the child's flexed arm, by prodding the abdomen (or asking the surgeon), and by opening the jaw.

Central nervous system responses obtainable in pupillary responses and lid reflexes are usually more informative than electroencephalographic signals, and autonomic responses such as sweating, vasomotion, and vagal activity are recognizable without the aid of instruments. Again we find that unassisted observation, if properly used, tells us a great deal and sometimes interesting items for which computers are not yet programmed, whether it concerns a fly that has lighted on an exposed kidney or a sudden rent in the aorta.

Monitoring apparatus: design and use

Numerous monitors are available, some of which are considered to be mandatory for all pediatric procedures; others are indicated for specific situations, and several are used only under exceptional conditions (Table 9-1). In the general use of monitoring instruments, one should follow the advice of Rowe (1973) and start by using those that are relatively simple to operate, reliable, and easily serviced. Monitors should be used only if they give information that is truly important, accurate, and reliable, without exposing the child to undue risk. Disadvantages and potential hazards to be considered when monitors are used are listed below*:

Exposure of child during establishment
Alarm, pain in establishment
Delay in starting operation
Injury
    Nasal bleeding, tracheitis, esophageal perforation
    Trauma to urethra, rectum
    Tissue injury, blood loss
    Vascular irritation, embolus
    Burns (heat, electric)
    Loss of digit, extremity, or life
Long-term immobilization of child
Interruption of rest
Instrumental error, breakdown
Error in interpretation
Distraction of anesthesiologist attention
Practice required on well patients to develop skill needed for use in critically ill

*From Smith, R. M.: Pediatric anesthesia in perspective; Sixteenth Annual Baxter-Travenol Lecture, Anesth. Analg. (Cleve.) **57**:634, 1978.

Table 9-1. Basic and supplementary monitoring approaches

MONITORING METHODS

I. Basic monitors

Eyes
Ears
Fingers
Anesthesia chart
Stethoscope
Blood pressure
Temperature

II. Supplementary monitors and measurements

Gas flow rates
Fluids given, urine output
Blood loss (measured)
Venous pH, Pco_2
Arterial Po_2, Pco_2
Electrocardiograph
Nerve stimulator
Central venous pressure
Tissue Po_2, pH
Serum Na, K, Ca^{++}, protein, osmolality
Coagulogram
Serial Hct
Inspired oxygen concentration
End-expired Pco_2
Right and left atrial pressures
Cardiac output
Pulmonary wedge pressure
Urine specific gravity, osmolality

From Smith, R. M.: Pediatric anesthesia in perspective; Sixteenth Annual Baxter-Travenol Lecture, Anesth. Analg. (Cleve.) **57**:634, 1978.

The introduction of more elaborate monitoring apparatus has met some resistance from those who have developed their technics without these instruments, have witnessed the errors attending their early usage, and remain critical. As a result, many older anesthesiologists make inadequate use of monitors. Younger individuals, with less clinical acumen, often seem to rely too heavily on instruments. However, they push on, learn rapidly, and soon are out ahead.

It is already apparent that skilled, reasonable use of physiologic monitors has unlimited potential. With the increasing capability, complexity, and cost of such instrumentation, it seems probable that availability of sophisticated monitoring facilities will be es-

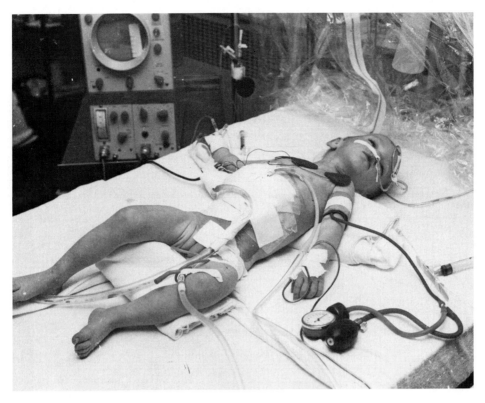

Fig. 9-5. Extensive monitoring often requires prolonged immobilization.

sential in the establishment of future pediatric centers.

Although many monitoring instruments have disadvantages, invasive monitors without exception carry real dangers and should only be used as temporary devices while continued effort is being made to replace them. Two of the least appreciated disadvantages of extensive monitoring are prolonged immobilization and the anguish that accompanies it (Fig. 9-5).

Essential monitors

Anesthesia chart. The anesthesia record, or chart, should rightfully be included among the anesthesiologist's essential monitoring guides (Fig. 9-6). It is seldom used to its potential for preanesthetic, anesthetic, and postanesthetic recording of the patient's subjective and objective reactions to the anesthetic and operation. Its use as a physiologic monitor has been described by Schnei-

der and associates (1976), who note improvements that could make the record more useful, such as built-in trend analysis and apparatus for continuous recording of data, which would make it unnecessary to rely on the conscientiousness of the anesthesiologist. Dillon (1957) has stressed the essential importance of the anesthesia chart as a medicolegal document.

In addition to the usual data noted in anesthesia records, it is helpful to show fluid exchange and temperature in specially designated columns. In pediatric charts it also is advisable to record the degree of evident anxiety of the child at the time of the preoperative visit, so that the effect of the medication can be evaluated.

Stethoscope. It is my firm conviction, and that of many others, that the stethoscope is the most important of all monitoring devices in pediatric anesthesia and that it should be used throughout all procedures in which gen-

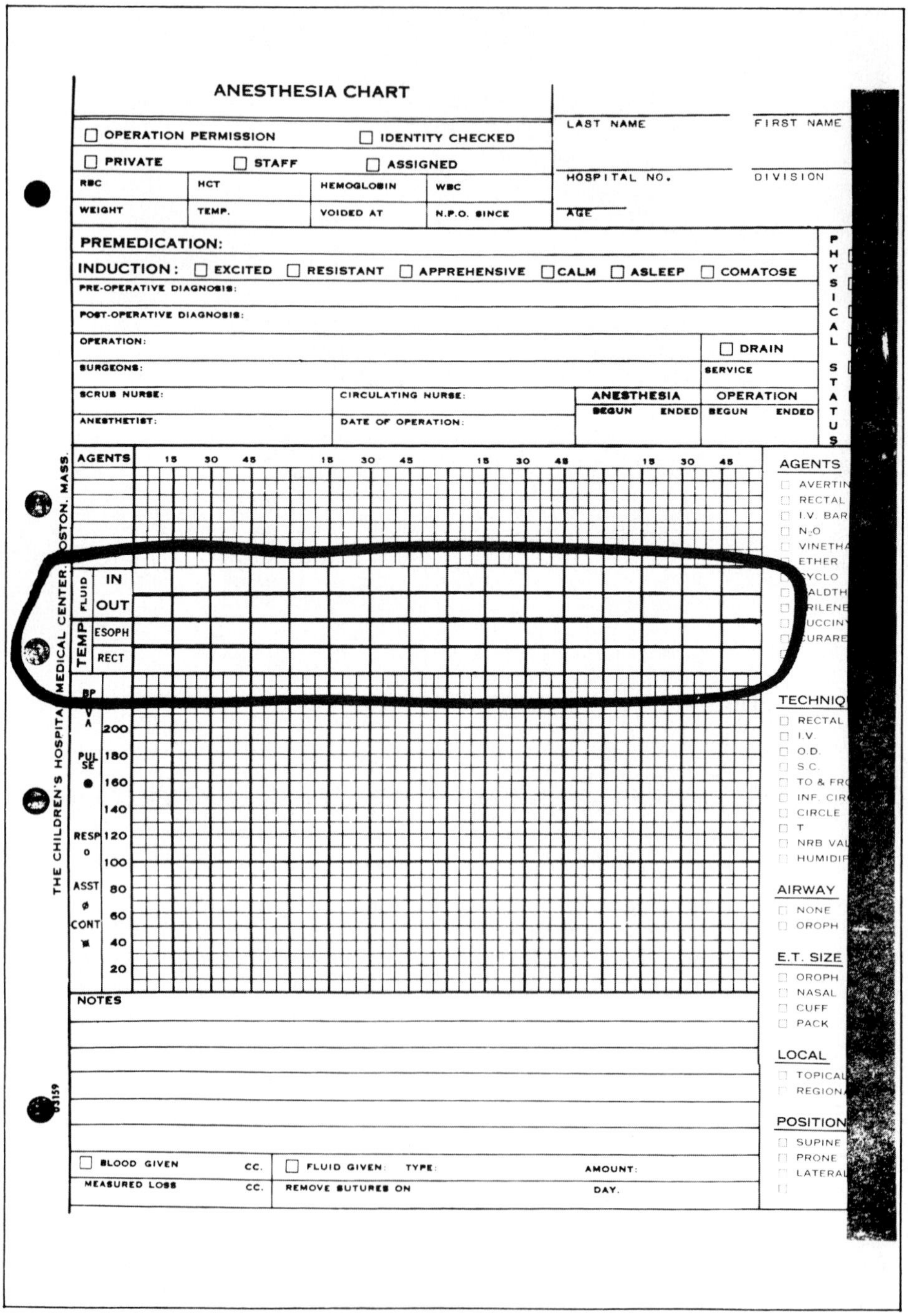
ANESTHESIA CHART

LAST NAME | FIRST NAME

HOSPITAL NO. | DIVISION

AGE

☐ OPERATION PERMISSION ☐ IDENTITY CHECKED

☐ PRIVATE ☐ STAFF ☐ ASSIGNED

RBC	HCT	HEMOGLOBIN	WBC
WEIGHT	TEMP.	VOIDED AT	N.P.O. SINCE

PREMEDICATION:

INDUCTION: ☐ EXCITED ☐ RESISTANT ☐ APPREHENSIVE ☐ CALM ☐ ASLEEP ☐ COMATOSE

PRE-OPERATIVE DIAGNOSIS:

POST-OPERATIVE DIAGNOSIS:

OPERATION: ☐ DRAIN

SURGEONS: SERVICE

SCRUB NURSE: CIRCULATING NURSE: ANESTHESIA BEGUN ENDED | OPERATION BEGUN ENDED

ANESTHETIST: DATE OF OPERATION:

PHYSICAL STATUS

AGENTS 15 30 45 15 30 45 15 30 45 15 30 45

FLUID IN OUT

TEMP ESOPH RECT

BP V A 200; PULSE ● 180; 160; 140; RESP ○ 120; 100; ASST ø 80; 60; CONT ✖ 40; 20

NOTES

☐ BLOOD GIVEN CC. ☐ FLUID GIVEN TYPE: AMOUNT:

MEASURED LOSS CC. REMOVE SUTURES ON DAY.

AGENTS: ☐ AVERTIN ☐ RECTAL ☐ I.V. BAR ☐ N_2O ☐ VINETHA ☐ ETHER ☐ CYCLO ☐ ALDTH ☐ RILENE ☐ UCCIN ☐ CURARE

TECHNIQ: ☐ RECTAL ☐ I.V. ☐ O.D. ☐ S.C. ☐ TO & FR ☐ INF. CIR ☐ CIRCLE ☐ T ☐ NRB VAL ☐ HUMIDIF

AIRWAY: ☐ NONE ☐ OROPH

E.T. SIZE: ☐ OROPH ☐ NASAL ☐ CUFF ☐ PACK

LOCAL: ☐ TOPICAL ☐ REGION

POSITION: ☐ SUPINE ☐ PRONE ☐ LATERAL

THE CHILDREN'S HOSPITAL MEDICAL CENTER, BOSTON, MASS.

03159

Fig. 9-6. The anesthesia chart should be considered one of the four essential monitoring devices of pediatric anesthesia.

eral anesthesia is used, with the exception of times when the chest is open and the anesthesiologist can visualize the action of heart and lungs directly.

Shortly after World War II, use of the precordial stethoscope became popular in the eastern United States, and it has since become the mark of the pediatric anesthesiologist. The simplicity, veracity, and versatility of this device have been widely attested to (Smith, 1953, 1962, 1978; Ploss, 1955; Dornette and Brechner, 1959; Dornette, 1963, 1973; Bosomworth and others, 1963; Bethune, 1965; Patterson, 1966).

Several variations in the design of the stethoscope are available for precordial use. Chestpieces include the standard and small sizes of a lightweight diaphragm model made for general use as well as the flat, heavy Littmann chestpiece* (Fig. 9-7). Other stethoscopes made particularly for anesthesia, such

*Distributed by 3M Co., St. Paul, Minn., as the Littmann acoustic pickup.

as the weighted Dupaco instrument,* also are available in child and adult sizes.

The difference between the performance of Dupaco and standard diaphragm stethoscopes is not easily distinguished. Dornette (1973) has noted that bell-shaped chestpieces, or accumulators, are better for low-pitched heart sounds and the diaphragm type is better for high frequency breath sounds. At The Children's Hospital Medical Center our preference for large-diaphragm stethoscopes is based on their wider area of reception and their flatter shape, which makes them more easily fixed to the chest, whether the child is in supine, lateral, or prone position.

Variations on the accumulator have been improvised to meet special purposes. During bronchography in darkened rooms, a stethoscope is mandatory, yet metal accumulators interfere with visualization and roent-

*Dupaco, 205 North Second Avenue, Arcadia, Calif.

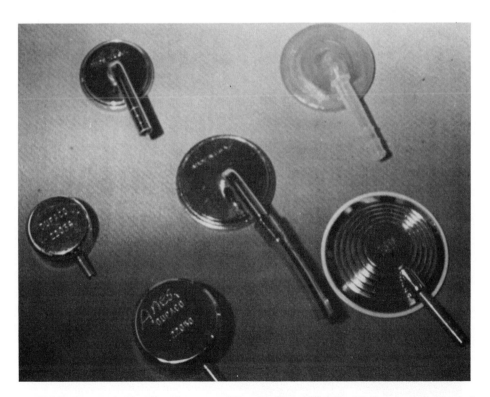

Fig. 9-7. Stethoscope chestpieces for precordial monitoring: child and adult Dupaco *(left diagonal)*, child and adult flat *(middle diagonal)*, plastic *(upper right)*, and Littmann *(lower right)*.

genography. Homemade diaphragm-type accumulators molded out of translucent acrylic have been substituted with success. Standard plastic accumulators are also available commercially (Fig. 9-7).

The heavy Dupaco accumulators slide off a child's chest and must be taped in place, but they rest easily in the suprasternal notch, where the signals are considerably less informative but still useful (Nelson, 1972).

The diasyst accumulator, designed by Cohen and Robbins (1966) to fit under blood pressure cuffs, conforms nicely to the chest of the small infant in whom standard chestpieces prove unsatisfactory. The diasyst can be used as an open-faced accumulator, but for use on uneven surfaces such as the bony thorax of a sick infant it is better to make a diaphragm for it by applying a thin sheet of plastic across its open face. Because of its atraumatic design, the diasyst is also valuable

as a precordial monitor for older children in prone position.

Before the stethoscope is fixed to a child's chest, the best site should be determined where both heart and lungs can be heard distinctly. This usually is at the border of the heart and lung at the left nipple line (Fig. 9-8).

An esophageal stethoscope is valuable when children are to be in prone position and when the precordium cannot be used because of operation or injury. It is also useful for most intrathoracic operations in children. One should avoid unnecessary use of esophageal stethoscopes in children, especially in infants, since their introduction and continued presence, in addition to an endotracheal tube and often an esophageal thermistor probe, adds to the incidence of local irritation and trauma.

Esophageal stethoscopes are available

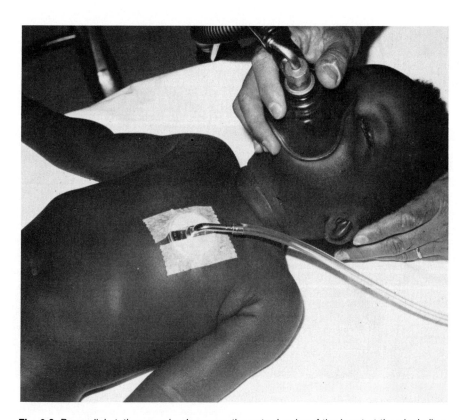

Fig. 9-8. Precordial stethoscope in place over the outer border of the heart at the nipple line.

commercially but at present only in French sizes 12 and 18. While size 12 French is suitable for infants, neither size is optimal for children between 3 and 12 years of age. Fortunately, esophageal stethoscopes can be made quite easily by cutting several small holes in a urethral catheter, slipping a piece of rubber dam over the terminal 2 or 3 inches, and tying it at both ends.

Numerous variations also are possible in stethoscope headpieces. When the binaural stethoscope is used continuously, the ears may become sore unless the headpiece is stretched apart so that the stethoscope hangs by gravity rather than by "ice tong" effect. The earpieces should be chosen to suit each individual. The Littmann stethoscope has particularly well designed earpieces. One can also relieve the strain by using one ear at a time or by using a monaural stethoscope. The original monaural earpiece described by Ploss (1955) had a molded plastic earpiece fitting only one ear. Other adaptations that have been made include using one standard earpiece fitted to a single piece of tubing, substituting the cone-shaped end of a rubber catheter, or simply using a short length of soft latex tubing for the earpiece. These have the advantage of fitting either ear and thus being interchangeable. A monaural device is considerably more comfortable, allows the use of one ear for communication with the surgical team, and is adequate for most situations. For operations on neonates, however, where heart and breath sounds are barely audible, the binaural stethoscope is definitely superior.

The "conjoined twin" stethoscope (Fig. 9-9) allowing two individuals to listen to the same signals has been a great help in teaching infant anesthesia.

Another attribute of the stethoscope is its ability to transmit sounds a considerable distance without appreciable loss of volume or character. Thus, it is possible to monitor a child during x-ray therapy by means of a 20-foot tubing between earpiece and chestpiece.

The standard stethoscope has only one real fault. Its signals are heard by only one person. If the anesthesiologist is not listening, the patient can regurgitate or aspirate or the heart may stop without being noticed. Although it is reasonable to expect the anesthesiologist to use the stethoscope continuously (except when heart and lungs can be watched during thoracotomy), it would be a great improvement to amplify stethoscopic sounds enough to be heard by the entire team. An instrument of this description has been under development by Hustead and could be an important step forward.

Other monitors, such as pulse detectors and the electrocardiograph, have been available for some time for visual or audible observation but are less versatile because they transmit a relayed signal limited to a single physiologic feature instead of a direct signal of several features.

Blood pressure apparatus. After years of trial and error, technics for measuring blood pressure have reached a most satisfactory state, combining adaptability to all ages, ac-

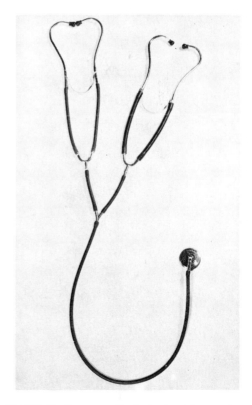

Fig. 9-9. Stethoscope with single chestpiece and two headpieces, an excellent teaching device.

curacy, simplicity, safety, economy, and patient acceptability. It is the one procedure that children frequently say they like.

It is particularly fortunate that these developments occurred, because the need for more accuracy in blood pressure determination was becoming evident, and the tendency toward use of intra-arterial cannulation was beginning to grow. With the accuracy of the present noninvasive apparatus, direct intra-arterial methods now can be restricted to use in exceptional procedures.

Major improvements have been made in both cuff and sensor. Blood pressure cuffs for infants have been improved by enlarging the inflatable portion so that it may be wrapped around the arm, allowing gentle, even compression of the brachial artery and thus replacing miniature inflatable bags that required excessive distension to obstruct arterial flow.

The width of the inflatable cuff is of considerable importance, and for children it has been generally believed proper for the width of the cuff to equal two-thirds the length of the humerus (Stephen and others, 1970). Pediatric cardiologists Park and associates (1976) declared that the standard width for children should be 20% greater than the diameter of the limb on which it is used. It is known that a cuff that is too narrow will give an erroneously high reading and one that is too wide will give an erroneously low one. Park and associates recommended cuffs measuring 3, 5, 8, 12, and 18 cm in width, the last for use on thighs. For our practice, two infant cuffs* made of latex have filled our needs in smaller patients—the first, for infants under 5 kg, has an inflatable portion 3.5 cm wide by 16 cm long and the second, for infants weighing 5 to 10 kg, has bag dimensions of 5.5 by 16 cm (Fig. 9-10). For older children and adolescents, the usual cloth-covered rubber bags are used, with widths of 7, 9, 12, and 18 cm.†

There has been little recent change in the

*Tillotson Rubber Co., Everett, Mass.
†W. A. Baum Co., Copiague, N.Y.

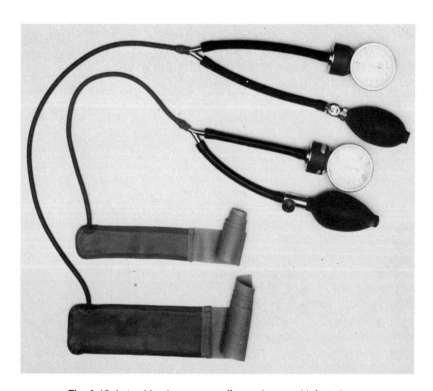

Fig. 9-10. Latex blood pressure cuffs: newborn and infant sizes.

design of the pressure gauge or manometer itself, but it is now an accepted practice to use the larger dial and fix the gauge to the anesthesia machine.

Greatest difficulty has been involved in finding satisfactory sensing devices to register the Korotkoff sounds. A standard stethoscope may be fixed to the arms of children who are 3 or 4 years of age, or a small diasyst sensor may be applied. In large, healthy patients undergoing relatively simple procedures it is reasonable to omit the stethoscope and simply measure systolic pressure by the bounce of the descending needle. For any major procedure, however, both systolic and diastolic pressures should be followed accurately. Attempts to find reliable pressure-sensing methods for infants have led to cumbersome and traumatic technics. Infrared sensors have caused serious burns, and arteriotomy has led to gangrene of fingers and forearms. Several satisfactory methods now exist, however, and one may no longer excuse oneself for omission of blood pressure recording on the ground of patient size.

In place of a stethoscope, one may use a second infant blood pressure cuff applied just distal to the regular cuff. If the inflation tube is connected to the stethoscope headpiece, the Korotkoff sounds may be detected clearly.

The greatest boon to infant blood pressure determination has been the development of the Doppler ultrasonic flowmeter* (Fig. 9-11) (Janis and others, 1970; Hernandez and others, 1971; Hochberg and Saltzman, 1971) and subsequently the Infrasonde sensor.† With these devices and correctly proportioned cuffs, one can follow systolic and diastolic pressures in infants of any size, even when they are awake and moving about in bed.

The Doppler sensor works on the principle that changes in arterial flow cause changes in the rate of reception of vibrating sound waves, the faster flow creating higher frequency (Poppers, 1971). The Infrasonde mechanism depends on vibration of the vessel wall rather than rate of blood flow. Sens-

---

*Parks Electronic, Beaverton, Ore.
†Marion Scientific Corp., Costa Mesa, Calif.

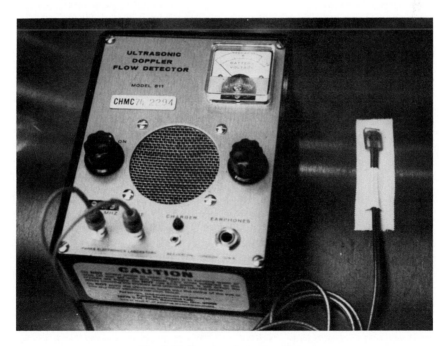

Fig. 9-11. Doppler ultrasonic sensor.

ing devices of either instrument may be fixed over the radial or other artery without incurring any hazard of laceration, burn, or electrical shock. Of the available devices, the Parks Doppler ultrasonic flowmeter, model 811, with loudspeaker, fits our situation most satisfactorily, acting as continuous monitor of heart sounds when not connected to blood pressure apparatus.

Several studies have shown noninvasive Doppler determination of blood pressure to be practically identical to intra-arterial determination at the same site (Kafka and Oh, 1971). However, central arterial pressure determinations show marked difference from peripheral Doppler pressure measurements in the presence of hemorrhage. Because of vasoconstriction, peripheral Doppler pressures begin progressive reduction at 25% loss of blood volume, while central pressure is sustained until 50% to 60% loss occurs (Harken and Smith, 1973). This finding justifies use of intra-arterial pressure determinations in the presence of deep hypothermia and shocklike states.

Blood pressure determination has been found to be of greater practical value during infant surgery than previously believed, and the recent technical improvements have been extremely helpful in estimating blood loss, anesthetic depth, and circulatory competence. As shown previously, arterial blood pressure is considerably lower in small infants (see Chapter 2). A starting blood pressure of 65 to 70 mm Hg does not necessarily signify danger, but any fall of 10 to 15 mm Hg should call for definitive action, such as reduction of anesthetic concentrations, administration of atropine, or replacement of blood. A Doppler apparatus with microphone sensor and loudspeaker* also serves as an excellent monitor for air embolism during neurosurgical operations when patients are in the sitting position (Michenfelder and others, 1972).

Temperature monitoring apparatus. In sharp contrast to monitoring of blood pres-

sure, methods for measurement and regulation of body temperature are still highly unsatisfactory. Much effort has been put into this area, yet inaccuracies and serious hazards are present in both recording and regulating devices (Battig, 1968; Smith, 1969; Crino and Nagle, 1968; Lebowitz, 1970).

The glass clinical thermometer is breakable and also must be shaken down or "reset" after each use, but it still has a place in anesthesia. At a wholesale price of 35 cents, it is one of the most accurate thermometers available and may be used for preoperative calibration of more elaborate instruments. It is also valuable for intraoperative spot checking and confirmation of other devices if positioned in nostril, mouth, axilla, or rectum and held by hand while testing. I have been unable to learn why these cannot be made of shatterproof glass.

Electronic thermometers are most widely used, the majority made on the basis of a Wheatstone bridge with thermistor probes that have a variety of sensing tips for use on skin surface, body cavities, or intramuscular areas (Leonard, 1966; Huber, 1973). Careless handling destroys accuracy promptly, but even when protected, both thermistor and readout box develop gross inaccuracy and must be calibrated for each use. Thus far, all available makes have failed to stand up to steady use and leave much to be desired.

Other temperature-measuring instruments consist of thermocouple sensing units with meter or digital readout. These are said to be more stable and have an advantage in that the sensing unit may be as small as the head of a pin (Dike and Machler, 1965). These devices are currently used for tympanic membrane thermometers as well as for application at usual sites (Benzinger, 1963, 1969).

It greatly increases the value of any monitor if an alarm can be incorporated into it. Alarm systems are available with both Wheatstone bridge–type* and thermocouple† apparatus, and their use is highly

---

*Versatone D8 Doppler, Medsonics, P.O. Box M, 9340 Pioneer Way, Mountain View, Calif.

*Yellow Springs Instrument Co., Yellow Springs, Ohio.
†Bailey Instruments Co., Inc., Saddle Brook, N.J.

advisable. To control temperature changes one should begin to act as soon as the temperature goes below 36° C (97° F) or above 38° C (100° F) (see Chapter 26).

The method of monitoring temperature depends on individual choice as well as the situation. The tympanic membrane is rated as the site for most accurate measurement of central arterial temperature. For investigational work this would be optimal, and many use it for routine clinical work, but the frequent appearance of blood on the sensing tip and the fear of electrical burns of the ear have discouraged some from using it (including me).

The generally accepted plastic thermistor probe can be used in nose, mouth, esophagus, and rectum with relative safety, but it

has been known to perforate or tear mucosa in each of these areas. Furthermore, the thermistor has caused burns of the perineum when used in the rectum in proximity to a cautery plate, apparently because of accumulation of charges along the thermistor wire (Bruner, 1967; Smith, 1969). For this reason it is important to avoid this situation and use a site more remote from the cautery plate or make sure that the thermistor wire makes no contact with the child's skin. The axilla is the safest location for thermistor placement, and in addition it is the only site that justifies reuse of the probe without sterilization. To obtain best results with this method, one should locate the sensing tip as near the axillary artery as possible (Fig. 9-12), taping the probe to the chest wall and bringing the arm

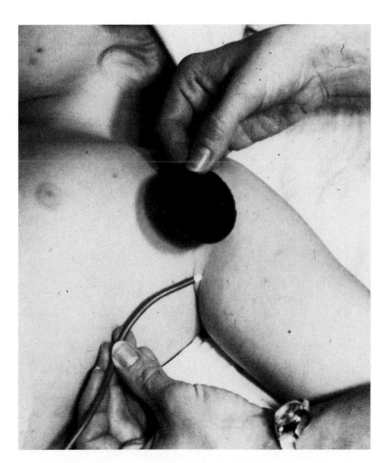

Fig. 9-12. The accuracy of axillary thermometry depends on the approximation of the thermistor to the axillary artery.

down close to the body. The standard plastic tip and the flat metal skin sensor are equally serviceable. Axillary temperature is often 0.7° to 1.0° C below core temperature at first but is within 0.5° C in 15 minutes. In small infants, it is more accurate, usually within 0.25° C of core temperature.

A desirable or safe range for a child's core temperature is approximately 36° to 38° C (97° to 100° F). As noted by scores of writers, hypothermia may be expected in any small infant who is brought into a cold operating room and exposed for preoperative preparation (France, 1957; Gough, 1960; Hercus, 1960; Stephen and others, 1960; Hackett and Crosby, 1960; Roe and others, 1966). Volatile skin-cleansing fluids have an additional ef-

fect, and the child's temperature may fall as low as 34° C (93° F) before the operation begins. To prevent this, the room is warmed to 27° C (80° F), humidity is increased, the baby's limbs are wrapped in sheet wadding, his body is covered as much as possible, and a stockinette hat is made for those with little hair. By far the most useful device for warming infants in the operating room is the twin-lighted infrared heating lamp* (Fig. 9-13). This bathes the baby in total instant warmth without subjecting the operating team to any discomfort and allows the surgeon access to the entire infant.

An infant's temperature often rises after he

*JH Emerson Co., Cambridge, Mass.

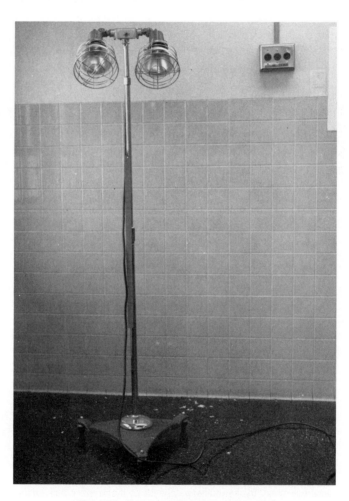

Fig. 9-13. Emerson infrared heating lamp.

is draped and the room becomes warmer. In many prolonged operations, however, several factors contribute to heat loss, including large wounds, exposure of abdominal or thoracic viscera, cool irrigating fluid, infusion of cold fluid and blood, hyperventilation with nonrebreathing systems, and use of peripheral vasodilating agents (halothane) and/or muscle relaxants. The effect of cooling from 36° to 33° C (96° to 92° F) results in depression of respiration and enzyme systems, greater absorption of inhalation anesthetics, and delayed recovery. Nevertheless, death due to unintentional hypothermia is unlikely except in one situation, i.e., where cold blood is given rapidly through an infusion in the arm.

Use of warming mattresses is generally advocated for smaller children (Goudsouzian and others, 1973), but most heating devices involve varying degrees of danger. It is certainly preferable to maintain body warmth by prevention of heat loss rather than by reliance on application of external heat whether from mattresses, lamps, or hot-air devices. If mattresses are to be used one must choose them with care. Small, poorly controlled units have caused severe burns.

In view of the fact that electronic thermometers and water-heating units are subject to major inaccuracy, two precautionary measures are advisable: (1) before any operation in which temperature change may be of particular danger, calibrate thermistor and readout box against a standard glass thermometer by simultaneous testing in a cup of water at body temperature, and (2) during operation, before taking any steps either to cool or warm a patient, recheck the child's temperature with a standard glass thermometer.

Several other precautions are necessary to avoid burning patients during anesthesia (Talbert, 1970). Water in heating units should not be heated above 39.5° C (103° F) at any time, and devices should be limited to this maximum. Poorly perfused tissues, whether due to hypothermia, generalized hypotension, or local pressure (especially with patients in lateral position), are more

easily damaged by heat or cold and should be more carefully protected (Morris and Kumar, 1972). All heating blankets should be covered by two layers of cotton blankets, and more should be added to protect areas under increased pressure. There are more accidents from burning than from overcooling. All are preventable, none excusable.

The danger of unintentional hypothermia is very common in anesthetized infants. While less common in older children and less marked, hypothermia is by no means rare. Hyperthermia, on the other hand, is rarely seen during anesthesia in children under 2 years of age. In older children, it occurs infrequently but has many possible causes. The management of both hypothermia and hyperthermia is discussed in Chapter 26.

Supplementary monitoring methods*

Many types of monitoring apparatus are adaptable for special supportive care during pediatric anesthesia. It is particularly in this area that increased capabilities must be measured against increased hazards.

Electrocardiograph. Although the electrocardiograph (ECG) is justly considered a standard monitor for adults, several disadvantages combine to detract greatly from its value in use with normal children. Children rarely develop significant intraoperative arrhythmias that are not evident by stethoscopic monitor, and the display of the tracing is usually behind the anesthesiologist so that he must turn his back to patient and surgeon when (and if) he observes it. Worse than that, since the tracing shows only electrical activity of the heart, a normal tracing may continue after hemorrhage has dropped the output to shock level. While giving false confidence in such circumstances, the ECG often distracts and disconcerts observers when abnormal tracings appear that have little significance. Finally, there is also a remote hazard of electrical trauma.

ECG is indicated when children are

---

*NOTE: More specialized monitoring methods are described in their specific area of use.

known to have arrhythmias or are at increased risk either because of their condition or the intended operation, e.g., eye operations, or because of bronchoscopy. Great improvement has been made in operating room ECGs; the present solid-state models with multichannel oscilloscope, battery pack, digital readout for pressure and pulse, and alarm systems are certainly more useful than early models, and freeze display and recording facilities have added further sophistication. For usual operating conditions, a small two-channel monitor for ECG and atrial pressure, mounted on the anesthesia machine, is suitable. Several manufacturers produce excellent apparatus. It is advisable to choose one make of apparatus rather than have an assortment of noninterchangeable equipment. For intracardiac operations, multichannel polygraphs are more versatile, with controls and display at the head of the operating table and a larger screen mounted overhead.

ECG apparatus used for children is adapted from standard devices simply by substitution of smaller electrodes, now disposable and expensive (another disadvantage of routine use). The arrhythmias encountered and their treatment are described in Chapter 26.

For general purposes, an audible signal denoting heart rate is of more practical value than an ECG tracing and is particularly indicated when vagal responses are expected. While most ECGs are equipped to produce this signal, devices intended specifically for this purpose (such as the previously mentioned Doppler flowmeter) are more informative.

For infants, a heart rate between 120 and 180 beats/min is acceptable if it is steady and rhythmic. Any rapid change within this range or rates outside of this deserve attention. Slower rates suggest vagal response to hypoxia; more rapid rates are less alarming but may suggest epinephrine release or supraventricular tachycardia. Heart rates in older children gradually decrease to adult norms of 70 to 90 per minute.

Central venous pressure. Measurement of central venous pressure (CVP) has relatively limited value in children and is subject to a variety of errors. However, when the apparatus is correctly functioning, CVP serves as a useful guide to right heart action and blood replacement during prolonged operations, especially when patients have reduced myocardial reserve, are receiving large amounts of blood, are prone, or are undergoing operations involving induced hypothermia or hypotension.

Cannulation of the veins of the upper extremity or neck is preferable for measurement of CVP, although the femoral vein can be used. There has been much early enthusiasm for percutaneous cannulation of the internal jugular vein by Seldinger technic (1953) and other technics, using either the high or low approach (Prince and others, 1976; Rao and others, 1977; Schwartz, 1977). The high incidence of hemorrhage and pneumothorax, and the occasional deaths, first gave convincing evidence that the low approach was unsafe and subsequently have made the use of the high approach appear questionable. It has been our preference to use brachial or external jugular veins by percutaneous technic, when possible, and otherwise to cannulate the brachial or internal jugular vein by direct vision through a small incision. As emphasized by Rowe (1973), the CVP apparatus must be adjusted precisely, with the zero line at the right atrial level, and interpreted with allowance for respiratory effects and age variations. Placement of the catheter tip must be checked by x-ray film or by passing it far enough to recognize right atrial configuration and then withdrawing it. Rowe also suggests that in the presence of abdominal distension, CVP measured via the inferior caval vein may give an erroneously high reading and the cephalic route is preferable. As noted by Haller (1969) and Talbert (1970), CVP is slightly reduced in younger children, but the responses are similar at all ages. Any sudden change should be viewed with alarm, the usual range being 3 to 10 mm Hg.

Right atrial pressure is easily measured by inserting a CVP catheter until appearance of the right atrial pressure curve, as is done to check catheter placement, but not withdrawing it. This measurement has been of use following shunt procedures for tetralogy of Fallot; a pressure of 25 mm Hg, regulated by fluid administration, has been used to "drive the heart" (Moffitt, 1962).

Left-heart function. Left atrial pressure is measured by means of a catheter inserted through the myocardial wall following open-heart procedures. In operations in which the chest is not opened, hemodynamics may be measured by means of the Swan-Ganz flow-directed catheter (Swan and others, 1970) to find right atrial pressure and left ventricular filling pressure (pulmonary capillary wedge pressure). Using the same catheter, one can determine the cardiac output by thermodilution technic (Weintraub and others, 1971; Gorlin, 1977). These procedures have become indispensible in cardiology and have increasing application in operative and postoperative pediatric surgery. They obviously involve more than average risk of significant complication and are reserved for patients who have borderline cardiac function. Noninvasive echocardiographic technics provide invaluable information concerning left ventricular function but as yet are not practical for intraoperative use (Buchbinder and Ganz, 1976).

Monitors of ventilatory function. For many years it has been possible to measure the rate of flow of anesthetic gases as they leave the anesthesia machine, and it is not difficult to determine the percentages of the resultant mixtures. It has recently become possible, by means of devices for continuous monitoring of partial pressure of inspired oxygen, to determine what the patient is inhaling with each breath. As noted in the review by Figallo and associates (1978), neither the analyzers based on the galvanic cell nor those based on the polarographic principle have reached a state of perfection, but both have definite practical value for clinical use.

While this is a forward step, what has been greatly needed for many years is a noninvasive method of continuous monitoring of arterial, or preferably tissue, oxygenation. Ear oximeters and similar devices have been of questionable value in nurseries and of very little use in the operating room. Percutaneous oxygen analyzers have now reached the stage where they give valuable information during intensive therapy of premature infants, and extension of their use into the operating room seems imminent. Of the many instruments already available, those made by Radiometer and Littin appear to be quite promising.

For clinical use at this time, mechanical ventilators give some idea of ongoing pulmonary function, but the most reliable guide is to measure gases in venous or arterial blood. It should be emphasized that venous blood often is adequate for evaluation of ventilation; the use of arterial puncture thus can be reserved for determination of partial pressure or saturation of oxygen.

Intermittent sampling of blood for gas and pH determination may suffice in operations of moderate length and/or stress, but arterial cannulation is preferable if more than four or five arterial samples are needed. The umbilical arteries may be used for sampling in neonates, but radial arteries are the site of choice under most circumstances. Percutaneous cannulation is accomplished with a 22-gauge Teflon needle in small neonates. Although a 22-gauge needle is preferable for all ages, a 20-gauge needle may be used in older patients. Presence of intact ulnar artery is determined by the Allen test or preferably by use of an ultrasonic flowmeter. Although some have experienced no complications in hundreds of cases and urge more frequent use of arterial cannulation (Furman and others, 1972; Ward and Green, 1965), the danger of infection, thrombosis, and loss of digits has been reported by others (Downs and others, 1973; Katz and others, 1974; Miyasaka and others, 1976) and convince us of the need for precautions and early removal (within 3 days). Lowenstein and associates (1971) have called attention to the danger of flushing arterial lines, a danger that is accentuated in the shorter arms of pediatric patients. Patency of the arterial line should be maintained by use of a suitable (Harvard) pump.

Maintenance of fluid and metabolic homeostasis. The essentials of fluid therapy, electrolyte balance, and blood replacement are discussed in Chapter 26. It is of primary importance in all operations to monitor all fluid components by measurement and recording of amount, type, and rate of exchange and to maintain careful observation for clinical signs of dehydration, hypovolemia, shock, pulmonary edema, congestive heart failure, hyponatremic hypervolemia, and acid-base imbalances. Catheterization of the urinary bladder is less often required in children, since renal complications are infrequent, but urinary output in open-heart procedures is of obvious significance. Urinary output of 0.5 to 1 ml/kg/hr is considered adequate (Filler and others, 1973).

The measurement of electrolytes and various blood components has definite indications in some instances, such as that of serum potassium in children with renal failure and blood sugar in diabetic children. Ionized calcium determination is gaining more importance in management of severely stressed patients (Hinkle and Cooperman, 1971; Radde and others, 1972; David and Anast, 1974).

The measurement of serum and urine osmolality is indicated in problems of fluid administration, especially after resuscitation (Finberg, 1967; Coran and others, 1971). While total protein and oncotic pressure determination have been advocated (Furman, 1971; Rowe, 1973), their usefulness has been less widely attested to. The electrode for muscle pH determination (Filler and Das, 1971) has also had limited use for operative procedures.

Selection of monitoring guides

Under present conditions of rapid change and variable situations it is inadvisable to make hard statements as to the necessity of one monitor or another. The anesthetic chart and blood pressure apparatus, as stated in Guidelines of the American Society of Anesthesiologists, are established requirements for all patients given general anesthesia. For pediatric patients, the precordial or esophageal stethoscope is of greater importance than any other monitor, but it is not so established in bylaws or regulations. While the need for temperature monitoring is generally accepted, ECG monitoring in children is still questioned by many, especially with increasing use of other pulse monitors. The application of more specialized methods of patient evaluation would be quite impossible to regulate by any generality at this time.

To return to our 4-year-old who was to undergo bilateral ureteral reimplant, one would certainly employ all the methods of clinical evaluation described in the first part of this chapter. Then, as shown in Fig. 9-6, the anesthesia chart would carry additional documentation of agents (concentrations or dosages and time of administration) and itemize surgical or anesthetic events, changes in patient condition, fluids administered and lost, and temperature. Monitors would include precordial stethoscope, blood pressure cuff with stethoscopic or ultrasonic sensor, thermistor (probe in esophagus or axilla), and ECG, the last being of least importance. With the child under intravenous anesthesia with muscle relaxants, mechanical ventilation would be used, and while not essential, one or two samples of venous blood might be used for determination of pH and P_{CO_2}. Blood loss should not be extensive. One particular complication to look for in genitourinary procedures has been that of rapid temperature elevation. While easily confused with early manifestation of malignant hyperthermia, it is almost sure to be caused by septic material released during surgical manipulation. The fluid allowance would be increased in this operation because of manipulation of abdominal viscera. Otherwise, the operation should not call for particularly sophisticated management. A nerve stimulator may be used for testing relaxation during and after termination of anesthesia, but its use is optional.

Additional measures of supportive care

It is often necessary to have one or two additional anesthesiologists on hand during part or all of the more demanding procedures. The chief responsibility of the primary anesthesiologist lies in direct care of the patient, and maintenance of the airway is always the overriding consideration. Other supportive functions should fall into place, with due consideration for prevention of iatrogenic complications.

In prolonged operations, increased danger from pressure, positioning, burns, and cautery must be considered. Great care must be taken to protect the eyes from pressure, exposure, or injury (Brooks, 1978). Rather than using ointments, it is preferable to tape lids together with atraumatic tape.

Ulceration of the nostril is easily caused by upward pressure of a nasogastric or nasotracheal tube, especially when the patient is prone or the head is covered by drapes. If any tube is passed through the nose, it should be taped to the upper lip, leaving the nostril in clear view.

If anesthesia masks are used throughout the entire procedure, strapping them to the face with tight rubber head straps can cause deep slough of nasal skin and cartilage. Two straps are sufficient, and the entire mask should be removed and the face massaged at intervals. If prone, the child's head should be lifted every 5 minutes to prevent local pressure damage.

Personnel fatigue should be avoided by maintaining intercommunication and occasional periods of relief. Toward the end of long procedures, increased danger of inattention may occur. The critical period has passed, the team is tired and relaxed, conversation diverts attention, and 15 to 20 minutes slip by before blood pressure is found at shock level because of unsuspected hemorrhage.

BIBLIOGRAPHY

Artusio, J. F., Corssen, G., Dornette, W. H. L., and Reves, J. G.: Monitoring depth of anesthesia, Clin. Anesth. 9:212, 1973.

Battig, C. G.: Electrosurgical burn injuries and their prevention, J.A.M.A. 204:1025, 1968.

Bedford, R. F., and Wollman, H.: Complications of percutaneous radial artery cannulation; an objective prospective study in man, Anesthesiology 38:228, 1973.

Benzinger, M.: Tympanic thermometry in surgery and anesthesia, J.A.M.A. 209:1207, 1969.

Benzinger, T. H.: Human thermostat, New York, 1963, McGraw-Hill Yearbook Science and Technology.

Bethune, R. W.: Precordial electrocardiograph stethoscope, Anesthesiology 26:228, 1965.

Bosomworth, P. P., Dietsch, J. D., and Hamelberg, W.: The effects of controlled hemorrhage on heart sounds, Anesth. Analg. (Cleve.) 42:131, 1963.

Brooks, G. Z.: Ocular injury during anesthesia; case reports and a review of the literature, Anesthesiol. Rev. 5:16, 1978.

Bruner, J. M. R.: Hazards of electrical apparatus, Anesthesiology 28:396, 1967.

Buchbinder, N., and Ganz, W.: Hemodynamic monitoring, Anesthesiology 45:146, 1976.

Churchill-Davidson, H. C.: A safe method of administering muscle relaxants, Fifteenth Clinical Conference in Pediatric Anesthesiology, Los Angeles, January 28-30, 1977.

Cohen, D. D., and Robbins, L. S.: Blood pressure monitoring in the anesthetized patient, Anesth. Analg. (Cleve.) 42:578, 1966.

Coran, A. G., Das, J. B., and Eraklis, A. J.: Use of osmometry in the preoperative and postoperative management of the newborn, J. Pediatr. Surg. 6:529, 1971.

Crino, M. H., and Nagel, E. L.: Thermal burns caused by warming blankets in the operating room, Anesthesiology 29:149, 1968.

David, L., and Anast, C.: Calcium metabolism in newborn infants, J. Clin. Invest. 54:287, 1974.

Dike, P. H., and Machler, R. C.: Thermometry. In Licht, S., editor: Therapeutic heat and cold, Baltimore, 1965, Elizabeth Licht, Publisher.

Dillon, J. B.: The prevention of claims for malpractice, Anesthesiology 18:794, 1957.

Dornette, W. H. L.: The stethoscope; the anesthesiologist's best friend, Anesth. Analg. (Cleve.) 42:711, 1963.

Dornette, W. H. L., and Brechner, V. L.: Instrumentation in anesthesiology, Philadelphia, 1959, Lea & Febiger, p. 80.

Dornette, W. S.: Monitoring in anesthesia; the signal to be monitored, Clin. Anesth. 9:19, 1973.

Downs, J. B., Fackstein, A. D., and Klein, E. F., Jr., and others: Hazards of radial artery catheterization, Anesthesiology 38:283, 1973.

Figallo, E. M., Smith, R. B., Pautler, S., and Reilly, K. R.: Continuous oxygen analyzers in clinical anesthesia; a review, Anesthesiol. Rev. 5:25, 1978.

Filler, R. M., and Das, J. B.: Muscle surface pH; a new parameter in monitoring of the critically ill child, Pediatrics 47:880, 1971.

Filler, R. M., Eraklis, A. J., and Das, J. B.: Fluids, electrolytes and intravenous nutrition. In Gans, S. L., editor: Surgical pediatrics, New York, 1973, Grune & Stratton, Inc.

Finberg, L.: Dangers to infants caused by changes in osmotic concentration, Pediatrics 40:1031, 1967.

Foote, G. A., Schabel, S. I., and Hodges, M.: Pulmonary complications of the flow-directed balloon-tipped catheter, N. Engl. J. Med. **290**:927, 1974.

France, G. C.: Hypothermia in the newborn; body temperatures following anaesthesia, Br. J. Anaesth. **29**: 390, 1957.

Furman, E. B.: Anesthesia for right hepatic lobectomy in a child; an exercise in blood volume management, Anesthesiology **35**:436, 1971.

Furman, E. B., Hairabet, J. K., and Romas, D. G.: The use of indwelling radial artery needles in a pediatric anaesthesia, Br. J. Anaesth. **44**:531, 1972.

Gorlin, R.: Practical cardiac hemodynamics, N. Engl. J. Med. **296**:203, 1977.

Goudsouzian, N. G., Morris, R. H., and Ryan, J. F.: The effects of a warming blanket on the maintenance of body temperatures in anesthetized infants and children, Anesthesiology **39**:351, 1973.

Gough, M. H.: Temperature changes during neonatal surgery, Arch. Dis. Child. **35**:66, 1960.

Guedel, A.: Inhalation anesthesia, New York, 1937, Macmillan, Inc.

Hackett, P. R., and Crosby, R. M. N.: Some effects of inadvertent hypothermia in infant neurosurgery, Anesthesiology **21**:356, 1960.

Haller, J. A., Jr.: Monitoring of arterial and central venous pressure in infants, Pediatr. Clin. North Am. **16**: 640, 1969.

Haller, J. A., Jr., and Talbert, J. L.: Surgical emergencies in the newborn, Philadelphia, 1972, Lea & Febiger.

Harken, A. H., and Smith, R. M.: Aortic pressure versus Doppler measured peripheral arterial pressure, Anesthesiology **38**:184, 1973.

Hercus, V.: Temperature changes during thoracotomy in children, infants and the newborn, Br. J. Anaesth. **32**:476, 1960.

Hernandez, A., Goldring, D., and Hartmann, A. F.: Measurement of blood pressure in infants and children by the Doppler ultrasonic technique, Pediatrics **48**:788, 1971.

Hinkle, J. E., and Cooperman, L. H.: Serum ionized calcium changes following citrated blood transfusion in anesthetized man, Br. J. Anaesth. **43**:1108, 1971.

Hochberg, H. M., and Saltzman, M. B.: Accuracy of an ultrasound blood pressure instrument in neonates, infants and children, Curr. Ther. Res. **13**:482, 1971.

Huber, F. C.: Principles of monitoring systems, Clin. Anesth. **9**:22, 1973.

Janis, K. M., Kemmerer, W. T., and Kirby, R. R.: Intra-operative blood pressure measurements in infants, Anesthesiology **33**:361, 1970.

Kafka, H. L., and Oh, W.: Direct and indirect blood pressure measurements in newborn infants, Am. J. Dis. Child. **122**:425, 1971.

Katz, A. M., Birnbaum, M., Moylan, J., and Pellett, J.: Gangrene of the hand and forearm; a complication of radial artery cannulation, Crit. Care Med. **2**:270, 1974.

Kitterman, J. A., Phibbs, R. H., and Tooley, W. H.: Catheterization of umbilical vessels in newborn infants, Pediatr. Clin. North Am. **17**:895, 1970.

Lebowitz, M. H.: Gangrene of a thumb following use of photo-electric plethysmograph during anesthesia, Anesthesiology **32**:164, 1970.

Leonard, P. F.: Principles of electricity. I. The electric meter and thermistor, Anesth. Analg. (Cleve.) **45**:246, 1966.

Lowenstein, E., Little, J. W., and Hing, H. L.: Prevention of cerebral embolization from flushing radial artery cannulae, N. Engl. J. Med. **285**:1414, 1971.

McKenna, T., and Wilton, T. N. P.: Awareness during endotracheal intubation, Anaesthesia **28**:599, 1973.

Michenfelder, J. D., Miller, R. H., and Gronert, G. A.: Evaluation of an ultrasonic device (Doppler) for the diagnosis of venous air embolism, Anesthesiology **36**: 164, 1972.

Miyasaka, K., Edmonds, J. F., and Conn, A. W.: Complications of radial artery lines in the pediatric patient, Can. Anaesth. Soc. J. **23**:9, 1976.

Moffitt, E. A., Kirklin, J. W., and Theye, R. A.: Physiologic studies during whole-body perfusion in tetralogy of Fallot, J. Thorac. Cardiovasc. Surg. **44**:180, 1962.

Morris, R. H., and Kumar, A.: The effect of warming blankets on maintenance of body temperature of the anesthetized paralyzed adult patient, Anesthesiology **36**:408, 1972.

Nelson, D. S.: A monaural stethoscope for anesthesiologists, Anesth. Analg. (Cleve.) **51**:177, 1972.

Park, M. K., Kawabori, I., and Guntheroth, W. G.: Need for an improved standard for blood pressure cuff size, Clin. Pediatr. **15**:784, 1976.

Patterson, J. F.: Stethoscope monitoring during anesthesia, Anesth. Analg. (Cleve.) **45**:572, 1966.

Ploss, R. E.: A simple constant monitor system, Anesthesiology **16**:466, 1955.

Poppers, P. J.: Indirect arterial blood pressure measurement by ultrasonography. In Mark, L. C., and Mark, S. H., editors: Highlights of clinical anesthesiology, New York, 1971, Harper & Row, Publishers, Inc.

Prince, S. R., Sullivan, R. L., and Hackel, A.: Percutaneous catheterization of the internal jugular vein in infants and children, Anesthesiology **44**:170, 1976.

Radde, I. C., Parkinson, D. K., Hoffken, B., and others: Calcium ion activity in the sick neonate; effect of bicarbonate administration and exchange transfusion, Pediatr. Res. **6**:43, 1972.

Rao, T. L. K., Wong, A. Y., and Salem, M. R.: A new approach to percutaneous catheterization of the internal jugular vein, Anesthesiology **46**:362, 1977.

Roe, C. F., Santulli, T. V., and Blair, C. S.: Heat loss in infants during general anesthesia, J. Pediatr. Surg. **1**:266, 1966.

Rowe, M. I.: Physiologic monitoring. In Gans, S. L., editor: Surgical pediatrics, New York, 1973, Grune & Stratton, Inc.

Schneider, A. J. L., Kreul, J. F., and Zollinger, R. M., Jr.: Patient monitoring in the operating room; an anesthetist's viewpoint, Med. Instrum. **10**:105, 1976.

Schwartz, A. J.: Percutaneous aortic catheterization; a hazard of supraclavicular internal jugular vein catheterization, Anesthesiology **46:**77, 1977.

Scott, S. M.: Thermal blanket injury in the operating room, Arch. Surg. **94:**181, 1967.

Seldinger, S. L.: Catheter replacement of the needle in percutaneous arteriography; new technique, Acta Radiol. **39:**368, 1953.

Smith, R. M.: Anesthesia for pediatric surgery. In Gross, R. E., editor: Surgery of infants and children, Philadelphia, 1953, W. B. Saunders Co.

Smith, R. M.: Signs of depth and danger, Int. Anesthesiol. Clin. **1:**153, 1962.

Smith, R. M.: Thermic emergencies in anesthesia, Hosp. Prac. **3:**68, 1968.

Smith, R. M.: Temperature monitoring and regulation, Pediatr. Clin. North Am. **16:**643, 1969.

Smith, R. M.: Pediatric anesthesia in perspective, Anesth. Analg. (Cleve.) **57:**634, 1978.

Snow, J.: On chloroform and other anesthetics, London, 1858, John Churchill.

Stephen, C. R., Ahlgren, E. W., and Bennett, E. J.: Elements of pediatric anesthesia, Springfield, Ill., 1970, Charles C Thomas, Publisher.

Stephen, C. R., Dent, S. J., Hall, K. D., and others: Body temperature regulation during anesthesia in infants and children, J.A.M.A. **174:**15, 1960.

Swan, H. J. C., Ganz, W., Forrester, J., and others: Catheterization of the heart in man with use of a flow-directed balloon-tipped catheter, N. Engl. J. Med. **283:**447, 1970.

Talbert, J. L.: Intraoperative and postoperative monitoring of infants, Surg. Clin. North Am. **50:**787, 1970.

Ward, R. J., and Green, H. D.: Arterial puncture as a safe diagnostic aid, Surgery **57:**672, 1965.

Ware, R. W.: New approaches to the indirect measurement of human blood pressure, Proceedings of Third National Biomedical Science Instrumentation Symposium, 1965.

Waters, D. J.: Factors causing awareness during surgery, Br. J. Anaesth. **40:**259, 1968.

Weintraub, W. H., Cuderman, B. S., Hunt, C. E., and others: Computer monitoring of cardiodynamics in the newborn, J. Pediatr. Surg. **6:**372, 1971.

Woodbridge, P. D.: Changing concepts concerning depth of anesthesia, Anesthesiology **19:**536, 1957.

Wright, B. D.: A new use for the Block-Aid monitor, Anesthesiology **30:**236, 1969.

Zahed, B., Sadove, M. S., Hatano, S., and Wu, H. H.: Comparison of automated Doppler ultrasound and Korotkoff measurements of blood pressure in children, Anesth. Analg. (Cleve.) **50:**669, 1971.

CHAPTER 10

Normal recovery

Operating room
Recovery room or postanesthesia room
Postoperative responsibility

Recovery begins as soon as the anesthesiologist stops active administration of anesthetic agents. It follows a definite progression, first in the *operating room,* where respiration is reestablished and tracheal extubation accomplished, then in the *recovery room,* where the patient regains full consciousness and cardiopulmonary stability (or in the *intensive care unit* for prolonged support), and finally in the *nursing division* or *ward,* where he recovers his strength and becomes ambulatory and ready for discharge. The management of ambulatory patients is described in Chapter 22.

Recovery involves as many dangers as induction, and the anesthesiologist has specific responsibilities in each phase. Two special disadvantages are characteristic of the recovery period: (1) the child must enter this phase with normal responses weakened by the foregoing operation and anesthesia, and (2) the greater hazard is that the supportive care of the anesthesiologist is being withdrawn, leaving the patient to provide his own cardiopulmonary effort and stability.

OPERATING ROOM

In the ascent from apnea and areflexia upward through stages of gagging, gasping, and excitement toward the normal state of conscious control, a child is exposed to a variety of potential disasters. To bring him through safely, an anesthesiologist needs knowledge, skill, speed, and good fortune. Prevention of both immediate and subsequent complications lies in attention to the numerous individual problems (Dripps, 1957).

Removal of gastric contents

While the child is still under general anesthesia and well relaxed one should decide whether to pass a tube into the stomach. Most neonates and many other patients come to the operating room with a nasogastric tube in place. The tube should have been tested earlier and should be kept open during the procedure. If not functioning properly it should be replaced. The passage of a nasogastric tube is necessary in many operations and may be accomplished at various other times, depending on its indication. In a great many pediatric procedures, gastric intubation is not mandatory but depends on the individual situation. If the operation was performed on an emergency basis, it is usually advisable to pass a nasogastric tube and remove it if the stomach appears to be empty. Some anesthesiologists believe that this procedure should be carried out on all children. At The Children's Hospital Medical Center, we examine the child's abdomen and frequently refrain from intubating the stomach if it is perfectly flat and there is no hollow note on percussion. Following inhalation anesthesia maintained by mask, a child may aspirate a small amount of gas that should be withdrawn, and considerably more may enter the stomach if forceful ventilation is necessary to overcome spasm or resistance. The greatest accumulation of gastric air occurs during attempts to resuscitate seriously depressed patients prior to tracheal intubation, a situation seen rarely at present.

216

With initiation of recovery from inhalation anesthesia with halothane and nitrous oxide, adequate spontaneous respiration should be established promptly, but the question may arise as to whether nitrous oxide or halothane should be discontinued first. Three considerations seem pertinent:

1. The fear of diffusion hypoxia (Fink, 1955) has decreased, and we no longer feel that early elimination of nitrous oxide is mandatory (Frumin and Edelist, 1969).
2. The incidence of atelectasis is increased when high concentrations of oxygen are used at the termination of anesthesia.
3. Premature awakening is more easily controlled by halothane than nitrous oxide.

Based on these factors, it seems reasonable to reduce both nitrous oxide and halothane simultaneously.

After use of relaxants and their reversal, there is a natural tendency to watch the child carefully until respiration first returns and then go on to other things. This is a dangerous error, for respiration may not be adequate for another 5 or 10 minutes, during which time severe hypoxia can develop.

Tracheal extubation

When endotracheal intubation has been used, extubation must be performed with care to avoid such complications as vocal cord spasm, apnea, aspiration of vomitus, and cardiac arrhythmias. The best time to extubate as well as the details of the actual extubation should be considered.

Time to extubate. Extubation in small infants who are still under anesthesia often is followed by apnea, which may lead to bradycardia and cyanosis. However, if the tube is left in place, it causes very little reaction. Therefore, in infants less than 2 to 3 months of age, extubation is delayed until they are fully awake. This means that the infant must actually open his eyes, the true sign of awakening that may not occur for at least 5 or 10 minutes after active movement of arms and legs has returned.

Older infants and children show less tendency toward sudden depression and show greater irritation from the tube when extubation is delayed (Koka and others, 1977). Consequently, most older children who are breathing normally are extubated as soon as they begin to show the return of reflexes. One important exception is the child who is suspected of having a full stomach. Such a child is allowed to awaken completely before extubation in order to give evidence of the full return of his gag reflex (see Chapter 22). There are a few other exceptions, such as the child whose jaws have been wired together or who has comparable danger of airway obstruction.

When a delay of not more than 10 or 20 minutes is expected, it seems safer to keep the child in the operating room rather than transport him to the recovery room for subsequent extubation.

Technic of extubation. The removal of the endotracheal tube must be carried out with as much attention to detail as was needed for intubation. Several steps are of importance (Figs. 10-1 to 10-4). As the child awakens, any stimulation may cause strong occlusion of the jaw, and consequently it is advisable to have an airway or bite block in place before any manipulation is started. The lungs are then inflated, and both sides of the chest are auscultated to test for full expansion and the presence of secretions. Secretions, if present, are removed by passage of a sterile suction catheter that does not take up more than half the lumen of the endotracheal tube.

It is desirable to have the patient sufficiently anesthetized to allow *direct examination of mouth and pharynx* at this time *using a laryngoscope for visualization.* Any material that is present can be promptly removed, and the usual blind jabbing will be eliminated. Finally, when the patient is breathing properly and the cuff of the endotracheal tube, if present, is deflated, the tube may be slipped out. Rather than using suction during extubation, as once believed proper, it is preferable to blow a strong flow of oxygen through the tube during extubation to force out secretions that may have accumulated between the tube and the tracheal wall. Use of suction at extubation reduces oxygen ten-

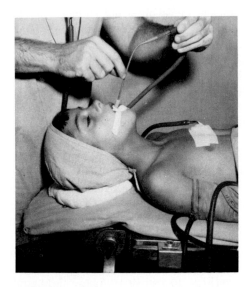

Fig. 10-1. The endotracheal tube and trachea are cleared with a small suction tube.

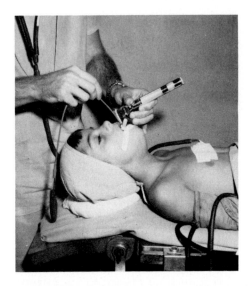

Fig. 10-2. While the child is still relaxed, the mouth and pharynx are examined with a laryngoscope, and material is cleared under direct vision.

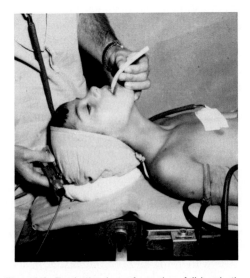

Fig. 10-3. Extubation is performed on full inspiration.

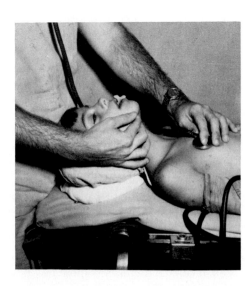

Fig. 10-4. Heart and lungs are checked immediately.

sion and stimulates laryngeal reflexes at the same time—a combination that has resulted in several deaths (Schumacher and Hampton, 1951; Branstater and Muallem, 1969).

The first moments following extubation are critical, especially in infants. If respiration is not resumed at once, preparation to take active steps must be made. If apnea is caused by momentary depression, this may be overcome simply by pressing on the child's chest. If spasm is not present, exchange will occur easily, and the patient usually will resume spontaneous respiration promptly. In case of spasm, oxygen can often be forced past the vocal cords by use of a bag and a mask. In severe laryngeal spasm this maneuver may not be effective. Consequently, as soon as spasm occurs it is wise to have an *assistant* prepare succinylcholine for immediate use while the anesthesiologist continues to attempt oxygenation. If given intravenously, 5 to 10 mg of succinylcholine (2 mg/kg) will be adequate to relieve spasm in a newborn at once and will be effective in 60 to 90 seconds if injected intramuscularly. If an intravenous infusion is not already in place, the intramuscular route may prove quicker than the intravenous route, since time must be taken for venipuncture. Following reestablishment of normal exchange, a careful check is made to look for gastric distension, pneumothorax, and airway secretions. Glottic spasm is discussed in more detail in Chapter 26.

Children frequently retch briefly on awakening and, although properly prepared, still may vomit enough to present some danger. Suction equipment must be immediately available and used with care and efficiency. Often it is sufficient to turn the child's head to the side to allow secretions to fall into the cheek for removal, or the child may be rolled on his side or face. Tipping the head of the table down is not especially helpful, and tipping it up is not safe. If vomiting is appreciable or if the stomach is distended, a large gastric tube is passed for evacuation.

While still on the operating table the child is undraped, placed in natural supine position, and briefly inspected for external injuries, loose or missing teeth, and distended stomach or bladder. Blood, skin-cleaning solutions, and other operative debris are removed, and the child is covered with a clean, warm blanket. Blood pressure, heart rate, color, blood replacement, and temperature should be checked before the child is taken from the operating room.

Anesthesiologists often take pride in having their patients wake up as the surgeon is tying his last knot. This may be a real asset if there is inadequate recovery care. However, prompt awakening often means early acute discomfort. If recovery care is adequate, it frequently is preferable to have the child sleep on for 15 or 20 minutes after the operation is finished. With the increasing tendency to reduce or eliminate preoperative medication, many patients now wake up without the benefit of either tranquilizer or analgesic. In the great majority of operations on children at least as young as 2 years of age, the anesthesiologist should make sure that enough medication has been given, either as premedication or during operation, to ease the early pain and anxiety on awakening. Morphine has long been the most reliable agent for this use. While some prefer to wait until the child shows the need for medication, both pain and anxiety are more easily prevented by medication than controlled after their onset. Reasonable precautions naturally should be taken for poor-risk patients.

The child is transported from the operating room either on a litter with guardrails or in his bed, properly positioned on his side or prone to provide maximum ventilatory safety (Fig. 10-5). Transportation of infants following operation demands the same strict attention to warmth and cleanliness that was observed before operation (Rickham, 1969; Haller and Talbert, 1972).

RECOVERY ROOM OR POSTANESTHESIA ROOM

The recovery room or postanesthesia room serves as an area of special care where the child's unsteady cardiovascular and respiratory systems become stabilized and the child regains complete consciousness. The

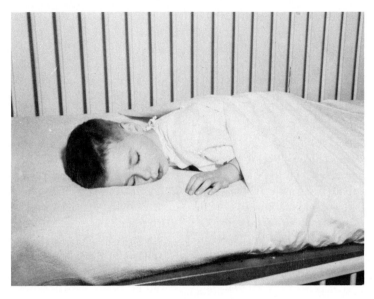

Fig. 10-5. Prone, or "T & A," position for transportation and recovery allows tongue to fall forward and secretions to escape.

recovery room has become a standard component of the operating room suite and should be immediately adjacent to it.

The organization of the recovery room will vary to suit the specific needs of the hospital and the type of surgery involved. Fairley (1969) recommends the provision of two recovery room beds for each operating room, a 24-hour total of two nurses for every three beds, and supervision by an anesthesiologist who directs respiratory care, resuscitation, pain medication, and discharge. Although the general concept of the recovery room is to treat all postoperative patients in the same area, in some hospitals it is more effective to set up special units for cardiac, neurologic, or other types of surgery.

The recovery room is equipped to give expert attention to all children who have had general anesthesia and to handle any emergency that may arise. Suction apparatus, laryngoscopes, endotracheal tubes, resuscitation equipment, ECG, cardiac defibrillator, monitors, heating and cooling apparatus, x-ray equipment, and a variety of drugs are required (see list below). A laboratory for immediate blood gas determination at any time of day or night is another essential component of this area, with competent personnel always available to operate it.

MEDICATION REQUIRED IN RECOVERY ROOM

Analgesics, sedatives, narcotics
Acetaminophen
Amobarbital (Amytal)
Aspirin
Diazepam
Edrophonium chloride (Tensilon)
Hydroxyzine
Meperidine
Morphine
Naloxone (Narcan)
Paraldehyde
Pentobarbital
Phenobarbital
Prochlorperazine dimaleate (Compazine)
Promethazine hydrochloride (Phenergan)
Trimethobenzamide hydrochloride (Tigan)

Antibiotics
Ampicillin (Polycillin)
Aqueous penicillin
Cephalothin (Keflin)
Chloramphenicol (Chloromycetin)
Clindamycin (Cleocin)
Gentamycin (Garamycin)
Kanamycin sulfate (Kantrex)
Methicillin sodium (Staphcillin)
Oxacillin
Procaine penicillin G (Bicillin C-R, Bicillin L-A, Wycillin)

Streptomycin
Sulfisoxazole (Gantrisin)
Tetracycline

Fluids

Ascorbic acid
Actifed syrup
Calcium gluconate
Calcium chloride
5% dextrose/¼N saline
5% dextrose/1N saline
50% glucose
Potassium chloride
Potassium phosphate
Sodium bicarbonate

Ointments

Desitin ointment
Nivea cream
Lidocaine jelly
Lidocaine viscous
Obtundia cream
Zinc oxide ointment

Miscellaneous

Bacitracin
Ilotycin
Neosporin
Panheprin
Tetanus toxoid

Initial care

When the child is brought to the recovery room, the anesthesiologist transfers him to his bed, positions him correctly, checks airway and ventilation, and inspects suction and oxygen equipment. The anesthesiologist reports to the nurse the child's condition, plus any special problems related to the events of the operation, and makes sure that suitable orders have been written. He remains with the child while the nurse checks heart rate, blood pressure, respiration, and temperature and does not leave until he is certain that the child is in reasonable condition and is well attended.

In the early postoperative period, a child's greatest problem often is that of airway obstruction. Recovery room attendants should be familiar with external signs of ventilatory inadequacy, should be skilled in the use of the stethoscope, and quick to act on the appearance of any form of hypoventilation. With small children, especially those who have had cleft-lip repair or other oral surgery, a traction suture placed in the tongue at the conclusion of operation provides recovery personnel with an excellent means of opening up the airway and stimulating respiration (Fig. 10-6).

Recovery room nurses also must be competent in early care of commonly encountered problems of excitement, pain, vomiting, temperature fluctuation, and delayed awakening, as well as less familiar complications such as pneumothorax, evisceration, or exsanguination.

Awakening responses

With present technics, awakening from anesthesia usually takes place within a few minutes after the end of operation. The time required before the child is truly alert will vary with premedication, anesthetic agent, and other factors but rarely exceeds 1 hour.

The child's postoperative awakening includes important medical and psychologic interactions. Many children wake up quietly, dozing at intervals, until they are fully responsive, without nausea, excitement, or other obvious disturbances. A large number of children, however, show active responses during awakening and present problems in diagnosis and/or management.

Often the first reaction seen is one of hyperactivity. Some children cry out loudly and beat around in the bed. This is the most common complication of the recovery period according to Downes and Nicodemus (1969), who found the highest incidence (13%) among healthy children 3 to 9 years of age.

An active, noisy child may invite immediate effective measures, such as heavy medication and restraints, but this kind of therapy can be lethal. While awakening excitement frequently may be related to drug response, other factors may enter the picture, playing either a contributing role or the predominant part. One must definitely exclude the presence of hypoxia before resorting to the use of depressant drugs.

Agitation caused by anesthetics may be variable in degree and duration, depending on the child, the drug, and the dosage. Studies have been made by Horne and Ahlgren (1973), Maguire and Aldrete (1975),

221

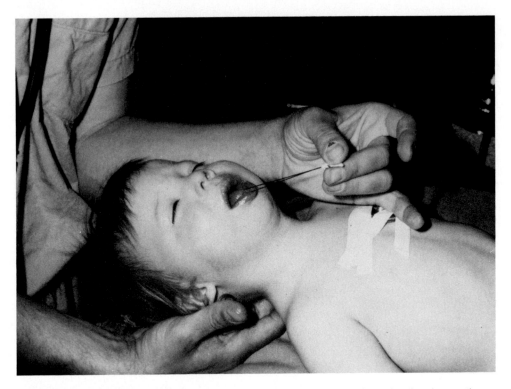

Fig. 10-6. A traction suture in the tongue serves as an excellent means of opening the airway, stimulating ventilatation, and preventing apnea.

and Steward (1977) comparing induction and recovery of children under halothane with those receiving enflurane. There was agreement that induction and recovery were more rapid with enflurane but that excitement during recovery also was significantly greater following enflurane anesthesia (possibly due to the more rapid awakening). Steward concluded that halothane was superior. While I agree, recovery from halothane still is far from ideal. Children often show pronounced excitement and shivering.

In 1955 Smith and associates observed a difference in the recovery from ether characterized by gross muscular clonus and the shivering more frequently seen following thiopental. Soliman and Gillies (1972), in their study of hyperactivity during recovery, made a similar differentiation, interpreting the hyperactivity seen following a variety of anesthetics as a natural process in the recovery of muscular function and shivering as being related primarily to altered response to temperature. Management of shivering is discussed in Chapter 26.

Barbiturates, cyclopropane, and halogenated agents have all been related to awakening delirium, usually of short duration and rarely remembered by the patients themselves. Following ketamine, however, hyperactivity may be prolonged, and in addition, patients have reported weird and upsetting experiences of partial consciousness that lasted many hours (Oduntan and Gool, 1970; Becsey and others, 1972). Children appear to have relatively few such reactions, but we have seen one in a 2-year-old child and possibly in an infant of 3 months.

As mentioned previously, much of this activity can be prevented by administration of sedatives or narcotics before, during, or after operation. If therapy is required following operation, one first makes sure that the child is breathing effectively and is well oxygenated. Then one can add thiopental (0.5 mg/kg) and induce another short nap, or one can use pentobarbital (1 mg/kg). Diazepam (Valium), though popular, is not predictable for such use and may cause delayed respiratory depression as well as vascular irritation when given intravenously unless administration is followed by immediate flushing (Schneider and Mace, 1974).

If medication is needed during the recovery of a child who has an infusion running, this is the preferred route to use. Giving painful, slowly effective, and poorly controlled medication at prolonged intervals is not rational when it is possible to titrate medication rapidly and painlessly by means of infusion.

The incidence of severe pain is closely associated with the surgical procedures involved. In pediatric surgery, pain medication is more frequently required following perineal procedures, operation for undescended testis, and orthopedic operations, particularly those requiring postoperative casts. Following thoracic and neurosurgical operations, pain is rarely severe enough to call for potent analgesics (Smith and others, 1961).

Of the several narcotics and analgesics available, morphine continues to be reliable and effective for control of both pain and excitement. Intravenous administration of 0.05 mg/kg is safe for normal children more than 9 to 12 months old and should be repeated according to individual requirement rather than given by any specified formula.

Greene (1971) has pointed to anticholinergic drugs as being responsible for early postoperative excitement and actual delirium. While scopolamine was indicted more frequently, atropine was named as the cause in an appreciable number of cases. The use of physostigmine was found to be highly effective in reversing both drugs when given in a dosage twice that of the original anticholinergic agent. It is highly probable that physostigmine will prove effective in reversing a number of other sedatives as well.

Continued uncontrollable activity in spite of sedation may suggest other causes. A healthy 5-year-old boy recently underwent strabismus correction of one eye. He received pentobarbital and morphine followed by nitrous oxide–halothane anesthesia. As he awoke, he screamed and thrashed, tearing at his bandaged eye and claiming total blindness. After 2 hours and three intravenous doses of meperidine, his mother was asked into the recovery room to help. He went to sleep in less than 2 minutes. His problems turned out to be his first separation from his mother, awakening in a strange room, and not having been adequately warned about the bandage on his eye. Warning the child of unexpected experiences has been discussed. The problem of awakening in a strange recovery room and the possibility of letting the mother into the recovery room are closely related and deserve more consideration.

As previously noted, emergence excitement is only one of many complications common to recovery. The management of vomiting, airway problems, hypothermia, and specific disease-related complications are discussed in Chapter 26 and elsewhere.

Orders for general care include the following:

1. **Position.** Usually on side or face down with shoulder support; position should be changed every 30 minutes.
2. **Vital signs.** Check pulse and respiration every 15 minutes for the first hour, every 30 minutes for the second hour, every hour for the following 4 hours, and every 4 hours thereafter. Check blood pressure at similar intervals.
3. **Temperature.** Check every hour for 4 hours or until stable and then every 4 hours.
4. **Oral intake.** Nothing by mouth if on gastric suction; otherwise liquids are allowed, progressing to semisolids and solids if the child is not nauseated.
5. **Fluids.** Blood is ordered to complete replacement of estimated loss; following this it is usually advisable to order enough 5% dextrose in ¼N saline solution to allow for half the daily fluid requirement (see Chapter 25). To prevent drowning of the patient by rapid infusion, the amount of fluid left in the container should not total more than 10 mg/kg; with infants the rate of administration is specified in drops per minute (usually 8 to 10).
6. **Sedation.** Small infants are denied sedation for fear of depression; from 6 months to 1 year of age, healthy infants may be given phenobarbital, 15 to 30 mg, if the drug is dissolved and administered rectally. Morphine or meperidine may be ordered for children at the age of 1 year. The first postoperative dose should be cut to half the regular dose; the regular dose of morphine is 0.75 mg/yr of age (up to 12 years) and of meperidine is 1 mg/kg. The

individual dose must be altered to conform to the child's condition. Narcotics should never be ordered "by the clock" but should be given only if needed.

As emphasized by Kornfield (1969), there are definite disadvantages as well as advantages to the recovery room concept. Children are not happy in the strange surroundings, their chief complaint often being that they want to go back to their beds. The emotional strain of awakening in a strange place has been said to be appreciable. Children also may be troubled by the sight of others in unpleasant attitudes, especially those who emerge from tonsillectomy unconscious with bloodied faces.

In our recovery room, nurses chart the course of each child's progress on a special form; one side relates to the serial observation of specific physical signs as well as the state of the airway and consciousness, and the other shows details of fluid balance (Fig. 10-7). With few exceptions, children are maintained in the recovery room for a minimum of 1 hour following any general anesthetic. By this time, they usually have awakened, have adapted to their surroundings, and have been given any required medication for discomfort. If cardiorespiratory functions have stabilized and no obvious problem exists, the anesthesiologist-in-charge reviews the records, rechecks the patient, and signs the discharge order.

Hospitalized children are transported by nurses or trained attendants to the nursing division, where suction equipment and oxygen again must be immediately available and nurses or attendants are ready to receive them. Care of ambulatory patients is described in Chapter 22.

POSTOPERATIVE RESPONSIBILITY

The anesthesiologist is responsible for the child until all danger of anesthetic complication is ended. The degree to which the anesthesiologist continues to control patient care following operation varies considerably and is usually related to his interest and ability. It is now a standard of the Joint Commission on Accreditation of Hospitals that the anesthesiologist make at least one postoperative visit and record a follow-up note. While this may satisfy regulations for a child following orchidopexy, daily visits for 10 or 12 days may be necessary after spinal fusion or a cardiac or neurosurgical procedure to ensure adequate ventilatory care, pain control, and freedom from hepatorenal complications. Precise notation of the anesthesiologist's findings and suggestions contribute equally to the patient's welfare and to the stature of the anesthesiologist.

The postoperative visits give the anesthesiologist his greatest opportunity to solidify personal relationships with child and parents, for it is then that he can do most to give the child a reasonable understanding of the whole hospital stay rather than leave him with a distorted, unpleasant picture in mind. The careful preoperative preparation and promise of painless procedure will bear sour fruit if the child is allowed to struggle through a harrowing recovery with no word of explanation or encouragement.

Should there be a complication of any kind, it is best to explain it to the parents with honesty and justify it if possible. If an anesthesiologist has established an understanding with patient and family before operation and has gained their respect, this will stand as the best possible means of avoiding any misunderstanding or litigation. A complication should be noted in the record to show that it was recognized, but definitive allocation of blame only invites hostile action.

Few realize the appreciation that parents feel for the anesthesiologist who will sit down and explain bothersome problems or simply develop a continuing relationship with a child. In such a relationship it is helpful to find out items that the child disliked so that they can be avoided (usually needles and the mask) and also to learn what, if anything, he had enjoyed, such as self-propelled go-carts and playroom activity.

The child who must return for repeated operations deserves most consideration and special effort to eliminate his particular dislikes. As a child recovers, one may find deeper reasons for his unhappiness, as in the case of the little 3-year-old who could not under-

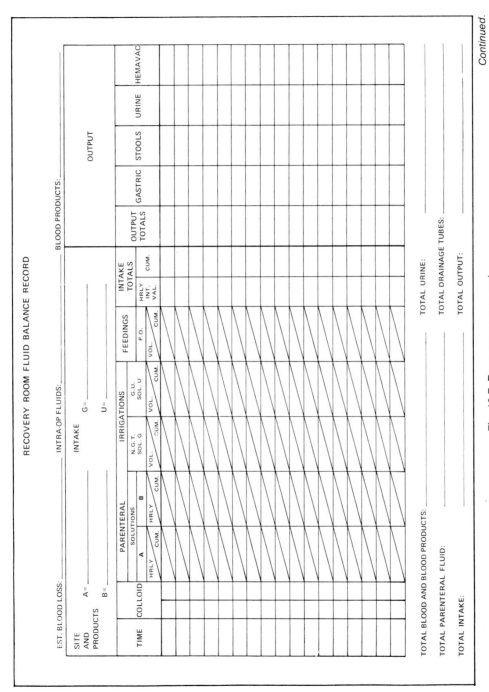

Fig. 10-7. Recovery room record.

Continued.

Schowengudt, C. G.: The recovery room. In Dornette, W. H. L., editor: Monitoring in anesthesia, Philadelphia, 1973, F. A. Davis Co.

Schweizer, O.: The recovery and intensive care unit; a clinical laboratory, Anesthesiology 32:246, 1970.

Shumacher, H. B., and Hampton, L. J.: Sudden death occurring immediately after operation in patients with cardiac disease, with particular reference to the role of aspiration through the endotracheal tube and extubation, J. Thorac. Cardiovasc. Surg. 21:48, 1951.

Smith, R. M., Bougas, T. P., and Bachman, L.: Shivering following thiopental and other anesthetic agents, Anesth. Analg. (Cleve.) 16:655, 1955.

Smith, R. M., Stetson, J. B., and Sanchez-Salazar, A.: Postoperative distress in children, Anesthesiology 22:145, 1961.

Soliman, M. G., and Gillies, D. M. M.: Muscular hyperactivity after general anesthesia, Can. Anaesth. Soc. J. 19:529, 1972.

Steward, D. J.: Enflurane for pediatric patients? Fifteenth Clinical Conference in Pediatric Anesthesiology, Los Angeles, January 28-30, 1977.

Wicklund, P. E.: Design of a recovery room and intensive care unit, Anesthesiology 26:667, 1965.

toward the area containing the median ante-brachial cutaneous, median, and musculocutaneous nerves, in that order (Fig. 11-1). Aspiration is attempted as the needle is advanced, and if blood is encountered, the needle is retracted and reinserted more cephalad. Paresthesias are not sought out, and solution should not be injected into these nerves. One half of the solution (1% lido-caine, 0.5 ml/kg [5 mg/kg]) is injected above or cephalad to the artery, where the remainder of the solution is injected to anesthetize the ulnar and radial nerves. A period of 15 to 20 minutes should be allowed for complete effect of the block.

Interscalene (Winnie) block. We have recently used interscalene brachial plexus block, described by Winnie (1970), for young patients with chronic renal failure who required establishment of an arteriovenous fistula in the arm. Axillary block has been avoided in these children for fear of damaging the axillary artery or compressing it by hematoma formation. The interscalene block is performed by locating the groove between the anterior and lateral scalene muscles at the level of Chassaignac's tubercle, introducing a 1½-inch 26-gauge needle caudally to penetrate the fascial sheath of the plexus, eliciting paresthesia, and then injecting 1% bupivacaine, 0.3 ml/kg (3 mg/kg).

Intravenous regional anesthesia

Probably the most practical block for hand, arm, or lower extremity is that established by intravenous injection of local anesthetic and first described by Bier in 1908, the intravenous regional, or Bier, block. This has been popularized by numerous reports in the last decade (Atkinson and others, 1965; Dunbar and Mazze, 1967; Gingrich, 1967; FitzGerald, 1976).

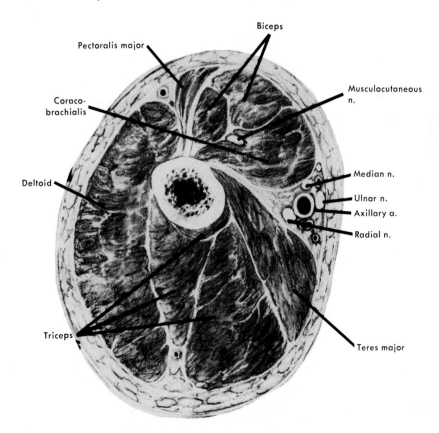

Fig. 11-1. Cross-section of arm showing nerve distribution at upper humeral level. (From Moore, D. C.: Regional block, Springfield, Ill., 1965, Charles C Thomas, Publisher.)

The standard technic consists of positioning a double pneumatic tourniquet on the arm or leg to be treated and then placing an intravenous infusion near the operative site. The limb is then exsanguinated by elevation, use of an Esmarch bandage, and inflation of the tourniquet that is more proximal to the body to twice the systolic pressure. The anesthetic, 0.5% lidocaine (without epinephrine), is then injected intravenously to a total of 3 mg/kg. A period of 10 minutes is allowed for fixation of anesthesia, and then the lower tourniquet is inflated and the upper, or proximal, one released. To prevent systemic effect, Dunbar and Mazze suggest that the second tourniquet should not be released less than 30 minutes after administration of the anesthetic, which is gradually taken up into the extravascular tissues.

It should be emphasized that while this block is the most easily performed, it carries the greatest incidence of complication, chiefly because of the escape or early release of the local anesthetic into the general circulation, the potential effect being seizures, cardiovascular collapse, or ventricular fibrillation. However, on the basis of 50 cases reported in 1976, FitzGerald suggests several modifications that may be made to simplify the procedure and adapt it for pediatric use. These include the use of one tourniquet instead of two for arterial occlusion, exsanguination of the limb by elevation without the use of an Esmarch bandage, and release of the tourniquet only 20 minutes after injection of the lidocaine anesthetic (0.5% lidocaine). Before attempting any of these simplifications, one should bear in mind Eather's warning of the danger of tourniquet failure, as well as the importance of preparation for treatment of toxic reactions. This type of block is not one to be performed in an unequipped area or private office.

Diagnostic and therapeutic block

Although seldom used for treatment of vascular disease, as in older patients, sympathetic nerve blocks may be used following fractures of arms or legs, following extensive soft-tissue damage, as in "wringer arm," or following injury to major vessels. After extensive surgical procedures on the limbs, stellate or lumbar sympathetic block may be performed to promote circulation and reduce edema formation. Technics are similar to those used in adults as described by Bonica (1953) and Moore (1957).* In actuality, it often is much more practical to perform low spinal anesthesia on a small child than it is to perform a lumbar sympathetic block. It entails far less needling, and the resultant block is more predictable and more rapidly effective. For the upper extremity, a stellate block is not difficult to perform, but in many situations axillary brachial block will prove as effective and probably entails fewer hazards.

Inoperable tumors are seen all too frequently in children, and here therapeutic blocks can be used with good effect. Ample sedation should be used before the block is performed, and light nitrous oxide or halothane anesthesia may be used as well. As recommended by Bonica (1953), a preliminary block with procaine should precede destructive blocks with alcohol or phenol.

ACUPUNCTURE

Along with many other claims made during the early enthusiasm over acupuncture was that children, having an active imagination and being easy to convince, would be excellent subjects for acupuncture. These claims do not seem to have been borne out in the Western world, and the use of acupuncture has found even less place in pediatric surgery than in adult surgery, where it is rarely seen.

BIBLIOGRAPHY

Amster, J. L.: Spinal anesthesia for poor pediatric surgical risks, Med. Rec. Ann. **144:**213, 1956.

Atkinson, D. I., Modell, J., and Moya, F.: Intravenous regional anesthesia, Anesth. Analg. (Cleve.) **44:**313, 1965.

Berkowitz, D., and Greene, B. A.: Spinal anesthesia in children; report based on 350 patients under 13 years of age, Anesthesiology **12:**376, 1951.

*As described in Chapter 19 (p. 473), there has been a sudden increase in the call for sympathetic blocks to treat sympathetic dystrophy following athletic strain in pediatric patients.

Bier, A.: Über einen neuen Weg local Anästhesie an den Gliedmassen zu erzeugen, Arch. Klin. Chir. **86:**1007, 1908.

Bonica, J. J.: The management of pain, Philadelphia, 1953, Lea & Febiger.

Chung, B., Naraghi, M., and Adriani, J.: Sympathomimetic effects of cocaine and their influence on halothane and enflurane anesthesia, Anesthesiol. Rev. **5:**16, 1978.

Clayton, M. L., and Turner, D. A.: Upper arm block in children with fractures, J.A.M.A. **169:**327, 1959.

Covino, B. G.: Local anesthesia, N. Engl. J. Med. **386:** 975, 1035, 1972.

DeJong, R. H.: Axillary block of the brachial plexus, Anesthesiology **22:**215, 1961.

DeJong, R. H.: Physiology and pharmacology of local anesthesiology, Springfield, Ill., 1970, Charles C Thomas, Publisher.

Dunbar, R. W., and Mazze, R. I.: Intravenous regional anesthesia; experience with 779 cases, Anesth. Analg. (Cleve.) **46:**806, 1967.

Eather, K. F.: Axillary brachial plexus block, Anesthesiology **19:**683, 1958.

Eather, K. F.: Regional anesthesia for infants and children, Int. Anesthesiol. Clin. **13:**19, 1975.

Ernst, F. W.: Guest discussion; regional anesthesia in children, Anesth. Analg. (Cleve.) **54:**389, 1975.

FitzGerald, B.: Intravenous regional anaesthesia in children, Br. J. Anaesth. **48:**485, 1976.

Foldes, F. F., Molloy, R., McNail, P. G., and others: Comparison of toxicity of intravenously given local anesthetic agents in man, J.A.M.A. **172:**1493, 1960.

Frederickson, E. L.: Quoted from a symposium on Ethrane and Forane, Anesthesiol. Rev. **2:**15, 1975.

Gingrich, E. F.: Intravenous regional anesthesia of the upper extremity in children, J.A.M.A. **200:**135, 1967.

Gray, H.: Anatomy of the human body, ed. 22, Philadelphia, 1930, Lea & Febiger.

Gray, T.: Study of spinal anesthesia in infants and children, Lancet **2:**913, 1909.

Harris, W. E., Slater, E. M., and Bell, H. M.: Regional anesthesia by the intravenous route, J.A.M.A. **194:** 1273, 1965.

Hassan, S. Z.: Caudal anesthesia in infants, Anesth. Analg. (Cleve.) **56:**686, 1977.

Hassan, S. Z., and Williams, J. R.: Spread of radiopaque solution in the epidural space of human neonate, J. Reprod. Med. **10:**31, 1973.

Johnston, R. R., Eger, E. E. II, and Wilson, C.: A comparative interaction of epinephrine with halothane, enflurane and isoflurane, Anesth. Analg. (Cleve.) **55:**709, 1976.

Junkin, C. I.: Spinal anesthesia in children, Can. Med. Assoc. J. **28:**51, 1953.

Leigh, M. D., and Belton, M. K.: Pediatric anesthesia, ed. 2, New York, 1960, Macmillan, Inc.

Levin, R. M.: Pediatric anesthesia handbook, Flushing, N.Y., 1973, Medical Examination Publishing Co., Inc.

Melman, E., Penuelas, J., and Marrufo, J.: Regional anesthesia in children, Anesth. Analg. (Cleve.) **54:** 387, 1975.

Moore, D. C.: Regional block, ed. 2, Springfield, Ill., 1957, Charles C Thomas, Publisher.

Moore, D. C., Bridenbaugh, D., Bridenbaugh, P. O., and Tucker, G. T.: Bupivacaine for peripheral block; a comparison with mepivacaine, lidocaine and tetracaine, Anesthesiology **32:**460, 1970.

Moore, D. C., and Toland, J. F.: Anesthesia for surgery of the nose, pharynx, larynx and trachea, Arch. Otolaryngol. **63:**275, 1956.

Patrick, R. T.: Correspondence, Anesth. Analg. (Cleve.) **54:**825, 1975.

Redo, S. F.: Surgery of the ambulatory child, New York, 1961, Appleton-Century-Crofts.

Robson, C. H.: Anesthesia in children, Am. J. Surg. **34:**468, 1936.

Ruston, F. G.: Epidural anesthesia in pediatric surgery, Anesth. Analg. (Cleve.) **36:**76, 1957.

Sadove, M. S., Wyant, G. M., Gittelson, L. A., and Kretchmer, H. E.: Classification and management of reactions to local anesthetic agents, J.A.M.A. **148:** 17, 1952.

Slater, H. M., and Stephen, C. R.: Hypobaric pontocaine spinal anesthesia in children, Anesthesiology **11:** 709, 1950.

Small, G. A.: Brachial plexus block anesthesia in children, J.A.M.A. **147:**1648, 1951.

Spiegel, P.: Caudal anesthesia in pediatric surgery, Anesth. Analg. (Cleve.) **41:**218, 1962.

Steinhaus, J. E.: Comparative study of experimental toxicity of local anesthetic agents, Anesthesiology **13:** 577, 1952.

Tandon, S. N., Monafo, W. W., and Tandon, N.: Analgesia by surface hypothermia, Anesthesiol. Rev. **5:** 34, 1978.

Touloukian, R. J., Wugmeister, M., Pickett, L. K., and Hehre, F. W.: Caudal anesthesia for neonatal anoperineal and rectal operations, Anesth. Analg. (Cleve.) **50:**565, 1971.

Wilton, T. N., and Wilson, F.: Neonatal anesthesia, Philadelphia, 1965, F. A. Davis Co.

Winnie, A. P.: Interscalene brachial plexus block, Anesth. Analg. (Cleve.) **49:**455, 1970.

Zsigmond, E. K., and Downs, J. R.: Plasma cholinesterase activity in newborns and infants, Can. Anaesth. Soc. J. **18:**278, 1971.

CHAPTER 12

Intravenous and intramuscular anesthesia

Advantages and disadvantages
Age limit for use of intravenous anesthesia
Indications for intravenous agents
Agents

The barriers between adult and pediatric anesthesia have been broken down in many areas, and the use of intravenous agents is an outstanding example. This change has been apparent in the United States but is considerably more obvious in England and France, where the intravenous approach has been more aggressively employed. In addition to the hesitance of American anesthetists to shift from mask to needle, an increasingly apparent drag on progress in this area has come from overprotective federal regulation of investigation and use of new drugs, especially in relation to children.

Intravenous drugs that have overcome these obstacles and have been more freely accepted for pediatric anesthesia include short-acting barbiturates, other less potent nonbarbiturate hypnotics, narcotics, and so-called dissociative and cycloplegic agents such as Innovar (consisting of fentanyl citrate plus droperidol) and ketamine. However, such foreign agents as propanidid and althesin are virtually unknown in the United States.

Although no investigator has concentrated exclusively on the pediatric use of intravenous agents, the extensive work of Dundee and his associates in the clinical and pharmacologic aspects of numerous intravenous agents provides invaluable guidance for use

with patients of all ages (Dundee, 1964, 1969; Clarke, 1969).

ADVANTAGES AND DISADVANTAGES

Intravenous anesthetics carry almost the same advantages for children as for adults. Once an infusion is established, induction is rapid and pleasant. The agents are nonflammable and generally free from metabolic disturbance and toxicity, and many of them reduce the incidence of postoperative excitement and nausea (Siker, 1965).

The disadvantages associated with most forms of intravenous anesthesia in pediatric work include greater difficulty in venipuncture, the child's dislike of needles, greater hazard of airway irritation and obstruction, and lack of controllability with consequent danger of overdosage. More definitive advantages and disadvantages may be related to specific drugs, e.g., the danger of using thiopental in patients with porphyria.

AGE LIMIT FOR USE OF INTRAVENOUS ANESTHESIA

Although there is no lower age limit for use of these agents, the less predictable response of neonates to all drugs is good reason to avoid intravenous administration in the very young. After a child reaches 6 months of age, his response is more predictable, but danger of respiratory depression and laryngotracheal irritation is still high. While it is possible to use this form of anesthesia in all ages, the disadvantages tend to outweigh the advantages until a child is 2 or 3 years old.

INDICATIONS FOR INTRAVENOUS AGENTS

Intravenous anesthesia may serve many purposes in children. Several that offer particular advantages may be grouped as follows:

For induction of anesthesia (as described in Chapter 7):
1. Patients who have infusions running upon arrival in the operating room
2. Critically ill patients
3. Retarded or unmanageable children

For very short procedures:
1. Cardioversion
2. Brief outpatient operations, suture removal, dental extraction, traction pin removal, etc.

For maintenance in longer procedures:
1. Orthopedic operations on limbs with the patient supine
2. Neurosurgical examinations or operations
3. Cystoscopy in females
4. Cardiac catheterization

For treatment of seizure disorders:
1. Status epilepticus
2. Encephalitis
3. Tetanus

AGENTS
Short-acting barbiturates

Intravenous anesthesia that has been given to children has consisted chiefly of the short-acting barbiturates, including hexobarbital (Evipal), methitural (Neraval), methohexital (Brevital), thiamylal (Surital), and thiopental (Pentothal). Most of these agents are remarkably alike, producing rapid induction of hypnosis with hardly any relaxation. These drugs are not classed as anesthetic agents and have even been termed "antanalgesic" by Dundee (1969), but simple procedures can be performed with barbiturates alone, and numerous operations can be performed with barbiturates fortified by nitrous oxide–oxygen mixtures.

The distribution and fate of short-acting barbiturates in adults have been extensively studied by Brodie (1952), Dundee and Barron (1962), Mark (1963), Saidman and Eger (1966) and others, but little investigation has been made of their fate in children other than the studies of Lindsay and Shepherd (1969).

For many years there was a reluctance to give intravenous barbiturates to children for fear of excessive respiratory depression and delayed awakening. Because of the child's proportionately greater amount of vessel-rich tissue, the uptake of drugs should be more rapid (Eger, 1974), the effect more quickly achieved, and metabolism, excretion, and recovery more prompt unless retarded by supplementary agents.

The predominant danger in younger patients receiving intravenous barbiturates lies in airway irritation, spasm, and obstruction, aggravated by the child's narrow air passages and increased incidence of respiratory infections, enlarged tonsils and adenoids, and asthmatic congestion.

Thiopental sodium. The virtual monopoly held by thiopental sodium (Pentothal) in the field of intravenous agents is partly because of its earlier production and more active promotion, but also because of its fewer side effects. Hiccoughs, sneezing, and other irregularities are rarely seen on induction, and there is no excitement or extrapyramidal activity. CSF pressure is reduced, making the agent useful in diagnostic and operative neurosurgical work (Dawson and others, 1971). Intraocular pressure also falls. Awakening is quiet, occasionally interrupted by shivering (Smith and others, 1955), and shows a low incidence of nausea.

Technics in the use of thiopental may be altered to suit the individual situation. The choice of premedication is an important variable. Atropine helps to reduce airway irritability but is not mandatory. Morphine should be given if operations involve considerable pain, but for many outpatient procedures elimination of supplemental drugs will reduce recovery time greatly.

For pediatric work, *thiopental is used in 2% or 2.5% solution*, as with adults. Administration of *4 mg/kg is suitable to induce sleep*. An initial 75% concentration of nitrous oxide is reduced to 66% after 5 or 10 minutes. Respiration is depressed early, but respiratory reflexes remain active, and use of an airway is likely to cause reaction unless topical anesthesia is added.

Eye signs are invaluable during thiopental–nitrous oxide anesthesia. Enough thiopental must be given to keep the eyes centered and fixed or the child will react to pain. With greater depth of barbiturate sedation, pupils constrict, but less than when caused by morphine overdosage. Thus, while the surgeon prepares the patient, increments of 1 or 2 mg/kg are added until the eyes are fixed, and close watch is kept as the first incision is made, after which responses tend to be less active. Obviously any movement will call for more sedation.

During the entire procedure a reasonable total dose of thiopental may be in the range of 20 mg/kg. This is generally sufficient for a 2- or 3-hour procedure and should be followed by prompt awakening. Usually one must give a large proportion of the total amount in the first 30 minutes, but the requirement falls off, with unused thiopental remaining. If more than 20 mg/kg is necessary, one can add more thiopental or supplement it with morphine or halothane, but this is rarely necessary. Since morphine can be reversed effectively, it is better for use toward the end of prolonged cases (Mark, 1971). The administration of thiopental and other sedatives and relaxants by continuous drip infusion increases the risk of overdosage and is especially undesirable for pediatric patients.

Supplementation with morphine (or other narcotics) throughout the whole operation enables one to use less barbiturate, provides more analgesia, and reduces airway irritability. If relaxants are used and the anesthetist is uncertain of adequate analgesic effect, this is an advisable move, but it prolongs recovery time, mixes agents and increases nausea.

When morphine is used, one may add 1 mg/25 kg shortly after induction and again at 30- to 45-minute intervals. Respiration may be slower with this method. With either technic, respiration must be carefully monitored and usually will need some manual assistance.

The respiratory depressant effect of thiopental is obvious but is seldom of importance unless it persists into the recovery period. Of more significance is the danger of vocal cord spasm caused by laryngotracheal irritability. Recourse to relaxant and intubation may be easier for the novice, but for outpatient and minor procedures it is often preferable to avoid intubation if possible.

If delayed awakening or respiratory depression occurs after operation, one should evaluate possible factors, especially if supplemental morphine or relaxants have been used. Before more drugs are added, a nerve stimulator will guide use of relaxant reversal. Slow, deep respiration and marked constriction of pupils suggest use of a morphine antagonist. In barbiturate excess, respiration is shallow, pupils are slightly constricted, and there is full muscular reaction to painful stimulation.

Numerous agents have been proposed to treat barbiturate overdosage. Ample opportunity for testing these agents has been available in poisoning and suicidal overdosage. Early trials of analeptic agents, such as succinate and ethamivan, were unsuccessful, and neither respiratory stimulant nor barbiturate antagonist was believed to exist. In the analeptic doxapram there is some evidence that in dosages of 0.5 to 1.0 mg/kg, the drug has few side effects and can hasten recovery from barbiturate overdosage (Siker and others, 1964). The action is probably due to baroreceptor stimulation rather than pharmacologic antagonisms (Gupta and Dundee, 1974), though central action was reported by Plaut and associates (1973). The clinical value of this agent is uncertain and has not been investigated in children.

Certainly any question of full stomach or preexisting airway obstruction or inflammation contraindicates use of thiopental for induction or for maintenance without intubation. In any child whose cardiovascular efficiency is reduced by anomalies, hypovolemia, or disease, thiopental may cause myocardial depression and hypotension and should be avoided. Porphyria, seldom encountered in the United States, is a specific contraindication to barbiturates (Dundee, McCleery, and McLaughlin, 1962).

Methohexital. Methohexital (Brevital), a methylated oxybarbiturate, differs from thiopental in several respects. It is more potent by a ratio of about 3 to 1 (Clarke and others, 1968), it is more rapidly eliminated, and it produces more undesirable side effects. The greater strength adds little to its value. Greater speed of recovery provides its principal indication, especially for outpatient work or for situations where very brief effect is wanted, as for cardioversion or electroconvulsive therapy. The comparative incidence of involuntary muscular movement, hiccough, and respiratory irregularity during induction is definitely greater with methohexital than with thiopental.

Methohexital is administered intravenously in 1% or 2% solution and has been used by intramuscular route without tissue damage (Miller and others, 1961). It is prepared by mixing 500 mg of powered agent in 50 ml of water to give a 1% concentration (10 mg/ml). An induction dose of 1 mg/kg and a maximum total dose of 4 to 6 mg/kg should provide satisfactory results.

Nonbarbiturate hypnotics

Several of the so-called tranquilizing agents have been administered intravenously for hypnotic effect during operation. Considerably less predictable than thiopental and having no analgesic action, these agents are sometimes used on the grounds of causing less cardiovascular depression than short-acting barbiturates (Etsten and Li, 1955).

Diazepam (Valium), currently popular as a sedative, and chlordiazepoxide (Librium), two benzodiazepine tranquilizers, have had a relatively favorable reception. Of the two, diazepam has been more successful, having several points in its favor. It produces relatively pleasant sedation or hypnosis with few side effects and more prompt recovery than most sedatives. Its action is due to depression of amygdala of the limbic system. It also acts on spinal internuncial neurons to give some degree of muscular relaxation. Although initially distributed with warnings that it should

not be used for young children (a standard production policy) nor for patients with seizure disorders, it soon proved to be the best drug yet known for the specific treatment of children with seizure disorders (Lombroso, 1966, 1974; Carter and Gold, 1977).

Diazepam is available as a viscid fluid for intravenous or intramuscular injection, supplied in 2-ml ampules containing 10 mg, at pH of 6.8 at 20° C. Intravenous administration of 10 mg will usually induce hypnosis in adults, but the requirement varies widely. For children a dose of 0.2 mg/kg is reasonable, to be followed by 0.1 mg/kg at 3-minute intervals until the child becomes relaxed and lightly asleep. This type of sedation serves nicely in older children during regional block or to help them tolerate ventilator therapy. It has been promoted enthusiastically for use in cardioversion, again on the premise that it causes less cardiac depression than barbiturates (Muenster and others, 1967). Abel and Reis (1971) found it valuable in quieting patients with impaired cardiac function following operation. They showed that with 0.1 mg/kg, blood pressure decreased, probably from reduction in peripheral resistance, but the accompanying increase in stroke volume preserved the integrity of the circulation.

Narcotics

Narcotics may be used in the pediatric age group in combination with various intravenous agents. Nitrous oxide, thiopental, and morphine now stand as three time-proven agents that are highly predictable and make a combination of great value. With the addition of d-tubocurarine, equally reliable, one can meet almost all demands. Complications arising from these agents are largely preventable in skilled hands and curable if they do occur. The single real disadvantage associated with all combinations of these agents is that of airway control. Ventilation is depressed by thiopental, slowed by morphine, and arrested by curare. Although it is seldom difficult to assist ventilation or intubate the trachea, this is not always desirable.

In sharp contrast, halothane still carries suspicion of toxic qualities but is superior to

243

most agents in preservation of ventilatory exchange.

Morphine is tolerated extremely well by infants and children. The lowered tolerance reported by Way and associates (1965), if significant at all, is limited to neonates. As previously noted, the intravenous addition of morphine during thiopental–nitrous oxide anesthesia adds analgesia and decreases airway irritability, often enabling one to avoid intubation. When intubation is employed, morphine supplementation enables one to maintain patients with similar thiopental–nitrous oxide combinations without relaxants. For normal children who have had thiopental induction (and intubation under relaxants if indicated) plus nitrous oxide–oxygen in a 2:1 ratio, 5 mg of morphine are diluted to 10 ml and administered in 0.5- to 1.0-mg doses early in the operation until the effect is obvious in constricting pupils, reduction of heart rate, and greater pulmonary compliance. The incidence of hypotension has been negligible when patients have been well ventilated and not subjected to excessive change in position during anesthesia.

Morphine, as employed by Lowenstein and associates (1969) in adults, has been of most critical value in management of infants and children with severe cardiac disease. Here thiopental is replaced by ketamine for induction (1 mg/kg), and morphine is added in increments of 0.1 mg/kg at 3-minute intervals until the infant is quiet and relaxed. Prompt reversal is always possible with naloxone (Narcan) in a dosage of approximately 0.002 mg/kg (0.1 mg/25 lb).

Several other narcotics may serve as intravenous analgesics during anesthesia. Meperidine (Demerol), in 1-mg/kg increments, and alphaprodine (Nisentil), in 0.4-mg/kg increments, have approximately the same effect, while fentanyl (Sublimaze), 0.0025 mg/kg, provides an equal effect of shorter duration. Fentanyl is more potent than morphine but acts in a similar manner. Droperidol (Inapsine) is a butyrophenone derivative that produces a prolonged state of detachment without actual sleep, thereby earning the term *neuroleptic*. When used alone as a premedi-

cant it causes increased anxiety and excessive pyramidal tract activity. It is an effective antiemetic and has alpha-adrenergic blocking action, which may counteract the vasoconstrictor effect of epinephrine.

The principal use of droperidol has been in combination with the short-acting narcotic fentanyl in a 50:1 ratio to form the mixture supplied under the name of Innovar. Useful qualities of Innovar include the effective analgesic action of fentanyl, 40 times as potent as morphine, and the sedative, or neuroleptic, effect of droperidol, which is said to render patients impervious to sensory or visual stimuli, such as amputation of an arm. Freedom from cardiovascular depression is a feature of Innovar that makes it useful in major cardiac operations, and it has some use in neurosurgical patients because of its lack of effect on CSF pressure.

In its usual application, Innovar containing 2.5 mg of droperidol and 0.05 mg of fentanyl per ml is used for induction and early establishment of anesthetic state, after which supplemental analgesia is provided by use of fentanyl alone. The usual initial dosage of Innovar for patients of all ages is 1 ml/10 kg. This is divided into three or four doses, each administered over 15 to 20 seconds elapsed time with an interval of 3 or 4 minutes between each fraction. The child drifts off quietly, but the problem of stiff thoracic cage may be troublesome and occasionally must be corrected with succinylcholine and tracheal intubation. As with adults, continuation of anesthesia is accomplished with nitrous oxide–oxygen and supplemental injections of fentanyl alone, since more droperidol is best avoided. Supplements of fentanyl should be made by diluting 1 ml of fentanyl (0.05 mg) to 10 ml and giving 0.5 to 1.0 ml (0.005 to 0.01 mg) as needed.

The analgesia provided by fentanyl should be adequate but is difficult for an anesthetist to evaluate, and several patients who appeared oblivious to their surroundings later gave painful reports of the procedure. Other disadvantages include the prolonged effect of droperidol, with extrapyramidal tract movements continuing for 8 to 10 hours after operation. The combining of two very different drugs to make a single agent is generally considered to be unwise (Foldes and others, 1970).

There seems to be no particular advantage in using Innovar in children when more reliable combinations are more easily administered, more economic, and more promptly excreted. However, Kay (1973) encourages its use from infancy, and Dawson, though more conservative, has found it valuable for older children.

Ketamine

In pediatric anesthesia, the importance of ketamine, introduced by Domino, Chodoff, and Corssen in 1965, is due in part to its potential value and in part to its potential danger, which is considerable because of misuse and misunderstanding as much as the drug itself. In spite of extensive preliminary trials, release for general use promptly showed initial evaluation to be unrealistic, and its rightful place is still uncertain.

Ketamine is a phencyclidone derivative, 2-(o-chlorophenyl)-2-(methylamino)-cyclohexanone, initially labelled CI-581. The features that attracted immediate interest were the rapid onset of hypnosis and analgesia after intramuscular or intravenous injection and the lack of cardiovascular or respiratory depression. Investigation of the action of ketamine suggests that it blocks afferent impulses in the diencephalon and associated pathways of the cortex, sparing the reticular formation of the brainstem, thus earning the label of dissociative anesthetic. Clinically it produces effective analgesia of somatic areas, so that skin, muscle, and bone may be operated on freely, but visceral pain is not obtunded. Preservation of gag reflex, laryngeal irritability, and continued muscle tension verging on rigidity are undesirable characteristics that limit the use of the agent markedly. Electroencephalographic evidence of seizure activity is often seen during ketamine anesthesia, and actual seizures have been observed, especially in patients with preexisting neurologic defects (Schwartz and others, 1974).

The troublesome hallucinations that discourage use of the drug in adults have been less frequent in children, but the awakening phase of children may entail considerable excitement (Wilson and others, 1970).

Ketamine increases CSF pressure significantly for 5 to 15 minutes (Gardner and others, 1971), but as shown by Dawson and associates (1971), this may be held within acceptable limits by pretreatment with thiopental.

The mechanism of cardiorespiratory stimulation has not been entirely clarified. Dowdy and Kaya (1968), Traber and associates (1970), and others have shown that there is a direct negative inotropic action on denervated heart. In the presence of intact sympathetic and autonomic nervous systems, however, a pressor effect causes increased blood pressure, heart rate, and cardiac output, a response present at all ages (Page and others, 1972). This serves as a most valuable adjunct in management of poor-risk patients but is a contraindication in the presence of hypertension or tachycardia. In their investigation of ketamine, Dowdy and Kaya also found evidence of antiarrhythmic activity.

Unchanged respiratory activity during ketamine anesthesia may be advantageous when it enables one to avoid endotracheal intubation, but presence of normal or increased laryngeal irritability is one of the drug's greatest drawbacks. Excessive salivation adds to dangers of gagging, obstruction, and aspiration.

Another important effect of ketamine is elevation of intraocular pressure. In a group of 15 children, Yoshikawa and Murai (1971) noted an average increase of 30%, maximum within 15 minutes after administration of ketamine and evident for approximately 30 minutes.

With the present concern over toxicity of anesthetic agents, ketamine has the advantage of a clean record with no known toxic effects on liver, kidney, or other organ systems.

Indications and contraindications. Because of its prompt action and effective analgesia, ketamine was originally believed to be especially valuable for treatment of burns, for outpatient procedures, and for eye examinations. Thanks to its remarkable analgesic effect and its usual cardiorespiratory support, ketamine has maintained its standing in burn treatment (Wilson and others, 1967), but unpredictable recovery time has made it a poor choice for outpatient procedures, and nystagmoid eye movements plus increased intraocular pressure limit its use for ocular work of any type.

However, new indications have been found for the drug that have unpredicted value. Poor-risk patients of all ages have been supported through induction or the entire operation by ketamine (Wilson and others, 1969). Infants with congenital cardiac defects undergoing operation (Nettles and others, 1973) or diagnostic catheterization studies (Szappanyos and others, 1969) have managed remarkably well under ketamine supplemented by limited amounts of relaxants (Stephen and others, 1970). Other poor-risk neonates have been maintained on ketamine during insertion of jugular feeding lines or more extensive procedures, but they must be watched with extreme care because of high incidence of respiratory irregularity and prolonged periods of apnea that may occur until several hours after operation.

In our experience at The Children's Hospital Medical Center, newborn twin boys were operated on for intestinal obstruction. Weighing 2.2 and 2.0 kg, they were given ketamine, 1 mg/kg, intravenously, and both had severely depressed respiration for 4 to 6 hours, other conditions being unremarkable.

It seems apparent from our experience and that of others that the reaction of small infants to ketamine is highly unpredictable and that it should be used only under great precautions. Janis and Wright (1972) reported reanesthetization of a 10-kg infant after halothane-ketamine anesthesia. Radnay and Badola (1973) described two infants who had seizures unexpectedly, and Sears (1971) enumerated several more who had severe laryngospasm, cardiac arrest, and vomiting followed by aspiration.

Ketamine has been useful in management

of small children who require daily x-ray therapy over periods that may last 2 or 3 weeks (Catton, 1973; Cronin and others, 1972; Bennett and Bullimore, 1973; Sanford and Jones, 1976). Continuation of spontaneous respiration during ketamine anesthesia permits anesthetists to withdraw 10 or 15 feet from the child, provided that adequate monitoring is observed. This technique still has dangers, however, primarily because of accumulation of secretions when a child is supine and partially covered by protective screens.

Dosage to provide immobility is also unpredictable. While *intramuscular administration of 6 to 10 mg/kg usually is sufficient*, recently a 7-kg infant at our hospital was quite unmanageable until her dosage was increased to 40 mg/kg.

The effect of ketamine on the airway underlies the most unsettled aspect of its use. Respiration continues to be active during ketamine anesthesia. Secretions are excessive but may be controlled by generous atropinization. Increased laryngotracheal reflexes are a constant concern, however, and must be avoided at all costs. This means that ketamine might be employed when a child is to lie facedown for 30 minutes, without endotracheal intubation. Another child, with burn contractures of the mouth and neck, might be anesthetized with ketamine for operations on face or body without intubation, provided that there is no abnormality that affects the lumen of the airway (Patterson, 1972). However, should a child have a large obstructing tongue, a tracheostomy scar suggesting a tracheal constriction, or any form of airway irritation, ketamine must be assiduously avoided. Use of ketamine in the presence of upper respiratory tract irritation, foreign body, cystic fibrosis, tumor, or other anatomic or pathologic lesion including asthma may induce severe prolonged choking and spasm, which have already caused several fatalities.

The administration of ketamine to patients who have recently ingested food, though permitted by some, is generally viewed to be highly dangerous and has demonstrated its fatal potentiality (Bosomworth, 1971). Full stomach should be included in the list of definite contraindications to ketamine.

Other contraindications, about which there is less confusion, are listed below and include children with neurotic tendency, history of seizures, increased intracranial pressure, or eyeball laceration and procedures involving marked blood loss.

Indications	Contraindications
Skin graft	Full stomach
Burn dressing	Respiratory infection, obstruction or other pathology (cystic fibrosis, tracheitis, asthma, old tracheotomy scar, etc.)
Superficial operations	
Cardiac catheterization	
Radiation therapy	
Induction of poor-risk cardiac patients	
	Increased intracranial pressure or eyeball trauma
	Neurotic or emotional tendency, seizure history
	Increased blood pressure
	Operation involving marked blood loss

The chief reason why the use of ketamine is limited almost entirely to children is the reduced incidence of hallucinogenic responses thus far observed in prepubertal children (Wilson and others, 1970). Dreams appear to be less upsetting to younger patients, as far as can be determined, though exceptions have occurred. Rees abandoned ketamine after witnessing a child repeatedly relive the horrors of an extensive body burn. Avoidance of ketamine during massive hemorrhage is advised, because its supportive vasotonic mechanism may hide evidence of actual blood loss until the response is exhausted, followed by sudden collapse (Zauder and Nichols, 1971).

Dosage and administration. Ketamine is supplied in 30-ml vials of 10-mg/ml and 50-mg/ml concentrations and in 5-ml vials of 100-mg/ml concentration. The solution pH is 3.5 to 5.5, but injection does not produce the burning or irritation characteristic of the alkaline barbiturates. The usual intravenous dose of 2 mg/kg produces a highly predictable response at all ages, patients usually becoming unconscious within 45 to 60 seconds and remaining so for 15 to 20 minutes. Intramuscular dosage is highly unpredictable. It seems advisable to start in the range of 6 mg/kg, since this may be sufficient for procedures involving minor stimuli. Wide variations have been encountered in intramuscular requirement. As previously noted, 40 mg/kg was necessary in one infant, and the resultant anesthesia was not prolonged.

In summary, ketamine has definite advantages and appears to be easy to use, but because of increased danger of respiratory complications and emotional disturbance, it is not suited to general use. Furthermore, it should only be administered by competent anesthetists in areas equipped for total anesthetic care.

Etoxadrol

Another dissociative agent resembling ketamine in action and in effect on brain monoamines is under investigation (Sung and others, 1973). This agent, etoxadrol, does not appear to have special value in children.

Intravenous steroids

Several steroid preparations have been employed in anesthesia. Hydroxydione (Viadril) enjoyed limited use between 1950 and 1960, but venous irritation was excessive. More recent additions include propanidid and althesin.

Propanidid. Propanidid (Epontol) is a derivative of eugenol (oil of cloves) and has been used in Europe since 1963. It provides hypnosis in a manner and potency similar to thiopental. Its outstanding feature is that it provides the fastest recovery of any of the currently used intravenous anesthetics. For this reason it is popular in busy outpatient clinics for brief operations, dental extractions, etc.

Propanidid has several limitations (Black and Clarke, 1971). Being a viscid fluid, it requires "solubilizing." This purpose is served by Cremophor El, a castor oil product that produces considerable vascular irritation. When used in moderate dosage (4 mg/kg), propanidid stimulates respiration, but larger doses produce coughing, motor twitching, and increasing cardiovascular depression (Gjessing, 1969; Evans, 1971; Rozenkranz,

1972). Recovery is prompt but often accompanied by vomiting. The agent seems to serve the anesthetist better than the patient, for reduced recovery time is bought at the expense of discomfort and increased risk.

A child's reaction to propanidid is similar to an adult's, but the incidence of complications related to venipuncture and vascular irritation usually is greater in smaller patients.

Althesin. Althesin is a mixture of two steroids, alphaxalone and alphadorlone acetate, in 3:1 proportion. Like propanidid, althesin is a viscid fluid, and Cremophor El is used to increase its solubility. Althesin is given to induce anesthesia or for procedures of 10 to 15 minutes' duration. Induction requires 40 to 120 ml/kg injected over 25 to 30 seconds (Swerdlow, 1973). It is pleasant, with a modest decrease in blood pressure similar to that of thiopental. With larger doses, however, hypotension is marked, and coughing, muscle twitching, and salivation parallel the dosage. A number of reports relate experiences of sudden onset of rash and severe bronchospasm, with one death (Avery and Evans, 1973). In spite of these faults, there appears to be continued interest in the drug in Europe. The report of Harrison (1973) that althesin blocks the development of malignant hyperthermia justifies further investigation, but routine use hardly seems reasonable.

BIBLIOGRAPHY

Abel, R. M., and Reis, R. L.: Intravenous diazepam for sedation following cardiac operations; clinical and hemodynamic assessments, Anesth. Analg. (Cleve.) **50**:244, 1971.

Avery, A. F., and Evans, A.: Reactions to althesin, Br. J. Anaesth. **45**:301, 1973.

Bennett, I. A., and Bullimore, I. A.: The use of ketamine hydrochloride anaesthesia for radiotherapy in young children, Br. J. Anaesth. **45**:197, 1973.

Black, G. W., and Clarke, R. S. J.: Recently introduced anesthetic drugs, Int. Anesthesiol. Clin. **9**:171, 1971.

Bosomworth, P. .B.: Ketamine symposium; comments by moderator, Anesth. Analg. (Cleve.) **50**:471, 1971.

Brodie, B. B.: Physiological disposition and chemical fate of thiobarbiturates in the body, Fed. Proc. **11**:632, 1952.

Carter, S., and Gold, A. P.: Status epilepticus. In Smith, C. A., editor: The critically ill child, ed. 2, Philadelphia, 1977, W. B. Saunders Co.

Catton, D. V.: Intramuscular ketamine-repeated injections, Can. Anaesth. Soc. J. **20**:227, 1973.

Clarke, R. S.: The eugenols—propanidid, Int. Anesthesiol. Clin. **7**:43, 1969.

Clarke, R. S., Dundee, J. W., Barron, D. W., and McArdle, L.: Clinical studies of induction agents. XXVI. The relation potencies of thiopentone, methohexitone and propanidid, Br. J. Anaesth. **40**:593, 1968.

Coppel, D. L., and Dundee, J. W.: Ketamine anaesthesia for cardiac catheterization, Anaesthesia **27**:25, 1972.

Corssen, G., Allard, R., Brosch, F., and Arbeuz, G.: Ketamine as the sole anesthetic in open heart surgery, Anesth. Analg. (Cleve.) **49**:1025, 1970.

Corssen, G., Gutierrez, J., Reves, J. G., and Huber, F. C., Jr.: Ketamine in the anesthetic management of asthmatic patients, Anesth. Analg. (Cleve.) **51**:588, 1972.

Cronin, M. M., Bousfield, J. D., Hewett, E. B., and others: Ketamine anaesthesia for radiotherapy in small children, Anaesthesia **27**:135, 1972.

Dawson, B., Michenfelder, J. D., and Theye, R. A.: Effects of ketamine on canine cerebral blood flow and metabolism; modification by prior administration of thiopental, Anesth. Analg. (Cleve.) **50**:443, 1971.

Domino, E. F., Chodoff, P., and Corssen, G.: Pharmacologic effects of CI-581, a new dissociative anesthetic, in man, Clin. Pharmacol. Ther. **6**:279, 1965.

Done, A. K.: Drugs for children. In Modell, W., editor: Drugs of choice 1970-1971, St. Louis, 1970, The C. V. Mosby Co.

Dowdy, E. G., and Kaya, K.: Studies of mechanism of cardiovascular responses to CI-581, Anesthesiology **29**:931, 1968.

Dowell, T.: Diazepam premedication in paediatric patients. In Knight, P. F., editor: Diazepam in anaesthesia, Bristol, 1968, John Write & Sons, Ltd.

Dundee, J. W.: Present position of new and established intravenous anesthetics; chairman's closing remarks, Int. Anesthesiol. Clin. **2**:793, 1964.

Dundee, J. W.: Current views on the clinical pharmacology of the barbiturates. In Clarke, R. S. J., editor: Newer intravenous anesthetics, Boston, 1969, Little, Brown & Co.

Dundee, J. W., and Barron, D. W.: The barbiturates, Br. J. Anaesth. **34**:240, 1962.

Dundee, J. W., McCleery, W. N. C., and McLaughlin, G.: The hazard of thiopental anesthesia in porphyria, Anesth. Analg. (Cleve.) **41**:567, 1962.

Eger, E. I. II: Anesthetic uptake and action, Baltimore, 1974, The Williams & Wilkins Co.

Etsten, B., and Li, T. H.: Hemodynamic changes during thiopental anesthesia in humans, J. Clin. Invest. **34**:500, 1955.

Evans, A. R.: Reaction to propanidid, Br. J. Anaesth. **43**:802, 1971.

Foldes, F. F., Shiffman, H. P., and Kronfeld, P. P.: The use of fentanyl, meperidine, or alphaprodine for neuroleptanesthetics, Anesthesiology **33**:35, 1970.

Gale, A. S.: Ketamine prevention of penile turgescence, J.A.M.A. **219:**1629, 1972.

Gardner, A. E., Olson, B. E., and Lichtiger, M.: Cerebrospinal fluid pressure during dissociative anesthesia with ketamine, Anesthesiology **35:**226, 1971.

Gibbs, L., Svigals, R. E., and Ricklan, M.: A double blind study of chlordiazepoxide as a preanesthetic agent in cardiac surgery, Anesth. Analg. (Cleve.) **50:**17, 1971.

Gjessing, J.: Hypotension, hypoventilation and delayed recovery after propanidid, Br. J. Anaesth. **41:**1012, 1969.

Gupta, P. K., and Dundee, J. W.: The effect of an infusion of doxapram on morphine analgesia, Anaesthesia **29:**40, 1974.

Harrison, G. G.: Althesin and malignant hyperexia, Br. J. Anaesth. **45:**1019, 1973.

Horton, J. N.: Adverse reaction to althesin, Anaesthesia **28:**182, 1972.

Hunter, A. S., Long, W. J., and Ryrie, C. G.: An evaluation of gamma-hydroxybutyric acid in paediatric practice, Br. J. Anaesth. **43:**620, 1972.

Janis, K. M., and Wright, W.: Failure to produce analgesia with ketamine in two patients with cortical disease, Anesthesiology **36:**405, 1972.

Johns, G.: Cardiac arrest following induction with propanidid, Br. J. Anaesth. **42:**74, 1970.

Johnstone, M., and Barron, P. T.: The cardiovascular effects of propanidid, Anaesthesia **23:**180, 1968.

Johnstone, R. E.: A ketamine trip, letter, Anesthesiology **39:**460, 1973.

Kay, B.: Neuroleptanesthesia for neonates and infants, Anesth. Analg. (Cleve.) **52:**970, 1973.

Kiyoshi, Y., and Yasuichi, M.: The effect of ketamine on intraocular pressure in children, Anesth. Analg. (Cleve.) **50:**199, 1971.

Lindsay, W. A., and Shepherd, J.: Plasma levels of thiopentone after premedication with rectal suppositories in young children, Br. J. Anaesth. **41:**977, 1969.

List, W. F.: Increased cerebrospinal fluid pressure after ketamine, Anesthesiology **36:**98, 1972.

Lombroso, C. T.: Treatment of status epilepticus with diazepam, Neurology **16:**629, 1966.

Lombroso, C. T.: The treatment of status epilepticus, Pediatrics **53:**536, 1974.

Lowenstein, E., Hallowell, P., Levine, F. H., and others: Cardiovascular response to large doses of intravenous morphine in man, N. Engl. J. Med. **281:**1389, 1969.

Mark, L. C.: Thiobarbiturates. In Papper, E. M., and Kitz, R. J., editors: Uptake and distribution of anesthetic agents, New York, 1963, McGraw-Hill Book Co.

Mark, L. C.: A rational approach to supplementation of nitrous oxide. In Mark, L. C., and Ngai, S. H., editors: Highlights of clinical anesthesiology, New York, 1971, Harper & Row, Publishers, Inc.

Miller, J. R., Stoelting, V. K., and Dann, M. W.: A preliminary report on the use of intramuscular metho-

hexital sodium (Brevital) for pediatric anesthesia, Anesth. Analg. (Cleve.) **40:**573, 1961.

Muenster, J. J., Rosenberg, M. S., Carleton, R. A., and others: Comparison between diazepam and sodium thiopental during D.C. countershock, J.A.M.A. **199:**758, 1967.

Nettles, D. C., Herrin, T. J., and Mullen, J. G.: Ketamine induction in poor risk patients, Anesth. Analg. (Cleve.) **52:**59, 1973.

Page, P., Morgan, M., and Loh, L.: Ketamine anaesthesia in paediatric procedures, Acta Anaesth. Scand. **16:**155, 1972.

Patterson, J. F.: Anesthesia in Vietnam, parts 1 and 2, Anesth. Analg. (Cleve.) **51:**306, 317, 1972.

Plaut, M. R., Gifford, R. R., and Jacobson, P. M.: Recovery from a central respiratory failure and administration of doxapram to a patient with a brainstem lesion, Anesthesiology **38:**596, 1973.

Price, H. L.: A dynamic concept of the distribution of thiopental in the human body, Anesthesiology **21:**40, 1960.

Radnay, P. A., and Badola, R. P.: Generalized extensor spasm in infants following ketamine anesthesia, Anesthesiology **39:**459, 1973.

Reier, C. E.: Ketamine—dissociative agent or hallucinogen? letter to the editor, N. Engl. J. Med. **284:**791, 1971.

Rozenkranz, I.: Cardiovascular collapse after propanidid, Br. J. Anaesth. **44:**1332, 1972.

Saidman, L. J., and Eger, E. I. II: The effect of thiopental metabolism on duration of anesthesia, Anesthesiology **27:**118, 1966.

Saidman, L. J., and Eger, E. I. II: Uptake and distribution of thiopental after oral, rectal, or intramuscular administration, Clin. Pharmacol. Ther. **14:**12, 1973.

Sanford, F. G., and Jones, C. W.: Immobilization for radiotherapy by ketamine; a case report, Anesthesiol. Rev. **3:**16, 1976.

Sari, A., Yoshiaki, O., and Takeshita, H.: The effect of ketamine on cerebrospinal fluid pressure, Anesth. Analg. (Cleve.) **51:**560, 1972.

Savege, T. M., Blogg, C. E., Foley, E. I., and others: The cardiorespiratory effects of althesin and ketamine, Anaesthesia **28:**391, 1973.

Schwartz, M. S., Virden, S., and Scott, D. F.: Effects of ketamine on the electroencephalograph, Anaesthesia **29:**135, 1974.

Sears, B. E.: Correspondence; complications of ketamine, Anesthesiology **35:**231, 1971.

Siker, E. S.: Postanesthetic respiratory depression, Anesth. Analg. (Cleve.) **44:**253, 1965.

Siker, E. S., Mustafa, K., and Wolfson, B.: The analeptic effects of doxapram hydrochloride on thiopentone-induced depression, Br. J. Anaesth. **36:**216, 1964.

Smith, R. M., Bachman, L., and Bougas, T.: Shivering following thiopental sodium and other anesthetic agents, Anesthesiology **16:**655, 1955.

Spoerel, W. E., and Kandel, P. F.: CI-581 in anaesthesia for tonsillectomies in children, Can. Anaesth. Soc. J. **17**:172, 1970.

Stephen, C. R., Ahlgren, A. W., and Bennett, E. J.: Elements of pediatric anesthesia, ed. 2, Springfield, Ill., 1970, Charles C Thomas, Publisher.

Sung, Y. F., Frederickson, E. L., and Holtzman, S. G.: Effects of intravenous anesthetics on brain monoamines in the rat, Anesthesiology **39**:478, 1973.

Swerdlow, M.: Althesin—a new intravenous anesthetic, Can. Anaesth. Soc. J. **20**:186, 1973.

Szappanyos, G. G., Bopp, P., and Fournet, P. C.: The use and advantage of "Ketalar" (CI-581) as anaesthetic agent in paediatric cardiac catheterization and angiocardiography, Anaesthetist **18**:365, 1969.

Traber, D. L., Wilson, R. D., and Priano, L. L.: Blockade of the hypertensive response to ketamine, Anesth. Analg. (Cleve.) **49**:420, 1970.

Way, W. L., Costley, E. C., and Way, E. L.: Respiratory sensitivity of the newborn infant to meperidine and morphine, Clin. Pharmacol. Ther. **6**:454, 1965.

Wilson, R. D., Nichols, R. J., and McCoy, N. R.: Dissociative anesthesia with CI-581 in burned children, Anesth. Analg. (Cleve.) **46**:719, 1967.

Wilson, R. D., and Traber, D. L.: Advances in anesthesia for plastic surgery in burns. In Fabian, L., editor: Clinical anesthesia; a decade of clinical progress, Philadelphia, 1971, F. A. Davis Co.

Wilson, R. D., Traber, D. L., and Evans, B. L.: Correlation of psychologic and physiologic observations from children undergoing repeated ketamine anesthesia, Anesth. Analg. (Cleve.) **48**:995, 1970.

Wilson, R. D., Traber, D. L., Priano, L. L., and others: Anesthetic management of the poor risk pediatric patient, Southern Med. J. **62**:767, 1969.

Wong, K. C., Martin, W. E., Hornbein, T. F., and others: The cardiovascular effects of morphine sulfate with oxygen and with nitrous oxide in man, Anesthesiology **38**:542, 1973.

Wyant, G. M.: Intramuscular Ketalar (CI-581) in paediatric anaesthesia, Can. Anaesth. Soc. J. **18**:72, 1971.

Yoshikawa, K., and Murai, Y.: The effect of ketamine on intraocular pressure in children, Anesth. Analg. (Cleve.) **50**:199, 1971.

Zauder, H. L., and Nichols, R. J.: Intravenous anesthesia, Clin. Anesth. **3**:318, 1969.

Zauder, H. L., and Nichols, R. J.: Intravenous anesthesia. In Fabian, L., editor: Clinical anesthesia; a decade of progress, Philadelphia, 1971, F. A. Davis Co., p. 317.

CHAPTER 13

Use of muscle relaxants

BACKGROUND

Muscle relaxants, whether used in the jungle (Gill, 1940) or in the operating room (Griffith and Johnson, 1942, 1951), have always been highly dramatic and uniquely interesting. The sudden, total effect and the pharmacologic mechanisms by which it is induced and reversed command respect and stimulate investigation.*

The introduction of relaxants into the practice of anesthesia aroused bitter dispute (Beecher and Todd, 1954). Objection to muscle relaxants was directed chiefly at the elimination of spontaneous respiration, the most valued sign of anesthetic depth, especially in children. This introduced the first "physiologic trespass" or intentional interruption of a basic function in anesthesiology. The mandatory use of tracheal intubation also worried many, as did the process of reversing relaxants.

In pediatric anesthesia there was less controversy but considerable indecision and changing of minds as to which agent was best. At present, the use of relaxants in all age groups is well established, and interest is focused on the role of succinylcholine in malignant hyperthermia and hyperpotassemia,

the relative values of d-tubocurarine, pancuronium, and metocurine, and the threatened disruption of previously accepted theories of relaxant action.

DEVELOPMENT OF CONCEPTS

The modern use of muscle relaxants was initiated by psychiatrists who curarized patients to reduce the muscle spasm of shock therapy. Observing this, Dr. Lewis Wright of E. R. Squibb Company encouraged several anesthesiologists to investigate the concept, and in 1942 Griffith and Johnson reported the first clinical application of curare* in surgical anesthesia. The next year Cullen described its administration to infants. The adoption of curare for both adults and infants spread throughout North America and England, being accepted more readily where surgeons depended heavily on cautery and welcomed a nonexplosive agent.

Reports on use of curare by Webster and Van Bergen (1949) and of curare and gallamine by Anderson (1951) suggested that children were normal subjects for these relaxants. Nevertheless, many operations were performed on infants with curare and oxygen alone on the assumption that they had analgesia. To examine this theory, Dr. Scott Smith (1947) induced colleagues to give him 500 units of Intocostrin (equal to 75 mg of d-tubocurarine), which had ample relaxant effect but provided no analgesia. Thereafter, it became mandatory to use an analgesic with curare.

---

*For excellent historical and scientific reading one should also refer to Bennett (1967), Betcher (1977), and Burnap and Little (1968).

*The term *curare* was loosely applied to several preparations prior to the standard preparation of d-tubocurarine.

It is interesting to note that in 1950 Rees explained in detail why ether was best for neonates and relaxants were contraindicated. Shortly thereafter Rees and associates established the startling concept of the relaxant technic for all pediatric procedures. This was first reported by Stead (1955), followed by the more familiar views of Rees in 1958 and 1960. The concept of the Liverpool group proved sound and established the safety and utility of the relaxant technic for pediatric anesthesia.

When succinylcholine was introduced,* the shorter duration of its effect made it appear safer for pediatric use. Instances of prolonged apnea (Kaufman and others, 1960; Churchill-Davidson, 1959) and severe bradycardia (Craythorne, Turndorf, and Dripps, 1960) followed, however, and once the routine reversal of *d*-tubocurarine was established, *d*-tubocurarine regained priority. In these changes, gallamine† followed *d*-tubocurarine in popularity—but at considerable distance.

During the past 30 years, several other relaxants have been tried and discarded. However, pancuronium, introduced by Baird and Reid in 1967, has gained a strong foothold in England and North America and has displaced *d*-tubocurarine in numerous institutions. Metocurine is a third nondepolarizing muscle relaxant with excellent clinical value (Goudsouzian and others, 1978), and it appears to be overtaking both *d*-tubocurarine and pancuronium.

RESPONSE OF INFANTS AND CHILDREN TO RELAXANTS

Much of the uncertainty about the pediatric application of relaxants has been because of the belief that the response of infants and children to both depolarizing and nondepolarizing agents was different from that of adults. Confusion still exists concerning the reason for this altered response, its degree, its duration, and, in fact, its existence. The studies on which present concepts are based are outlined below.

Stead (1955) was the first to suspect that the response to muscle relaxants was not the same for all ages. He reported that neonates were more tolerant than adults to succinylcholine and required twice the relative dose in mg/kg to produce comparable respiratory depression. On the same basis, he found infants to be more sensitive than adults to *d*-tubocurarine, their response suggesting that of patients with myasthenia. This report suggested greater safety in the use of succinylcholine.

Telford and Keats (1957), measuring succinylcholine requirement (mg/kg/min) during operation, reported tolerance to succinylcholine in children to be maximum at birth and to decline to adult levels by 14 to 16 years of age (Fig. 13-1).

Bush and Stead (1962), with increasing experience, pointed out the dangers of suxamethonium (succinylcholine), including altered response to repeated administration, uneven muscle relaxation, and phase II block, and attested to the reliability of *d*-tubocurarine. The authors reported that the neonate required only half the normal dose of *d*-tubocurarine by weight but that this sensitivity decreased and disappeared by the second month of life. At this time, *d*-tubocurarine was recommended as the better agent for children (Bush, 1963).

Churchill-Davidson and Wise (1963), using electromyography, found the newborn resistant to decamethonium, requiring two to three times the adult dose (mg/kg) to paralyze thenar muscles.

On further investigation, Churchill-Davidson and Wise (1964) stated that the average dose of *d*-tubocurarine required for paralysis of the hand muscles in the infant corresponded closely to the equivalent dose (mg/kg) for an adult but that respiratory depression was significantly greater in the infant.

Reversal of *d*-tubocurarine in the neonate was found to be prompt with either neostigmine or edrophonium (Tensilon) but often was only temporary with edrophonium.

Lim and associates (1964) evaluated relax-

---

*Succinylcholine was known to pharmacologists in 1906 but was not used in clinical anesthesia until 1949.
†Gallamine was first used in 1949.

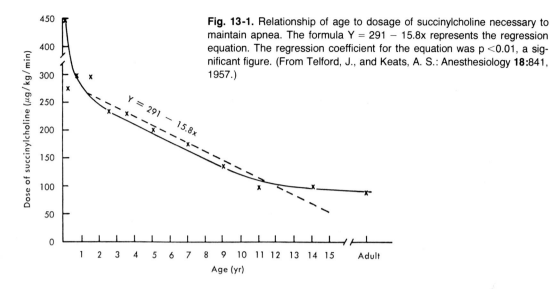

Fig. 13-1. Relationship of age to dosage of succinylcholine necessary to maintain apnea. The formula $Y = 291 - 15.8x$ represents the regression equation. The regression coefficient for the equation was $p < 0.01$, a significant figure. (From Telford, J., and Keats, A. S.: Anesthesiology **18**:841, 1957.)

ant response by measuring mean CO_2 expiration. They reported that younger children metabolized succinylcholine more rapidly but that the drug produced more pronounced relaxation in infants under 1 year old than in older patients.

Further electromyographic investigation carried out by Nightingale and associates (1966) and Long and Bachman (1967) gave evidence of tolerance of the young child to succinylcholine when given in a dosage of 0.3 mg/kg but not when given in a dosage of 0.5 mg/kg. The intensity and duration of action of a 0.3-mg/kg dose, as measured by action potentials, was found to increase steadily in patients studied between 4 months and 13 years of age.

Walts and Dillon (1969, 1969a) also compared duration of response of infant and adult to muscle relaxants, but they did it with reference to body surface area, using *d*-tubocurarine (4 mg/m²) and succinylcholine (40 mg/m²) in fixed dosages. Their results showed prolonged duration of infant response to *d*-tubocurarine but similar response of infant and adult to succinylcholine.

Goudsouzian and associates studied the dosage and duration of pancuronium (1974) and *d*-tubocurarine (1975) by constructing dose-response curves based on body weight, with twitch response being plotted against

the log dose of relaxants on log-probit paper. Their conclusions were that (1) children were *less* sensitive to both *d*-tubocurarine and pancuronium than adults when dosage was based on body weight, (2) there was greater variability of response in the youngest infants tested, (3) pancuronium was approximately 5.5 times as potent as *d*-tubocurarine in infants and children, (4) recovery from both *d*-tubocurarine and pancuronium was more rapid in children than in adults, and (5) recession of neuromuscular blockade was slower following *d*-tubocurarine than following pancuronium.

Cook and Fischer (1975), comparing infants 1 to 10 weeks old, children 3 to 7 years old, and adults, found that infants required higher dosages of succinylcholine than children, and children higher dosages than adults, to produce the same degree of neuromuscular blockade. They related the difference to the relatively greater fluid volume of younger subjects.

Another study by Cook and Fischer (1978) using train-of-four analysis showed that a paralyzing dose of succinylcholine (1.5 mg/kg) produced a phase I neuromuscular block, not a phase II block as previously contended, and that recovery time was not prolonged when compared with older children.

Thus, because of changing methods of evaluation, there is no clear agreement among investigators. From a practical point of view it appears that a tolerance to succinylcholine may exist throughout childhood, while any sensitivity to nondepolarizing agents is present only in the first month of life.

The reasons for the infant's altered responses to relaxants, if existent, are not clear. The responses to depolarizing and nondepolarizing agents are so different that interest in the comparison has greatly diminished, and any theory basing both responses on the same factor seems untenable.

Among the theories considered for the difference in response of child vs adult are altered uptake of drugs (Kalow, 1963), difference in the transport and distribution among neuromuscular end-plates (Katz and Papper, 1963), difference in the structure of end-plates (Zachs, 1964), variations in enzymatic activity (Hodges, 1955; Kaufman and others, 1960; Lehmann and others, 1957; Zsigmond and Patterson, 1967), and variations in elimination of the drugs. Thus far, few of these areas have been studied. Anatomic development of the end-plate has been worked out carefully (Drachman, 1963). It is known that the neonate has a full complement of muscles, nerves, and end-plates, but the individual structural development may not be complete until 2 years of age. Alteration of response could be involved here. Cholinesterase activity has been demonstrated in the midfetal period, and Drachman (1963) used d-tubocurarine effectively in chick embryos with predictable response even at this age. Thus, all the essential structural units appear to be present at birth.

The sensitivity to d-tubocurarine, if it does truly exist, appears to parallel the early physiologic changes of neonates in adapting to extrauterine life. It might be related to renal or hepatic development rather than to changes of the neuromuscular structure.

Clarification of succinylcholine tolerance should lie in other directions. The relative size of fluid compartments may play an important part in distribution of relaxants to end-plates. The initial preponderance of the extracellular space at birth and the gradual shift to intracellular preponderance is in line with the gradually diminishing succinylcholine tolerance (Kalow, 1963).

The enzymatic breakdown of succinylcholine naturally deserves scrutiny in relation to altered succinylcholine effect. Increased tolerance to depolarizing drugs would suggest increased cholinesterase activity. Evidence appears to destroy this hypothesis, however. Cholinesterase levels in infants have been found to be slightly reduced, with mean levels of 59 units for mature newborns as compared with the adult mean of 85 units (Lehmann and others, 1957). Normal response has been found in adults with cholinesterase levels of 60 or below, and hence the enzyme concentration does not appear to explain the child's altered reaction.

Zsigmond and Patterson (1967) questioned the clinical observations of the infant's tolerance to succinylcholine. In their study of the potency of plasma cholinesterase activity, they found the absolute activity of plasma cholinesterase in infants to be only one third of that in adults. Again we are left with inconclusive and contradictory evidence, and it appears that a more satisfactory explanation will be found to be related to a gradually altering relationship between end-plates, muscle mass, and body fluid compartments.

Absence of fasciculation is characteristic of the myasthenic and also parallels the absence of shivering in the neonate. This could demonstrate either immature or pathologic neuromuscular development. The marked cardiac slowing seems to be evidence of parasympathetic predominance thought to be peculiar to the infant.

Failure in the search for explanation of different relaxant responses has been associated with decreasing evidence of importance of this question. This may explain the lack of attention paid to specific action of pancuronium in younger patients.

In most respects, the older child's reaction to relaxants resembles that of adults, as described by Foldes (1957, 1959, 1966) and Kaufman (1971).

ADVANTAGES AND INDICATIONS

The advantages of relaxant agents are well established. In addition to complete relaxation unrelated to generalized depression, they include nonflammability, direct route of administration without dependence on ventilation, rapid effect, freedom from metabolic or toxic effects, little if any effect on myocardium or the peripheral vascular system, and absence of epinephrine sensitivity (Gray and Nunn, 1971; Feldman, 1973).

The same advantages exist for children as for adults, but the need for relaxants is less marked. Abdominal relaxation is usually adequate with halogenated agents without supplemental use of relaxants. Indications for relaxants in children include tracheal intubation and other short-term use for brief periods of relaxation during abdominal closure or fracture reduction or for relief of laryngeal spasm or convulsion. In addition, relaxants are used for longer periods in combination with thiopental, nitrous oxide, and narcotics as noted below.

The combined use of halogenated agents and relaxants for maintenance involves increased risk but in skilled hands produces excellent operating conditions.

The versatility of relaxants has been demonstrated by those who have adapted it to practically all pediatric procedures. Usually, however, relaxants are reserved for procedures in which they prove a significant advantage. Excluding those administered for intubation, relaxants are probably involved in about 10% to 15% of pediatric anesthetic procedures in the United States; halothane plays a much heavier role.

In our practice at The Children's Hospital Medical Center, intramuscular injection of succinylcholine (1.5 mg/kg) is the standard method for intubation of neonates, with only oxygen used for supplementation. Succinylcholine is added to halothane for intubation in approximately 30% of older children. Intermittent intravenous injection of succinylcholine is administered during bronchoscopic procedures and occasionally for surgical operations, and "drip succinylcholine" is used only once or twice a year.

Among the nondepolarizing agents, we naturally have had greatest experience with *d*-tubocurarine and have found it reliable for a wide variety of clinical uses in healthy infants and children. Pancuronium has been chosen recently for use in small infants with hypotensive tendency, while metocurine has been adopted for the major part of our work, particularly in long or difficult procedures.

AGENTS

Clinical experience with muscle relaxants in children has been confined chiefly to succinylcholine, *d*-tubocurarine, gallamine, pancuronium, and metocurine. Investigational work has centered on the same group, with the addition of decamethonium, on which many of Churchill-Davidson's studies have been based.

Succinylcholine

Pediatric anesthesiologists should know succinylcholine (succinyldicholine, suxamethonium [British], Anectine) well, first because of its several useful qualities and second because of its interesting and dangerous side effects.

Administered by either intravenous or intramuscular route, succinylcholine is rapidly hydrolyzed by pseudocholinesterase to succinylmonocholine, a less powerful muscle relaxant, and then to succinic acid and choline (Foldes and Rhodes, 1953; Litwiffer, 1969; Gray and Nunn, 1971).

Intravenous administration of succinylcholine initiates a depolarizing neuromuscular block that occurs within 10 to 20 seconds and lasts 3 to 10 minutes, depending on the dosage (Kalow and Gunn, 1959).

Atropine is necessary prior to intravenous succinylcholine to prevent vagal bradycardia, which is said to be especially dangerous following a second dose of relaxant. It has been customary to order atropine (0.02 mg/kg) 45 to 60 minutes prior to anesthesia. To avoid this injection and the resultant dry mouth, it is preferable to wait and inject the atropine by either intravenous or intramuscular route immediately after the child has been put to sleep.

Following intravenous administration of succinylcholine, fasciculation will occur in teenagers and adults and may cause muscle pain unless blocked by previous administration of 2 or 3 mg of *d*-tubocurarine or 0.5 to 1 mg of pancuronium. Fasciculation is mild in small children following intravenous succinylcholine and is absent in infants (Bush and Roth, 1961).

Intramuscular use of succinylcholine has several advantages for both anesthesiologist and child. Obviously it is easier to administer, and fasciculations rarely, if ever, occur. Sudden apnea and rapidly developing hypoxia are avoided, for relaxation increases gradually over approximately 2 minutes, allowing the infant to ventilate spontaneously even though too weak to resist intubation. The muscarinic effect of succinylcholine is reduced, and atropine is not essential. In fact, *one should not* use simultaneous intramuscular injections of atropine and succinylcholine, because both drugs have initial vagotonic action that can be dangerous if effective at the same time.

Many of the variable responses to succinylcholine have been traced by Kalow and Gunn (1959) and Whittaker (1970) to genetically related differences in the activity of pseudocholinesterase (PCE). The test for PCE potency, measured in percent of PCE inhibition by dibucaine and termed the dibucaine number (DN), was devised by Kalow and Genest (1957). The DN for atypical PCE was found to be 20 and that for typical PCE to be 80.

Dosage. For succinylcholine, a dose of 1.5 mg/kg (0.7 mg/lb) of lean body weight is practical by any route in children of any age. Although neonates have been shown to tolerate higher dosage than older patients, occasionally it may be safer to reduce their dosage to 1.0 mg/kg for the following reasons: (1) neonates requiring surgery often are sicker than the average pediatric patient, (2) one does not need full relaxation for intubation of neonates, and (3) there is less danger of severe bradycardia with the reduced dosage.

Healthy older children may receive dosages on an adult scale of 1.5 mg/kg. If atropine has been given in adequate amount (0.02 mg/kg) within 30 minutes, it is better to be generous with succinylcholine in older children and avoid the problems of incomplete relaxation. If repeated administration of succinylcholine is planned, increments of one-fourth to one-third the original amount may be given when indicated by returning muscle tone. Some advise repeating atropine prior to a second administration of succinylcholine, but this does not appear necessary if the initial dose still carries adequate effect.

In a study of intramuscular administration of succinylcholine in children, Glowacki and associates (1958) found surprisingly similar results with doses of 0.5, 0.75 and 1.0 mg/lb, the average onset of apnea being 2.2, 2.1, and 2.0 minutes and duration of depression averaging 10.2, 10.0, and 12.8 minutes, respectively. When using intramuscular succinylcholine for intubation, one usually does not wait for complete respiratory arrest but preferably for reduction of resistance while some exchange is still present (McCaughey, 1962).

Disadvantages and contraindications. The known complications involving succinylcholine have increased steadily since its introduction (see below). All relaxants expose the patient to hypoxia if the anesthesiologist should be unable to establish an airway or should fail to ventilate adequately. Infants have numerous pathologic anomalies near the upper airway, including cystic hygroma, harelip, Pierre Robin syndrome, and choanal atresia. As stated by Beldavs (1962), harelip does not contraindicate use of a relaxant, but Pierre Robin syndrome should.

SUCCINYLCHOLINE (ANECTINE) (DEPOLARIZING AGENT)

Contraindications

Possible intubation problem
Gastric distension
Suspected malignant hyperthermia
Severe tissue destruction with denervated muscle mass (burns, large wounds)

Neuromuscular pathology (spinal cord injury or disease, myopathies, myotonia, ptosis)

Renal failure with high serum potassium level

Atypical or low acetylcholinesterase level

Pheochromocytoma

Technic*

Effective pretreatment with vagolytic agent given within 45 minutes prior to intravenous use of succinylcholine

Dosage

Birth to 1 month old: intramuscular or intravenous route, 1.5 mg/kg

Over 1 month old: intravenous route, 1.5 mg/kg; intramuscular route, 2.0 mg/kg

Subsequent dosage: one third to one fourth of the initial dose

Complications

Bradycardia, arrhythmia, arrest

Prolonged apnea

Elevation of serum potassium level

Prolonged local or general spasticity

Initiation of malignant hyperthermia

Increased intraocular, intracranial, or intragastric pressures

Among several complications of succinylcholine, prolonged apnea was first noted and was blamed on overdosage, phase II block (Churchill-Davidson, 1959), and pseudocholinesterase deficiency (Kaufman and others, 1960). Bradycardia due to unopposed muscarinic effect of succinylcholine was reported by Leigh and associates (1957) and Craythorne, Turndorf, and Dripps (1960). Usually of short duration, these vagal responses occasionally are enough to cause complete asystole. As is well known, atropine reduces this response but must be administered in adequate dosage (0.02 to 0.03 mg/kg) within 45 minutes beforehand to be effective.

Succinylcholine has an important effect on intraocular, CSF, and intragastric pressures (Craythorne, Rottenstein, and Dripps, 1960). Pandey and associates (1972) found that patients with mean intraocular pressure of 15.5 mm Hg (SD 4.67) showed a mean rise of 17.9 and 19.9 mm Hg in nonintubated and intubated patients, respectively, all pressures re-

*In exceptional situations, an infusion of succinylcholine may be used by intermittent drip technic, 100 mg of succinylcholine in 500 ml of crystalloid making a suitable 0.02% solution.

turning to or below initial levels within 6 minutes. These figures are representative for normal adults and children. The elevation of pressure can be reduced by 75% to 80% by prior administration of nondepolarizing agents. Indications and restrictions for succinylcholine during ocular surgery are discussed in Chapter 20. The effect of succinylcholine and other agents on intracranial pressure is described in Chapter 18.

Several studies have been made on the effect of succinylcholine on the child's intragastric pressure. Resting intragastric pressure in children has been reported to be slightly higher than in adults. Salem and associates (1972) found the mean intragastric pressure of children to be 13.8 cm H_2O, and Roe (1962) and La Cour (1969) reported 11.9 and 7.0 cm H_2O, respectively, as the mean pressure for adults. Following succinylcholine, however, strenuous fasciculation in adults led to marked elevations, while 20 children under 5 years of age studied by Salem showed no rise but an actual reduction of intragastric pressure. Although absence of fasciculation in children makes the greatest difference, sedation with various combinations of thiopental, morphine, and halothane plus the conservative dosage of succinylcholine (1 mg/kg) used by Salem may have modified his results to some extent. He advises use of succinylcholine for children with full stomach and concludes that prior use of nondepolarizing agents is not indicated.

Such studies on normal children may appear reassuring, but I believe that muscle relaxants are not safe in the presence of an overfilled stomach. The pressure is there already, and if one removes esophageal tone by use of a relaxant, the gastric content may suddenly appear in the hypopharynx, Sellick maneuver notwithstanding. Management of the full stomach is discussed in Chapter 22.

Any patient with a myoneural disorder should be evaluated with particular care before use of succinylcholine. The myotonias show hypersensitivity to succinylcholine and may show prolonged spasticity (Cohen, 1966; Baraka and others, 1970). Myotonic dystrophy, myotonia congenita, and paramyotonia congenita fall within this group (Kaufman and others, 1960; Genever, 1971).

Generalized rigidity following first administration of succinylcholine is often seen, making intubation and ventilation extremely difficult (Cody, 1968). Sustained flexor spasm following administration of succinylcholine is definitely suggestive of either presence of a chronic muscular disorder or onset of malignant hyperthermia (Patterson, 1962; Britt and others, 1973).

Denervation sensitivity. In children with burns or other injuries involving tissue destruction or denervated muscle masses, a perplexing situation has gradually taken shape. In 1959 Finer and Nylen noticed multiple fatalities in children undergoing burn treatment. McCaughey (1962) and Bush (1964), adding experiences of their own, brought widespread attention to this problem. Accumulated evidence pointed to sudden release of potassium immediately after succinylcholine injection in patients whose injuries were at least 1 week old. Doubters were silenced by evidence produced by Tolmie and associates (1967), who documented significant changes in electrocardiogram and plasma potassium in one subject during three cardiac arrests (Fig. 13-2).

Extensive investigation of this problem

now reveals a clinical picture of denervated muscle that, as first demonstrated by Rosenblueth and Cannon in 1939 and subsequently confirmed by Thesleff (1960, 1961), becomes sensitive to stimulation at any area and releases potassium from the entire muscle instead of the end-plate.

It has been found that in addition to burns (Schauer and others, 1969), any extensive tissue damage, as well as tetanus, acute and chronic paraplegia, and myoneural diseases, carries the same risk of sudden elevation of potassium (Paton, 1956; Birch, 1969; Mazze and others, 1969; Stone and others, 1969; Tammisto and others, 1969; Cooperman and others, 1970; Smith and Grenvic, 1970; Tobey, 1970). Consequently, succinylcholine is contraindicated in any patient who has sustained significant myoneural dysfunction. During the first week after the initial injury, the risk does not reach the maximum degree but varies enough to be prohibitive and persists until the healing phase is well established. In our experience, patients with cerebral palsy have shown no abnormal response to muscle relaxants of any kind.

Further investigation of potassium metabolism has shown that succinylcholine causes an immediate, brief elevation of serum potassium level in normal subjects, usually not more than 0.5 to 1 mEq/L, or 25% over resting value (Roth and Wuthrick, 1969; Stovner and others, 1972). Patients with moderate preoperative hyperpotassemia, as in uremia, are at risk because this 25% elevation may put them in a markedly dangerous zone. They do not have the elevation of 5 to 10 mEq/L seen in the traumatized group. Serum potassium levels above 5.5 mEq/L are considered abnormal, while those above 9.0 mEq/L may be fatal. The highest levels measured in patients with subsequent recovery have been near 18 mEq/L.

The use of d-tubocurarine to suppress the potassium flux of succinylcholine was demonstrated in dogs by Klupp and Kraupp (1954) and in man by Birch and associates (1969) as well as Miller and Way (1971). For explanation of the movements of potassium and their prevention by curare and other agents,

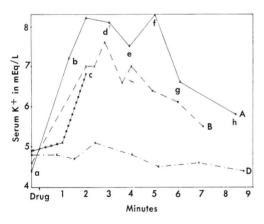

Fig. 13-2. Serum potassium after intravenous injection of 60 mg succinylcholine *(curve A)*, 40 mg succinylcholine *(curve B)*, 40 mg succinylcholine *(curve C)*, and 100 mg gallamine *(curve D)*. (From Tolmie, J. D., Joyce, T. H., and Mitchell, G. D.: Anesthesiology **28:** 467, 1967.)

investigators are studying cell membrane stability, transmembrane potentials, and cholinergic receptors (Smith and Corbascio, 1965; Kendig and others, 1972; Gronert and others, 1973; Gronert and Theye, 1974). In contrast to succinylcholine, it has been shown by List (1967) and others that thiopental, Innovar, ether, halothane, gallamine, curare, and pancuronium cause prompt reduction of serum potassium, with gradual return toward normal.

Succinylcholine also appears to be involved in the initiation of malignant hypothermia, but the mechanism is less clearly defined (Thut and Davenport, 1966). This problem is discussed in Chapter 26.

d-Tubocurarine

Once the most radical and exotic drug used in anesthesia, d-tubocurarine (DTC) now ranks as a relatively conservative agent that has stood the test of time and has few unpredictable qualities.

DTC is a naturally occurring alkaloid prepared from *Chondodendron tomentosum* vines of the Amazon basin. Its site of action at the myoneural junction was established by Claude Bernard in 1849. This concept stood unchallenged until the recent proposal of a prejunctional site by Standaert and Riker (1967), Galindo (1970), and others, who produced evidence that both depolarizing and nondepolarizing muscle relaxants act on the neural part of the junction and the nerve itself in smaller concentrations than those that block transmission. As yet, this concept has not gained wide acceptance.

DTC acts as a nondepolarizing or competitive neuromuscular blocking agent, causing a phase II block that is reversible by anticholinesterase drugs. The uptake, distribution, and excretion have been examined by Kalow (1953), Marsh (1951), Paton (1956), Eger (1974), Cohen (1974, 1975), and others.

Curare is effective by intravenous or intramuscular route. The maximal response following intravenous administration occurs in approximately 60 to 90 seconds in adults, whereas that following intramuscular injection occurs in 6 to 8 minutes. Duration of effect varies with the number of injections and total dose administered. The first effective dose usually lasts approximately 20 minutes in older children and adults. Because of reduced circulation time, the uptake and effect by both intravenous and intramuscular routes are more rapid in infants and children. *When using intravenous DTC in neonates, one should expect immediate onset of apnea.*

Kalow (1953) showed that following intravenous administration, DTC diffuses rapidly into tissues, muscle concentration exceeding that of blood within 3 minutes. The drug was found to undergo partial metabolism, leaving 33% to be excreted unchanged in urine.

The fact that DTC has an alternate route of excretion via the biliary system allows use of the drug in patients with reduced renal function.

DTC is characterized as having ganglionic blocking and histaminogenic action, with resultant hypotensive effect. Hypotensive and bronchospastic responses do occur in pediatric age groups but do not exclude the drug from use in asthmatic patients, in whom it is often employed during mechanical ventilation in treatment of status asthmaticus.

Dosage, duration, and deactivation are predictable, and the agent is definitely nontoxic. In conditions where sensitivity is increased, as in myasthenia, the agent is not absolutely contraindicated. Overdosage causes prolonged apnea but seldom causes other side effects.

For pediatric use, DTC has been valuable in intravenous combinations with thiopental and morphine, or with halogenated agents plus nitrous oxide, in a great many procedures that require relaxation and are expected to last more than 30 minutes.

Indications for use of DTC in our hands formerly included (1) open-heart surgery and other types of intrathoracic operations requiring controlled respiration, especially those with right-to-left shunts, (2) extensive abdominal procedures including hepatic resection, renal transplant, and excision of Wilms' tumor, (3) spinal fusion, and (4) neurosurgical operations, particularly when hyperventilation is required.

At present, our use of DTC is being considerably constricted because of the rather frequent incidence of hypotension and the less frequent incidence of bronchospasm associated with the drug. As mentioned earlier, pancuronium now is used when we wish to raise the arterial pressure, and metocurine is used when we wish to maintain the arterial pressure unchanged.

DTC has played an increasingly important role in mechanical ventilation of postoperative and nonsurgical patients by providing enough depression to allow takeover of respiratory control. This use of curariform drugs is not new. Crude extracts of curare, or "woorara," were tried on tetanus patients in 1859 by the English physician Spencer Wells (Burnap and Little, 1968), and in 1889 Farquharson listed 33 patients treated for various spastic conditions, with less than perfect results.

Dosage. The dosages used for DTC in children depend on several variables, including (1) whether DTC is to be supplemented by ether, halothane, or other agents that will reduce DTC requirement, (2) whether DTC is used to supply relaxation for intubation or is to be initiated after intubation with other agents, and (3) whether one believes that neonates are more sensitive to the drug. Dosages suggested for practical use are shown below. Some reduction is made for neonates, but our observations suggest greater duration rather than greater intensity of relaxant effect in neonates.

d-TUBOCURARINE, GALLAMINE, PANCURONIUM, METOCURINE (NONDEPOLARIZING MUSCLE RELAXANTS)

General contraindications

Possible intubation difficulty
Gastric distension
Neuromuscular pathology
Malignant hyperthermia

Additional contraindications to gallamine and pancuronium

Renal failure
Hypertension
Tachycardia

Dosages

d-Tubocurarine:
  Initial dose for intubation, all ages: 0.5 mg/kg IV
  Initial dose following intubation with succinylcholine: 0.25 mg/kg IV
Gallamine:
  Initial dose for intubation: 2 mg/kg IV
  Initial dose following intubation with succinylcholine: 1.5 mg/kg
Pancuronium:
  Initial dose for intubation: 0.1 mg/kg IV
  Initial dose following intubation with succinylcholine: 0.06 mg/kg
Metocurine:
  Initial dose for intubation: 0.25 mg/kg IV
  Initial dose following intubation: 0.15 mg/kg IV
Subsequent dosages of all agents: one fifth to one fourth of initial dose as required

Reversal

Atropine, 0.02 mg/kg, with neostigmine (Prostigmin), 0.06 mg/kg; neostigmine may be repeated if first dose is inadequate

Technic. A practical method for use of DTC is to induce sleep with thiopental (4 mg/kg) supplemented by a 2:1 mixture of nitrous oxide and oxygen, then intubate with succinylcholine (1.5 mg/kg IV), and about 1 minute later give the first dose of DTC. With the child already intubated and relaxed, one may reasonably start with half the standard intubation dose and use 0.25 mg/kg, with the expectation of repeating this within 5 minutes when the succinylcholine wears off.

Some experts object to mixing different types of relaxants in this way and insist on waiting until the patient reacts before adding curare, in spite of frequent incidence of bucking, salivation, and possible extubation before control is regained. We prefer to avoid these responses and give the long-acting agent without waiting for evidence of need. A third alternative is to avoid succinylcholine entirely and use DTC from the outset. This requires the full intubation dose of curare (0.5 mg/kg). The first choice, to intubate with succinylcholine and add curare before the child begins to react, has been most satisfactory in our experience.

During maintenance, 66% nitrous oxide is probably sufficient analgesic, but supplementation with thiopental for sedation, or preferably morphine for analgesia, is reasonable for added security. Indications of their need are sensed chiefly by rising blood pressure and heart rate, as well as increasing resistance to inflation of the lungs and/or returning motor activity. Such supplementation is also helpful in avoiding sudden awakening that may be embarrassing when DTC fortified only by nitrous oxide is being used. Morphine also carries over to reduce pain and excitement during recovery.

A clinical problem with DTC may arise if relaxation starts to wear off when only 10 or 15 minutes of surgery remain. If one adds DTC, it may delay recovery. Alternatives are (1) use of slightly shorter acting gallamine, (2) use of succinylcholine, which is often done but has the theoretical disadvantages of setting up a prolonged block, (3) use of hyperventilation, (4) addition of narcotics or barbiturates, or (5) supplementation with halothane. Of these, the last two seem most practical.

Reversal of DTC and other nondepolarizing agents was once thought dangerous (Pooler, 1957; Riding and Robinson, 1961), but refraining from their use led to increased incidence of complications (Salanitre and Rackow, 1961). It is now widely believed that reversal should be carried out even when spontaneous respiration appears effective, since residual relaxant still may be present. This is our belief.

Neostigmine has been the most reliable agent used for reversal of neuromuscular block (Gray and Nunn, 1971). Alternatives include edrophonium (Tensilon), galanthamine, germine diacetate, and pyridostigmine bromide.

Dosage of neostigmine apparently does not demand precision; experts use the same amount regardless of the time elapsed since administration of relaxant or the degree of functional return. For adult use, the combination of atropine, 1 mg, and neostigmine, 5 mg, is easily remembered and may be reduced to suit any size. In actuality, infants often require relatively larger doses. The minimal dose for neonates at our institution has been atropine, 0.2 mg, and neostigmine, 0.15 mg, and an additional 0.10 mg of neo-

stigmine has often been needed. Conversely, adults seem to require less neostigmine than this rule suggests. The dosage that we suggest is shown on p. 260.

For evaluation of relaxant reversal in older children, one relies on signs used with adults, i.e., movement of all limbs with normal strength of hand grip, wide opening of eyes without wrinkling forehead, deep breathing, especially with measurement of breathing against resistance (Bendixen and Bunker, 1962), head raising, and voluntary protrusion of the tongue (Bendixen and others, 1959; Nielsen and Bennike, 1965).

The use of peripheral nerve stimulation for intraoperative evaluation of neuromuscular block is strongly advocated by Churchill-Davidson (1972) but disparaged by Gray and Nunn (1971). Some of those who favor its use now find the train-of-four modification more practical, since it does not require previous establishment of a control state (Ali and others, 1970; Goudsouzian and others, 1975). Undoubtedly nerve stimulation is used more frequently to test return of function at the end of operation and is the primary method of distinguishing between phase I and phase II block when return of function is delayed.

Judging the reversal of muscle relaxants in small infants may present some difficulty. The presence of crying, generalized body activity, and ability to hold up the unsupported head are useful guides (Smith, 1966a; Ryan, 1975; Ryan and Goudsouzian, 1975).

Dangers and disadvantages. The greatest danger associated with DTC is that of hypoxia during operation or recovery. In normal patients this is simply a matter of inadequate support by the anesthetist.

Patients with airway obstruction or in whom endotracheal intubation may be difficult, or those with full stomach, stand in extreme danger of rapid hypoxic death if curarizing agents are used and the anesthetist is unable to intubate or ventilate.

Increased sensitivity to DTC, such as seen in myasthenic patients and others with myoneural diseases, does not add significantly to risk if the presence of sensitivity is recognized. With reduced dosage, muscle relaxants still may be employed, provided that the usual ventilatory support is available.

Postoperative respiratory depression is especially common in infants who have become cold during operations, and prompt warming is one of the essentials in reestablishment of function.

Factors affecting action of nondepolarizing relaxants. As noted in reviews by Foldes (1959), Katz and Katz (1966), Cohen (1966), Miller (1975), and others, the action of these agents may be influenced by several variables, including body temperature, acid-base balance, antibiotics, tumor and other disease, cancer-controlling agents, cholinesterase inhibitors, and cardioactive agents. The increased neuromuscular depression caused by supplemental inhalation agents is well documented.

Many of these alterations are seen in pediatric anesthesia. Muscle relaxants induce body cooling by reduction of muscle metabolism. Bigland and associates (1958) established the concept that cooling decreased curare requirement and rewarming would lead to increased relaxant effect. This was not evident clinically, for warming hypothermic curarized infants has usually produced better muscle power. More recently, the traditional concept was opposed by contradictory data (McKlveen and others, 1973).

The acid-base balance has been shown to affect relaxant reversal. DTC reversal is favored by slightly alkalotic arterial pH, gallamine by an acidotic pH.

Prolongation of relaxant effect by intraperitoneal instillation of different antibiotic agents is well known (Doremus, 1959). Pittinger and Long (1959) listed neomycin, dihydrostreptomycin, streptomycin, polymyxin B, and kanamycin as sharing this effect. It was further noted that intraperitoneal administration of streptomycin can produce precipitous hypotension and that although neostigmine antagonizes the blocking effect of neomycin, dihydrostreptomycin, and streptomycin, it tends to *prolong* the effect of polymyxin B and kanamycin.

The use of calcium gluconate to assist re-

versal in these situations has been suggested (Corrado, 1963). Fortunately, the prolongation of effect is not always seen. In our experience, intraperitoneal neomycin has been administered during operation in several different patients, with no alteration of relaxant effect.

Gallamine

In the search for a nondepolarizing muscle relaxant that did not cause histamine release or ganglionic blockade, gallamine (Flaxedil) was developed and has played a secondary role. Its action is generally similar to that of DTC but is of shorter duration and somewhat less predictable. The response in infancy has not been studied in detail; it is weaker, the dose (1.1 mg/lb [2 mg/kg]) being five times that of DTC. Although absence of ganglionic blocking effect protects patients from hypotension, the tachycardia that gallamine may initiate may be more difficult to control and in our experience led to death of a patient in status asthmaticus. The greatest weakness of the drug is that reversal is favored by the presence of acidosis (Baraka, 1967; Katz and Papper, 1963).

Pancuronium

Of the several nondepolarizing neuromuscular blocking agents developed during the past 30 years, pancuronium was the first to present a real challenge to DTC. Pancuronium bromide, a bisquaternary ammonium steroid, was introduced in England in 1967 by Baird and Reid, who reported it to be five times more potent than DTC and to lack both ganglionic blocking action and histamine response. These characteristics were confirmed by subsequent observers in Europe (McDowell and Clarke, 1969; Fastner and Agoston, 1970; Sellick, 1970) and in the United States (Foldes, 1971; Katz, 1971; Stoelting, 1972). Lund and Stovner (1970) found 1 mg of pancuronium to be equipotent to 5.6 mg of DTC, while Nightingale and Bush (1973) reported a 1:6.2 ratio.

Pancuronium is used by intravenous route in dosages varying from 0.01 mg/kg (Saxena and Bonta, 1970) to 0.2 mg/kg (Beam, 1973).

The speed of onset is reported by some to be faster than that of DTC, but most time comparisons appear debatable thus far, because the elapsed time necessary prior to intubation has been stated to be anywhere between 20 seconds (Bennett and others, 1973) and 90 seconds (Sellick, 1970).

Duration of action is affected not only by dose but even more by associated sedatives and anesthetics. Prior use of succinylcholine or supplemental halothane extends its duration by approximately one third, supplementation by methoxyflurane by one half, and supplementation by ether or enflurane by two thirds. Without supplementation, a full dose (0.08 mg/kg) of pancuronium is effective for 25 to 90 minutes.

Distribution and neuromuscular blocking action of pancuronium are thought to be similar to that of other nondepolarizing relaxants.

The predominant value of pancuronium lies in the absence of ganglionic blocking action, with resultant lack of depressant effect on the cardiovascular system (Loh, 1970; Baird, 1970; Waud and Waud, 1975).

Although DTC rarely causes hypotension in pediatric patients, it is more common in geriatric patients (Levin and Dillon, 1971), and the effect is markedly increased when associated with halothane (McDowell and Clarke, 1969; Katz, 1971a) or hypovolemia. Pancuronium, like gallamine, may initiate hypertension and tachycardia, which may be of considerable danger to patients with weak hearts. This response is said to be entirely blocked when halothane is used with pancuronium; however, pancuronium is still to be avoided in patients with hypertensive heart disease.

Since patients with renal failure cannot excrete pancuronium effectively, it should be avoided. Patients with liver disease require increased dosage but are not harmed by the drug.

Speirs and Sim (1972) demonstrated that not enough pancuronium passes the placenta to affect the neonate.

Side effects, disadvantages, and dangers. Pancuronium has few major weaknesses.

Tachycardia, if persistent, as well as hypertensive responses may be damaging to weakened overactive hearts. Beam (1973) reported a heart rate of 210 beats/min lasting for 51 minutes, and as stated, others have found great variability in the intensity and duration of neuromuscular block depending on premedicant and supplemental anesthetic drugs.

As with DTC, the action of pancuronium may be prolonged by several antibiotic agents and is intensified if used in myasthenic patients.

Dangers involving inadequate support during induced apnea and injudicious use in patients with airway problems are similar to those with other muscle relaxants.

The child's response to pancuronium has had less extensive investigation. However, Bennett and associates (1971) reported on its use in 100 infants and children, Nightingale and Bush (1973) compared the action of DTC and pancuronium in 244 children, and Yamamoto (1972) has published a similar study.

Bennett, using doses of 0.1 mg/kg and 0.15 mg/kg, with only atropine for premedication and without other relaxants, found pancuronium effective and devoid of both histaminic response and ganglionic blockade. Although he reported good predictability, he later remarked that the duration of block may be modified greatly by supplemental use of premedicants, succinylcholine, or inhalation agents. Undesirable side effects noted were profuse salivation and sweating.

Nightingale and Bush (1973) figured comparable pediatric doses of DTC and pancuronium to be 0.8 mg/kg and 0.13 mg/kg, respectively. With these doses they found that 88% of patients could be intubated 1 minute after receiving curare and stated that speed of onset and degree of block were similar for the two agents, but DTC again showed more histamine response and hypotension.*

The marked hypertension noted following pancuronium, more pronounced in younger children, was reason to state that the agent

*Most references give 2 minutes as the time for intubation after pancuronium.

should be avoided in pheochromocytoma, adrenogenital syndrome, and hypertension caused by renal disease.

Data have been presented to show that incremental doses of pancuronium may bring increasing cumulative action, but the data of other workers show no cumulative effect, and we are left in another controversy. If using incremental dosage, one should certainly bear this possible complication in mind. Incremental doses usually are approximately one fifth of the initial dose.

A definitive study of the neuromuscular effects of pancuronium in infants and children was reported by Goudsouzian and associates (1974). This study included 17 patients from 6 weeks to 7 years of age. Patients were stabilized on 1% to 2% halothane; then, following incremental doses (0.02 to 0.06 mg/kg) of pancuronium, twitch response was measured for percent depression. With initial doses, the response was variable, but at 0.06 mg/kg, 95% to 100% depression always occurred. By comparison with adult responses described by Katz (1971) and Miller and associates (1972), the authors concluded that children (of all ages) were more resistant than adults to pancuronium.

For reversal, Goudsouzian found that atropine, 0.02 mg/kg, and neostigmine (Prostigmin), 0.08 mg/kg, were effective in all cases. Reversal of pancuronium, if carried out as with DTC, has been predictable and reliable, but it is advisable to wait until 40 minutes after the last administration of pancuronium to attempt it.

Although Nightingale and Bush state that pancuronium is the relaxant of choice for children with cardiac disease, the Rees group that they represent still is said to prefer DTC for standard procedures (Bush, 1974).

Metocurine

Metocurine (dimethyltubocurarine) was described as clinically useful in 1948 by V. K. Stoelting and associates but was largely overlooked until attention was redirected to it by R. K. Stoelting (1974), Donlon and associates (1974), and Goudsouzian and associates (1975). Metocurine is a potent nondepolariz-

ing neuromuscular blocking agent with a definite advantage in having no release of histamine and no alteration of cardiovascular activity. Goudsouzian and associates (1978) report it to be twice as potent as d-tubocurarine in children, while previous work has shown pancuronium to be four times more potent than metocurine (Goudzouzian and others, 1974) (Fig. 13-3). No alteration of response was found by these workers in neonates, infants, or children.

The dosage for metocurine was found to be variable in smaller infants, as with other relaxants. Incremental doses of 0.05 mg/kg were tried, and 90% twitch depression was gained with the third dose, spaced 5 to 8 minutes apart. Onset of neuromuscular block is similar to that of d-tubocurarine, and duration and recovery time are also similar, while duration and recovery under pancuronium were found to be shorter. Reversal of metocurine is accomplished as with other nondepolarizing agents and has not been a source of difficulty. Cardiac arrhythmias have not been noticed at any phase of metocurine use.

It has been our clinical impression that

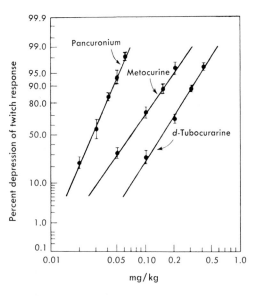

Fig. 13-3. Comparative dose-response curves for pancuronium, metocurine, and d-tubocurarine in infants and children. (From Goudsouzian, N. G., Liu, L. M., and Savarese, J. J.: Anesthesiology **49:**266, 1978.)

metocurine is remarkably well suited to use in pediatric anesthesia and is especially valuable in the care of sicker infants.

BIBLIOGRAPHY

Ali, H. H., Utting, J. E., and Gray, C.: Stimulus frequency in the detection of neuromuscular block in humans, Br. J. Anaesth. **42:**967, 1970.

Anderson, S. M.: Use of depressant and relaxant drugs in infants and children, Lancet **2:**965, 1951.

Baird, W. L. M.: Clinical experience with pancuronium, Proc. R. Soc. Med. **63:**697, 1970.

Baird, W. L. M., and Reid, A. M.: The neuromuscular blocking properties of new steroid compound, pancuronium bromide, Br. J. Anaesth. **39:**775, 1967.

Baraka, A.: Effect of carbon dioxide on gallamine and suxamethonium block in man, Br. J. Anaesth. **39:**786, 1967.

Baraka, A., Haddad, C., Afifi, A., and Baroody, M.: Control of succinylcholine-induced myotonia by d-tubocurarine, Anesthesiology **33:**669, 1970.

Beam, L. R.: Pancuronium bromide side effects, J.A.M.A. **223:**1044, 1973.

Beecher, H. K., and Todd, D. B.: A study of deaths associated with anesthesia and surgery, Ann. Surg. **140:**2, 1954.

Beldavs, J.: Intramuscular succinylcholine for endotracheal intubation in infants and children, Can. Anaesth. Soc. J. **6:**141, 1959 and **9:**306, 1962.

Bendixen, H. H., and Bunker, J. P.: Measurement of inspiratory force in anesthetized dogs, Anesthesiology **23:**315, 1962.

Bendixen, H. H., Surtees, A. D., Oyama, T., and Bunker, J. P.: Postoperative disturbances in ventilation following use of muscle relaxants in anesthesia, Anesthesiology **20:**121, 1959.

Bennett, A. E.: How "Indian arrow poison" curare became a useful drug, Anesthesiology **28:**446, 1967.

Bennett, E. J., Bowyer, D. E., Giesecke, A. H., Jr., and Stephen, C. R.: Pancuronium bromide; a double blind study in children, Anesth. Analg. (Cleve.) **52:**17, 1973.

Bennett, E. J., Daughety, M. J., and Bowyer, D. E.: Pancuronium bromide; experiences in 100 pediatric patients, Anesth. Analg. (Cleve.) **50:**798, 1971.

Betcher, A. M.: The civilizing of curare; a history of its development and introduction into anesthesiology, Anesth. Analg. (Cleve.) **56:**305, 1977.

Bigland, B., Goetzec, B., Maclagan, J., and Zaimis, E.: The effect of lowered muscle temperature on the action of neuromuscular blocking drugs, J. Physiol. **141:**425, 1958.

Birch, A. A., Jr., Mitchell, G. D., Playford, G. A., and Lang, C. A.: Changes in serum potassium response to succinylcholine following trauma, J.A.M.A. **210:**490, 1969.

Britt, B. A., Kalow, W., Gordon, A., and others: Malignant hyperthermia; an investigation of five patients, Can. Anaesth. Soc. J. **20:**431, 1973.

Burnap, T. K., and Little, D. M., Jr.: The flying death; classic papers and commentary on curare, Int. Anesthesiol. Clin. **6:**491, 1968.

Bush, G. H.: The use of muscle relaxants in infants and children, Br. J. Anaesth. **35:**552, 1963.

Bush, G. H.: The use of muscle relaxants in burnt children, Anaesthesia **19:**231, 1964.

Bush, G. H.: Personal communication, 1974.

Bush, G. H., and Roth, F.: Muscle pains after suxamethonium chloride in children, Br. J. Anaesth. **33:**151, 1961.

Bush, G. H., and Stead, A. L.: The use of d-tubocurarine in neonatal anaesthesia, Br. J. Anaesth. **34:**721, 1962.

Churchill-Davidson, H. C.: The causes and treatment of prolonged apnea, Anesthesiology **20:**535, 1959.

Churchill-Davidson, H. C.: In Wylie, W. D., and Churchill-Davidson, H. C., editors: A practice of anaesthesia, ed. 3, Chicago, 1972, Year Book Medical Publishers, Inc.

Churchill-Davidson, H. C., and Wise, R. P.: Neuromuscular transmission in the newborn infant, Anesthesiology **24:**271, 1963.

Churchill-Davidson, H. C., and Wise, R. P.: The response of the newborn infant to muscle relaxants, Can. Anaesth. Soc. J. **11:**1, 1964.

Cody, J. R.: Muscle rigidity following administration of succinylcholine, Anesthesiology **29:**159, 1968.

Cohen, E. N.: Patients with altered sensitivity. In Foldes, F. F., editor: Muscle relaxants, Philadelphia, 1966, F. A. Davis Co.

Cohen, E. N.: Uptake and elimination of skeletal muscle relaxants. In Scurr, C., and Feldman, S., editors: Scientific foundations of anaesthesia, Chicago, 1975, Year Book Medical Publishers, Inc.

Cook, D. R., and Fischer, C. G.: Neuromuscular blocking effects of succinylcholine in infants and children, Anesthesiology **42:**662, 1975.

Cook, D. R., and Fischer, C. G.: Characteristics of succinylcholine neuromuscular blockade in neonates, Anesth. Analg. (Cleve.) **57:**63, 1978.

Cooperman, L. H., Strobel, G. E., Jr., and Kennell, E. M.: Massive hyperkalemia after administration of succinylcholine, Anesthesiology **32:**161, 1970.

Corrado, A. P.: Respiratory depression due to antibiotics; calcium in treatment, Anesth. Analg. (Cleve.) **42:**1, 1963.

Craythorne, N. W., Rottenstein, H. S., and Dripps, R. D.: The effect of succinylcholine on intraocular pressure in adults, infants and children during general anesthesia, Anesthesiology **21:**59, 1960.

Craythorne, N. W., Turndorf, H., and Dripps, R. D.: Changes in pulse rate and rhythm associated with the use of succinylcholine in anesthetized children, Anesthesiology **21:**465, 1960.

Cullen, S. C.: The use of curare for the improvement of abdominal muscle relaxation during inhalation anesthesia, Surgery **14:**261, 1943.

Donlon, J. V., Ali, H. H., and Savarese, J. J.: A new approach to the study of four nondepolarizing relaxants in man, Anesth. Analg. (Cleve.) **53:**934, 1974.

Doremus, W. P.: Respiratory arrest following intraperitoneal use of neomycin, Ann. Surg. **149:**546, 1959.

Drachman, D. B.: The developing motor-endplate; pharmacological studies in the chick embryo, J. Physiol. (Lond.) **168:**707, 1963.

Eger, E. I. II: Muscle relaxant uptake and elimination. In Eger, E. I. II, editor: Anesthetic uptake and excretion, Baltimore, 1974, The Williams & Wilkins Co.

Farquharson, R. W.: Guide to therapeutics and materia medica, ed. 4, Philadelphia, 1889, Lea Bros. & Co.

Fastner, Z., and Agoston, S.: A new neuromuscular blocking agent, pancuronium bromide (Pavulon); pharmacological and clinical studies, Clin. Trials J. **7:**254, 1970.

Feldman, S.: Muscle relaxants; major problems in anesthesia, vol. 1, Philadelphia, 1973, W. B. Saunders Co.

Finer, B. L., and Nylen, B. O.: Double cardiac arrest with survival, Br. Med. J. **1:**624, 1959.

Foldes, F. F.: Muscle relaxants in anesthesiology, Springfield, Ill., 1957, Charles C Thomas, Publisher.

Foldes, F. F.: Factors which alter the effects of muscle relaxants, Anesthesiology **20:**464, 1959.

Foldes, F. F.: The choice and administration of muscle relaxants, Clin. Anesth. **2:**33, 1966.

Foldes, F. F., editor: Muscle relaxants, Philadelphia, 1966a, F. A. Davis Co.

Foldes, F. F.: Studies of pancuronium in conscious and anesthetized man, Anesthesiology **35:**496, 1971.

Foldes, F. F., and Rhodes, D. H., Jr.: Role of plasma cholinesterase in anesthesiology, Anesth. Analg. (Cleve.) **32:**305, 1953.

Galindo, A.: Depolarizing neuromuscular block, J. Pharmacol. Exp. Ther. **178:**339, 1970.

Genever, E. E.: Suxamethonium-induced cardiac arrest in unsuspected pseudohypertrophic muscular dystrophy, Br. J. Anaesth. **43:**984, 1971.

Gill, R. C.: White water and black magic, New York, 1940, Henry Holt & Company.

Glowacki, E. T., Austin, S., and Greifenstein, F. E.: Intramuscular doses of succinylcholine as an adjunct in anesthesia, Anesth. Analg. (Cleve.) **37:**211, 1958.

Goudsouzian, N. G., Donlon, J. V., Savarese, J. J., and Ryan, J. F.: Reevaluation of dosage and duration of action of d-tubocurarine in the pediatric age group, Anesthesiology **43:**416, 1975.

Goudsouzian, N. G., Liu, L. M., and Savarese, J. J.: Metocurine in infants and children, Anesthesiology **49:**266, 1978.

Goudsouzian, N. G., Ryan, J. F., and Savarese, J. J.: The neuromuscular effects of pancuronium in infants and children, Anesthesiology **41:**95, 1974.

Gray, T. C., and Nunn, J. F.: General anaesthesia, Borough Green, Kent, 1971, Butterworth & Co., Publishers, Ltd.

Griffith, H. R.: The evolution of the use of curare in anesthesiology, Ann. N.Y. Acad. Sci. **54:**493, 1951.

Griffith, H. R., and Johnson, E.: The use of curare in general anesthesia, Anesthesiology **3:**418, 1942.

Gronert, G. A., Lambert, E. H., and Theye, R. A.: The response of denervated skeletal muscle to succinylcholine, Anesthesiology **39:**13, 1973.

Gronert, G. A., and Theye, R. A.: Effect of succinylcholine on skeletal muscle with immobilization atrophy, Anesthesiology **40:**268, 1974.

Hodges, R. J. H.: Suxamethonium tolerance and pseudocholinesterase levels in children, proceedings of World Congress of Anesthesiologists, Scheveningen, The Netherlands, September 5-10, 1955, pp. 247-251.

Kalow, W.: Urinary excretion of d-tubocurarine in man, J. Pharmacol. Exp. Ther. **109:**74, 1953.

Kalow, W.: Relaxants. In Papper, E. M., and Kitz, R. J., editors: Uptake and distribution of anesthetic agents, New York, 1963, McGraw-Hill Book Co.

Kalow, W., and Genest, K.: A method for the detection of atypical forms of human serum cholinesterase; determination of dibucaine numbers, Can. J. Biochem. **35:**339, 1957.

Kalow, W., and Gunn, D. R.: The relation between dose of succinylcholine and duration of apnea in man, Anesthesiology **20:**505, 1959.

Katz, R. L.: Clinical neuromuscular pharmacology of pancuronium, Anesthesiology **34:**55, 1971.

Katz, R. L.: Modification of the action of pancuronium by succinylcholine and halothane, Anesthesiology **35:**602, 1971a.

Katz, R. L., and Katz, G. J.: Complications associated with the use of muscle relaxants. In Foldes, F. F., editor: Muscle relaxants, Philadelphia, 1966, F. A. Davis Co.

Katz, R. L., and Papper, E. M.: The effect of alkalosis in the action of neuromuscular blocking agents, Anesthesiology **24:**18, 1963.

Kaufman, L.: Anaesthesia for the older child. In Gray, T. C., and Nunn, J. F., editors: General anaesthesia, Borough Green, Kent, 1971, Butterworth & Co., Publishers, Ltd.

Kaufman, L., Lehmann, H., and Silk, E.: Suxamethonium apnoea in an infant; expression of familial pseudocholinesterase deficiency in three generations, Br. J. Med. **1:**166, 1960.

Kendig, J. J., Bunker, J. P., and Endow, S.: Succinylcholine-induced hyperkalemia; effects of succinylcholine on resting potentials and electrolyte distributions in normal and denervated muscle, Anesthesiology **36:**132, 1972.

Klupp, H., and Kraupp, O.: Über die Freisetzung von Kalium aus der Muskulatur unter der Einwirkung einiger Muskelrelaxantien, Arch. Int. Pharmacodyn. Ther. **98:**340, 1954.

La Cour, D.: Rise in intragastric pressure caused by suxamethonium fasciculations, Acta Anaesth. Scand. **13:**255, 1969.

Lehmann, H., Cook, J., and Ryan, E.: Pseudocholinesterase in early infancy, Proc. R. Soc. Med. **50:**147, 1957.

Leigh, M. D., McCoy, D. D., Belton, M. K., and Lewis, G. B.: Bradycardia following intravenous administration of succinylcholine chloride to infants and children, Anesthesiology 18:608, 1957.

Levin, N., and Dillon, J. B.: Cardiovascular effects of pancuronium bromide, Anesth. Analg. (Cleve.) 50: 808, 1971.

Levy, G. L.: Pharmacokinetics of succinylcholine in newborns, Anesthesiology 32:551, 1970.

Lim, H. S., Davenport, H. T., and Robson, J. G.: The response of infants and children to muscle relaxants, Anesthesiology 25:161, 1964.

List, W. L.: Serum potassium changes during induction of anaesthesia, Br. J. Anaesth. 39:480, 1967.

Litwiffer, R. W.: Succinylcholine hydrolysis; a review, Anesthesiology 31:356, 1969.

Loh, L.: The cardiovascular effects of pancuronium bromide in man, Anaesthesia 25:356, 1970.

Long, G., and Bachman, L.: Neuromuscular blockade by d-tubocurarine in children, Anesthesiology 28:723, 1967.

Lund, I., and Stovner, J.: Dose-response curves for d-tubocurarine, alcuronium and pancuronium, Acta Anaesth. Scand. (Suppl.) 37:238, 1970.

Marsh, D. F.: The pharmacology of calabash curare, Ann. N.Y. Acad. Sci. 54:307, 1951.

Mazze, R. I., Escue, H. M., and Houston, J. B.: Hyperkalemia and cardiovascular collapse following administration of succinylcholine to the traumatized patient, Anesthesiology 31:540, 1969.

McCaughey, T. J.: Hazards of anaesthesia for the burned child, Can. Anaesth. Soc. J. 9:220, 1962.

McDowell, S. A., and Clarke, R. S.: A clinical comparison of pancuronium and d-tubocurarine, Anaesthesia 24:581, 1969.

McKlveen, J. R., Sokoll, M. D., Gergis, S. D., and Dretchen, K. L.: Absence of recurarization rewarming, Anesthesiology 38:153, 1973.

Miller, R. D.: Factors affecting the action of muscle relaxants. In Katz, R. L., editor: Monographs in anesthesiology. Volume 3: Muscle relaxants, New York, 1975, Excerpta Medica.

Miller, R. D., and Way, W. L.: Inhibitions of succinylcholine-induced increased intragastric pressure by non-depolarizing muscle relaxants and lidocaine, Anesthesiology 34:185, 1971.

Miller, R. D., Way, W. L., Dolan, W. M., and others: The dependence of pancuronium- and d-tubocurarine–induced neuromuscular blockades on alveolar concentrations of halothane and forane, Anesthesiology 37:573, 1972.

Nielsen, E., and Bennike, K.: The head-lift test after administration of d-tubocurarine, Acta Anaesth. Scand. 9:13, 1965.

Nightingale, D. A., and Bush, G. H.: A clinical comparison between d-tubocurarine and pancuronium in children, Br. J. Anaesth. 45:63, 1973.

Nightingale, D. A., Glass, A. G., and Bachman, L.: Neuromuscular blockade by succinylcholine in children, Anesthesiology 27:736, 1966.

Pandey, K., Badola, R. P., and Kumar, S.: Time course of intraocular hypertension produced by suxamethonium, Br. J. Anaesth. 42:191, 1972.

Paton, W. D. M.: Mode of action of neuromuscular blocking agents, Br. J. Anaesth. 28:470, 1956.

Patterson, I. S.: Generalized myotonia following suxamethonium, Br. J. Anaesth. 34:340, 1962.

Pittinger, C. B., and Long, J. P.: Potential dangers associated with antibiotic administration during anesthesia and surgery, Arch. Surg. 79:207, 1959.

Pooler, H. E.: Atropine, neostigmine and sudden death, Anaesthesia 12:198, 1957.

Rees, J. G.: Anaesthesia in the newborn, Br. Med. J. 2:1419, 1950.

Rees, J. G.: The child as a subject for anaesthesia. In Evans, F. T., and Gray, T. C., editors: Modern trends in anaesthesia, New York, 1958, Harper & Row, Publishers, Inc.

Rees, J. G.: Paediatric anaesthesia, Br. J. Anaesth. 32: 132, 1960.

Riding, J. E., and Robinson, J. S.: The safety of neostigmine, Anaesthesia 16:346, 1961.

Roe, R. B.: The effect of suxamethonium on intragastric pressure, Anaesthesia 17:179, 1962.

Rosenblueth, A., and Cannon, W. B.: Effects of preganglionic denervation on superior cervical ganglion, Am. J. Physiol. 125:276, 1939.

Roth, F., and Wuthrick, H.: The clinical importance of hyperkalaemia following suxamethonium administration, Br. J. Anaesth. 41:311, 1969.

Ryan, J. F.: Use of muscle relaxants in pediatric anesthesia, Int. Anesthesiol. Clin. 13:1, 1975.

Ryan, J. F., and Goudsouzian, N. G.: Muscle relaxants in pediatric anesthesia. In Katz, R. L., editor: Monographs in anesthesiology. Volume 3: Muscle relaxants, New York, 1975, Excerpta Medica.

Salanitre, E., and Rackow, H.: Respiratory complications associated with the use of muscle relaxants in young infants, Anesthesiology 22:194, 1961.

Salem, M. R., Wong, A. Y., and Lin, Y. H.: The effect of suxamethonium on the intragastric pressure in infants and children, Br. J. Anaesth. 42:166, 1972.

Saxena, P. R., and Bonta, I. L.: Mechanism of selective cardiac vagolytic action of pancuronium bromide; specific blockade of cardiac muscarinic receptors, Eur. J. Pharmacol. 11:332, 1970.

Schauer, P. J., Brown, R. L., Kirksey, T. D., and others: Succinylcholine-induced hyperkalemia in burned patients, Anesth. Analg. (Cleve.) 48:764, 1969.

Sellick, B. A.: Pancuronium bromide; clinical experience of a new muscle relaxant, Proceedings of the Fourth World Congress on Progress in Anesthesiology, Tokyo, 1970.

Smith, N. T., and Corbascio, A. N.: The hemodynamic effects of potassium infusion in dogs, Anesthesiology 26:633, 1965.

Smith, R. B., and Grenvic, A.: Cardiac arrest following succinylcholine in patients with central nervous system injuries, Anesthesiology 33:558, 1970.

Smith, R. M.: Pediatric patients, Clin. Anesth. 2:34, 1966.

Smith, R. M.: Pediatric patients. In Foldes, F. F., editor: Muscle relaxants, Philadelphia, 1966a, F. A. Davis Co.

Smith, S. M.: The use of curare in infants and children, Anesthesiology **8**:176, 1947.

Speirs, I., and Sim, A. W.: The placental transfer of pancuronium bromide, Br. J. Anaesth. **44**:370, 1972.

Standaert, F. G., and Riker, W. F.: The consequences of cholinergic drug actions on motor nerve terminals, Ann. N.Y. Acad. Sci. **144**:517, 1967.

Stead, A. L.: The response of the newborn infant to muscle relaxants, Br. J. Anaesth. **27**:124, 1955.

Stoelting, R. K.: The hemodynamic effects of pancuronium and d-tubocurare in anesthetized patients, Anesthesiology **36**:612, 1972.

Stoelting, R. K.: Hemodynamic effects of dimethyl-tubocurarine during nitrous oxide–halothane anesthesia, Anesth. Analg. (Cleve.) **53**:513, 1974.

Stoelting, V. K., Graf, J. P., and Vieira, Z.: Dimethyl ether of d-tubocurarine iodide as an adjunct to anesthesia, Proc. Soc. Exp. Biol. Med. **69**:565, 1948.

Stone, W. A., Beach, T. P., and Hamelberg, W.: Succinylcholine danger in the spinal cord injured patient, Anesthesiology **32**:168, 1969.

Stovner, D., Endresen, R., and Bjelke, E.: Suxamethonium hyperkalaemia with different induction agents, Acta Anaesth. Scand. **16**:46, 1972.

Tammisto, T., Brander, M., and Airaksinen, M.: Hypoxia and suxamethonium-induced muscle injury, Br. J. Anaesth. **41**:276, 1969.

Telford, J., and Keats, A. S.: Succinylcholine in cardiovascular surgery of infants and children, Anesthesiology **18**:841, 1957.

Thesleff, S.: Effects of motor innervation on the chemical sensitivity of skeletal muscle, Physiol. Rev. **40**:734, 1960.

Thesleff, S.: Nervous control of chemosensitivity in muscle, Ann. N.Y. Acad. Sci. **94**:535, 1961.

Thut, W., and Davenport, H. T.: Hyperpyrexia associated with succinylcholine-induced muscle rigidity; a case report, Can. Anaesth. Soc. J. **13**:425, 1966.

Tobey, R. E.: Paraplegia, succinylcholine, and cardiac arrest, Anesthesiology **32**:359, 1970.

Tolmie, J. D., Joyce, T. H., and Mitchell, G. D.: Succinylcholine danger in the burned patient, Anesthesiology **28**:467, 1967.

Walts, L. F., and Dillon, J. B.: The response of newborns to succinylcholine and d-tubocurarine, Anesthesiology **31**:35, 1969.

Walts, L. F., and Dillon, J. B.: Clinical studies of the interaction between d-tubocurarine and succinylcholine, Anesthesiology **31**:39, 1969a.

Waud, B. E., and Waud, D. R.: Physiology and pharmacology of neuromuscular blocking agents. In Katz, R. L., editor: Monographs in anesthesiology. Volume 3: Muscle relaxants, New York, 1975, Excerpta Medica.

Webster, C. F., and Van Bergen, F. H.: Pentothal-curare mixture with endotracheal N_2O and O_2 in infants, Bulletin of University of Minnesota Hospital, Minn. Med. Found. **20**:525, 1949.

Wells, T. S.: Three cases of tetanus, in which "woorara" was used, Int. Anesthesiol. Clin. **6**:474, 1968.

Whittaker, M.: Genetic aspects of succinylcholine sensitivity, Anesthesiology **32**:143, 1970.

Yamamoto, T., Baba, H., and Shiratsuchi, T.: Clinical experience with pancuronium bromide in infants and children, Anesth. Analg. (Cleve.) **51**:919, 1972.

Zachs, S. I.: The motor endplate, Philadelphia, 1964, W. B. Saunders Co.

Zsigmond, E. K., and Patterson, R. L.: Plasma cholinesterase activity of neonates and infants, paper delivered at annual convention of the American Medical Association, Atlantic City, N.J., June 1967.

CHAPTER 14

Hypotensive technics

Development of hypotensive technics
Applications and rationale of induced
  hypotension
Agents and technics in controlled hypotension

General and plastic surgery
  Excision of hepatic tumors, hepatectomy
  Excision of pheochromocytoma (Katz and Wolf,
  1971)
  Extensive plastic procedures in highly vascular
  areas

Cardiovascular surgery
  Control of hypertension in repair of coarctation of
  aorta
  Deep hypothermic arrest for open-heart repair in infants

Orthopedic surgery
  Hip replacement
  Spinal fusion

Miscellaneous
  Jehovah's Witness problems

The intentional reduction of blood pressure has had several applications in adult surgery and because of the continuing enthusiasm of Enderby and a few other individuals has maintained a definite though minor role in anesthesiology. The use of deliberate hypotension for pediatric procedures has been more limited because the hazards are relatively high, and for many years it was restricted to exceptional situations. More recently, greater surgical endeavors, increasing problems in obtaining replacement blood of adequate quantity and quality, and less conservative pediatric anesthesiologists have brought about increased use of hypotensive methods (see below). At present, anesthesiologists are in a rather dangerous position. Now that the effectiveness of the procedure has been demonstrated, we are pressured from many sides to employ this method in order to save blood or facilitate the work of the surgeon. At the same time we are deeply concerned by our lack of knowledge of the hemodynamics involved and by unexpected complications that must be eliminated before widespread use of the technic can be justified.

CONDITIONS FOR WHICH INDUCED HYPOTENSION HAS BEEN ADVOCATED IN CHILDREN

Neurosurgery
  Clipping of cerebral aneurysm
  Excision of intracranial tumors
  Control of acute hypertensive crises

DEVELOPMENT OF HYPOTENSIVE TECHNICS

As a background to the theory and practice of induced hypotension, review articles by Larson (1964) and Bodman (1967) are outstanding and should be required reading for anyone entering the field.* As they point out, induced hypotension to facilitate surgery was used as early as 1912. As a working concept, however, the major impetus came shortly after World War II, when five different methods were promoted within 5 years, and early applications were widespread and often extreme. The development of the methods suggests the progress in the understanding of the underlying problems.

Arteriotomy. In 1946, to facilitate neurosurgery Gardner introduced the method of

---

*Valuable additional material is found in a symposium on deliberate hypotension, Br. J. Anaesth., July 1975, and in a review article of sodium nitroprusside by Tinker, J. H., and Michenfelder, J. D.: Anesthesiology 45:340, 1976.

arterial cannulation and withdrawal of blood before operation and retransfusion afterward. This induced all of the physiologic distortions of shock, and in addition, faulty arteriotomy caused the loss of several hands.

Hypotensive spinal anesthesia. Using a more rational approach, Gillies of Edinburgh (1949) induced autonomic ganglion block, vasodilation, and hypotension by means of high spinal anesthesia, a method subsequently advocated by Greene in the United States (1958). Although this technic was effective, extended application of it led to wide abuse (Little, 1955) and gradual abandonment. Neither of the above methods had application in children.

Adrenergic blocking agents. The "lytic cocktail" of Laborit and Huguenard (1951) combined promethazine (Phenergan), chlorpromazine (Largactil), and diethazine hydrochloride (Diparcol) and produced sufficient release of vasomotor tone to reduce both blood pressure and body temperature. Prolonged effect and poor control limited the usefulness of the mixture, but chlorpromazine was retained on individual merits, chiefly to promote cooling (Dundee and others, 1954).

The beta-adrenergic blocking agent propranolol came into use more recently in hypotensive work to control the tachycardia associated with ganglionic blocking agents (Hellewell and Potts, 1966).

Ganglionic blocking agents. Following Gillies' demonstration of the effectiveness of autonomic block by direct anatomic approach, it would seem a natural step to accomplish the same end by intravenous infusion of ganglionic blocking agents. However, as told by Leigh (1975), the first ganglionic blocking drugs to be used for intentional hypotension were found during the search for antagonists for a depolarizing muscle relaxant, decamethonium. While Organe, Hunter, Davison, and others made important initial contributions, Enderby in 1950 plunged into full-scale pursuit of the concept, enthusiastically promoting a series of ganglionic blocking agents that proved both effective and practical and had successful applica-

tion in pediatric anesthesia. The most widely accepted were pentolinium (Enderby, 1954), trimethaphan (Magill and others, 1953; Nicholson and others, 1953), and hexamethonium (Enderby, 1961).

Ether, halothane, and curare gradually became recognized as effective primary or secondary agents for induction of hypotension, their action originally being attributed to ganglionic blocking action (Johnstone, 1956; Sleath and Archer, 1967).

Sodium nitroprusside. Sodium nitroprusside (SNP), a drug acting entirely on smooth-muscle fibers, was first administered for control of hypertensive heart disease but proved too evanescent. Moraca and associates (1962) reported its successful application in anesthesia, but during the next 10 years attention was directed chiefly toward the succession of methonium compounds. Between 1970 and 1975 interest returned to SNP. The withdrawal of hexamethonium and pentolinium from production has left SNP and trimethaphan in major roles.

Total circulatory arrest. A concept not usually mentioned in discussions of hypotensive technics has been that of total circulatory arrest. While 40% reduction of blood pressure achieved by vasodilating drugs proved adequate for many operations on vascular tissues, several procedures involving the heart and great vessels required the elimination of all blood flow. The step-by-step development of cardiopulmonary bypass and induced hypothermia gradually brought about the realization of this impossible dream, enabling surgeons to work in an immobile, bloodless field for 60 to 90 minutes. This technic is described in more detail in subsequent chapters.

APPLICATIONS AND RATIONALE OF INDUCED HYPOTENSION

The concept of induced hypotension is confusing, because it has been developed more on the basis of results than reason. Surgeons find it easier to operate if there is less blood in the field, and the economy of blood transfused has additional advantages. Any of several methods may be used to lower blood pressure and achieve these two goals.

Unfortunately, it is not yet clear which hemodynamic factor is most important in meeting the surgeon's demands. If it is reduction of systolic pressure, the level to which it must be reduced to make an appreciable difference to the surgeon is variable and difficult to determine. It is not known what degree of hypotension each organ can tolerate or what signs of stress one should monitor during such procedures. Among the hemodynamic factors thought to be of importance are heart rate, arterial systolic, mean, and diastolic pressure, central venous pressure, ventricular and atrial preload and afterload, peripheral venous compliance, arterial impedance, flow distribution, cardiac output, cardiac index, transmural myocardial pressure, available oxygen, cerebral blood flow, coronary blood flow, and coronary sinus oxygen content.

As a few answers begin to appear, more questions arise. After learning the importance of such variables, we must find the added significance of the rate of pressure change and of the duration of lowered pressures.

AGENTS AND TECHNICS IN CONTROLLED HYPOTENSION
General anesthetics and muscle relaxants

The ganglionic blockade provided by ether anesthesia has been used for reduction of intraoperative hypertension such as that seen in coarctation of the aorta, but the agent now is obsolete. d-Tubocurarine also may be of assistance in lowering systemic pressure but does not produce sufficient reduction to be of value as a primary agent for this purpose.

Halothane. Halothane has played a more significant role and may have increasing potential in view of changing concepts of the danger of myocardial depression (Bland and Lowenstein, 1976; Hamilton, 1976). The principal hypotensive action of halothane has been shown to be direct, dose-related depression of myocardial contractility, with resultant decrease in stroke volume, cardiac output, and cardiac index (Prys-Roberts and

others, 1974; Gersh and others, 1972). Although halothane was initially believed to cause definite peripheral vascular dilation and reduction of peripheral resistance (Johnstone, 1956), this has been found to be an inconstant response (Severinghaus and Cullen, 1958). An increase in pulmonary artery pressure and right atrial pressure and increased pulmonary vascular resistance appear to be more predictable responses to halothane.

Halothane has been used for profound hypotension in several fields of adult surgery, including gynecology (Linacre, 1961), neurosurgery (Hugosson and Högström, 1973), and general and plastic surgery (Prys-Roberts and others, 1974).

The use of halothane for profound hypotension has been less extensive in pediatric anesthesia. This probably is because of the increased concentration of halothane required to produce hypotension in children and the higher incidence of bizarre arrhythmias seen in children in such circumstances. Because of the adaptability of halothane to pediatric anesthesia and its easy controllability, there would seem to be advantages in its application for induction of moderate degrees of hypotension in the younger age group.

If used for this purpose, one should omit atropine and probably morphine, since both cause tachycardia, thereby sustaining cardiac output and arterial pressure. Because MAC for halothane (and other agents) is higher in younger individuals and because children generally are more resistant to induced hypotension, one might expect that higher concentrations of halothane would be needed when dealing with children. Without atropine, however, the hypotensive response to halothane occurs much sooner, and one should begin with concentrations of 1% or 2%, watching the blood pressure closely while increasing the anesthetic. Bradycardia may appear suddenly, leading to severe fall in cardiac output and pressure, especially since respiration will be assisted or controlled. If attained gradually, a 25% reduction of mean arterial pressure (MAP) is probably allowable, although experience has not been sufficient to justify the statement of a definite policy.

In the use of halothane for hypotension, bradycardia should be expected to be a prominent feature and may be an essential step in attaining an MAP of 60 to 65 mm Hg. Should further reduction of pressure or the appearance of arrhythmias cause alarm, recovery should be accomplished by reducing the halothane concentration and increasing oxygenation and *not* by using atropine at this time. Atropine, given at the height of vagal response, often produces wild and dangerous arrhythmias. It should be given to prevent rather than treat vagal responses.

Toward the end of the operation, as in most forms of induced hypotension, normotension should be regained before the wound is closed so that all bleeding points may be identified.

As yet, halothane has not been cleared of the condemnation of Prys-Roberts and associates (1974) for unaltered or increased impedance to ventricular ejection and progressive impairment of myocardial contractility. Halothane is currently being used as a secondary agent in concentrations of 1% to 2%, with the greater effect being produced by SNP or, until recently, pentolinium.

Trimethaphan. Trimethaphan camphorsulfonate, also called trimethaphan camsylate and trimetapan and marketed as Arfonad (Roche), was first used clinically by Magill and associates (1953). It is a short-acting ganglionic blocking agent that also acts by relaxing smooth muscle of arterioles and causes histamine release, with further increase of hypotensive effect (Payne, 1963; Adams and others, 1973). Trimethaphan is best administered by intravenous drip. It is packaged in ampules containing 500 mg in 10 ml and is used in 0.1% solution for adults. As reported by Anderson (1955), normotensive children are more resistant, and we have found it advisable to use a 0.4% solution (500 mg in 125 ml) in 5% dextrose or saline.

Since trimethaphan is rapidly effective, operations may proceed normally until 10 minutes prior to the need for pressure reduction, when the drip is started at 1 mg/kg/min and regulated as needed after 1 to 2 minutes of trial.

In dealing with children, one should not lower arterial pressure more rapidly than 5 mm Hg/min. Overshoot will be slight with trimethaphan, but one usually aims at 70 or 80 mm Hg systolic and slows the drip at 10 mm Hg above that level. If the solution is discontinued, pressure rises promptly, so control must be maintained.

Although the agent is more suited to short-term use, it has been employed for prolonged neurosurgical procedures. Trimethaphan has served us chiefly for clipping cerebral aneurysms and for reduction of hypertension during repair of coarctation of the aorta. Bennett and Dalal (1974) reported on the use of trimethaphan for this purpose. For reduction of MAP to levels of 50 to 60 mm Hg, others have used trimethaphan in craniofacial repair, spinal fusion, and a variety of orthopedic, plastic, and general surgical operations.

Similar to other ganglionic blocking agents, trimethaphan causes reduction of cardiac output. When it was used in conjunction with halothane, Jordan and associates (1971) found an 11.8% reduction of cardiac output, and Didier and associates (1965) reported a 50% reduction in cardiac index. Histamine release is evident occasionally in local skin reactions and renders the agent less suited to use with asthmatic children.

Tachyphylaxis is probably the most troublesome feature associated with trimethaphan (Kilduff, 1954). It is seen frequently and may require rapidly increasing dosage during the course of the procedure. In such cases, supplemental halothane may help in controlling the tachycardia. If a constant drip of trimethaphan is used, one may be misled into giving much more trimethaphan than necessary, since the requirement may level off after a short time. For this reason, the drip should be discontinued at 15- to 20-minute intervals to allow evidence of returning blood pressure before continuing.

At termination of operation and discontinuation of trimethaphan, normal pressure usually is regained within 10 to 15 minutes but if delayed may be restored by use of vasopressor drip of 0.01% phenylephrine (Neo-Synephrine), which must be given slowly to prevent initiation of bleeding. The infusion should be removed at the end of operation to avoid inadvertent addition of more agent.

Over the years of continued use, trimethaphan has appeared to cause fewer serious complications than comparable hypotensive agents and for this reason continues to play an appreciable role in controlled hypotension.

Hexamethonium bromide. Hexamethonium bromide (Bistrium), a ganglionic blocking agent, was one of the principal drugs used during the height of the enthusiasm for hypotensive technics in the early 1950s. Complications that damaged the reputation of the technic were due as much to unrestricted use as to the faults of the drug or technic (Little, 1955; Enderby, 1961).

The principal hemodynamic effect of hexamethonium bromide was thought to be reduction of cardiac output, followed by hypotension. Onset of hypotension was relatively slow, requiring 10 to 15 minutes. Because of the occasional hypersensitive response, it was advisable to use a test dose of 5 mg (for adults) and then, if response was normal, to follow with 25 to 30 mg (0.3 mg/kg), which would be expected to keep the arterial pressure at 65 to 70 mm Hg for 30 to 45 minutes. Recovery was gradual, requiring 3 to 4 hours, during which time patients were kept horizontal and relatively immobile. Tachycardia was extremely common, with the rapid rate boosting cardiac output and compensating for decreasing output and vasodilation and consequently preventing the intended hypotension. Propranolol was used effectively to control the tachycardia but might cause precipitous fall in pressure and often delayed recovery of normotension.

Hexamethonium bromide was useful, however, and was reasonably well tolerated by children. It was especially effective in controlling hypertension during repair of coarctation of the aorta, as was trimethaphan.

For reasons not altogether clear, it was withdrawn from production in 1965.

Pentolinium tartrate. Another ganglionic blocking agent, pentolinium tartrate (Ansolysen), five times more potent and somewhat longer acting, displaced hexamethonium bromide in common usage but was said by Payne (1971) to have no obvious advantage over it. In the hands of more discerning clinicians, pentolinium (and patients) suffered considerably less abuse than had hexamethonium bromide. It was used extensively in England by Enderby and his followers (1950, 1954) and by other disciples in the United States (Eckenhoff and Rich, 1966; Davis and others, 1974; Fahmy and Laver, 1976).

The withdrawal of pentolinium from commercial production in 1974 came as an unpleasant surprise to many clinicians and investigators who continued to rate it as the best in the field. Since pentolinium is still being studied and discussed and is being used by those who have hoarded private supplies, it can be described in the present tense.

The hemodynamic effect of pentolinium, like that of hexamethonium bromide, consists primarily of reduction of arterial pressure due to decreased cardiac output. The speed of onset is not great, but the fluctuation of pressure is such that administration in divided dosage is advisable to avoid overshoot or sudden premature recovery.

Neither hexamethonium bromide nor pentolinium cause histamine release or tachyphylaxis, but in both, the ganglionic blocking action often causes troublesome tachycardia and interferes with the desired reduction of pressure. For this reason, preoperative use of atropine is usually omitted, and propranolol may be given either before or during operation. Salem and associates (1974) found this helpful, using 0.05 to 0.07 mg/kg. Others prefer to avoid propranolol; Katz (1974) believes that it alters and prolongs the action of other drugs, while Szyfelbein and Ryan (1974) prefer to use fentanyl to prevent or treat the tachycardia, finding it effective, of short duration, and reversible.

As with other hypotensive agents, pentolinium can be varied in the degree to which it is extended. If used conservatively, carrying systolic pressures from levels above 120 mm Hg down to 100 mm Hg, risk should be negligible, and there would be little need for additional or invasive monitoring. Unfortunately, the improvement in the surgical field does not parallel the degree of pressure reduction and may not be appreciable until MAP is decreased to 80, 70, 60, or 65 mm Hg.

If pentolinium is used as the sole hypotensive agent, it is questionable whether MAP should be carried below 60 or 65 mm Hg for long operations. With the addition of halothane, hypothermia, and hemodilution, as advocated by Furman (1977), and scrupulous application of continuous arterial oxygenation and carbon dioxide content, base excess, hematocrit, red cell mass, and ionized calcium, plus administration of 100% oxygen and measurement of central venous pressure and urinary output, it appears possible to carry children for several hours with MAP below 60 mm Hg.

For the average clinician, it probably would be sufficient and definitely safer to aim for an MAP between 60 and 70 mm Hg using 1.0% to 1.5% halothane as a supplement to the ganglionic blocker, to maintain FI_{O_2} at 0.7, and to measure blood gases and arterial pressure by cannulation and urinary output by catheter. Central venous pressure sometimes is helpful but seldom is mandatory.

The dosage of pentolinium varies with each writer, but that of 0.3 mg/kg is most often quoted for adults. Salem and associates (1974) report use of 0.15 to 0.3 mg/kg, and Furman (1977), 0.15 mg/kg. The approach of Szyfelbein and Ryan (1974), who used repeated increments of 0.25 mg in neonates to 1 mg in older children, with 4- to 5-minute intervals to observe response, appears more controlled than single-dose methods (see suggested dosage programs below). Once a suitable level is reached, it should be possible to retain it at an even plane by adjustment of halothane concentration, with the initial pentolinium remaining active for 3 to 4 hours.

SUGGESTED DOSAGE PROGRAMS FOR HYPOTENSIVE TECHNICS IN CHILDREN

Trimethaphan (Arfonad)

Drip administration of 0.1% to 0.4% solution, as needed, to gain and hold MAP at 60 to 65 mm Hg

Aid reversal with 0.01% phenylephrine drip, as needed

Hexamethonium bromide (Bistrium)

Test dose: 0.1 mg/kg
Wait 5 minutes
Full dose: 0.5 mg/kg

Pentolinium tartrate (Ansolysen)

Single-dose technic: 0.15 to 0.3 mg/kg
Divided doses, at 5-minute intervals:
Neonate: 0.5 mg, 0.25 mg, 0.25 mg, 0.25 mg
6-yr-old: 0.5 mg, 0.5 mg, 0.5 mg, 0.5 mg
12-yr-old: 1.0 mg, 1.0 mg, 1.0 mg, 1.0 mg
Adult: 2.0 mg, 1.0 mg, 1.0 mg, 1.0 mg

Sodium nitroprusside (Nipride)

Microdrip of 0.01% SNP to reduce MAP to 60 to 65 mm Hg; hold by maintaining slower rate or by adjusting supplemental halothane; reverse by discontinuing agent
Rate of drip:
0.5 to 3 g/kg/min, normal
3.5 to 10 g/kg/min, abnormal
Over 10 g/kg/min, dangerous
Total estimated dose (rate × predicted duration) should not exceed 3.5 mg/kg (Davies and others, 1975)

Pentolinium has been used for a variety of pediatric procedures, and many successes have been claimed. Viguera and Terry (1966) reported it to have been invaluable in the removal of a huge facial tumor in a 9-month-old infant. Salem and associates (1974) have been strong advocates, using it for neurosurgical, orthopedic, plastic, and general surgical procedures to facilitate surgery and save blood and to avoid confrontation by Jehovah's Witnesses. Fahmy and Laver (1976), in a thorough investigation of hypotensive agents, rated pentolinium at the top, citing three important advantages: (1) a stable heart rate and right ventricular pressure can be established before surgery is begun, (2) the heart rate and right ventricular pressure give a reliable indication of blood flow, and (3) relative changes in myocardial oxygen consumption can be monitored by multiplying the heart rate by the arterial systolic pressure.

On the negative side, there are contraindications and complications. Contraindications to the use of ganglionic blocking agents are listed below and are self-explanatory. Disadvantages and actual complications associated with pentolinium have chiefly been due to excessive hypotension and inability to reverse it over many hours. The cardiovascular accidents that have been seen in the elderly are not apt to occur in children. Some who have used pentolinium for spinal fusion have abandoned it, either because it lacked appreciable advantage (Stiles, 1976) or because the prone position was thought to be incompatible with hypotension (Relton and Conn, 1963; Salem and others, 1976). A survey by Salem and associates (1976), reporting complications in the use of hypotensive technics in children, revealed the varied possibilities for disaster, mainly due to loss of control and prolonged hypotension, and included four preventable deaths.

CONTRAINDICATIONS TO THE USE OF INDUCED HYPOTENSION

Anemia
Hypovolemia
Hypothyroidism
Malnutrition
Cerebrovascular disease
Ischemic heart disease
Peripheral vascular disease
Severe obstructive lung disease
Renal impairment or hypertension

Special contraindications to the use of SNP

Vitamin B_{12} deficiency
Leber's optic atrophy
Tobacco amblyopia

Sodium nitroprusside [$Na_2Fe(CN)_5$]. The prominent place that SNP now holds in the field of induced hypotension, the recently recognized danger of its toxicity, and the uncertainties still involved in the concept of induced hypotension suggest more detailed consideration of SNP and its use.

The progression of SNP to its present position was a gradual one. The drug was described by Playfair in 1849, and its hypotensive effect is said to have been known by Claude Bernard of that era. Its pharmacologic action was reported by Hermann in 1886, its toxicity by Johnson in 1929, and its metabolism by Lang in 1933. Page tested the drug in extensive clinical trials, using it for control of acute hypertensive episodes (1951), for which it still is used, and for continuous control of hypertension (Page and others, 1955), for which the brief action of SNP proved impractical.

The application of SNP for induced hypotension during anesthesia was reported by Moraca and others (1962). Being light-sensitive, SNP required last-minute preparation and special handling. Because of this awkwardness and the continued popularity of the methonium compounds, there was little initial enthusiasm for SNP, but increasing problems with the methonium compounds and improved packaging of SNP (Nipride, Roche) reversed the situation in the early 1970s. For a short time, the controllability of SNP and its supposed freedom from toxicity encouraged wide use. Its further application for the reduction of left ventricular filling pressure and afterload in patients with acute myocardial infarction and cardiac failure has considerably increased the scope of its usefulness (Guiha and others, 1974; Franciosa and others, 1972). The appearance of fatal complications, however, has caused general concern and tightened restrictions on its use.

As presently packaged in dihydrate form for medical use, SNP is a reddish brown powder that dissolves in water, showing a faint brownish tint, and turns blue when exposed to light or when mixed in an alkaline solution, the ferric ion being reduced to the ferrous form. It is emphatically stated that the compound should be dissolved in 5% dextrose and water solution, that nothing else is to be added to the solution, that both the powder and the solution should be carefully protected from light, and that the solution should be discarded within 4 hours after mixing or before that time if it shows bright red, green, or bluish discoloration.

The action of SNP is not that of a ganglionic blocking agent. SNP acts directly on peripheral vessels, with the depression of tonic smooth-muscle fibers causing vascular dilation and reduction of arterial systolic and diastolic pressures as well as venous and pulmonary arterial pressures. According to Jack (1974), this is due to the nitroso group (—NO), which inhibits both the influx and the intracellular activation of calcium ions.

In sorting out the various hemodynamic effects of SNP, we find that most observers are impressed with cardiac output as a measure of efficiency, and many observers feel that SNP is superior in this feature. Whereas ganglionic blocking agents all reduce cardiac output, Styles and associates (1973) find it unchanged by SNP, and Wildsmith and associates (1973), Katz and Wolf (1971a), and Lawson and associates (1976) find it increased to as much as 20% above control levels. A different view is expressed by Laver and Bland (1975) who point out that the vasodilation of SNP produces lower afterload by reducing arterial impedance and lower preload by increasing venous compliance, and that by application of the Frank-Starling definition of ventricular function, cardiac output under SNP may increase, remain constant, or even decline.

Of greater importance than cardiac output is the relationship between the oxygen requirement and the available oxygen at hypotensive levels. By measuring cardiac output and oxygen saturation in patients under SNP, Styles and associates (1973) calculated that available oxygen remained unchanged during SNP hypotension. Other variables of obvious importance include coronary perfusion, myocardial oxygen consumption, and cerebral blood flow. Ivankovich and associates (1976) reported increased cerebral blood flow during SNP infusion, while Katz and Wolf (1971a) have stressed the advantage of improved renal perfusion with increased urine output.

The hypotensive response to intravenous SNP is rapid, profound, and evanescent, thereby making it the most finely controllable of the hypotensive agents. In "normal" patients, the arterial pressure may be varied at will by altering the rate of the SNP infusion, and it returns to control level within 2 or 3 minutes after the infusion is discontinued. From the viewpoint of the surgeon this is just right, but in the dim light of present physiologic understanding one is less certain. Rapid hemodynamic changes are rarely desirable, and Rolleson and Hough (1969) have reported signs of myocardial ischemia with sudden reduction of arterial pressure. Furthermore, any agent having sudden, potent effect lends itself more easily to errors of administration. Complications in patients who do not react normally to SNP present another critical factor that is described below.

Special contraindications. In general, the indications and contraindications for the use of SNP are similar to those for the ganglioplegic agents. Because of the major peripheral action of the drug, some believe that SNP should not be used in the treatment of compensatory hypertension, i.e., arteriovenous shunts and coarctation of the aorta (drug insert, Roche). Since Bennett and Dalal (1974) have reported favorably on this application, the situation remains in question.

Because of SNP's cyanide content, Davies and associates (1975a) warn of the specific contraindication of SNP for patients with Leber's optic atrophy and those with tobacco amblyopia. Both diseases are known to involve metabolic disorders with resultant high levels of blood cyanide.

Administration. Mindful of the restrictions, one can proceed with use of the drug. A vial containing 50 mg of the powdered compound is opened, and 2 or 3 ml of dextrose in water are added to dissolve the powder. This solution is then added to 500 ml of 5% dextrose in water to make a 0.01% (100 μg/ml) solution. This is mixed for intravenous infusion and should be regulated accurately by a mechanical pump or microdrip apparatus that will be maintained for the sole purpose of administering SNP. The solution is carefully protected from light.

The problem of dosage of SNP seems to be its most dangerous feature. Before a potent drug is given by intravenous route, three essentials should be established: (1) the proper concentration of solution, (2) the rate of administration, and (3) the maximum safe total dose. In the case of SNP, none of these essentials appears clearly defined. In the 0.01% solution generally recommended for adults, small children must receive 0.2 to 0.5 ml/min. Such amounts are difficult to measure accurately, and error may cause serious overdosage, but more dilute solutions may cause overhydration. We leave it at 0.01%.

The rate of administration, according to the package insert, may be 0.5 to 8 μg/kg/min, which leaves considerable latitude. The initial rate of infusion suggested by Palmer and Lassiter (1975) is narrowed down to 0.5 to 1.5 g/kg/min, with 1.0 serving as a conservative place to start. At this rate, SNP should show initial effect in 1 to 2 minutes and may be regulated to reduce MAP to 65 mm Hg over a period of about 10 minutes. As soon as a steady rate of infusion has been established, one should estimate the rate of SNP requirement and also the expected total dose. While there is much disagreement here also, Davies and associates (1975) contend that rates exceeding 10 μg/kg/min are dangerous and call for discontinuation of the drug. The allowance by McDowall and associates (1974) of 26 μg/kg/min is looked on as far too much.

The total predicted dose may be calculated as the product of the rate of administration and the surgeon's estimate of the operating time. Here the limit of SNP is often loosely set at 3 to 3.5 mg/kg without respect to time. While Lawson and associates (1976) would prefer 10 mg/kg as the maximum, Tinker (1976) reported that Michenfelder has found that the maximum safe SNP dose for dogs may be as little as 1 mg/kg/4 hr. In this we heed the cries of the wounded and regard 3.5 mg/kg as our safe limit for total dosage.

Estimates of suitable dosages for children have varied. Lawson and associates (1976) constructed a nomogram based on age/weight ratio. McHugh and associates (1978) subsequently warned that this gave dangerously high dosages. In their work, they found that either age or weight could be used as the basis of a more reliable formula. Their formulas were as follows:

$$\text{SNP } (\mu g/min) = 5.17 + 5.02 \times \text{age (yr)}$$
$$\text{SNP } (\mu g/min) = -1.43 + 1.94 \times \text{weight (kg)}$$

Several procedures are followed as a means of reducing the duration of use of SNP and the concentration used. The drug is withheld until the operation is underway, atropine and morphine are omitted to prevent tachycardia, and halothane is used to provide an appreciable part of the hypotensive effect.

Accurate monitoring is needed during SNP hypotension. Measurement of blood pressure by oscillometer or Doppler apparatus is considered adequate by some and might be for pressure reduction of under 25%, but for moderate or profound degrees of hypotension intra-arterial cannulation would appear preferable. This involves appreciable risk and is one of the reasons why induced hypotension should not be used without definite justification. Arterial cannulation is needed during deep hypotension for frequent determination of blood gases as well as for following arterial pressure. In addition, the usual stethoscope and thermometer are obligatory, and urethral catheter, ECG, and central venous pressure line are helpful. All of these monitors fall far short of desired methods of evaluating oxygen delivery and tissue perfusion. The electroencephalograph has had surprisingly little application during hypotension, although Prior (1971) has worked on a method of estimating cerebral function during anesthesia and hypotension.

During all phases of the hypotensive procedure one guards particularly against hypoxia (see list of signs on p. 278). Rapid induction can cause myocardial ischemia, which may be suspected if there is ECG evidence of inverted T waves and runs of ventricular extrasystoles. Other signs of hypoxia include dilated pupils, hypovolemia, and severe alkalosis. Pa_{O_2} should be maintained above 100 mm Hg, pH between 7.35 and 7.45, and Pa_{CO_2} between 25 and 35 mm Hg.

277

SIGNS SUGGESTING HYPOXIA OR CYANIDE POISONING DURING INDUCED HYPOTENSION

Tachycardia, bradycardia, arrhythmias
Metabolic acidosis
High dose requirement
Increased mixed venous oxygen content
Decreased arterial–mixed venous oxygen difference
Dilated pupils
High blood cyanide content
Marked hypothermia

ANTIDOTES FOR CYANIDE POISONING

Sodium nitrite: 5 mg/kg in 20 ml water over 3 to 4 minutes (Greiss and others, 1976)
Amyl nitrite: inhale every 2 minutes
Sodium thiosulfate: 2 mg/kg
Hydroxocobalamin (Cottrell, 1978)

Naturally, the degree of hypotension affects the physiologic risk. If MAP is not carried below 65 mm Hg, a time limit should not be necessary. If the pressure is reduced below this approximate level, the duration should be limited in proportion to the reduction. As with comparable drugs, it is advisable to regain normal pressure before the wound is closed to prevent postoperative bleeding.

To terminate hypotension, SNP is discontinued. Blood pressure should return to control level within 5 minutes if fluid replacement and other supportive measures have been adequate. Patients are maintained in horizontal position for 3 or 4 hours before being allowed to move about and are not released from the hospital for 24 hours.

Complications. For several years, SNP was believed to be devoid of major toxicity. Side effects were seen infrequently, consisting of nausea, vomiting, twitching, sweating, and apprehension, all of which were believed to be results of overdosage that could be relieved by decreasing the rate of SNP infusion. Chronic overdosage is reputed to have caused hypothyroidism in one patient (Katz and Wolf, 1971a).

During 1974 and 1975, three deaths due to SNP were reported by Jack (1974), Davies and associates (1975a), and Merrifield and Blundell (1974), and severe metabolic acidosis was reported by McDowall and associates

(1974) and MacRae and Owen (1974). Investigation of these incidents by Toronto workers Davies and associates (1975a) and Greiss and associates (1976) led to the concept that individuals might respond to SNP by any one of four different ways. Under usual conditions, normal patients who are given 0.01% SNP show rapid fall in MAP (to 50 or 60 mm Hg), which will be maintained easily on 3 to 3.5 μg/kg/min and return to initial level promptly on discontinuation of the drug.

The first abnormal response, thought to be tachyphylaxis, is found in patients whose arterial pressure falls with initial administration of SNP but, on continuation of the drug, rises within 30 to 40 minutes, to be controlled only by increasing dosages. This has been seen several times and is believed to be due to the initial presence of adequate tissue rhodanase and sodium thiosulfate, followed by early depletion of one, probably the thiosulfate. When this response develops gradually, Davies and associates have been successful in treating the condition with intravenous administration of 150 mg of sodium thiosulfate in a period of 15 minutes and subsequently proceeding with SNP.

The second abnormal response is seen in patients whose arterial pressure falls with administration of SNP but who require a high dose from the start (over 3.5 μg/kg/min).

The third abnormal response consists of such resistance to SNP that hypotension is unobtainable by this means, even with greatly increased dosage. Davies and associates believe that patients who show either of the last two responses are in danger of developing metabolic acidosis and cyanide poisoning, and they recommend discontinuation of the drug.

While Lawson and associates (1976) disparage the views of Davies' group on toxicity and tachyphylaxis, these views have been confirmed by the investigation of Posner and associates (1976). Tachyphylaxis has also been reported by Amaranth and Kellermeyer (1976), and the potential danger of cyanide poisoning during SNP administration is generally acknowledged, impressing one with the responsibility for watching for signs of such toxicity and being prepared to treat it should it develop.

Intravenous nitroglycerine. The apparent usefulness of SNP, coupled with its inherent dangers, made the next step to the use of intravenous nitroglycerine rather obvious. Nitroglycerine has been thoroughly investigated and widely employed for relief of vasoconstriction, is rapidly metabolized without toxic products, is predictable, and is usually well tolerated (Stetson, 1978). Overdosage produces unpleasant pounding headache and flushing, which are of relatively short duration.

The intraoperative use of nitroglycerine began in 1968 in conjunction with myocardial vascularization procedures. Viljoen of Cleveland Clinic used both intramuscular and intravenous routes of administration to ensure myocardial flow during and after surgery. With continuing experience in the use of the agent for deliberate intraoperative hypotension, Fahmy (1978) has found several advantages in nitroglycerine when compared with SNP. Slightly slower response allows greater control and smoothness of initiation and maintenance, and higher mean and diastolic pressures at equal systolic pressure provide greater myocardial perfusion.

In clinical use of intravenous nitroglycerine, Fahmy has employed a 0.01% solution of the drug in 0.9% saline solution, starting the infusion at a rate of 20 μg/min until arterial systolic pressure reaches 75 torr and then reducing the rate to hold the pressure at that level. At termination of the infusion, recovery of preoperative pressure has required approximately 10 minutes as compared with the 5 minutes usually required after use of SNP. As yet there has been little recorded experience with intravenous nitroglycerine in pediatric age groups; however, the more resilient vessels of younger patients should provide additional safety for use of the agent.

BIBLIOGRAPHY

Adams, A. P., Clarke, T. N. S., Edmonds-Seal, J., and others: Effects of sodium nitroprusside on myocardial contractility and haemodynamics, Br. J. Anaesth. **45:**120, 1973.

Amaranth, L., and Kellermeyer, W. F.: Tachyphylaxis to sodium nitroprusside; clinical reports, Anesthesiology **44:**345, 1976.

Anderson, S. M.: Controlled hypotension with Arfonad in paediatric surgery, Br. Med. J. **2:**103, 1955.

Bennett, E. J., and Dalal, F. Y.: Hypotensive anesthesia for coarctation; a method of prevention of postoperative hypertension, Anaesthesia **6:**20, 1974.

Bland, J. H. L., and Lowenstein, E.: Halothane-induced decrease in experimental ischemia in the nonfailing heart, Anesthesiology **45:**287, 1976.

Bodman, R. I.: Controlled hypotension. In Hewer, C. L., editor: Recent advances in anaesthesia and analgesia, Boston, 1967, Little, Brown & Co.

Boyan, C. P., and Brunschwig, A.: Hypotensive anesthesia in radical pelvic and abdominal surgery, Surgery **31:**829, 1952.

Cottrell, J. E.: Prevention of nitroprusside-induced cyanide toxicity with hydroxocobalamin, N. Engl. J. Med. **298:**809, 1978.

Davies, D. W., Greiss, L., Kadar, D., and Steward, D. J.: Sodium nitroprusside in children; observations on metabolism during normal and abnormal responses, Can. Anaesth. Soc. J. **22:**553, 1975.

Davies, D. W., Kadar, D., Steward, D. J., and others: A sudden death associated with the use of sodium nitroprusside for induction of hypotension during anesthesia, Can. Anaesth. Soc. J. **22:**547, 1975a.

Davis, N. J., Jennings, J. J., and Harris, W. H.: Induced hypotensive anesthesia for total hip replacement, Clin. Orthop. **101:**93, 1974.

Didier, E. P., Claggett, O. T., and Theye, T. A.: Cardiac performance during controlled hypotension, Anesth. Analg. (Cleve.) **44:**379, 1965.

Dundee, J. W., Mesham, P. R., and Scott, W. E. B.: Chlorpromazine and the production of hypothermia, Anaesthesia **9:**296, 1954.

Eckenhoff, J. E., Enderby, G. E., Larson, A., and others: Pulmonary gas exchange during deliberate hypotension, Br. J. Anaesth. **35:**750, 1963.

Eckenhoff, J. E., and Rich, J. C.: Clinical experiences with deliberate hypotension, Anesth. Analg. (Cleve.) **45:**21, 1966.

Enderby, G. E. H.: Controlled circulation with hypotensive drugs and posture to reduce bleeding in surgery; preliminary results with pentamethonium iodide, Lancet **1:**1145, 1950.

Enderby, G. E. H.: Pentolinium tartrate in controlled hypotension, Lancet **2:**1097, 1954.

Enderby, G. E. H.: Halothane and hypotension, Anaesthesia **15:**25, 1960.

Enderby, G. E. H.: A report on mortality and morbidity following 9,107 hypotensive anaesthetics, Br. J. Anaesth. **33:**109, 1961.

Eppens, H.: Sodium nitroprusside in hypotensive anaesthesia, correspondence, Br. J. Anaesth. **45:**124, 1974.

Fahmy, N. R.: Nitroglycerine as a hypotensive drug during general anesthesia, Anesthesiology **49:**17, 1978.

Fahmy, N. R., and Laver, M. B.: Hemodynamic response to ganglionic blockade with pentolinium during N_2O-halothane anesthesia in man, Anesthesiology **44:**6, 1976.

Franciosa, J. A., Guiha, N. H., Limas, C. J., and others: Improved left ventricular function during nitroprusside infusion in acute myocardial infarction, Lancet **1:**650, 1972.

Furman, E. B.: Anesthetic management and blood conservation during scoliosis surgery, paper presented at spring session of American Academy of Pediatrics, New Orleans, April 17, 1977.

Gardner, W. J.: The control of bleeding during operations by induced hypotension, J.A.M.A. **132:**572, 1946.

Gersh, B. J., Prys-Roberts, C., Reuben, S. R., and Schulz, D. R.: The effects of halothane on the interactions between myocardial contractility, aortic impedance, and left ventricular performance. II. Aortic input impedance, and the distribution of energy during ventricular ejection, Br. J. Anaesth. **44:**767, 1972.

Gillies, J.: Anaesthesia for the surgical treatment of hypertension, Proc. R. Soc. Med. **42:**295, 1949.

Greene, N. M.: Hypotensive spinal anesthesia, Baltimore, 1958, The Williams & Wilkins Co.

Greiss, L., Tremblay, N. A. G., and Davies, D. W.: The toxicity of sodium nitroprusside, Can. Anaesth. Soc. J. **23:**480, 1976.

Guiha, N. H., Cohn, J. N., Mikulic, E., and others: Treatment of refractory heart failure with infusion of nitroprusside, N. Engl. J. Med. **291:**587, 1974.

Hamilton, W. K.: Do let the blood pressure drop and do use myocardial depressants, editorial, Anesthesiology **45:**273, 1976.

Harp, J. R., and Wollman, H.: Cerebral metabolic effects of hyperventilation and deliberate hypotension, Br. J. Anaesth. **45:**256, 1973.

Hellewell, J., and Potts, M. N.: Propranolol in hypotension, Br. J. Anaesth. **41:**28, 1966.

Hermann, L.: Ueber die Wirkung des Nitroprussidnatriums, Arch. Physiol. **39:**419, 1886.

Holmes, F.: Induced hypotension in orthopedic surgery; hexamethonium bromide in 407 orthopedic operations, J. Bone Joint Surg. **38:**846, 1956.

Hugosson, R., and Högström, S.: Factors disposing to morbidity in surgery of intracranial aneurysms with special regard to deep controlled hypotension, J. Neurosurg. **38:**561, 1973.

Hunter, A. R.: Hexamethonium bromide, Lancet **1:**251, 1950.

Ivankovich, A. D., editor: Nitroprusside and other short-acting hypotensive agents, Int. Anesthesiol. Clin., volume 16, 1978.

Ivankovich, A. D., Miletich, D. J., Albrecht, R. F., and Zabed, B.: Sodium nitroprusside and cerebral blood flow in the anesthetized and unanesthetized goat, Anesthesiology **44:**21, 1976.

Jack, R. D.: Toxicity of sodium nitroprusside, correspondence, Br. J. Anaesth. **46:**2, 1974.

Johnson, C. C.: The actions and toxicity of sodium nitroprusside, Arch. Int. Pharmacodyn. Ther. **35:**480, 1929.

Johnstone, M.: The human cardiovascular response to Fluothane anaesthesia, Br. J. Anaesth. **28:**392, 1956.

Jordan, W. S., Graves, C. L., Boyd, W. A., and others: Cardiovascular effects of three techniques for inducing hypotension during anesthesia, Anesth. Analg. (Cleve.) **50:**1059, 1971.

Katz, R. L.: Sodium nitroprusside in children, Twelfth Clinical Conference in Pediatric Anesthesiology, Los Angeles, January, 1974.

Katz, R. L., and Wolf, C. E.: Pheochromocytoma. In Mark, L. C., and Ngai, S. H., editors: Highlights of clinical anesthesiology, New York, 1971, Harper & Row, Publishers, Inc.

Katz, R. L., and Wolf, C. E.: The use of sodium nitroprusside for controlled hypotension and treatment of hypertensive emergencies. In Mark, L. C., and Ngai, S. H., editors: Highlights of clinical anesthesiology, New York, 1971a, Harper & Row, Publishers, Inc.

Kilduff, C. J.: The use of Arfonad in controlled hypotension, Lancet **1:**337, 1954.

Laborit, H., and Huguenard, P.: L'hibernation artificielle par moyens pharmacodynamiques et physiques en chirurgie, J. Chir. (Paris) **67:**631, 1951.

Lang, K.: Die Rhodanbildung im Thierkörper, Biochem. Z. **259:**243, 1933.

Larson, A. G.: Deliberate hypotension, Anesthesiology **25:**683, 1964.

Laver, M. B., and Bland, J. H. L.: Anesthetic management of the pediatric patient during open-heart surgery, Int. Anesthesiol. Clin. **13:**149, 1975.

Lawson, N. W., Thompson, D. S., Nelson, C. L., and others: A dosage nomogram for sodium nitroprusside-induced hypotension under anesthesia, Anesth. Analg. (Cleve.) **55:**574, 1976.

Leigh, J. M.: The history of controlled hypotension, Br. J. Anaesth. **47:**745, 1975.

Linacre, J. L.: Induced hypotension in gynaecological surgery, Br. J. Anaesth. **33:**45, 1961.

Little, D. M.: Induced hypotension during anesthesia and surgery, Anesthesiology **16:**320, 1955.

Lowson, J. A.: Sodium nitroprusside in hypotensive anaesthesia, correspondence, Br. J. Anaesth. **44:**908, 1972.

MacRae, W. R., and Owen, M.: Severe metabolic acidosis following hypotension induced with sodium nitroprusside, Br. J. Anaesth. **46:**795, 1974.

Magill, I. W., Scurr, C. F., and Wyman, J. B.: Controlled hypotension by a thiophanium derivative, Lancet **1:**219, 1953.

McDowall, D. G., Keaney, N. P., Turner, J. M., and others: The toxicity of sodium nitroprusside, Br. J. Anaesth. **46:**327, 1974.

McHugh, R. D., Berry, F. A., Jr., and Longnecker, D. E.: Dose requirements of sodium nitroprusside during anesthesia in children, abstract, annual meeting of the American Society of Anesthesiologists, Chicago, 1978.

Merrifield, A. J., and Blundell, M. D.: Toxicity of sodium nitroprusside, Br. J. Anaesth. **46:**324, 1974.

Moraca, P. P., Bitte, E. M., Hale, D. E., and others: Clinical evaluation of sodium nitroprusside as a hypotensive agent, Anesthesiology **23:**193, 1962.

Nicholson, M. J., Sarnoff, S. J., and Crehan, J. P.: Intravenous use of thiophanium derivative (Arfonad RO 2-2222) for production of flexible and rapidly reversible hypotension during surgery, Anesthesiology **14:**215, 1953.

Page, I. H.: Treatment of essential and malignant hypertension, J.A.M.A. **147:**1311, 1951.

Page, I. H., Corcoran, A. C., Dustan, H. P., and others: Cardiovascular actions of sodium nitroprusside in animals and hypertensive patients, Circulation **11:**188, 1955.

Palmer, R. F., and Lassiter, V. C.: Sodium nitroprusside, N. Engl. J. Med. **293:**294, 1975.

Payne, J. P.: The circulatory effect of halothane, Proc. R. Soc. Med. **56:**92, 1963.

Payne, J. P.: Ganglionic blockade. In Gray, T. C., and Nunn, J. F., editors: General anaesthesia, Borough Green, Kent, 1971, Butterworth & Co., Publishers, Ltd.

Posner, M. A., Rodkey, F. L., and Tobey, R. E.: Laboratory report; nitroprusside-induced cyanide poisoning; antidotal effect of hydroxocobalamin, Anesthesiology **44:**330, 1976.

Prior, B.: A cerebral function monitor, Br. J. Med. **2:**736, 1971.

Prys-Roberts, C., Gersh, B. J., Baker, A. B., and others: The effects of halothane on the interaction between myocardial contractility, aortic impedance, and left ventricular performance. I. Theoretical considerations and results, Br. J. Anaesth. **44:**634, 1972.

Prys-Roberts, C., Lloyd, J. W., Fisher, A., and others: Deliberate profound hypotension induced with halothane; studies of dynamics and pulmonary gas exchange, Br. J. Anaesth. **46:**105, 1974.

Relton, J. W. A., and Conn, A. W.: Anaesthesia for the surgical correction of scoliosis by the Harrington method in children, Can. Anaesth. Soc. J. **10:**603, 1963.

Rolleson, W. N., and Hough, J. M.: An examination of some electrocardiographic studies during hypotensive anaesthesia, Br. J. Anaesth. **41:**561, 1969.

Ryan, J.: Personal communication, 1974.

Sadove, M. S., Wyant, G. M., and Gleave, G.: Controlled hypotension; a study on Arfonad (RO 2-2222), Anaesthesia **8:**175, 1953.

Salem, M. R., Bennett, M. B., Rao, T. L. K., and ElEtr,

A. A.: An examination of complications related to hypotensive anesthesia, paper presented at Annual Meeting of American Society of Anesthesiologists, San Francisco, October 11, 1976.

Salem, M. R., and Ivankovic, A. D.: The place of beta-adrenergic blocking drugs in the deliberate induction of hypotension, Anesth. Analg. (Cleve.) **49:**427, 1970.

Salem, M. R., Wong, A. Y., Bennett, E. J., and others: Deliberate hypotension in infants and children, Anesth. Analg. (Cleve.) **53:**975, 1974.

Salem, M. R., Yonook, K., and Shaker, M. H.: The effect of inspired oxygen concentration on jugular bulb oxygen tension during deliberate hypotension, Anesthesiology **33:**358, 1970.

Schlant, R., Tsagaris, T., and Robertson, R.: Studies on the acute cardiovascular effects of intravenous sodium nitroprusside, Am. J. Cardiol. **9:**51, 1962.

Severinghaus, J. W., and Cullen, S. C.: Depression of myocardium and body oxygen consumption with Fluothane, Anesthesiology **19:**165, 1958.

Sleath, G. W., and Archer, L. T.: Halothane for controlled hypotension in back surgery, Can. Anesth. Soc. J. **14:**407, 1967.

Stetson, J. B.: Intravenous nitroglycerine; a review, Int. Anesthesiol. Clin. **16:**261, 1978.

Stiles, C. M.: Personal communication, 1976.

Styles, M., Coleman, A. J., and Leary, W. P.: Some hemodynamic effects of sodium nitroprusside, Anesthesiology **38:**173, 1973.

Szyfelbein, S. K., and Ryan, J. F.: Use of controlled hypotension for primary surgical excision in an extensively burned child, Anesthesiology **41:**501, 1974.

Taylor, T. H., Styles, M., and Lamming, A. J.: Sodium nitroprusside as a hypotensive agent in general anaesthesia, Br. J. Anaesth. **42:**859, 1970.

Tinker, J. H., and Michenfelder, J. D.: Pharmacology, toxicology and therapeutics, review article, Anesthesiology **45:**340, 1976.

Vesey, C. J., Cole, P. V., Linnel, J. C., and others: Some metabolic effects of sodium nitroprusside in man, Br. Med. J. **2:**140, 1974.

Viguera, M. C., and Terry, R. N.: Induced hypotension for extensive surgery in an infant, Anesthesiology **27:**701, 1966.

Viljoen, J. F.: Anaesthesia for internal mammary implant surgery, Anaesthesia **23:**515, 1968.

Wildsmith, J. A. W., Marshall, R. L., Jenkinson, J. L., and others: Haemodynamic effects of sodium nitroprusside during nitrous oxide–halothane anaesthesia, Br. J. Anaesth. **45:**71, 1973.

Wilson, J.: Leber's hereditary optic atrophy; a possible defect of cyanide metabolism, Clin. Sci. **29:**505, 1965.

PART TWO

CLINICAL MANAGEMENT OF SPECIFIC ANESTHETIC PROBLEMS

Anesthesia for infants under one year of age

If the essence of a substance has been defined as the "crucial element," it is entirely fitting that the management of the newborn infant should be called the "essence" of pediatric anesthesia. Certainly, the fundamental reason for the existence of pediatric anesthesia as a separate discipline lies in the strikingly different problems encountered in this age group.

Many anesthesiologists primarily skilled in adult technics find the normal 6-year-old child something of a challenge and a 3-year-old definitely out of their field. While the differences found at these age levels are appreciable and the hesitation well-founded, the differences are of a relative degree and somewhat predictable. In approaching even a normal neonate, however, one steps into an entirely new situation. Whether one is dealing with a 5-pound neonate with a myelomeningocele, a 2-week-old infant with choanal atresia, or simply a 3-pound premature infant in need of a circumcision, the problems encountered in this age group are so foreign, not only in relation to size but in altered physiologic patterns, unusual lesions, and varied pharmacologic responses, that it is impossible to predict or to imagine how they will react until one actually finds out by firsthand experience.

Anesthesiologists entering this field should familiarize themselves with the general features of the situation and know something of the development of infant anesthesia, the surgical problems, the risks involved, and the many individual physiologic peculiarities of infants before undertaking their management.

If the management of infants is the essence of pediatric anesthesia, it should follow that progress in pediatric anesthesia is measured by progress in the care of infants. In 1912 the statement was made that "any pediatric operation lasting more than 15 minutes is destined to failure." The progress that has occurred since then started rather gradually. Ramstedt devised his pyloromyotomy in 1912, but at that time and for many years thereafter, surgeons preferred to use local anesthesia for this and other considerably more complicated abdominal procedures. It was not until 20 years later that the tempo began to speed up. In the United States, early attempts at major surgery in infants were made using cyclopropane by mask with to-and-fro technic, and in Britain, Ayre (1937) developed the T-tube rebreathing system, used with endotracheal intubation and ether for neurosurgical and harelip operations.

The next two decades were spent searching for agents, technics, equipment, monitoring methods, intravenous support, and antibiotics until, approaching 1970, it became possible for reasonably skilled anesthesiologists to take a 2500-gram neonate through a 3- or 4-hour operation with some assurance, using any one of a number of agents and technics. Surgical mortality was known to be highest in the neonate, but death became a rarity in the operating room and occurred chiefly in the postoperative period because of respiratory complications, errors in hydration, intestinal obstruction, and infection.

During the last decade we have seen a tremendous convergence of clinical and scientific interest in the newborn, particularly the high-risk newborn, attended in intensive care facilities by teams of dedicated neonatologists backed by cardiologists, respiratory physiologists, hematologists, nephrologists, and geneticists.

Surgeons and anesthesiologists, who were the prime factors in overcoming the problems of tracheoesophageal fistula and omphalocele, are apt to be pushed aside until the infant has been examined by the neonatologist, catheterized by the cardiologist, and processed by computerized hematology. Any surgeon or anesthesiologist who expects to participate in more than purely technical aspects of the care of these infants must keep informed on the rapidly evolving concepts and skills of the new and more specialized fields.

As anesthetic risks, infants are assumed to be weak and to bear high operative mortality, but the variety and magnitude of operations that they can tolerate are impressive. Although infant surgery was once limited to emergency procedures and those necessary to correct life-threatening lesions, these restrictions now apply chiefly to premature babies, those of 1000 grams representing our new frontier. For other infants, the field has widened greatly. Certainly the most remarkable procedure to date is the repair of congenital heart lesions under induced arrest of ventilation and circulation, with the most brazen disrespect for physiologic barriers ever demonstrated in human surgery.

DUAL RESPONSIBILITY OF THE ANESTHESIOLOGIST IN NEONATAL SURGERY

An anesthesiologist lives by the skill with which he can match the permissible extent of surgery with his ability to ensure the patient's total recovery. He bears a dual responsibility in facilitating the work of the surgeon while supporting the life of the patient. This is especially evident in dealing with infants.

Responsibility to the surgeon

The surgeon presents the anesthesiologist with two major requests: he wishes to perform a particular operation and he requests suitable operating conditions.

Surgeons who operate on children today expect to invade any part of the body, and few expect to make any compromise to reduce either time or trauma. To illustrate the numerous anesthetic and surgical problems encountered in infant surgery, a tabulation is shown listing 1000 operations performed at The Children's Hospital Medical Center on infants under 1 year of age (Table 15-1).

The *surgeon's requirements for suitable operating conditions may be stated as follows:* (1) adequate exposure of the operative site, (2) an immobile subject with adequate relaxation, (3) sufficient time to operate properly, and (4) survival of the child, with minimal side effects. In addition, the surgeon may make other requests, such as having the infant returned to the mother without upsetting the breast-feeding routine.

Responsibility to the infant

To serve the infant properly, the anesthesiologist must administer sufficient anesthesia to enable him to tolerate incision and disturbing reflex stimulation. Most of the anesthesiologist's efforts, however, will be devoted to supporting the infant. The outstanding features are protective:

1. Prevention of pain and harmful reflexes
2. Prevention of cooling and acidosis

Table 15-1. Operations performed on 1000 infants under 1 year old at The Children's Hospital Medical Center, January 1978 to March 1979

Thoracic and cardiovascular lesions

Mediastinal abscess	1
Lobar emphysema, lobectomy	3
Vascular ring	3
Patent ductus arteriosus	36
Coarctation of aorta	2
Aortic stenosis	1
Pulmonic stenosis	2
Atrial septal defect	7
Ventricular septal defect (uncomplicated)	25
Tetralogy of Fallot (shunts)	9
Tetralogy of Fallot (total repair)	25
Endocardial cushion defect	4
Single ventricle	3
Transposition of great arteries (TGA)	12
TGA with other lesions	4
Total anomalous pulmonary venous return (TAPVR)	2
Hypoplastic left heart	6
Truncus arteriosus	2
Ebstein's anomaly	1
Ectopia cordis	1
Double outlet right or left ventricle	2
Complex combined intracardiac defects	33
	184

General surgical lesions and procedures

Hernia, hydrocele, undescended testes	138
Pyloric stenosis	33
Duodenal atresia	3
Meconium ileus	1
Malrotation of intestine	2
Ruptured esophagus	2
Gastric perforation	2
Ruptured spleen and liver	1
Biliary atresia	4
Meckel's diverticulum	1
Omphalomesenteric duct	2
Enterocolitis	6
Hirschsprung's disease (pull through)	2
Appendicitis	1
Imperforate anus	3
Miscellaneous forms of intestinal obstruction	22
Adrenal tumor	1
Pancreatectomy	1
Neuroblastoma	4
Wilms' tumor	1
Sacrococcygeal teratoma	2
Exstrophy of bladder	1
Nissen diaphragmatic plication	4
Diaphragmatic hernia	5
Eventration of diaphragm	4
Tracheoesophageal fistula, esophageal atresia	4
Simple esophageal atresia	1
Omphalocele	4
Gastroschisis	4
Miscellaneous colostomies, closures, esophageal dilatations, rectal biopsies, and secondary closures of omphalocele	32
Miscellaneous operations on body surface	42
	333

Plastic surgical procedures

Cleft lip repair	29
Cleft palate repair	5
Skin grafts to burns and scars	9
Plastic to webbed fingers	1
Repair of lacerated tongue	1
Macrostomia repair	1
Craniofacial repair, Crouzon's syndrome	1
Miscellaneous outpatient procedures	19
	67

Genitourinary procedures

Hypospadias repair	4
Nephrectomy	1
Pyeloplasty	1
Excision of testicular tumor	1
Excision of renal tumor	1
Repair of ureteropelvic obstruction	4
Repair of posterior urethral valve	1
Ureteral taper	1
Repair of torsion of testis, megaureter, penile web, ureterocele, reflux, urinary anomaly (1 each)	7
Circumcision, meatal dilatation	28
Cystoscopy	3
Cystogram and cystoscopy	5
Kidney biopsy	1
	58

Neurosurgical lesions and procedures

Craniosynostosis repair	14
Ventriculoperitoneal shunts and shunt revisions	55
Excision of meningocele	6
Excision of lipomeningocele	5
Excision of encephalocele	1
Excision of myelomeningocele	24
Removal of cervical tumor	1
Excision of tumor of scalp	1
Excision of frontal cyst	1
Repair of facial nerve	1
Drainage of brain abscess	1
Control of subdural hemorrhage	1
Repair of depressed skull fracture	3
Correction of AV malformation	2
Cerebellar ataxia—pneumoencephalogram	1
Excision of lumbosacral sinus	1
Excision of occipital sinus	1
	120

Orthopedic lesions and procedures

Reduction of congenital dislocated hip and cast changes	60
Club foot corrections and casts	19
Excision of accessory digit	4
Osteotomy	3
Spinal fusion	3
Change spica casts under anesthesia	6
Adductor release	8
Muscle biopsy	7
Repair of trigger thumb	2
Drainage of septic hip	2
	114

Continued.

Table 15-1. Operations performed on 1000 infants under 1 year old at The Children's Hospital Medical Center, January 1978 to March 1979—cont'd

Otolaryngologic lesions and procedures		Ophthalmic lesions and procedures	
Laryngoscopy, bronchoscopy	33	Excision of orbital tumor	1
Tonsillectomy	1	Cataract extraction	3
Excision of cyst of mouth	1	Goniotomy	2
Excision of nasopharyngeal tumor	4	Resection and recession	1
Excision of oronasal fistula	1	Eye examinations under anesthesia	4
Drainage of retropharyngeal abscess	2	Repair of laceration of globe	1
Laser excision of subglottic hemangioma	2	Excision of cyst of lid	1
Removal of foreign body from trachea	2	Repair of laceration of lid	1
Removal of foreign body from pharynx	1	Excision of chalazion	1
Removal of foreign body from esophagus	2	Lacrimal duct probing	15
Tracheostomy	1		30
Myringotomy and placement of tubes	38		
Repair of choanal atresia	4	**Dental surgery**	
	92	Excision of ranula	2

3. Prevention of injury to eyes and lungs by high concentration of oxygen
4. Prevention of distension of gas-filled spaces with nitrous oxide
5. Prevention of overhydration
6. Prevention of excess handling and contamination

SPECIAL CHARACTERISTICS OF THE NEONATE

Many of the features of the neonate are described in Chapter 2 in a discussion of individual systems. It seems reasonable to group them all together at this time and consider the neonate as a single entity.

Outstanding factors frequently mentioned as complicating the infant's operative course are the increased incidence of hypothermia, hypoxia, atelectasis, metabolic acidosis, hypoglycemia, and retrolental fibroplasia, most of these being augmented by the presence of prematurity. There are several other features of the neonate's constitution that threaten his existence (see list opposite). To discuss them in detail is impractical, but it is important to point them out and suggest that they be investigated by any anesthesiologist who expects to care for neonates during and after major operations. Several deserve further emphasis. In addition to standard pediatric texts, *Care of the High-Risk Neonate* edited by Klaus and Fanaroff (1973) is recommended for information in this area.

CHARACTERISTICS OF NEWBORN AND PREMATURE INFANTS

Central nervous system

Bilirubin toxicity*
Intraventricular hemorrhage*
Seizures
Depression of respiratory center (apnea)*

Cardiorespiratory

Shunting
Cardiac failure
Atelectasis
Hypoxia
Respiratory distress syndrome*

Hematologic

Anemia of the newborn
Anemia of prematurity*
Left shift of dissociation curve
Reduced functional residual capacity
Reduced pulmonary compliance

Hepatorenal

Decreased metabolism of drugs and bilirubin
Decreased glomerular filtration, concentrating power, and excretion of large molecules

Ocular

Susceptibility to retrolental fibroplasia*

Metabolic

Increased tendency toward:
  Metabolic acidosis*
  Hypothermia
  Hypoglycemia
  Hypocalcemia

Increased incidence of generalized infection

High incidence of multiple congenital anomalies*

*Items of particular concern in premature infants.

The neonate's *cardiovascular system*, especially when overloaded with blood drained from the placenta, is often on the verge of congestive failure (Nadas and Fyler, 1972). The presence of congenital lesions, such as ventricular septal defect or coarctation of the aorta, augment this effect, and prematurity hastens its onset (Liebman and Whitman, 1973). The strain of hypoxia and/or asphyxia further weakens the heart, intracardiac left-to-right shunting increases, and unpredictable and often disadvantageous changes may occur in the patency and direction of flow of the ductus arteriosus (Rudolph, 1973). Relatively hypotensive at birth, infants exposed to stress easily develop shock unless treated promptly.

Disorders of the *respiratory system*, including airway and intrapulmonary problems, and early hemodynamic alterations present the greatest difficulties in the neonate. Narrow airways, small alveoli, decreased surfactant, and zero transpulmonary pressure at functional residual capacity (FRC) combine to make atelectasis one of the most common complications of the early recovery period.

The normal degree of shunting, calculated to be approximately 20% of cardiac output at birth, may be 40% or 50% in the presence of major cardiac defects or respiratory distress syndrome.

The limited function of the *kidney*, as previously described, reduces the infant's ability to excrete large water loads and drugs such as penicillin that are composed of large molecules. Immature renal function and enzymatic functions play a large part in the prolonged depression that may follow heavy sedation of the mother during labor. Fortunately, renal function appears less severely affected by prematurity than other organ systems.

The infant's inability to maintain his *body temperature* has been generally recognized, but the full effect of cold on the infant's body mechanisms has not been determined. Neonates are now intentionally cooled to 20° C for cardiac operations and recover nicely if properly handled, but when cooled unintentionally without suitable safeguards they show prolonged depression, metabolic acidosis, hypoglycemia, drug overdosage, and other physiologic derangements.

Full-term infants with a blood glucose level below 40 mg/dl and premature infants with a blood glucose level below 20 mg/dl are considered to be hypoglycemic. *Hypoglycemia* occurs more frequently in low birth weight infants. Two thirds of them are boys, and contributing factors may be a diabetic mother, reduced glycogen stores, hypothermia, anoxia, acidosis, and/or respiratory distress. Since severe hypoglycemia leads to brain damage, prompt recognition and correction are essential.

Hypocalcemia is less frequent but by no means a rarity and should be suspected in infants who have required resuscitation, especially following the use of bicarbonate or citrated blood. Since it is the ionized portion of calcium that is effective, one should not be misled by normal levels of total serum calcium. It should be noted that following intravenous administration of calcium gluconate with transfusion of citrated blood there is an immediate reduction of ionized calcium (Maisels and others, 1974) (Fig. 15-1).

Hyperbilirubinemia, whether due to increased destruction of red blood cells or to reduced ability of the liver to metabolize bilirubin, is another subtle danger, rendered more difficult to evaluate by the advent of light therapy, which reduces the superficial jaundice more readily than the bilirubin concentration of serum. Serum bilirubin levels over 12 to 14 mg/dl or persistence of jaundice after 10 days of age are considered abnormal for full-term neonates, while concentration of 6 mg/dl in premature infants is considered to be the safe upper limit (Odell and others, 1973).

Hematologic features of fetal blood are adapted to increase of uptake of oxygen by red cells. This is accomplished by increased concentration of 2,3-DPG and shift of the dissociation curve to the left. After birth, this becomes a disadvantage to the infant, who now needs improved delivery of oxygen to tissues. Iron content with moderate anemia

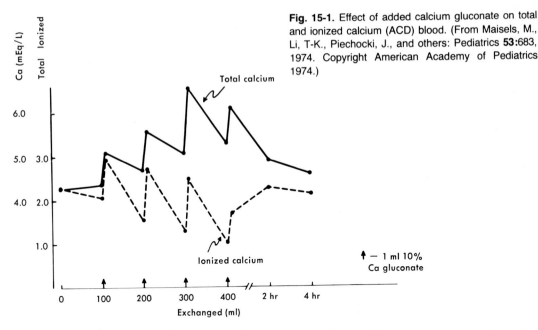

Fig. 15-1. Effect of added calcium gluconate on total and ionized calcium (ACD) blood. (From Maisels, M., Li, T-K., Piechocki, J., and others: Pediatrics **53**:683, 1974. Copyright American Academy of Pediatrics 1974.)

Table 15-2. The changing etiology of neonatal septicemia

	1927-1957	1953-1968
Number of cases	170	240
β-hemolytic streptococcus	28.2%	6.6%
Staphylococcus	15.8%	11.3%
Enterococcus	—	7.4%
E. coli	34.0%	33.3%
Klebsiella, Aerobacter	<1%	17.9%
Pseudomonas	7.6%	9.2%
Proteus	—	2.0%
Mixed	3.5%	1.6%
Other	9.4%	10.8%

From Fanaroff, A. A., and Klaus, M. H.: Neonatal infections. In Klaus, M. H., and Fanaroff, A. A., editors: Care of the high-risk neonate, Philadelphia, 1973, W. B. Saunders Co.

of infancy often is more critically reduced in premature infants, occasionally to 6 or 7 g/dl (Stockman and others, 1977).

While the foregoing complications are primarily due to inborn neonatal frailties, several serious hazards are largely of iatrogenic origin.

Contamination and *cross-infection* are major threats to all hospitalized infants and are a greater danger in smaller infants. The type of the principal offending organisms undergoes continual change; presently gram-

negative organisms are more difficult to control than gram-positive.

Infants are more susceptible to infection of all types, including bacterial, fungal, viral, and parasitic, and have especially low resistance to organisms that thrive in moist environments, such as *Monilia* and *Pseudomonas*, the latter being one of the more familiar inhabitants of ventilating devices. Table 15-2 shows the incidence of the changing prevalence and nature of neonatal organisms as summarized by Fanaroff and Klaus (1973). Anesthesiologists should observe at least those rules of cleanliness that would be required in a newborn nursery.

Retrolental fibroplasia and oxygen toxicity

The use of oxygen becomes a matter of greater concern, for it must be administered in strictly individualized concentrations. While the extremely hypoxic infant may require administration of 100% oxygen, the danger of retrolental fibroplasia (RLF) must be considered in any neonate receiving over 20% oxygen. Vascularization of the retina is usually complete at birth, and fully developed infants should not be subject to RLF (Patz, 1969). Premature infants, however, may require protection until 3 months after birth. For these patients, it was formerly believed that administration of oxygen at concentrations under 60% was safe. It has been found more recently that less severe forms of RLF may occur after brief exposure to 40% oxygen (Aranda and others, 1971), and even infants with cyanotic heart disease may develop RLF. Arterial oxygen tension of 100 mm Hg is presently believed to be the upper limit of safety until infants are mature. With these factors in mind, it seems reasonable to avoid use of more than 50% oxygen in normal neonates under 2 weeks of age and in premature infants until 3 months of age if they are judged to have normal lung function and oxygenation. During anesthesia equal amounts of nitrous oxide and oxygen are used unless there is evidence of hypoxia or reduced oxygen uptake.

The direct effect of high concentration of oxygen on the lung over a prolonged period can cause irreversible irritation of alveolar tissue. However, the most common result of high concentration of oxygen during infant anesthesia is postoperative atelectasis, often consisting of total collapse of one lung. To prevent atelectasis, it is advisable to add air to the inspired mixture prior to the completion of any infant anesthesia.

Nitrous oxide becomes undesirable in lesions involving potential distension of the gut, as in diaphragmatic hernia, intestinal obstruction, or omphalocele (Eger, 1974). In preparation for these situations it is advisable to have E tanks containing air mounted on anesthesia machines used for neonates. In our institution we have replaced cyclopropane hangers and mounts with those for air.

Overhydration

The admonition to avoid *overhydration* is quite serious in view of the increasing belief that infants can tolerate larger water loads than previously believed possible. Until there is a better understanding of infant fluid metabolism and more agreement on therapy, one should not adopt any single rule of quantity allowance. The essential point to bear in mind is that the amount needed by neonates varies greatly in relation to their lesions. The

fluid allowance for a normal neonate should be reduced for infants with cardiac failure or intracranial lesions but increased for those with intestinal obstruction and doubled or tripled for those with gastroschisis or necrotizing enterocolitis (see Chapter 25).

Infant's response to surgery and anesthesia

In Chapter 2 and elsewhere, numerous references are made to the altered functions and responses of the infant that may have bearing on the anesthetic management. For the sake of convenience, it seems reasonable to review the more important features.

Although it seems improbable that a neonate senses pain in the same manner as older individuals, the marked responses often observed are indications for the use of some form of analgesia for all potentially painful procedures (Smith and Smith, 1972).

In spite of the *reduced observable reaction to operative stimuli in infants*, they require higher concentrations of anesthetic agents to attain surgical planes of anesthesia. MAC for all agents studied is highest in infants and declines throughout life (p. 10).

The *response to stress in young infants* is characterized more by release of norepinephrine than epinephrine (as in adults), while in minor stress, as of simple operations, the increase in plasma free fatty acids shows more consistent response than that of either catecholamine (Talbert and others, 1967).

Lactate and pyruvate concentrations, as studied in infants by Yamazaki and associates (1975), showed similar responses to halothane and ether anesthesia as seen in adults, halothane causing no elevation and ether showing significant rise after 60 minutes followed by plateau effect.

Altered response to pharmacologic agents is most to be expected in the first few months of life and is largely due to immature hepatorenal systems, immature enzyme activity, and relative fluid overload.

Premature infants

In the foregoing material many generalizations are made in reference to premature infants. In view of the growing concern over these patients, more specific consideration seems in order.

The term "premature" suggests something quite different from "full term." Actually, of course, there is little difference between an infant weighing 2500 grams and one weighing 2400, for gradients develop gradually. With greater deficits of age or weight, the handicaps become more obvious, those under 1200 grams having shown extremely low survival rates.

For statistical purposes, some line of demarcation is necessary in management of small infants. Prior to 1961, the term "premature" was used to designate any live infant weighing 2500 grams or less at birth (Gross and other surgeons often used the more convenient limit of 5 pounds). In 1961, however, the World Health Organization and the American Academy of Pediatrics adopted the term "low birth weight baby" for those infants and designated as "premature" only those live infants who had been born less than 37 weeks after the beginning of gestation. The continued reference to weight as the determining factor is understandable but confusing.

In spite of the attention centered on these small infants, there has been relatively little documentation of actual anesthetic or surgical management. Gross's series of 159 operations on premature infants prior to 1959, with 54% survival, stands up well against later work, and his record was made without present methods of postoperative respiratory care or intravenous alimentation.

In 1965 Fonkalsrud and associates reported 48.6% survival in 175 premature infants operated on between 1950 and 1965, comparing this with 83.3% survival on 245 full-term neonates.

During 1975 and 1976, out of 25 premature infants operated on at our hospital, there was a 52% survival rate.

While the failure to meet Gross's record is difficult to explain, several minor points may have had some effect: (1) generalized sepsis has been a prominent feature in all reports, and the changing flora of hospital in-fections could account for the persistence of this problem; (2) prior to 1960 infants with diaphragmatic hernia were usually those who had survived several days and were more viable than those now brought to operation during the first day of life; (3) the increasing incidence of necrotizing enterocolitis, one of the most lethal of all neonatal problems, adds to the recent mortality; and (4) one can also assume that whatever the current type of operation, the teaching hospital will be the recipient of the more complicated cases that will bear the highest mortality.

In our series of 25 cases, it is interesting to note that the smallest infants (under 1500 grams, 5 out of 7 survived) fared considerably better than the larger ones (8 out of 18 survived).

Special management considerations. As previously noted and as shown in the list of characteristics on p. 288, any alteration in response typical of the full-term newborn will be increasingly evident in the premature infant. Several factors are of particular importance to the anesthesiologist. The central nervous system is subject to seizure activity and is probably the origin of the apneic spells that endanger smaller infants. As noted by Klaus and Fanaroff (1973), increasing frequency and duration of these spells is an ominous sign. Intracranial hemorrhage occurs without specific cause in many premature infants, but the incidence increases sharply with hypoxia or other types of stress.

The more rapid development in these infants of hypothermia, hypoxia, and metabolic acidosis, as well as hypoglycemia and hypocalcemia, is well recognized.

The absence of surfactant in small premature infants, in addition to their narrow airways, sets the stage for atelectasis, one of the most common postoperative complications of the neonate. Among the many hazards of prematurity, the worst probably include infection, respiratory distress syndrome, the combined incidence of multiple congenital anomalies, and the iatrogenic complications of oxygen toxicity and retrolental fibroplasia.

In spite of the infant's altered response to pain, there is general agreement that all infants should be rendered analgesic during surgical procedures. Surgeons who attempt gastrostomy or establishment of alimentation lines on struggling infants should realize that such stress may induce intracranial hemorrhage, hypoxia, and metabolic acidosis. During general anesthesia blood pressure is apt to be between 50 and 60 mm Hg, and clinical signs are difficult to follow. Airway obstruction is particularly troublesome during all phases of induction, maintenance, and recovery because of small airways, poor respiratory control, active laryngotracheal responses, and flexibility of the thoracic cage. Moment-to-moment attention is mandatory for several hours after recovery from anesthesia.

Persistence of increased risk. Although respiratory distress syndrome seldom appears after the first few weeks of life, the danger of retrolental fibroplasia may persist until 2 or 3 months of age. It has been apparent in their clinical management that infants born prematurely continue to show abnormal response to anesthesia for as much as 6 months after birth. For this reason we designate any premature infant as at increased risk until he is 6 months of age and shows reasonable progress in growth and development. Evidence of abnormal anesthetic response has consisted of hypotension, abnormal respiratory control, and delayed recovery from anesthesia. Steward (1977) has delineated these observations more accurately and reports that premature infants show reduced FRC for at least 1 month and reduced compliance for as much as 6 months after birth.

The "physiologic anemia" of the newborn seen in normal neonates also occurs in premature infants, but with much greater speed and to a greater extent. At birth, the hematocrit may be high, but infants operated on for herniorrhaphy at 1 month usually show levels between 25% and 30% and occasionally much lower. This "anemia of prematurity," like that of the newborn, has not been adequately explained, nor has it been shown what, if any, harm it conveys to the patient. As stated by Stockman and associates (1977), it is difficult to determine whether the fall in hemoglobin is "physiologic" and at what point the infant is in fact "anemic." Anesthesiologists, faced with this situation and the existing information, must plan management on the basis of each situation. Oski (1973) has stated that anemia is not clinically evident until hemoglobin falls to 5 or 6 g/dl. We believe that a hematocrit of 25% is acceptable if other circumstances are favorable.

PREOPERATIVE MANAGEMENT
Transportation and preliminary care

As soon as the need for operation is suspected in a neonate, a decision must be made as to where the procedure should be performed. With increasing centralization of definitive neonatal care facilities and modernization of transportation, performance of unusual pediatric operations by unqualified teams is usually avoidable. The anesthesiologist at the primary-care hospital should have a voice in the decision on moving the infant in relation to the following considerations:

1. The adequacy of anesthetic, surgical, and postoperative facilities at the primary hospital (of the three, the last is most often lacking)
2. The availability of better care facilities and transportation
3. The ability of the infant to survive transportation
4. The eventual salvageability of the infant

Transportation of poor-risk neonates has undergone great improvement (Segal, 1972). Ambulances have been replaced by vans for short distances (Morse, 1973) and by helicopters and fixed-wing planes for long-distance service (Hackel, 1975). These are now constructed to provide room for incubator, two attendants, and equipment, with suitable lighting and control of temperature, noise, and excess motion. The equipment should approximate that of a small intensive care unit and include the items shown in the list on p. 294. The transport incubator, as emphasized by Hackel (1975), should meet special requirements for visibility and supportive treatment (see design criteria on p. 294). It should allow not only clear view of the infant within but also should provide enough warmth to allow the child to be unhampered by heavy wrapping. As noted by Rickham (1970), it is usually advisable to transport infants lying on their sides.

Personnel responsible for care of infants during transportation obviously must be trained in the particular skills required for such mobile emergency service, preferably physicians with experience in neonatal care, resuscitation, and airway maintenance.

EQUIPMENT FOR INFANT TRANSPORT VEHICLE

Effective suction apparatus with at least 20 each of sizes 6, 8, and 10 French vented suction catheters, sterile

Oxygen source

Resuscitation equipment: airways, laryngoscope, endotracheal tubes, bag-and-mask apparatus

Drugs for resuscitation

Apparatus for intravenous and intra-arterial catheterization, supportive fluids

Monitoring devices: stethoscope, blood pressure and temperature monitors, cardiac monitor and readout, alarm-controlled apnea monitor

Ventilator, equipped for CPAP technic

Equipment for thoracotomy

DESIGN CRITERIA FOR TRANSPORT INCUBATOR*

1. Ability to provide a neutral thermal environment
2. Easy access to the infant for intensive care, including assisted ventilation
3. Monitoring of heart rate, inspired oxygen, core and/or skin temperature, and blood pressure
4. A fail-safe humidified oxygen/air delivery system with a 3-hour capability
5. Adequate lighting of the unit under all conditions
6. Portable lightweight rechargeable power units for the heating, lighting, and monitoring systems with adequate power for 3 hours
7. Means of safely stabilizing the unit in the incubator to prevent injury during sudden changes in speed or altitude

Reception at hospital center, resuscitation, and evaluation

Infants may arrive at the major center in critical condition, some having required endotracheal intubation and resuscitation en route. An essential part of the management is to alert the receiving hospital of the in-

---

*From Hackel, A.: A medical transport system for the neonate, Anesthesiology **43:**258, 1975.

fant's transfer and condition so that suitable personnel and equipment may be standing by when the infant arrives.

On admission, necessary steps will first be taken to restore ventilation, circulation, and warmth. With the exception of infants having diaphragmatic hernia, who may be sent to x-ray and operating room, most infants are transferred to the newborn nursery for further evaluation and preoperative preparation. Special measures often indicated are determination of arterial oxygen tension, provision of accurately measured oxygen concentration, establishment of nasogastric sump suction and lines for intravenous feeding and arterial monitoring, and administration of vitamin K and definitive therapeutic agents, the correction of hypoglycemia being among the most important.

The anesthesiologist may be expected to take part in any supportive treatment during this period. For greater coverage of neonatal care, the material by Gregory (1975), Klaus and Fanaroff (1973), and Swyer (1969) offers excellent information.

For the sick neonate who is frequently found to be cold, hypoxic, and acidotic, the provision of warmth and oxygen is more easily accomplished than the correction of acidosis. Acid-base problems are discussed in detail in Chapter 25 but deserve brief mention here.

Correction of acidosis. The marked degree of metabolic (and respiratory) acidosis shown by smaller and weaker infants has been of concern to all and is a major determining factor in their recovery. Srouji (1967), Raphaely and Downes (1973), and others have emphasized the importance of this factor, urging that operation should be delayed until these values are brought back toward normal by prompt correction with sodium bicarbonate or tris(hydroxymethyl)aminomethane (THAM). The following formulas for correction of acidosis with sodium bicarbonate frequently have been advised:

When pH is between 7.3 and 7.1:

$$mEq\ NaHCO_3 = base\ deficit\ \times$$
$$kg\ body\ weight \times 0.3$$

When pH is less than 7.1:

$$\text{mEq NaHCO}_3 = \text{base deficit} \times \text{kg body weight} \times 0.6$$

The modification of the first formula, as noted by Dibbins and Kiesewetter (1969), is because in severe acidosis the volume requiring buffering is that of the total body water, represented by the figure 0.6, which is substituted for 0.3, which represents the extracellular space.

Unfortunately, there has been increasing evidence that sudden changes in serum pH, even in the proper direction, may cause hyperosmolality (Finberg, 1967) and lead to intracranial hemorrhage, a relatively frequent finding in neonates so treated. Simmons and associates (1974) have been so distressed by the incidence of intracranial hemorrhage that they have adopted the following regulations: "Bicarbonate is never given by rapid push and is always diluted with water at least 1:200 (600 mOsm per liter), and total sodium administration is restricted to less than 8 mEq per kilogram per day."

This concern, plus lack of evidence of discrete gain by rapid buffering, has influenced many to attempt to make initial correction of acidosis by improving ventilatory exchange, using buffering agents in a supplementary role, if at all. In their management of neonates with diaphragmatic hernia, illustrated by correction of severe base deficit by ventilation and operation alone, Rowe and Uribe (1971) have demonstrated remarkable success in definitive therapy without buffering (p. 321).

Before operation, the anesthesiologist should reevaluate any newborn with particular attention to the unique features of this group. They include weight, gestational age, birth history, Apgar score, temperature, ventilatory adequacy (with blood gases, if indicated), general activity and coordination, bilirubin, blood glucose, type of cry, and fluid intake and output.

Signs of increased risk include birth weight below 2500 grams or gestational age less than 37 weeks denoting prematurity, weak cry or abnormal neuromuscular activity suggesting central nervous system lesion, blood glucose level below 30 mg/dl, bilirubin level over 6 mg/dl in premature infants or over 12 to 14 mg/dl in full-term infants, arterial pH under 7.15, and Pa_{CO_2} over 65 mm Hg.

OPTIMAL TIME FOR OPERATION

Infants having such lesions as cleft lip, cystic hygroma, or a small meningocele require operation early in infancy, but the best time for the child to undergo the procedure is open to question. There is a tradition among surgeons that operative viability is greater in the first 3 days of life than at any time in the next 5 to 6 weeks (Clatworthy, 1970). Based largely on clinical impression, Lynn (1963) has even constructed a theoretical "vitality curve" to illustrate this concept.

When one considers the extensive adaptations that the neonate makes in respiratory, cardiac, and renal function in the first 10 days of life, it is hard to see why an infant should be thought to be a better risk immediately after birth. Woolley (1972) sagely comments that an infant either does or does not need surgery during the first 6 weeks of life, and it should not be pushed into the first 3 days at risk of inadequate preparation nor delayed to 6 weeks for fear of poor patient response. Our own experience in operations performed in the fourth week for hernia, harelip, and pyloromyotomy (no deaths in 7000 cases) sheds some doubt on Lynn's curve, which bottoms out at 4 weeks.

Preparation of anesthetic facilities and equipment

In a planned approach for neonatal surgery, *warming the operative suite* is often the first step to be taken. Although some surgeons resist such attempts, Roe and associates (1966) stress its importance, and Martin (1975) stated that room temperature should be 80° F (26° C) during procedures on infants. Our aim is to have the room temperature at about 75° F, depending on supplemental measures for assistance. As described previously, these include wrapping the infant's limbs in sheet wadding, covering the head with a stockinette cap, using a circulating water mattress or infrared lamp, humidifying anesthetic gases, and avoiding deep relaxation (Smith, 1969; Goudsouzian and others, 1973; Farman, 1962).

Regardless of whether the infant is expected to need general or only local anesthesia, *apparatus for general anesthesia, intubation, and resuscitation* is prepared for all infants about to undergo general surgery. One may choose between circle or nonrebreathing technics (see Chapter 6), but infants should no longer be expected to breathe against valves spontaneously without assistance. Humidification of nonrebreathing apparatus is recommended here, more for prevention of heat loss than for prevention of tracheal drying.

It is always of primary importance to *prepare effective suction apparatus and to provide suction catheters small enough to pass through chosen endotracheal tubes.* Masks, airways, stethoscopes, and other equipment for infant anesthesia are described in Chapter 6.

Many anesthesiologists fail to realize the *danger of contamination* when dealing with small infants. Neonates have reduced resistance to most of the common infectious organisms. Greater use of penicillin in mothers has reduced the incidence of streptococcal infections in infants but has increased that of staphylococcal and gram-negative infections (Fanaroff and Klaus, 1973). Stethoscopes, blood pressure cuffs, and other equipment that is usually believed to be innocuous must be considered to be possible sources of contagion unless suitably cleaned or covered. Objects touching an infant should be clean and, where possible, should be sterile, especially those entering the infant's mouth (this rules out the use of one's fingers as a pacifier or to pry open a child's mouth in the process of tracheal intubation).

As the last step before the anesthesiologist takes charge of the neonate, it should be a standard procedure for him to scrub his hands thoroughly.

Neonates are usually brought into the operating room in the enclosed, warmed bassinettes in which they were transported from the nursing division and are not removed until the surgeons are present and ready to operate. Before the infant is removed from the bassinette, blood pressure apparatus and stethoscope are applied and arms and legs are wrapped in sterile sheet wadding to prevent loss of body heat. Most neonates will come to the operating room with a nasogastric tube in place. It is checked for placement and patency and *left open to drain.*

Operating lights and infrared lamp serve to warm the area where the infant is to be placed on the operating table. During preparation of the wound area, the lights are kept focussed on the child but away from his eyes. He is covered as much as possible, and exposure is limited to the areas that are being worked on.

The choice of anesthesia will depend partly on the child's size and partly on the intended operation. The choice usually is between local infiltration, nitrous oxide and halothane, and nitrous oxide–relaxant combinations.

Local infiltration anesthesia was used frequently during the developmental stages of pediatric surgery and still offers definite advantages, especially for abdominal procedures in very small, weak premature infants, as described on p. 232. Using 0.5% procaine (Novocain) or 0.25% lidocaine (Xylocaine), one can inject 3 ml of either agent per kilogram body weight for local infiltration. Details concerning local anesthetic agents are described in Chapter 11. Actual limits of safety have been difficult to determine for small infants, and it is preferable to reduce administration where possible. Greater safety is also to be expected when agents are administered in divided doses and when they are injected into areas having reduced rate of uptake.

It is always necessary to fit the anesthetic to the infant. Increasing the anesthetic to suit the developing premature infant and the neonate requires several gradations, as described in the discussion of anesthesia for intestinal obstruction below.

Among the general anesthetic agents that

have been used for neonates, ether required considerable skill, especially during induction, and was gladly abandoned in favor of cyclopropane, which offered less irritation and more rapid control, with the additional advantage of maintaining peripheral circulation more effectively. Halothane has succeeded both, providing even smoother induction than cyclopropane, but when used with infants it requires increased caution, for once induction has been accomplished there is greater danger of myocardial depression. Generous atropinization (0.1 to 0.2 mg) is advised for neonates to prevent early appearance of bradycardia and resultant reduced cardiac output. With this precaution, halothane should remain the inhalation agent of choice in infant anesthesia, since enflurane and isoflurane are more irritating and more depressing to respiration. Particular attention must be paid to heart rate and blood pressure when any fluorinated anesthetic is used.

Nitrous oxide is singularly ineffective in small infants and, though valuable for supplementary analgesia, is of little use for induction (see Chapter 7). For these infants it is most effective to start with a mix of 2-liter flows of oxygen and nitrous oxide and 1% halothane. Babies become quiet very soon and appear to be anesthetized on 1.0% or 1.5% halothane, but they often react smartly to incisions unless the concentration is increased to 2.0% or 2.5% for a short period. Subsequent halothane concentration, with assisted spontaneous ventilation, will probably be between 1.0% and 2.0% and should provide adequate analgesia and relaxation while the infant is at a level allowing him to maintain flexor tone in his arms.

Muscle relaxants may be used successfully for most procedures in the neonatal period but occasionally mandate the use of endotracheal intubation that would not otherwise be needed. Relaxants also cause great heat loss and involve problems of delayed return of full ventilation, especially in premature infants or those who have become hypothermic. The differing views on infant's responses to relaxants have been described (Chapter 13) and leave one with some uncertainty in regard to dose and duration, but when relaxants are administered with proper precautions they prove reliable and effective.

When used intravenously, succinylcholine in a dose of 2 mg/kg produces immediate relaxation and apnea, with some risk of bradycardia unless prevented by atropine. As described in Chapter 13, the intramuscular use of succinylcholine has the advantage of allowing one to choose a safe time to intubate before the onset of apnea and also avoids the hazard of bradycardia. Dosage of 1.5 mg/kg usually provides sufficient relaxation for easy intubation without ever producing apnea, although there is considerable variation in the infant's response.

d-Tubocurarine has been used extensively in England and America and will serve in many instances. The reputed sensitivity of neonates to d-tubocurarine has led some to reduce initial dosage to 0.25 mg/kg, but in our experience it has been more satisfactory to use 0.5 mg/kg as an intubating dose, given intramuscularly in one dose or intravenously in two doses separated by a 2-minute interval. The hypotensive effect often seen in the use of this agent has influenced us to use it less frequently for neonates. The change has mainly been in favor of metocurine.

Both gallamine and pancuronium should provide greater circulatory support than d-tubocurarine, but in our hands occasional unpredictable tachycardia has been troublesome. Because of added difficulties in reversal, gallamine appears to have fallen into general disuse. Administration of pancuronium in a dose of 0.1 to 0.15 mg/kg, as advised by Bennett and associates (1973), should be effective, but duration and reversal have appeared to be more variable than desired. As stated in Chapter 13, the practice of reversing all nondepolarizing relaxants is definitely recommended.

The possibility of using ketamine for infants undergoing operations of lesser magnitude, such as insertion of cannulae or unilateral herniorrhaphy, would seem reasonable were it not for the fact that ketamine may act as a marked respiratory depressant in small infants, causing repeated spells of apnea. This response has been noted in several instances and has been sufficient to discourage our use of it for infants expected to breathe spontaneously after operation. Other disadvantages related to ketamine are the continued motion and lack of relaxation, which make it unsatisfactory for many procedures, and the dangerous hypotensive response that may be evoked when ketamine is used for patients who have been receiving halothane (Bidwai and others, 1975).

However, ketamine proves highly valuable for induction of poor-risk infants, especially those having cardiac lesions involving right-to-left shunts, hypotension, or decreased pulmonary flow. Here ketamine gives much needed support during induction, and respiratory depression is prevented by routine postoperative ventilatory assistance.

Innovar has been used sparingly in small infants. Though recommended by Kay (1973), the prolonged depressant effect of droperidol (Inapsine) and the lack of easy controllability are not in its favor.

Endotracheal intubation of neonates should not be considered to be mandatory simply because of their age or size. However, since so many of them either are in critical condition or are undergoing one of the more hazardous operations, intubation will be indicated in the majority of cases.

The maintenance of anesthesia should consist of giving no more anesthetic than is necessary and concentrating on supportive features of ventilation, the proper amount of oxygenation, warmth, and sufficient (but not too much) fluid replacement.

It is extremely difficult to know what is happening to a 5-pound infant who is hidden under a mass of drapes with several surgeons obstructing the only area that is exposed. One must make the most of the few clinical signs that are available and use those monitors that can give significant information without adding greater risk.

The anesthesiologist usually can uncover enough of the infant's head to observe circulation and color and can estimate muscle tone

by exposing or feeling one of the infant's arms. In most of the operations performed on neonates under halothane it is possible and desirable to keep the infant in a light enough plane of anesthesia to maintain definite flexor tone in his biceps (see Fig. 9-3). The anesthesiologist must listen for both breath sounds *and* heart sounds at all times rather than rely on either one alone. For this purpose a binaural stethoscope is preferable. Blood pressure *is* a reliable sign, and a Doppler sensor may be used instead of intra-arterial cannulation. CVP measurement is seldom indicated during infant operation except for intracardiac procedures, but the ECG, while not of real value for monitoring arrhythmias during these operations, is indicated for infants whose heart sounds might become inaudible during unusual stress of blood loss or manipulation. Thus, while ECG would not be indicated during pyloromyotomy, it certainly would be during repair of diaphragmatic hernia.

When several monitors are being used, a second anesthesiologist should be available to watch and maintain them. Otherwise, increasing use of monitors results in decreasing attention to the patient.

Maintenance of body warmth and fluid replacement have been stressed repeatedly and are mentioned briefly here. In addition to the standard warming devices, the use of a stockinette cap is a help to babies with little hair, and humidification prevents heat and moisture loss from the respiratory tract. The maintenance of as much muscle tone as allowable during the procedure also helps to reduce heat loss. When halothane is used, the degree of relaxation can be controlled to meet the varying needs of the surgeon during operation, and the infant will not remain flaccid throughout the entire procedure.

The intravenous infusion often is the most difficult part of an operation and must be in secure working condition prior to the initial incision. The infusion should be placed in clear view and within easy reach of the anesthesiologist.

Toward the end of operation, the anesthesiologist promotes return of activity and spontaneous respiration by reducing the anesthetic and reversing the relaxants. To prevent atelectasis, one may intermittently disconnect the endotracheal tube or remove the mask and ventilate the infant with room air, using manual compression of the chest if the baby is still apneic.

Extubation of all neonates and other infants under 6 months old is not performed until they are warm, show effective cardiovascular function, are breathing actively, are moving all extremities, and actually *open their eyes*. Premature extubation of small infants frequently is followed by return of respiratory depression.

When the infant is to be supported by respiratory assistance, it is usually preferable to use a nasotracheal tube strapped securely to the face without pressure on the nostrils, its proper depth confirmed by immediate postoperative x-ray.

ANESTHETIC MANAGEMENT DURING OPERATIONS CHARACTERISTIC OF THE NEONATE AND SMALL INFANT

The general measures that have been outlined pertain to most small infants regardless of the operation they are undergoing. The following discussion concerns the particular areas of importance in several of the most characteristic and/or the most unique surgical conditions of infancy. It is assumed that readers will have glanced at the foregoing part of this chapter as well as parts dealing with infants in the chapters on physiology, induction, intubation, and maintenance. Rather than a repetition of such details here, chief emphasis is placed on special features of care relating to individual situations.

Intestinal obstruction

Many of the smallest infants requiring operation are those who have intestinal obstruction that may be due to annular pancreas, intestinal atresia or stenosis, duplication of intestine, meconium ileus, tumors, enterocolitis, or other lesions (Gross, 1953; Mustard and others, 1969; Potter and Craig, 1976).

The actual causes of the intestinal obstruction may differ considerably, but the problems of management are so similar that they can be described in one group. Unfortunately another feature of intestinal obstruction in infancy, regardless of its cause, is its tendency to recur, requiring one or often several reoperations, with the infant in ever-increasing distress.

Diagnosis of obstruction is made on the basis of vomiting, distension, absence of bowel sounds, and radiologic evidence of gas-filled loops of bowel. A single film of the infant's chest and abdomen is generally most helpful (Fig. 15-2).

Inability to retain food or fluid becomes dangerous more rapidly in younger patients, and if vomiting and toxicity are added, the progress of dehydration, metabolic acidosis, and inanition accelerates accordingly. There are also severe ventilatory complications, for the distended bowel forces the diaphragm into a high, fixed position, markedly reducing ventilation and offering increased risk of aspiration and subsequent atelectasis and pneumonia (Sunshine and Lewis, 1973).

Prompt surgical relief is imperative but should be preceded by thorough evaluation of the child's condition and initiation of corrective fluid and electrolyte therapy, as described in Chapter 25. Some relief of distension can be gained by passage of an effective nasogastric sump suction catheter (Replogle and Reyes, 1972).

Surgical repair of neonatal intestinal obstruction involves varied problems in opening of the abdomen, correction of the causative factor, and abdominal closure. Most infants will show some degree of distension; occasionally it will be extreme. When there is high duodenal obstruction, however, as in annular pancreas, the abdomen may be quite flat.

Repair of the obstructing lesion may require mere freeing of minor adhesions but is more apt to call for resection of a portion of duplicated intestine or a large segment of necrotic bowel and establishment of a colostomy. Peritoneal closure often is facilitated by operative relief of the distension, one no-

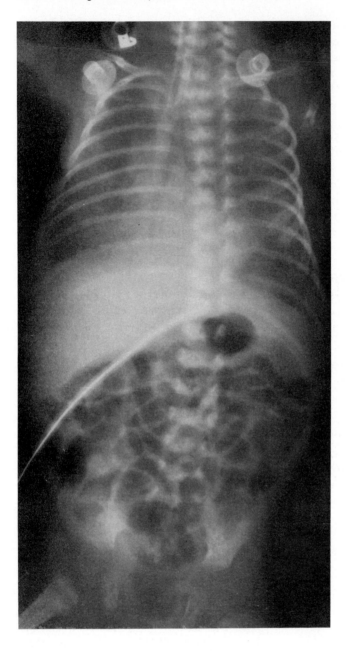

Fig. 15-2. Single film of an infant's chest and abdomen is an important element in preoperative evaluation.

table exception being the infant with meconium ileus, where the gluey meconium is seldom removable and peritoneal closure must be accomplished over a bulging intestine (Fig. 15-3). Another exception is the infant with necrotizing enterocolitis, who is too sick to tolerate bowel resection and a similar difficult closure will be necessary.

The operative time required for work of this nature may be less than an hour for the simpler procedures, but the resection and repair of several segments of bowel followed by colostomy may easily consume 4 or 5 hours.

The *anesthetic management* of small infants with intestinal obstruction is especially interesting. In order to suit the anesthetic to the needs of child and surgeon, one may

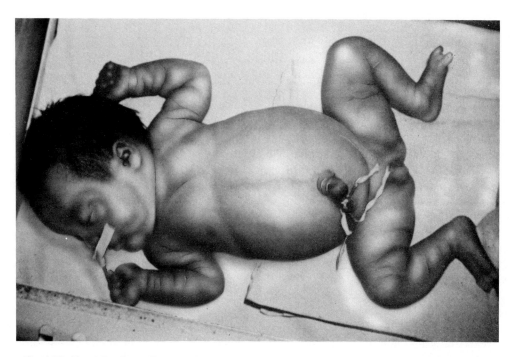

Fig. 15-3. Meconium ileus. Preoperative nasogastric suction and awake intubation are indicated. The distended abdomen will not be relieved by operation, and closure will require full relaxation.

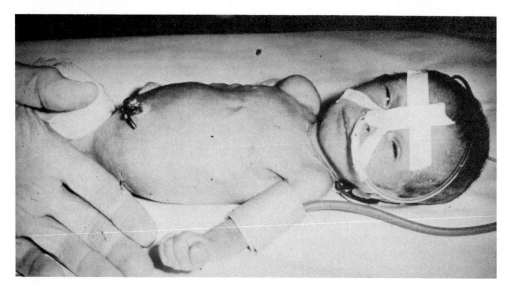

Fig. 15-4. A weak 2-lb baby with duodenal atresia. Abdomen is not distended, and local anesthesia may be sufficient.

require almost every combination of infant technic.

When the baby lies weak and uncomplaining, general anesthesia will probably not be necessary (Fig. 15-4). An infusion, if not already running, can be started under *local anesthesia* and the arms and legs restrained by sheet wadding and tape.

As described in Chapter 11 and the foregoing section of this chapter, local anesthesia consisting of 0.5% procaine, 2 or 3 ml/kg, can be injected along the site of incision and where the towel clips are to be placed. The anesthesiologist will monitor the infant continuously. Weaker babies will show little sign of disturbance and may profit by administration of oxygen, if hypoxic, or a mixture of nitrous oxide and oxygen for support and mild analgesia. Sucking on a rubber nipple is often enough to satisfy the little ones during operations under local anesthesia.

In slightly stronger babies this approach may be satisfactory until closure of the abdomen, when addition of halothane (1% to 2%) may be necessary. For such brief use, administration using a lightly fitting mask should be adequate.

Infants who are active, cry spontaneously, and resist being handled offer greater difficulty. The use of restraints and local anesthesia is the safest method if the operating team has not had previous experience with such undersized patients. If available, however, general endotracheal anesthesia affords the surgeon much better working conditions.

Although I believe that awake intubation of infants is seldom desirable, the presence of intestinal obstruction and distension in neonates does seem a just indication for its use. While very small infants are more difficult to intubate, their virtual immunity to postintubation tracheitis is reassuring. The technic of intubation is described in detail in Chapter 8.

Immediately after intubation, the anesthesia apparatus is attached and the chosen agents are administered. Our choice is usually between halothane–nitrous oxide and DTC or metocurine–nitrous oxide combinations for infants of this size. During operation, while the infant is partially eviscerated, the diaphragm moves easily, and light inhalation anesthesia is adequate.

One may reasonably wish to omit the supplemental use of nitrous oxide for fear of increasing preexisting distension. Another analgesic should then be added to supplement relaxants and possibly halothane as well, for the increased concentration of halothane that will be required may cause hypotension. Ketamine is a possible alternative, but the hazard of postoperative respiratory depression is a disadvantage. It would be preferable to reduce halothane to minimal analgesic concentration and provide the necessary relaxation with intravenous muscle relaxants. Whether using halothane or relaxants, if nitrous oxide is omitted one should replace it with air or helium to reduce the danger of oxygen toxicity in susceptible infants. If neither is available, the hazard of nitrous oxide distension certainly can be assumed to be less than that of RLF.

If halothane is used for maintenance, one should start with 0.5% concentration, increasing it to 1.0%, 1.5%, or 2.0% with assisted ventilation until the desired level is denoted by adequate abdominal relaxation balanced by effective cardiac activity (strong, regular heart sounds, heart rate of 120 to 190 per minute, and blood pressure of 60 to 80 mm Hg). Deep relaxation is not desirable, and infants should be maintained at a plane light enough to allow definite flexor tone in biceps muscles. It must not be assumed that these infants will maintain adequate spontaneous respiration. Spontaneous respiration is preferable to controlled respiration, but the anesthesiologist should expect to supply a minimum of assistance at all times in such a manner as to reduce or eliminate the work of inspiration and add resistance during expiration to provide positive end-expiratory pressure (PEEP) and prevent reduction of FRC. When relaxants are used, controlled respiration obviously will be required.

Monitoring of clinical signs is absolutely mandatory during such operations on infants. One must insist on hearing *both* the heart and breath sounds at all times, since it is easy to be misled by listening to heart or respiration alone. Blood pressure must also be followed closely, and hypotension (below 60 mm Hg) should serve as an indication for reduction of halothane, administration of additional fluids, or other measures. Under halothane and *d*-tubocurarine, most small infants have an increased tendency toward hypotension that will be augmented in the presence of hypovolemia. Administration of blood or colloid, 2 ml/kg, followed by response in blood pressure further suggests the presence of hypovolemia and the need for more replacement. Hypotension under halothane also may be due in part to vagal action that should be corrected by administration of atropine (0.1 or 0.2 mg by either intravenous or intramuscular route).

As the abdomen is opened, some relaxation is helpful but not imperative. After the bowel has been exteriorized, surgical relaxation is not needed, and the child can breathe without marked diaphragmatic resistance.

During intestinal repair, manipulation of the bowel will increase loss of tissue fluid, and added replacement will be needed in the form of albumin and balanced electrolyte solutions in proportion to the duration of operation and condition of the child. Serum protein and electrolyte levels are determined prior to operation and at intervals during operation in more critical situations. ECG may help to evaluate potassium and calcium balance (Drop and Laver, 1975).

Blood replacement may be required if the infant becomes hypotensive or if several anastomoses are necessary. In intestinal procedures where measurement of blood loss is difficult, the traditional rule of 10 ml of blood per pound of body weight (20 ml/kg) for a safe, effective replacement is often very nearly what is needed.

Intestinal obstruction has been one of the major causes of death in infant surgery, death usually coming 10 to 14 days after operation with increasing malnutrition and terminal pneumonia. This picture has been greatly improved since the development of parenteral alimentation by Dudrick and associates (1968), Filler and associates (1969), and others. Death now is limited primarily to infants who were diagnosed late and who required excision of more than 80% of small and large bowel.

With duodenal atresia and other forms of high intestinal obstruction, distension may not even be present before operation, and in most other varieties preoperative distension is relieved by surgery. With meconium ileus and necrotizing enterocolitis, however, the bowel often remains distended, and ab-

dominal closure can be facilitated by generous relaxation provided either by continued use of d-tubocurarine, or, when halothane is used, by supplemental doses of succinylcholine (0.5 mg/kg preceded by initial administration of atropine, 0.1 mg).

Among infants operated on for intestinal obstruction, those with high intestinal lesions may be among the smallest. Among the sickest will be infants with *necrotizing enterocolitis* and those who have suffered *intestinal perforation in utero* and whose entire bowel may be gangrenous at operation. Some of these return for repeated operations, in progressively worsening condition, supported for weeks by ventilators and parenteral alimentation. These infants require a minimum of anesthesia, with efforts being directed toward supportive care with abundant preoperative plasma, blood, and antibiotics.

At the end of all operations on small infants, as well as on all patients with intestinal obstruction, the nondepolarizing relaxants are reversed if they have been used, and the child is allowed to wake up, move his arms and legs, and *open his eyes* before the endotracheal tube is removed. If extubation is performed while children are depressed, cold, or still asleep, apnea may ensue. After extubation the child is covered, allowed to cry, and observed until his condition justifies his removal to recovery facilities.

Intestinal obstruction due to imperforate anus

Male infants with imperforate anus may require operation soon after birth for relief of obstruction. In female infants, the usual presence of a rectovaginal fistula in association with imperforate anus prevents development of distension, and the operation is usually postponed until several weeks later. Anesthetic requirements will vary depending on the degree of distension and whether the operation is a simple perineal anoplasty, a temporary colostomy, or an extensive abdominoperineal repair. Although most of the problems are predictable, it is worth repeating that significant loss of blood should be expected during any perineal operation. Furthermore, while blood loss may be minimal during performance of the original colostomy, *subsequent closure of the colostomy frequently demands blood replacement*, and the procedure should not be started until reliable infusion has been established and blood has been prepared for transfusion. This is one of the most difficult rules to impress upon inexperienced individuals. Convincing evidence was gained from a series reported by Davenport and Barr (1963) showing greater blood loss during colostomy closure than during repair of patent ductus arteriosus.

Omphalocele and gastroschisis

Omphalocele, as the name implies, is a herniation of the abdominal viscera into the base of the umbilical cord (Fig. 15-5). It is thought to occur once in 6000 to 10,000 live births and to be caused by the more rapid growth of the viscera than the peritoneal cavity during the sixth to tenth week of fetal life. The resultant defect is a striking globular enlargement of the umbilical cord, varying from approximately 2 to 20 cm in diameter. It contains representative portions of small and large bowel, spleen, stomach, and liver, held tightly enclosed in a thin-walled, avascular sac consisting of peritoneum and amniotic membrane. The defect in the abdominal wall often is as large as the omphalocele at its greatest dimension, but it may be considerably smaller, the viscera apparently being extruded through a narrow stalk into a portion of cord that stretches to the size of a grapefruit.

Infants born with free eviscerated bowel were formerly believed to have an omphalocele that had ruptured in utero. While this may occur, free eviscerated bowel in neonates more frequently represents an unrelated anomaly termed *gastroschisis* (Moore and Stokes, 1953). In gastroschisis the viscera are extruded, but without any covering membrane they fall loosely over the infant's abdomen. The defect in the abdominal wall through which the viscera pass lies beside the umbilical stalk, which, as seen in Fig. 15-6, remains uninvolved.

A large, intact omphalocele is impressive,

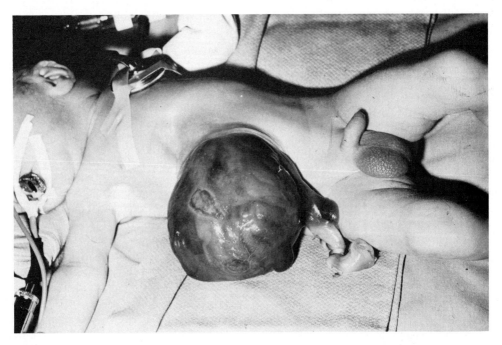

Fig. 15-5. Newborn with large omphalocele, sac intact. Umbilical cord is seen emerging from mass. The major problem will be replacing the viscera in the small abdominal cavity.

but gastroschisis usually creates more problems. Without the protective sac, more rapid loss of plasma and body heat can occur, and the unprotected gut is exposed to infection, formation of adhesions, and subsequent intestinal obstruction.

Surgical correction of both omphalocele and gastroschisis is directed toward placing the extended organs inside the peritoneal cavity and bringing the abdominal wall together over them. Since the infant's abdomen developed with the viscera outside, the usual space was not provided to contain them, and the rectus muscles remain contracted and firm.

While small gastroschisis defects rarely occur, the size of omphaloceles varies considerably. Small omphaloceles occasionally are seen that can be closed in anatomic layers with little difficulty. To close a large defect, whether an omphalocele or gastroschisis, the surgeon must force the organs into the unprepared abdomen with considerable pressure, pushing the diaphragm high into the chest and at the same time compressing the inferior vena cava, thus impeding the venous return from the legs. The resultant respiratory embarrassment and/or reduction of venous return can be lethal if the surgeon persists in his attempt to accomplish a complete closure of muscle, fascia, and skin.

The alternative formerly necessary in such cases was for the surgeon to stretch the skin over the protruding viscera to make a thin-walled sac and to attempt an anatomic closure months later (Gross, 1948). Unfortunately, such delayed repairs often involved greater difficulties.

These problems once constituted a challenge for anesthesiologist and surgeon equal to those of tracheoesophageal fistula and diaphragmatic hernia. Fortunately, the situation was greatly relieved by the development of the staged closure by Schuster in 1967. This consists of suturing a strip of plastic mesh (Dacron-reinforced Silastic sheeting) to the rectus muscle on each side of the abdomen and suturing them together to enclose the herniated viscera securely without restricting ventilation or circulation (Fig. 15-7).

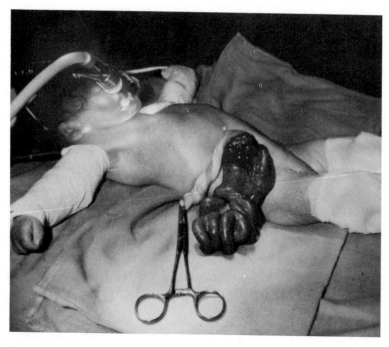

Fig. 15-6. Gastrochisis, sometimes called ruptured omphalocele, but umbilical cord is intact. Heat loss, rapid dehydration, and infection are added to problems of omphalocele.

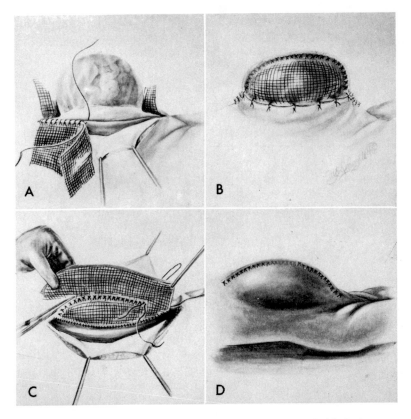

Fig. 15-7. Staged omphalocele repair. **A,** Suturing mesh to rectus muscle. **B,** Mesh closure completed. **C,** Rectus muscle has stretched, allowing reduction of size of mesh. **D,** First skin closure, to be followed by complete removal of mesh with normal abdominal contour. (From Schuster, S. S.: Surg. Gynecol. Obstet. **125:**837, 1967.)

The mesh sac thus formed stretches the rectus muscles enough to allow the surgeon to tighten the sac and reduce its size (without anesthesia) at 3- or 4-day intervals. Final closure of muscle layers and skin, requiring general anesthesia and considerable relaxation, can be made in 10 to 14 days. Use of this method has eliminated most of the problems of pressure and respiratory obstruction that threatened the infant, has increased the survival rate of infants with large omphaloceles, and has been especially valuable in the treatment of gastroschisis, from which recovery had been relatively uncommon (Bill, 1969).

Although the staged repair has been a major advance, recovery still may be prolonged and frequently is complicated by ileus, adhesions, and intestinal obstruction, for which additional operations may be necessary. Survival depends on nursing care and often on ventilatory support and intravenous hyperalimentation.

Recently a significant reduction in the use of the staged mesh closure has come with the finding that by forceful stretching of the rectus muscles during primary repair, the abdominal wall can be extended enough to allow complete layered closure of moderately sized lesions.

Special anesthetic considerations. Fortunately there is never delay in making the diagnosis of omphalocele. Preliminary care and transportation of these infants should be carried out promptly. These infants frequently require transferral to a suitably equipped hospital, but unless they are protected, they will become dangerously hypothermic and dehydrated. Although sclerema is seldom seen now, these infants were ideal candidates for this complication. The defect must be covered with sterile saline sponges and then with towels, plastic drapes, or silver foil to prevent heat loss. A nasogastric sump tube is inserted, and the child is transported in a warmed bassinette to the area where he will be prepared for operation.

A reliable intravenous infusion is essential in all of these procedures. Although excessive abdominal pressure is less frequently encountered when one is using modern methods of closure, it is still advisable to place the infusion in one of the upper extremities so that it cannot be obstructed by pressure on the inferior vena cava either during or after operation. As will be noted later, such an infusion will carry fluids to the chambers of the heart with little admixing, and additional care must be taken to avoid the use of cold or acid blood or other potentially dangerous agents.

Although the extruded bowel may be no greater than a walnut, operation almost always requires general endotracheal anesthesia with nasogastric tube and standard noninvasive monitoring apparatus. Intubation may be performed without anesthesia or relaxant, but since the intestine is not under pressure before operation, use of intramuscular succinylcholine is advantageous for more active infants.

During the course of operation the anesthesiologist's principal concerns are the preservation of ventilation and the replacement of fluid. Actually, the problem of evaluating respiratory depression is least difficult in the larger defects, where it is obvious that a staged closure will be necessary. Then either halothane or muscle relaxants may be used, and the infant should not need postoperative respiratory assistance.

At the present time it is the defect of moderate size that presents the greatest difficulty in management and evaluation.

Here a primary closure is of sufficient advantage to justify considerable effort, but the effort should be provided by the surgical team rather than the infant. During any closure the anesthesiologist and surgeon must work together to evaluate the degree of abdominal pressure that the infant can tolerate. Use of a muscle relaxant will facilitate the work of the surgeon but will make it impossible to judge the adequacy of spontaneous exchange. Although one can still estimate the degree of respiratory restriction by resistance to manual ventilation, it is safer to use halothane and retain some evidence of what the infant can do for himself.

Since closure will require some tension in most of these intermediate-sized defects, postoperative ventilatory assistance for 12 to 24 hours may be indicated. Whether extubation is performed early or late, prior to removal of the tube one must be sure that the infant is warm and well hydrated, that the anesthetics have been cleared and relaxants reversed, that the child moves and breathes actively, and that he has actually awakened and has spontaneously opened his eyes.

Conservative treatment. By painting intact omphaloceles with alcohol or mercurochrome several times a day for several weeks, Grob (1963), Bill (1969), and others have found that in even the largest of the lesions the skin will gradually fill in from the periphery, force the viscera back into the abdomen, and completely close the lesion.

Dressings of plastic material kept moist and sterile by Neosporin spray have been used for defects that were not suitable previously for surgical closure and others in which previously attempted surgical closures had broken down.

The postoperative care of all infants following omphalocele repair is extremely demanding. The nasogastric tube is left in place, and the infant is maintained on carefully regulated parenteral alimentation for days or sometimes weeks before he can be fed by mouth.

ESOPHAGEAL ATRESIA, TRACHEOESOPHAGEAL FISTULA, AND RELATED ESOPHAGEAL ANOMALIES

The first attempts to perform intrathoracic operations on sick newborns were concentrated on those with esophageal atresia. The solutions to the problems met in correcting these lesions represent some of the great achievements of pediatric anesthesia and surgery. In spite of intensive efforts, there were no survivals until 1939, when both Leven of St. Paul and Ladd of Boston succeeded with their complicated multistaged procedures. The modern era of primary end-to-end esophageal anastomosis was opened in 1941 by Haight of Detroit. At this time, most operations of this type were accomplished without benefit of endotracheal intubation and with little knowledge of monitoring, intravenous support, antibiotics, or postoperative care. Each procedure was a major event, demanding the undivided attention of the institution's top-ranking surgeon and anesthesiologist and the all-out effort of supporting residents and nurses. Every survivor was a personal victory for each person involved.

During the intervening 40 years considerable experience was gained. Large series of operations have been reported by several surgeons: Gross (1953), 224 cases; Waterston and associates (1962), 218 cases; Haight (1969), 288 cases; and Koop and associates (1974), 354 cases. Parallel opportunity in anesthesia management, as reported by Wilton (1952), Zindler and Deming (1953), Kennedy and Stoelting (1958), Johnston and Conn (1966), Calverley and Johnston (1972), and others, has changed the picture to one of considerable standardization and predictability, with 100% survival expected in infants that do not have added handicaps. Attention now may be focussed on particular areas where complications may be reduced and survival of poor-risk infants can be improved.

For excellent coverage of these considerations, the articles by Koop and associates (1974) and Calverley and Johnston (1972) are highly recommended.

Embryology, types, and incidence of esophageal anomalies

The embryologic origin of esophageal atresia is uncertain, but it is believed to be caused by pressure of anomalous vessels passing across the esophagus during the third to sixth week of fetal life. The incidence of esophageal atresia is approximately 1 in 4000 live births (Haight, 1969).

Several types of esophageal atresia are well known. Anesthesiologists should be aware of the different variants, for the management differs in relation to the particular lesion involved. The presence or absence of a fistula between trachea and esophagus is of obvious importance. In addition, it is essential to know whether the fistula connects the trachea to the upper or lower segment of the esophagus or if the esophagus is intact but has a tracheoesophageal fistula (TEF) (anatomic H-fistula, or Gross type F).

Unfortunately, reclassification and regrouping of esophageal anomalies by several writers have been quite confusing. The six variants described by Gross (1953) are shown in Fig. 15-8. There is general agreement that

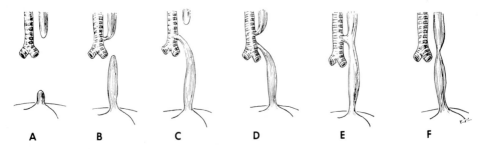

A	B	C	D	E	F

Fig. 15-8. Types of congenital abnormalities of the esophagus. **A,** Esophageal atresia, no esophageal communication with the trachea. **B,** Esophageal atresia, the upper segment communicating with the trachea. **C,** Esophageal atresia, the lower segment communicating with the back of the trachea. Over 90% of all esophageal malformations fall into this group. **D,** Esophageal atresia, both segments communicating with the trachea. **E,** Esophagus has no disruption of its continuity but has a tracheoesophageal fistula. **F,** Esophageal stenosis. (From Gross, R. E.: The surgery of infancy and childhood, Philadelphia, 1953, W. B. Saunders Co.)

the most common type is that designated by Gross as type C, esophageal atresia with fistula between trachea and distal segment of the esophagus, which includes 80% to 90% of the cases in all groups reported. The relative incidence of the remaining 10% to 20% has varied among different writers, but the intact esophagus with TEF and the isolated esophageal atresia without fistula (Gross types E and F) have appeared to be considerably more common than the others.

Diagnosis

The presence of hydramnios during pregnancy should alert the obstetrician to the likelihood of some form of intestinal obstruction in the fetus. The existence of esophageal atresia should be discovered at birth by routine testing of esophageal patency using a soft rubber catheter. Details of the exact nature of the defect may then be determined by radiography, preferably by use of an opaque rubber catheter that will coil in the blind upper pouch of the esophagus. If more detail is necessary, Koop and associates (1974) advise barium, stressing the danger of oily or water-soluble materials.

If the diagnosis is missed at birth, most infants with esophageal defects will soon show signs of gagging and coughing on secretions that they cannot swallow, with resultant respiratory distress and cyanosis, and, unless treated promptly, the rapid progression of pneumonia and death. Unlike most forms of esophageal deformity, the H-type lesion, involving a fistula without esophageal atresia, causes no swallowing problem, and the diagnosis may not be made for several months or years, until suggested by recurrent respiratory problems of a less intense nature.

Preoperative evaluation and preparation

An initial consideration in evaluating infants with esophageal atresia is whether operation can be performed before the lungs have become contaminated by aspiration. Although operation for these infants has not been treated on an emergency basis since the pioneer phase, when possible it may be advantageous to prepare a fresh, unfed neonate for operation within 2 or 3 hours after delivery, not as a lifesaving procedure, as for infants with diaphragmatic hernia, but as a method of optimum care. Any infant who has been fed or who is more than a few hours old will miss this opportunity.

All infants with esophageal anomalies must undergo usual preoperative care, with particular attention to recognition of complicating factors that may interfere with survival, among which Calverley and Johnston (1972) give priority to prematurity, congenital anomalies, and pulmonary complications.

The incidence of prematurity or weight under 2500 grams in association with esophageal atresia has exceeded 50% in our experience, considerably more than with any other lesion. Unless extremely small, however (weighing under 1500 grams), these infants have not presented particular difficulty on the basis of their size or maturity. The major significance of prematurity should be to alert one to the increased probability of finding important unrelated anomalies.

Several studies of TEF have stressed the importance of complicating congenital defects, which they estimated were responsible for approximately 30% of the TEF deaths. In view of the improved operative management of TEF, it is probable that such anomalies now contribute more than 50% of the mortality.

The variety of associated defects has been great, and those of the cardiovascular and gastrointestinal systems outnumber all others. Although the incidence of intestinal anomalies has nearly equalled that of the cardiac defects, in our experience *the presence of unsuspected cardiac defects has been and still is the greatest threat to the life of the infant with TEF.* The presence of a major cardiac lesion frequently is not evident during the first few days of life, allowing the infant to tolerate anesthesia and operation without complication. Their recovery is retarded, however, and is mistakenly believed to be due to some surgical problem until cardiac failure becomes obvious, at which time the infant is found to have transposition of the great vessels or coarctation of the aorta or combinations of several major defects.

To emphasize the importance of associated cardiac defects in infants with TEF, data of Greenwood and associates (1976) are shown below in which 14.7% of the 326 infants with TEF operated on at this hospital were found to have cardiac lesions. The mortality of those with cardiac malformations was 79% as compared with 22.7% mortality in infants without cardiac defects.

CARDIAC ANOMALIES ASSOCIATED WITH TRACHEOESOPHAGEAL FISTULA*

Total number of infants with tracheo-esophageal and esophageal atresia	326
Cardiac anomalies	
Ventricular septal defect	17
Coarctation of the aorta	3
Tetralogy of Fallot	6
Atrial septal defect	5
Other	17
TOTAL	48 (14.7%)

Efforts to reduce the high mortality in infants with cardiac malformations should be centered on earlier diagnosis of the condition and avoidance of fluid overload.

Among gastrointestinal lesions of importance, imperforate anus is well known and usually diagnosed at birth. Pyloric stenosis, however, has occurred in increased frequency, often as a complicating factor in recovery from operation.

Two complications of primary importance in TEF that are caused by the lesion itself are *pneumonitis* and *gastric distension*. Pneumonitis and right upper lobe pneumonia are almost impossible to prevent, since tracheal soiling is caused by spillover from the blind upper pouch of the esophagus and also by gastric reflux through the fistula. The use of antibiotics to control the pulmonary infection is a standard procedure, as is the immediate placement of a sump suction drain in the upper pouch. Closure of the TEF is considered to be of sufficient value to justify per-

forming ligation under high-risk conditions when total esophageal repair cannot be undertaken. For several years it was a general practice to perform initial ligation of the fistula under local anesthesia in premature infants and delay esophageal repair until the infant reached the weight of a normal neonate (Holder and others, 1962).

Although it has been customary to position infants in a semisitting position before closure of the fistula, Koop and associates (1974) have favored keeping them with head elevated but facedown for better control of tracheal secretions.

Gastric distension, while more easily managed than pneumonia, presents a more acute hazard, since passage of air through the fistula often so dilates the stomach that the diaphragm is immobilized and ventilation is seriously embarrassed (Fig. 15-9). Babies should be inspected for the presence of this situation on admission, since immediate relief by gastrostomy or even by needle aspiration may be necessary.

Since gastric distension may occur at any time, and since gastrostomy is usually needed for postoperative feeding, it is advantageous to perform the gastrostomy soon after the infant's admission and then continue with other therapy prior to the esophageal repair. Gastrostomy should require little relaxation and 15 or 20 minutes of operating time. Local infiltration anesthesia is adequate and may actually be preferable if the infant has pneumonia or if the fistula is unusually large, as described below. There is considerable variation in the indications and the timing of gastrostomy. Some surgeons perform the procedure routinely on admission of the infant, whereas others combine it with the total repair if it had not been necessary previously.

Surgical problems in repair of tracheoesophageal fistula and esophageal atresia

It is of utmost importance for the anesthesiologist and the surgeon to know the problems and needs of each other, for both are working in the same small area and often

*Adapted from Greenwood, R. D., Rosenthal, A., and Nadas, A. S.: Cardiovascular anomalies associated with congenital diaphragmatic hernia, Pediatrics **57:**92, 1976.

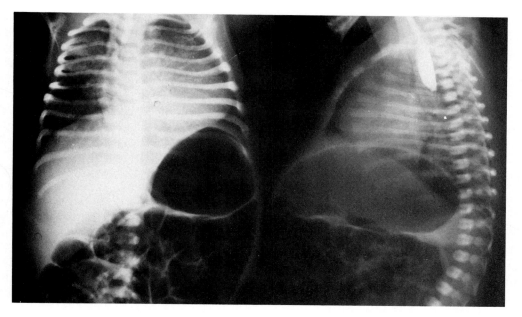

Fig. 15-9. Gastric distension, in Type C lesion, may need prompt relief. (Courtesy Dr. Arnold Colodny, Boston, Mass.)

must interfere with each other's progress. Communication and cooperation are absolute necessities.

Although there are variations in several surgical details, the infant is always positioned lying on his left side. Incision is made under the right scapula and well across the midaxillary line at the fourth intercostal interspace, allowing the surgeon to approach the vagus nerve, esophagus, trachea, and fistula by either the retropleural or transpleural route. In spite of somewhat greater technical difficulty, the retropleural route is generally favored at present, since the complications of postoperative leakage or breakdown of the esophageal anastomosis are less often fatal.

As previously mentioned, the first operation may consist only of exposing and tying off the fistula, since this may be a lifesaving procedure. Although this operation may require 1 or 2 hours, the stress and risk imposed on the infant are considerably less than in the total repair.

When total repair is performed, the fistula will be divided surgically and closed before the esophageal repair is undertaken. While the fistula seldom is difficult to locate, one or both of the esophageal stumps may require considerable dissection before they are identified and prepared for anastomosis. Until he begins the anastomosis, the surgeon will have retracted the right lung and compressed the trachea from time to time but will not have required absolute diaphragmatic paralysis. For the repair, however, he will want, and should have, total immobility of the diaphragm until he is quite satisfied that the repair is complete. The anesthesiologist should know that there are few sutures of more critical importance than those that a surgeon places in performance of primary esophageal anastomosis. Under the best circumstances, suturing the two ends of the esophagus is an exacting procedure, but when the ends must be pulled together and sutured under tension, the difficulty is considerably greater and the average surgeon may require 20 or 30 minutes for the anastomosis.

When the distance between the upper and lower esophageal segments is excessive, or in other situations where the original anastomosis has broken down, a more extensive repair may be necessary involving intra-thoracic transposition of the transverse colon. This procedure is usually postponed until the infant weighs 6 or 7 kg and is in optimum condition. (Eraklis and Gross, 1966; Soave, 1972).

Repair of the H-fistula is completely different inasmuch as no esophageal anastomosis is required and division of the fistula is usually accomplished through an incision in the neck.

Anesthetic management of tracheoesophageal atresia

The anesthesiologist participates in preoperative care, especially where directed toward improving respiration. Occasionally a very small or sick infant will require preoperative intubation and supportive ventilation. The high incidence of *congenital cardiac lesions seen in association with TEF and the difficulty in their early diagnosis should be strong deterrents to aggressive fluid therapy.* Intravenous fluids, given at a rate of 4 ml/kg/hr, should be sufficient under most circumstances, with additional allowances for measured loss by sump drainage, gastrostomy, and operative blood loss.

The usual concern for oxygenation, warmth, and cleanliness is maintained during all phases of transport and preparation. Preoperative administration of atropine seems definitely advisable in order to reduce secretions and prevent vagal response to halothane.

As previously described, several different operations may be performed on infants with tracheoesophageal fistula, each requiring different anesthetic management. For *gastrostomy* it is often sufficient to use local infiltration and restraints, but general endotracheal anesthesia may be used in strong active babies. Nitrous oxide, oxygen, and halothane make a satisfactory combination. Whether local or general anesthesia is used, these infants are monitored by a skilled anesthesiologist with stethoscope, blood pressure apparatus, and thermometer. More elaborate devices should not be needed. All of these

infants will have previously established infusions and sump suctions in place. For *ligation of the TEF without esophageal anastomosis,* it has been not only possible but preferable to use local infiltration in some instances where an unusually large fistula made anesthesia difficult. More often, however, the surgeon will need a quieter patient, and general endotracheal anesthesia, with either halothane or intravenous agents, is used. Little relaxation will be required, blood should not be needed, and ECG, intra-arterial cannulation, and CVP line are not recommended, since the attention and time they require and the hazard imposed are not justified by the information they provide. For *total primary repair of TEF* and for *colon transposition,* greater outlay of supportive and monitoring technics will be required, for in these procedures respiratory and cardiac function are frequently embarrassed by surgical manipulation. In addition, the magnitude of the operations far exceeds the others in respect to blood loss and duration of surgery. An ECG is useful when cardiac sounds become difficult to hear, and in the presence of major cardiac defects arterial cannulation may be helpful. Some infants will still carry umbilical infusion lines.

An esophageal stethoscope should not be used in infants with esophageal atresia, but the left precordium should be free for application of a standard stethoscope. This must be carefully wedged under the infant and fixed firmly, for it is apt to be pushed away from the chest. The stethoscope is vitally important in this operation, for it effectively measures cardiac output, ventilation, and the presence of secretions, all of which are of more than usual concern to the anesthesiologist.

Awake intubation may be accomplished in weak infants, but one must take particular care to avoid any tracheal manipulation in addition to that required for the operation. Thus, the use of intramuscular succinylcholine and oxygen has additional advantage here.

Except for rare cases where postoperative ventilatory support is anticipated, oral intubation is chosen and a tube that allows a slight leak on moderate positive pressure is used (size 3.0 or occasionally 3.5 mm ID).

As previously mentioned, the presence of a large fistula can be troublesome at the outset, shunting air and anesthetic gases from trachea to esophagus and stomach. Prior to performance of gastrostomy this will cause marked gastric distension. If gastrostomy has been established, gases simply pass on through. In such cases the infant may be allowed to breathe spontaneously while the fistula is ligated under local infiltration anesthesia, or one may begin by awake intubation and pass the tip of the endotracheal tube beyond the tracheal opening of the fistula. When this method is chosen, one runs the increased chance of passing the tube into the right bronchus and occluding the left. Consequently it is wise to cut an extra hole near the tip of the tube on the left side, so that gases may reach the left lung. After the fistula has been divided, the tube should be withdrawn enough to assure good ventilation to both lungs.

For maintenance of anesthesia there is no single agent or technic of choice. A 50% nitrous oxide and oxygen base with added halothane or relaxant and either a T-system or a circle system modification may be used with good results. One must be able to control the level of anesthesia and produce a quiet chest and diaphragm without cardiovascular depression. Our current approach is to use light halothane and nitrous oxide, with substitution of a relaxant should blood pressure become depressed by halothane. d-Tubocurarine has been our choice, though pancuronium and metocurine now are preferred.

During the course of the operation, secretions may block the trachea, and one must be able to use suction effectively at any time. For this purpose a straight endotracheal adapter is definitely indicated. Surgical manipulation of the lungs, trachea, and esophagus may also cause complete airway obstruction at frequent intervals, usually at its worst during division of the fistula. The anesthesiologist must protect the infant in such situations but occasionally must allow the surgeon

intervals of trespass when they are mandatory for the procedure. In order to provide the best anesthetic and supportive care, the anesthesiologist must stand and watch the progress of the operation, noting the effectiveness of the heart beat, the filling or compression of the lungs, the amount of retraction being employed, and the loss of blood. During both transpleural and retropleural operations it should be evident whether the right lung is expanded or deflated. In spite of surgical retraction, the anesthesiologist should be able to maintain expansion of at least one third of the right lung.

If halothane has been administered by controlled ventilation, awakening often is delayed unless the halothane is discontinued fully 10 to 15 minutes prior to completion. If nondepolarizing relaxants have been used, they should be reversed. Most of these infants should be expected to breathe adequately without the added risks of mechanical ventilation.

Postoperative care is of great importance in these infants. Fluids are limited until it is certain that the infant has no cardiac lesions. Intravenous and gastrostomy routes are both maintained. Oral feedings are started after the esophageal anastomosis has had a chance to heal (3 to 5 days).

Major complications to be feared are continuing pneumonia, pneumothorax, atelectasis, and leakage or breakdown of the wound. Esophageal stricture at the site of repair may be mild or may require repeated dilation under general anesthesia.

CONGENITAL DIAPHRAGMATIC HERNIA

The neonate with a large congenital diaphragmatic hernia (CDH) presents a combination of features of outstanding interest to both anesthesiologist and surgeon. This problem represents one of the few surgical emergencies of the newborn period, often demanding immediate supportive therapy and definitive surgery. Mortality is high even under optimal conditions, and several features in management are currently under debate. In the event of survival, however, the reward is great, for once CDH is corrected there usually is little residual functional impairment.

Estimates of the incidence of CDH have varied from 1 in 600 to 1 in 18,000 live births but average about 1 in 5000 (Gravier and others, 1971). There is closer agreement in data concerning the male to female ratio, which is reported consistently at 2:1 (Bock and Zimmerman, 1967; Bell, 1973).

The embryologic development of CDH has been studied by several workers (Kitagawa and others, 1971; Reid, 1967; Gray and Skandalakis, 1972). The normal diaphragm is formed by the fusion of several components (septum transversum and pleuroperitoneal, mediastinal, and intercostal lumbar muscular components) during the eighth to tenth week of fetal life. Initially these septa are composed of membranous folds of pleura and peritoneum that later become reinforced by muscle fibers. The anterior portion of the diaphragm is formed before the posterior, for a time leaving the posterolateral area of each pleural cavity in free communication with the peritoneal cavity through the pleuroperitoneal canal (foramen of Bochdalek). A smaller retrosternal foramen (of Morgagni) also allows passage between pleural and peritoneal cavities during diaphragmatic development. Under normal circumstances the foramen of Morgagni closes first, and then the right and finally the left foramen of Bochdalek close. Failure of the fusion of the muscular elements, whether due to growth disturbance, pressure, or trauma, results in persistence of the foramen in the affected area.

In addition to the above types of hernias, there may be agenesis of one or both leaves of the diaphragm.

Although prematurity and various associated congenital defects often further incapacitate the infant, the chief elements of danger lie in the size of the defect, its position, the presence or absence of a sac, and the consequent amount of viscera occupying the chest. If the hernia is one of minor degree, the infant may show few signs at birth, and the real diagnosis be made only after recurrent bouts of respiratory or gastrointestinal

distress. If the herniation is extensive, filling one side of the chest and crowding the other (Fig. 15-10), the infant may become severely hypoxic immediately after birth and die within a few hours in spite of all known approaches. At present, approximately half of the infants brought to pediatric centers for treatment of diaphragmatic hernia are critically hypoxic.

As shown below, the diaphragmatic hernias most frequently seen in infants are those through the left or right posterolateral foramen of Bochdalek (Fig. 15-11). Together these account for approximately 80% of all diaphragmatic lesions, with the left outnumbering the right by a ratio of 5:1. The left Bochdalek hernias are also larger, usually involving at least one third of the diaphragm. Since Bochdalek hernias have no sac, the left chest often is jammed full of stomach, spleen, small and large bowel, and part of the liver. Hernias through the right foramen of Bochdalek are considerably smaller, because the diaphragm and right pleural cavity are protected by the broad dome of the liver. Morgagni, or retrosternal, hernias are usually small and have a sac that acts to limit the extent of visceral herniation, but because of their proximity to the heart they may impede cardiac output. Larger hiatus hernias, on the other hand, rarely interfere with cardiac or respiratory function at birth but eventually cause gastric irritation.

RELATIVE INCIDENCE OF DIAPHRAGMATIC LESIONS IN CONGENITAL DIAPHRAGMATIC HERNIA*

Left posterolateral (left Bochdalek)	69
Right posterolateral (right Bochdalek)	13
Esophageal hiatus	5
Diaphragmatic	4
TOTAL	91

The effect of a large diaphragmatic hernia on an infant is not evident until birth, but the crowding of the pleural cavity throughout fetal development prevents the development of the ipsilateral lung, which at birth appears one quarter of its normal size and

*Data from Gross, R. E.: The surgery of infancy and childhood, Philadelphia, 1953, W. B. Saunders Co.

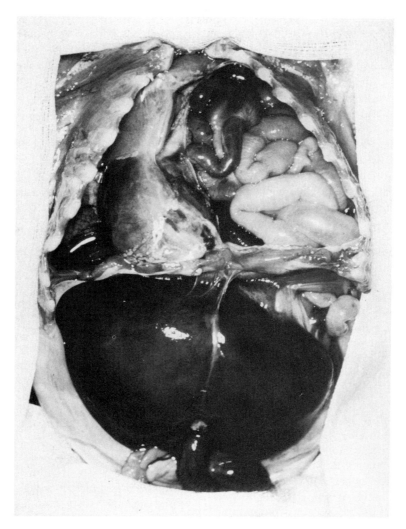

Fig. 15-10. Diaphragmatic hernia at postmortem examination showing obliteration of left pleural cavity and severe compression of the heart and right lung. (Courtesy Dr. Arnold Colodny, Boston, Mass.)

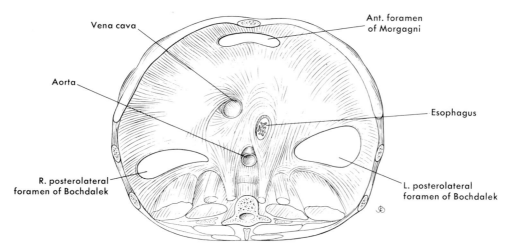

Fig. 15-11. Diagram (from below) showing sites of congenital diaphragmatic hernia.

totally unexpanded, averaging 8 to 10 grams as compared with the normal 30. While not actually rudimentary, as it is frequently termed, it is hypoplastic. As shown by Areechon and Reid (1963) and by Real and Esterly (1973), there may be a reduction in bronchial and bronchiolar branching, with the total number of bronchiolar generations being reduced from the usual 22 to only 16 or 18. A less marked reduction in number of alveoli also takes place.

While the reduction of size and structure of the smaller lung is of some importance, the main burden placed on the infant is by way of the right-to-left shunting and consequent difference between alveolar and arterial oxygen tension (A-aDo₂).

Further cardiorespiratory restriction is caused by displacement of the heart and mediastinum away from the side of the hernia. The resultant growth of the contralateral, or "good," lung is so affected that its average weight, as shown by Snyder and Greaney (1965), is usually 10% below normal.

An added feature of prime importance is the increased tendency of each lung, and more often the contralateral one, to develop pneumothorax (Sunshine and Lewis, 1973). This has been one of the outstanding causes of mortality in CDH (Woolley, 1976).

The additional problems imposed by other congenital defects may deal the fatal blow to a child with CDH. Greenwood and associates (1976) found a 23% incidence of significant cardiac defects in 48 infants recently operated on for CDH at our institution, and they stressed the importance of early recognition, most accurately accomplished by echocardiography and/or cardiac catheterization.

Diagnosis

The birth of an infant with a large diaphragmatic hernia calls for prompt recognition and efficient treatment if his life is to be saved (see summary of diagnosis and treatment opposite). Anesthesiologists should be alert to the fact that this is a true surgical emergency. Immediately after delivery the

CARDIAC ANOMALIES ASSOCIATED WITH CONGENITAL DIAPHRAGMATIC HERNIA*

Total of infants with congenital diaphragmatic hernia	48
Cardiac anomalies	
Ventricular septal defect	2
Common atrium, ventricular septal defect	1
Ectopic heart, tricuspid atresia, ventricular septal defect	1
Tetralogy of Fallot	2
Tetralogy of Fallot, atrial septal defect	1
Atrial septal defect, patent ductus arteriosus	1
Coarctation of the aorta	1
Pulmonic stenosis	1
Inferior caval obstruction	1
TOTAL	11 (23%)

infant may appear normally oxygenated and make energetic attempts to breathe. Failure to ventilate adequately will soon be obvious, as *cyanosis* rapidly increases and the heart begins to slow. If, after the upper airway has been cleared and oxygen has been administered, the infant's color and normal heart rate are restored, one should immediately think of diaphragmatic hernia as a possible diagnosis. Observance of a *flat, scaphoid (boat-shaped) abdomen* adds to the probability of this diagnosis, which can be confirmed by *auscultation (absent breath sounds on side of hernia)*, and *x-ray film showing loops of bowel in the chest* (Fig. 15-12).

DIAGNOSIS AND TREATMENT OF DIAPHRAGMATIC HERNIA
Diagnosis
Increasing cyanosis after birth
Scaphoid abdomen
Absent breath sounds, left or right side
X-ray film showing intestinal loops in chest

Treatment
Suction mouth and pharynx
Ventilate carefully
Intubate trachea
Insert nasogastric suction catheter
Warm, transport
Correct acidosis (±)
Operate

*Adapted from Greenwood, R. D., Rosenthal, A., and Nadas, A. S.: Cardiovascular anomalies associated with congenital diaphragmatic hernia, Pediatrics **57**:92, 1976.

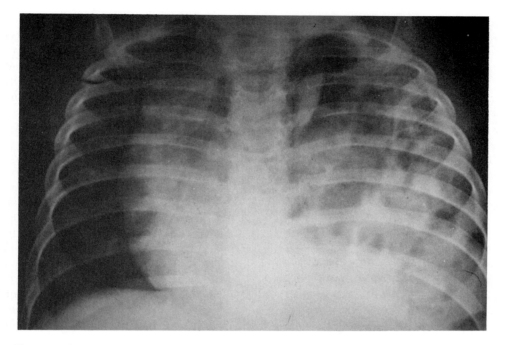

Fig. 15-12. Diaphragmatic hernia. X-ray film shows loops of intestine in the left side of the chest, displacement of the heart to the right, and compression of the right lung.

Treatment

The first evidence of inadequate ventilation calls for immediate *clearing of the airway by suction catheter*, preferably aided by laryngoscope, followed by mask administration of *oxygen*. This should be performed with the aid of a precordial stethoscope using minimal effective assistance in order to avoid inducement of pneumothorax. Repeated appearance of cyanosis should be an *indication for endotracheal intubation* without anesthesia, followed by *passage of a nasogastric tube*, thereby reducing intrapleural pressure. Gentle respiratory assistance will then be resumed under continual guidance by stethoscope, as the infant is carried through x-ray examination and transported to the operating room.

Immediate thoracotomy has been advised for relief of intrapleural pressure in situations where the infant appears to be moribund, but we have not attempted this maneuver.

Minimal preoperative preparation should include examination of the head, neuromuscular system, body cavities, chest, and abdomen, a total body x-ray film, and drawing of blood for complete blood count and crossmatching. Arterial blood for determination of blood gases may be drawn at the start of operation.

At this point, some prefer to delay operation until the infant's ventilatory state and acid-base balance have been evaluated and correction has been attempted by administration of sodium bicarbonate (Boles and others, 1971; Raphaely and Downes, 1973). It has been our practice, as well as that of others (Rowe and Uribe, 1971; Baffes, 1969), to operate at once when infants show signs of respiratory distress.

Following administration of vitamin K, the infant is taken into the operating room and placed on the table using standard methods of maintaining cleanliness and preserving body heat. The application of necessary monitors quickly follows: precordial or esophageal stethoscope, blood pressure cuff (with Doppler sensor), thermistor, and ECG. If

317

the infant had an umbilical catheter in place on admission, it is used for sampling and pressure determination but not for administration of any material. If the infant is in serious condition, time is not taken to establish a new arterial line until after operation. If the infant is not in distress, we do not believe that arterial cannulation is justified.

A reliable infusion must be started prior to operation and should be placed in the arm, as in the case of omphaloceles, since a tight abdominal closure may interfere with venous return.

Up to this point, the anesthesiologist will have used 100% oxygen in obviously hypoxic infants but oxygen diluted with nitrous oxide in others to prevent damage to eyes and lungs. To control the infant and afford some analgesia, halothane may be added in small increments until the infant is quieted. Should more than 1.5% or 2.0% be required for relaxation, it is advisable to add d-tubocurarine in an initial dose of 1.0 mg followed by 0.5 mg supplementation, which will allow reduction of halothane concentration.

If the infant has been brought in from another institution with an endotracheal tube already in place, experience has taught us to remove it and insert one of known dimensions and patency. This is considered mandatory if the original tube is a tapered Cole tube, which is especially apt to become obstructed during transportation and is unsuitable for postoperative ventilatory assistance even when patent.

For repair of diaphragmatic hernia the infant is positioned on the operating table with the affected side slightly elevated. Although a transthoracic incision has been advocated by a few surgeons, there is now almost universal acceptance of the transabdominal approach for repair of Bochdalek hernias, since this enables the surgeon to correct the intestinal malrotation that is found in 50% of cases and allows him better opportunity to perform the difficult feat of returning the viscera into the reduced space of the peritoneal cavity.

A 6- to 8-cm subcostal wound allows the surgeon access to the underside of the diaphragm. When the surgeon starts to extract the stomach and other organs from the chest, the infant may show a shocklike reaction with apnea and sudden drop in heart rate and cardiac output. The surgeon must desist immediately in such situations and allow time for the infant to recover before proceeding. Atropine (0.1 mg) by intravenous route may be helpful here.

Throughout the entire operation, and especially in such critical moments, the anesthesiologist must refrain from using forceful ventilatory assistance. As discussed later, the use of a manometer to guide external pressure is misleading, and one must judge by breath sounds, color, and blood gas determination, when available. Following complete removal of abdominal viscera from the chest, major reflex responses should not recur. Although one should not expect improved ventilation of the hypoplastic lung, compliance of the contralateral lung and cardiac output often are significantly increased.

Repair of the diaphragmatic defect requires complete immobilization for 5 to 45 minutes, depending on the size of the defect. When the entire side of the diaphragm is absent, it may be necessary to replace it with a mesh implant, which will require more prolonged control.

Closure of the abdomen following diaphragmatic repair presents much the same problem as in infants with omphalocele in that the peritoneal cavity may not be large enough to receive the viscera without the application of excessive force. Here again, by manual stretching of the rectus muscles the closure usually can be made without recourse to use of the plastic bag or silo and staged closure frequently needed for closure of large omphaloceles. In some cases the anesthesiologist must contend with moderate respiratory restriction for which ventilatory assistance will be required for 2 or 3 days.

In management of infants during closure, the anesthesiologist has two alternatives: (1) he may maintain spontaneous respiration, thereby rendering closure difficult but ensuring adequate ventilation, or (2) he can provide complete relaxation to facilitate the repair, hoping that respiration will be adequate when the relaxant wears off. This is a matter to be decided by personal preferences. If one favors the latter, as I do, one must be sure to stay with the infant and support respiration until there is no longer any doubt of the adequacy of ventilation. If respiration remains inadequate, a decision must be made whether to reopen the wound and use a staged repair or to maintain the infant on a mechanical ventilator. Because of increased incidence of pneumothorax in infants with diaphragmatic hernia, use of mechanical ventilation carries additional hazard; however, in many of the poor-risk neonates now being treated, such assistance is necessary even when ventilatory exchange is not restricted by the surgical repair.

One of the major lessons learned about CDH in recent years was the danger of pneumothorax in the postoperative period. For this reason, it is now a standard practice to leave a drainage tube in one or both pleural cavities and obtain x-ray films of the chest immediately after operation and at least once daily thereafter until the hypoplastic lung has shown substantial expansion. If there is sudden change in pulse or respiration in the postoperative period, pneumothorax should be suspected at once, x-ray films obtained, and the chest aspirated or the faulty tube replaced, as indicated. The necessary equipment should be kept in readiness at the bedside at all times. The early postoperative course is critical for 48 to 72 hours or more, after which time there should be some expansion of the hypoplastic lung. Studies by Chatrath and associates (1971), Reid (1967), and Wohl and associates (1977) have shown that the lungs of most of the children who have survived show little or no reduction in function, although the hypoplastic lung remains structurally deficient in the maximum number of bronchial generations and, to a lesser extent, the number of alveoli.

Special management considerations

Infants with CDH probably present the single greatest challenge to pediatric anesthesiologists and surgeons. They require immediate diagnosis so that correct resuscitation and preparation may be provided.

Mortality in infants under 3 days old. A sharp decline in survival rates between 1950 and 1965 was puzzling at first but proved to be due to the fact that many of the sickest infants had not lived long enough to reach the surgeons and were not included in estimations of survival. When it was realized that better methods of diagnosis and resuscitation were adding these extremely high-risk infants to the picture, it became obvious why the rate of success had decreased. Now, when survival of infants with CDH is discussed it is essential to distinguish between those whose symptoms were not immediately evident and those whose symptoms were severe enough to require treatment during the first 1 to 3 days of life. It is now clearly evident that the infant who does not require operation until he is 3 days old should have a 100% chance of survival, whereas the 1- to 3-day-old infant will face some increased mortality and those under 1 day of age will only survive if an extreme effort is made. It is this last group that naturally commands the most attention at present and that the following remarks are chiefly concerned with.

The importance of *prompt diagnosis* has been stressed, as has subsequent need of airway clearance and assisted respiration with 100% oxygen followed by endotracheal intubation. The first costly error often made is use of excessive pressure in inflating the infant's lungs during resuscitation. This is an understandable mistake, since many infants born with respiratory distress syndrome require additional pressure, and these infants are seen more frequently than those with CDH. Ten seconds taken to listen to both sides of an infant's chest are enough to determine whether his life depends on reducing or increasing the force of ventilatory assistance. If breath sounds are audible on one side and not the other, ventilatory force should be reduced to the minimum required to maintain normal heart beat, in spite of some degree of continuing cyanosis.

The *danger of injuring the lungs by excess pressure* during the operation has been

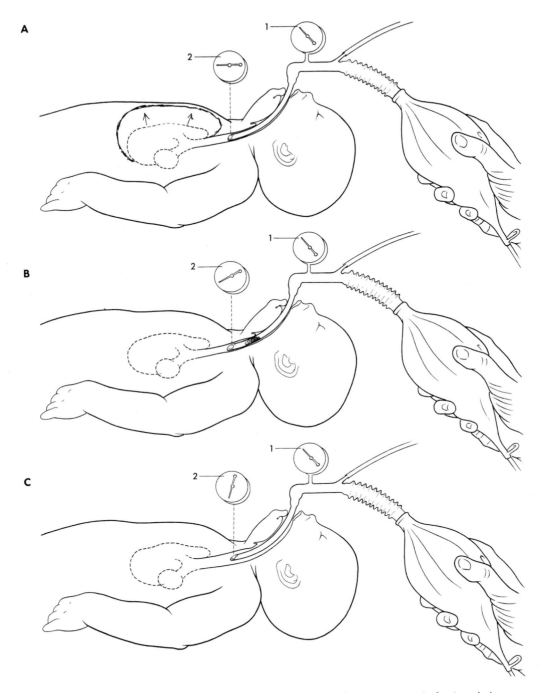

Fig. 15-13. Diagram showing futility of limiting inflation pressure by measurement of external airway (bag) pressure. External pressure measured by in-line manometer *(1)* may be moderately reduced by passing air through an infant endotracheal tube, **A,** or greatly reduced by the presence of a major obstruction, **B,** or by a large leak around the tube, **C.** Readings at *(2)* represent intrathoracic pressures measured by esophageal balloon.

stressed repeatedly in previous reports, and there has been strong feeling that one should never attempt to expand the hypoplastic lung after the viscera have been removed from the chest. Many writers, including Creighton and associates (1966), Smith (1969), and Boles and associates (1971), have further stated that one should monitor the external force being used and have stated set limits of 15 or 20 cm H_2O that should not be exceeded. While it is true that the lung may be damaged by forceful attempts to expand it, it is also true that the infant becomes much stronger as soon as the hypoplastic lung does expand, and it seems reasonable to make a guarded try to initiate the process of expansion under direct vision.

Measurement of ventilating pressure. Fear of inducing pneumothorax by excessive ventilating pressure led to the concept that inflating, or bag, pressure should be measured by an in-line pressure gauge, and should be limited to 15 or 20 cm H_2O. While the attempt to prevent excessive pressure was commendable, the assumption that intrathoracic pressure could be monitored by measuring external, or bag, pressure was wrong and potentially dangerous. As indicated in Fig. 15-13, if one could measure the pressure at both ends of the endotracheal tube of an anesthetized patient, pressure measured at *1*, in the external airway, could easily be damped before reaching *2*, in the thorax, if there were constriction, obstruction, or kinking of the endotracheal tube or if the tube were so small that there was a large leak around it. Two other situations invalidating the external monitor as an indicator of intrathoracic pressure would be any very rapid rate of respiration or the presence of decreased pulmonary compliance, which would retard the flow of gases through the narrowed air passages. On the other hand, the use of a balloon or tambour inserted in the esophagus for monitoring intrathoracic pressure would be quite advantageous, and a limit of 15 to 20 cm H_2O pressure would have some merit.

Correction of metabolic acidosis. A point of considerable disagreement today is whether one should attempt to correct metabolic acidosis prior to operation or proceed directly with reduction of the hernia. Many of these infants show arterial pH of less than 7.0, Pa_{CO_2} above 60 torr, and Pa_{O_2} below 40

torr and may also be hypothermic. One reported by Raphaely and Downes (1973) was found to have a pH of 6.68, Pa_{CO_2} of 114 torr, and Pa_{O_2} of 18 torr. By establishing arterial lines one can follow changes in blood gases while an effort is made to titrate the metabolic acidosis with repeated administration of sodium bicarbonate or THAM. As shown in Fig. 15-14, Rowe and Uribe (1972) demonstrated that acidosis could be markedly improved by operation alone, without prior use of alkalinizing drugs. These authors also stated that the use of an alkalinizing agent, by artificially inducing improved blood gases, deprives the physician of an excellent sign of the infant's true state of health. As yet, there are insufficient data to prove that one method is better than the other.

Measurement of arterial gases and shunting. The monitoring of blood gases to determine the degree of hypoxia, acidosis, and shunting has been used chiefly to evaluate the progressive condition of the individual patient.

Raphaely and Downes (1973) extended the use of such measurements by showing that the amount of change in shunting following operation could be used as valid prediction of

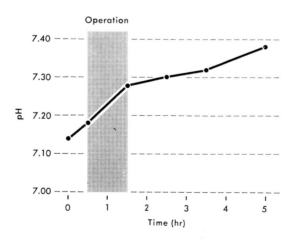

Fig. 15-14. Chart of arterial pH of infant with diaphragmatic hernia, pH shown rising over 5-hour period without buffering. (From Rowe, M. I., and Uribe, F. L.: Surgery **70**:758, 1971.)

survival under current methods of treatment. In an investigation of 58 infants they showed that those survived whose mean A-aDo$_2$ showed a significant reduction after operation, while those whose A-aDo$_2$ remained high (350 to 650 torr) did not survive. In the opinion of the authors, survival of these patients could only be expected with the application of a membrane oxygenator or other more advanced devices than presently employed.

Pharmacologic control of pulmonary circulation. A major advance and a new direction of approach has been made with the recognition of the role of pulmonary hemodynamics in infants with CDH and with attempts to alter them by pharmacologic therapy.

Prior to 1970, improvements in diagnosis, early treatment, and supportive care brought many poor-risk infants through surgical repair of the diaphragm and early hours of recovery only to die 24 to 48 hours later, seemingly because of cardiac failure, acidosis, and hypoxia.

In studies of infants with CDH, Murdock and associates (1971) reported a marked difference between oxygen saturation of the radial artery and the abdominal aorta, demonstrating large and variable degrees of shunting. Cardiac catheterization studies by Dibbins and Weiner (1974) and by Collins and associates (1977) showed that most of the right ventricular outflow of infants with CDH is forced through the contralateral, or expanded, lung, causing unilateral pulmonary circulatory overdistension, resultant right-to-left shunting within the lung or across the foramen ovale or ductus arteriosus, virtual return to fetal circulation, and resultant hypoxia and death. Since complete obliteration of the ductus has been shown to cause death by diastolic hypertension, it is essential to maintain a variable degree of patency of the ductus, avoiding both excessive and inadequate pulmonary perfusion pressure.

The use of pulmonary vasodilators in conjunction with dopamine to maintain cardiac output, as reported by Dibbins and Weiner (1974) and again by Dibbins (1976), has introduced the most delicate touch thus far developed in the care of the critically ill infant with CDH. Chlorpromazine in doses of 1 mg/kg was used to decrease pulmonary vascular resistance by local alpha blockade, and dopamine, in doses of 10 μg/kg/min, was used to increase myocardial contractility by direct beta stimulation. The logic of this approach is convincing, and our own use of the method proved to be lifesaving for the first infant on whom we tried it.

ANESTHESIA FOR INFANTS ONE MONTH TO ONE YEAR OF AGE

After the neonatal stage, the infant becomes an easier subject and the lesions become less exotic. Herniorrhaphy then becomes the most common procedure performed, followed closely by pyloromyotomy and a variety of others, including harelip repair, excision of cystic hygroma, neurosurgical repair of hydrocephalus, subdural hematoma, or meningocele, and those for intrathoracic pathology including vascular ring, hamartoma, and various congenital cardiac lesions.

With the exception of the last category, which are described in the next chapter, most of the above procedures are tolerated well by infants, provided that reasonable precautions are observed. In general, inhalation and intravenous agents are used with nonrebreathing or closed circle apparatus without recourse to methods of exceptional complexity. With precise observation of minutiae and the ability to avoid complications, results can be achieved equal to those in other age groups.

Inguinal herniorrhaphy

The fact that inguinal hernia is so frequently seen in infants and that the mode of repair is relatively simple has led many to believe that it is an operation to be undertaken in community hospitals or as an outpatient procedure. This may be reasonable when the infant is strong, the hernia small, the hematocrit normal, the surgeon able to perform a precise, delicate job in less than 10 minutes, and, as usual, the anesthesiologist highly skilled. However, there are several factors that may alter the situation considerably. Because of the large number of these operations and the many hazards in store for the unwary, this simple procedure deserves extra consideration.

Under ideal conditions, a small infant may be fed by breast or bottle at 6:00 AM, be brought to the hospital and operated on as an outpatient, and be home again by noon. Anesthetic management would consist of 3-hour denial of oral intake, administration or omission of atropine as preferred, and administration of nitrous oxide, oxygen, and halothane by mask. Supplemental aids would consist of a precordial stethoscope, blood pressure apparatus, oropharyngeal airway, and pad under the infant's shoulders.

Conditions are seldom ideal, however. Inguinal hernia occurs much more frequently in infants who are premature or have other forms of integumental weakness; the hernia may be large, bilateral, or incarcerated, and the hematocrit is more often below 30% than above. The operation is often attempted by surgeons with little pediatric experience. In teaching hospitals it is assumed to be the rightful property of the youngest surgical initiate.

The surgeon's requirements are not many, but he needs to have the infant immobile and relaxed, and he prefers to have the patient recover promptly.

A reasonable anesthetic approach for all such procedures might be to use awake intubation and halothane, nitrous oxide, and oxygen for maintenance, but there are often better methods by which to meet special conditions.

When the patient is a 2-pound survivor of 3 weeks of intensive therapy for respiratory distress and an open-heart repair, one does not relish the thought of an unsuccessful herniorrhaphy. Depending on the size of the hernia and the quality of the available facilities, one should consider transportation, postponement, or the use of local infiltration, caudal block, ketamine, Innovar, inhalation, and/or relaxants with endotracheal intubation or inhalation without intubation. Few

surgeons are now willing to work on infants under local anesthesia.

Although ketamine might seem an excellent choice, it may act as a strong respiratory depressant in small infants and is best avoided unless one plans to use postoperative ventilatory assistance. In spite of advocates of regional and intravenous technics, the choice usually centers on inhalational approaches.

No rules can be made for problems of this nature. The infant should be treated by the best individuals available and the decisions left to them. If both anesthesiologist and surgeon are highly skilled, halothane, nitrous oxide, and oxygen by mask would seem best for the infant, whereas in less skilled hands endotracheal intubation would be added.

Other less serious situations often arise, the most frequent being that of low hematocrit. When an infant's repeat hematocrit is 26% to 30% and the child has no other contraindications to operation, the surgeon often has reason to believe that the danger of operation would be less than that of transfusion or of strangulation of the hernia while waiting for an acceptable blood count. Unless the hematocrit is less than 26%, this belief probably has some justification. After the risks that are being accepted are pointed out, it is reasonable to proceed if the team is capable and sets out with the understanding that only one side will be repaired if the infant shows signs of stress.

Herniorrhaphy on a premature neonate can be performed under local infiltration and should be if the child is weak and the anesthetist inexperienced; however, the operation will be more difficult to perform. For anesthesiologists and surgeons of moderate ability, the most conservative management probably is awake intubation followed by 50% nitrous oxide and oxygen topped by halothane. Maintenance of the airway is difficult without intubation. While intubation and especially extubation may initiate their own problems, they are more easily handled than intraoperative airway obstruction. For the skilled anesthesiologist, however, an endotracheal tube simply adds unnecessary manipulations, prolonging both induction and recovery. The shoulders should be raised to provide maximal air exchange, and an oropharyngeal airway usually is needed to keep the tongue from cleaving to the roof of the mouth. Then, enough anesthesia to keep the infant from moving is all that is necessary.

Children bearing increased risk of any sort are not good candidates for outpatient surgery. Once again, warning should be taken in the case of any infant who was born prematurely, for it has been our experience that they tolerate anesthesia and operation poorly until they are several months old.

Infantile hypertrophic pyloric stenosis

Pyloric stenosis was stated by Gross in 1953 to be the condition most frequently requiring operation during infancy. In spite of 1787 operations performed at our hospital at that time and another 1320 between 1953 and 1977, the procedure has fallen into second place, herniorrhaphy having taken a strong lead. Nevertheless, repair of pyloric stenosis has always seemed the most satisfying operation in pediatric practice, since it involves a quick, uncomplicated, lifesaving procedure for infants who are otherwise sound and healthy. Furthermore, there is enough internal medicine to lend some intellectual challenge, and the actual management offers an opportunity for both anesthesiologist and surgeon to demonstrate the advantage of technical finesse. Finally, for those about to take oral examinations in anesthesiology, one can count on being questioned about pyloric stenosis.

Incidence. According to several sources cited by Daly and Conn (1969) and Benson (1969), the incidence of pyloric stenosis varies from 1 in 250 to 1 in 500 live births in the Western world; in black populations the incidence is 1 in 2000. The 4:1 ratio of male to female incidence is well established, and there has been a striking tendency toward increased incidence in infants whose parents had the lesion as well as in first-born children. In 1974 an allegation was made by Johnstone of Rochester, N.Y. that infants operated on for pyloric stenosis or inguinal

hernia had an increased incidence of asthma later in childhood. This was investigated in Boston by Ballantine and associates (1975) and in Toronto by Jones and associates (1976) with completely negative findings.

Pathology. The lesion itself consists of an increase in the number of smooth-muscle fibers of the pylorus, as well as considerable edema of the pyloric mucosa and submucosa, and is detectable microscopically at birth.

As stated by Benson (1969), the onset of symptoms may occur at birth, occasionally as early as the fourth or fifth day, or as late as the fifth month, but the average is 3 weeks. As the lesion becomes clinically evident, it attains the size and consistency of an olive and on cross-section is avascular, white, and rubbery-firm. Increasing obstruction of the gastric outlet first delays and then prevents digestion of food and fluids, with resultant distension and projectile vomiting following feeding, loss of gastric secretions with their high chloride content, and development of hypochloremic alkalotic dehydration associated with weight loss, anemia, and progressive inanition.

Vomitus may contain specks of blood but should not contain any bile, in spite of the fact that jaundice is occasionally observed without obvious explanation. A characteristic symptom is the visible pattern of peristalsis passing from left to right across the abdomen. In a great majority of cases, an experienced pediatric surgeon can make a definite diagnosis by palpating the tumor. Others depend on x-ray examination with the use of a barium meal, thereby complicating the situation considerably for the anesthesiologist.

The diagnosis of pyloric stenosis usually can be made in the early stages of the process, but one still finds exceptions where an infant has become severely dehydrated and anemic, with such serum electrolyte dislocations as sodium, 125 mEq/L, chloride, 85 mEq/L, and potassium, 2.0 mEq/L. Infants who are diagnosed early should have a minimum of 4 to 8 hours of hydration prior to operation. A baby that is severely dehydrated may require 3 or 4 days for safe replacement of fluids, electrolytes, proteins, and blood. Details concerning such therapy are described in Chapter 25.

Surgical requirements. The standard pylorus-splitting operation introduced by Ramstedt in 1912 is actually so simple that an extended dissertation hardly seems necessary. Because it is performed so frequently, however, and on infants with such promising postoperative possibilities, several details of the surgical and anesthetic management of the infant seem worthwhile.

Until recently some surgeons preferred to perform this operation under local anesthesia in order to return the infant to the mother's breast with minimal delay. At present, few are willing to work on an infant that is not well relaxed, much less one that is squirming about under restraints. Consequently, the need for general anesthesia is usually taken for granted. Positioning the infant so that the right upper quadrant protrudes out toward the surgeon is also expected and requires some practice.

The Ramstedt incision rarely exceeds 5 cm in length, and the abdominal wall in these lean infants rarely exceeds 5 mm in thickness. After the peritoneum has been opened, there will be a probing for the pyloric tumor, its duration inversely proportional to the experience of the surgeon. These moments or minutes will be happier if the infant is nicely relaxed. When the tumor is located and pulled up through the small incision there will be considerable tension on the stomach regardless of the degree of relaxation. Should the stomach not be empty at this time, regurgitation could hardly be avoided.

Once the tumor is thus delivered and firmly grasped, little more relaxation is needed. The surgeon incises the tumor and then splits it down to the pyloric mucosa. During this brief time the blood vessels visible in the operating field often appear increasingly dusky. This should not be ignored, but if the child's color is normal elsewhere, the local cyanosis usually can be ascribed to the constricting effect of the small wound on the exposed viscera. Surgical closure is relatively

brief, for it usually involves only two or three sutures in the peritoneum, two or three in the muscular layers, and two or three more in the skin.

Anesthetic management. The anesthesiologist has a particular responsibility for these infants. Pyloromyotomy, like herniorrhaphy, may be attempted in situations where either the personnel or the equipment is inadequate. A critically ill, but potentially intact, infant should be provided with optimal treatment. Too frequently, a child with pyloric stenosis is added hurriedly to a surgeon's crowded schedule, accepted as an emergency by the anesthesiologist, and submitted to operation at a greatly increased risk. Medical therapy for pyloric stenosis often constitutes an emergency, but surgery never.

Regardless of the time of day or night, definite information is necessary, and special care must be taken. Before an infant is accepted for pyloromyotomy, the following information should be obtained:

1. Birth weight, weight prior to the onset of vomiting, and present weight
2. Duration of active vomiting and its character, frequency, and usual quantity
3. Intake over this period, general effect on urination and stooling, and last voiding
4. Hospital course, laboratory blood and electrolyte data as indicated, and therapy administered to date
5. If severely dehydrated, the presence of coma or other neurologic signs

It is assumed that an anesthesiologist should know enough to evaluate these findings and call for further examination or treatment as needed.

In the anesthetic management of infants with pyloric stenosis, *there is one all-important measure that must be performed before induction of anesthesia—thorough emptying of the stomach* (Fig. 15-15).

The obstructed gastric outlet invariably dams up a potentially lethal quantity of fluid in the stomach, in the presence of which any form of anesthesia is contraindicated. Once the stomach is effectively emptied, one has relatively little to fear. The infant may be brought to the operating floor with a naso-

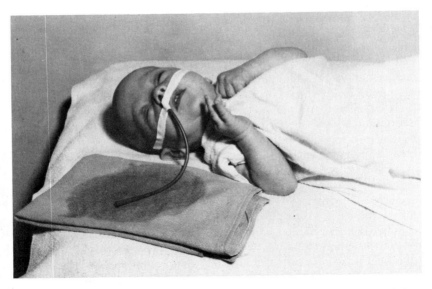

Fig. 15-15. Pyloric stenosis. The stomach must be emptied before anesthesia, preferably by means of sterile rubber urethral catheter, size 10 or 12 French, with several extra holes cut in it.

gastric tube already inserted. Since this often is a small-bore plastic tube, it should be removed. The anesthesiologist should be absolutely sure that an adequate tube has been passed into the stomach. A rubber urethral catheter, size 12 French with several additional holes, is recommended. This is inserted through the nose (preferably) or through the mouth, often with voluminous results, the gastric content often exceeding 100 ml. The tube is strapped securely in place, and if the returns have shown barium, curds, or other solids, the stomach is gavaged until clear, if possible. I prefer to leave the tube in place throughout the operation, because I have encountered no increased tendency for the infant to aspirate, as adults do, and I like to keep an escape line open should more secretions appear.

These infants should be in relatively good condition by the time of operation, even those initially dehydrated having been allowed time for replenishment. If the child has had adequate preoperative fluids, an infusion should not be mandatory during the brief operative procedure unless the diagnosis is uncertain or there are other extenuating circumstances. Atropine is definitely recommended.

As previously mentioned, the anesthetic requirements of the surgeon are immobility and preferably some relaxation, but less than that needed for herniorrhaphy.

There is little doubt today that halothane is the agent of choice for pyloromyotomy. Rapid, easy induction without requiring enough agent to depress cardiac output, easy control, and prompt recovery fit the situation nicely. There are those, however, who prefer intravenous and even regional technics. For uncomplicated pyloromyotomy, the use of such technics would seem to offer little benefit while subjecting the infant to increased manipulation.

Airway management is of primary concern in the care of infants with pyloric stenosis. There is widespread feeling that they require endotracheal intubation because of gastric retention. On the basis of over 2000 cases, however, I contend that endotracheal intubation is not mandatory if the stomach has been rinsed clear and effectively emptied. In such cases, it has been our practice to use mask anesthesia, thus avoiding those infrequent but inevitable complications seen with any unnecessary maneuver. It is to be emphasized, however, that in the event that barium or other solids are found in the stomach and have not been completely removed, endo-tracheal intubation is definitely indicated.

When mask anesthesia is employed, a mask with a cushioned rim will fit snugly over the nasogastric tube if held correctly. A headstrap is not used. The infant's chest is elevated on a folded towel so that the head can be extended, and an oropharyngeal airway is inserted as soon as the baby is asleep. The anesthesiologist keeps one hand on the breathing bag to maintain the needed amount of positive pressure.

As with other infants, 50% oxygen and 50% nitrous oxide with increments of halothane up to 3.0% usually suffice. When the infant is quiet and movable, he is tilted slightly onto his left side and a pad is inserted under his lower ribs to facilitate surgery.

Supportive and monitoring requirements are not extensive. Body heat may be maintained by wrapping the limbs or by use of a heating lamp or water mattress, but unless the room is very cold there should not be significant loss of temperature. Stethoscope, blood pressure apparatus, and thermometer should supply ample information without ECG or other instruments. A certain nicety of touch is required to maintain ventilatory exchange without provoking mechanical or reflex obstruction, or to overcome it should it be encountered. When it is obviously caused by light plane of anesthesia or mesenteric reflex, one can usually rely on gentle assistance of inspiratory efforts until the spasm clears, and one can always produce relaxation by administration of succinylcholine (1 mg/kg by intravenous or intramuscular route).

When the surgeon pulls the tumor up through the wound, the anesthesiologist should lift the mask to look for signs of regurgitation (I have yet to see any). Moderate relaxation is required until the peritoneum is closed. At that time the anesthesia may be reduced. Otherwise the operation may be completed while the infant is still in surgical anesthesia. One of the principal advantages of avoiding intubation lies in the ability to have the child awake as soon as the last suture is placed and to not have to go through

reversal of muscle relaxants after the operation is over. The nasogastric tube is removed as soon as the child wakes up.

If preanesthetic passage of the nasogastric tube brings back milk curds or traces of barium, endotracheal intubation is clearly indicated. Preferences and methods for intubation are outlined in Chapter 8. The presence of a few bits of detritus, though undesirable, hardly represent a "full stomach," and neither awake intubation nor rapid intravenous induction is necessary. Intramuscular administration of succinylcholine, 1.5 mg/kg, has been most advantageous in our experience, and halothane is our next choice. Two indications for endotracheal intubation, in addition to inability to clear the stomach completely, are an inexperienced surgeon and the possibility of a more extensive operation than pyloromyotomy. With intubation, there will be less difficulty in maintaining the airway during operation but greater heat loss and some delay before the infant is ready to return to the recovery unit.

As emphasized by Conn (1963) and Bennett and associates (1968), particularly close watch must be maintained over these infants for several hours after operation, especially if they have become chilled, for they have a tendency to become apneic even after awakening and crying. Although this has been related to their metabolic alkalosis, other factors probably contribute, since apnea has similarly been noted following herniorrhaphy and harelip repair in infants of the same age.

Oral feedings are started 8 hours after surgery. Some vomiting often occurs at first, but soon subsides, and the infants are usually discharged on the first or second postoperative day.

Biliary atresia

Anesthesiologists may be presented with the problem of severely jaundiced infants with true biliary atresia. These infants often live for months, occasionally for several years, before eventual hepatic failure. Various procedures to create biliary drainage have been attempted over the past 30 years, but all were unsuccessful with the exception of Kasai's operations (1974), which as noted by Koop (1976) proved to be of help only to infants with stenosis rather than atresia of bile ducts.

Before the threat of litigation became so evident, we anesthetized these severely jaundiced infants with ether, cyclopropane, or halothane, feeling confident in the belief that the jaundice was due to obstruction rather than hepatitis. Although there have been no complications suggesting anesthetic toxicity, it is now believed advisable to avoid agents associated with liver toxicity and to substitute muscle relaxants and nonhalogenated analgesics.

Hirschsprung's disease

The basic pathology underlying congenital megacolon, or Hirschsprung's disease, is a ganglionosis, or total absence of ganglion cells, in the intrinsic nerve supply of the sigmoid colon and occasionally of more proximal segments of large bowel. The normal nerve supply, consisting of Auerbach's plexuses and Meissner's plexuses that together form the myenteric nerve complex of the bowel, usually becomes an increasingly diffuse network in the descending and terminal bowel. Its absence, which occurs in approximately 1 in 10,000 infants, causes a condition resembling spasm of the area lacking cells, while the normal bowel proximal to the spastic portion undergoes tremendous distension, with retention of feces and intestinal obstruction or, in less serious cases, prolonged bouts of constipation.

Operation is performed for immediate relief by colostomy in acute situations, but definitive surgery is the performance of excision of the aganglionic portion and replacement by normal bowel that is freed and advanced toward the rectum in one of several variations of the "pull through" operation introduced by Swenson in 1950 (Benson, 1979).

The disease is usually evident soon after birth and is suspected when infants fail to gain weight, have abnormal stooling, and have doughy, distended bellies. Definitive diagnosis is made by biopsy of the rectal wall by perineal approach.

The principal corrective procedure is extensive and involves abdominal maneuvers to mobilize the normal colon, as well as perineal procedures to remove the aganglionic portion, or to make the alternative anastomoses involved in Soave or Duhamel procedures.

Children requiring the pull-through procedure are often in a state of severe malnutrition and require extensive corrective therapy before being subjected to such a severe onslaught. Among major considerations for preoperative repair are blood volume, hemoglobin, protein, and vitamin deficiencies.

For the operation itself, one should be prepared for a 6- to 8-hour procedure, during most of which the surgeon not only will expect profound relaxation but also will be manipulating bowel and other viscera more than in almost any other operation. Thus, there will be an appreciable blood loss, but the third-space loss here will be at the maximum level.

An anesthetic technic should be employed that affords relaxation without depression, and thus the nondepolarizing relaxants have an advantage. Monitoring of arterial pressure by cuff is adequate, but arterial gases may be desirable, and arterial cannulation is justifiable, as is CVP measurement, though neither seem irreplaceable. The essential monitors, as usual, are stethoscope, blood pressure apparatus, thermometer, and, in this case, urethral catheter.

Fluid replacement, at approximately 8 ml/kg/hr, should include water, glucose, electrolytes, albumin, and red blood cells either as whole blood or as a blood product.

In relation to the specific pathology and the handling of the gut, the child will have a sump suction tube draining the upper gastrointestinal tract, and one should consider the advisability of avoiding nitrous oxide to prevent intestinal distension, although this measure does not appear to play a significant part.

At least two infusions should be employed. Since the child's legs will be fixed in stirrups for most of the procedure, the infusions are best placed in the arms or hands.

The greatest danger during this long operation is the development of shock, which may appear at any time because of altering effects of blood and fluid loss, hypothermia, and heavy surgery. In addition to replacement of losses, one of the best measures for regaining normal balance is total cessation of surgery for a period of 5 minutes or more, with removal of retractors and maximum obtainable reduction of stress.

Neuroblastoma

As stated by Gross (1953), next to leukemia, neuroblastomas are the most common neoplasm of infancy and childhood. In a series of 96 cases, Gross found 57% in the abdomen and 23% in the central nervous system. By far the greatest number occurred in the first year of life. Since they arise from the posterior elements of abdomen and thorax and grow to large proportions, removal is difficult and hemorrhage often extensive.

Anesthetic management requires full relaxation, nasogastric suction, and provision for massive blood loss and its replacement. Since removal of the tumor often interferes with venous return from the lower body and limbs, the arms should be used for at least one large-bore cannula.

One should be aware that release of epinephrine from these tumors may cause sudden changes in blood pressure or cardiac rhythm. Unlike the aberrations seen in pheochromocytoma, neither complication has been particularly troublesome in our experience.

Sacrococcygeal teratoma

Among the unusual types of pathology seen in neonates, that of sacrococcygeal teratoma bears special cause for concern because of its potential size (Fig. 15-16) and its misleading tendency to develop anterior to the sacrum, reaching extensive proportions without external manifestation. Thus, two aspects are of unusual importance: first, to be prepared for tremendous and rapid loss of fluid and blood (intraoperative exsanguination has

been reported in several), and second, the absolute necessity for continuous observation of the operative field by the anesthesiologist, since the quantity of blood loss is as unpredictable as the time at which it may occur. As with operations carrying the threat of extensive hemorrhage, infusions are established in the arms, with generous quantities of fresh blood standing by.

Another feature worth considering in operations on large external tumors is the advisability of elevating the tumor and allowing the contained blood to drain back into the effective circulating volume both for the purpose of reducing blood loss and facilitating the operation. In doing this, one must weigh the possibility of overloading the circulation and of disseminating carcinomatous cells, since some of the tumors have malignant potential (Exelby, 1972).

Tumors about the face and neck

Cystic hygromas, hemangiomas, and other lesions may occur in the region of the neck and face and often endanger the airway (see Figs. 8-14 and 8-15). In such situations endotracheal intubation may be indicated prior to anesthesia. Obviously, relaxants should not be used when there is danger of airway obstruction. While older children tolerate awake intubation poorly, this is often successful in small infants with airway problems. In massive obstructing tumors, it may be necessary to perform tracheostomy at the beginning or conclusion of the operation. In either case, an endotracheal tube should be in place before the tracheostomy is performed. Maintenance of anesthesia for removal of these large tumors involves several hazards, especially when they occur in the neck. Vagal reflexes are active, and severe arrhythmias, including cardiac arrests, have been known to occur. Surgical manipulation may cause dislocation of the endotracheal tube, and many of these tumors may cause severe blood loss.

Genitourinary operations

During recent years there has been a pronounced increase in the number and variety

329

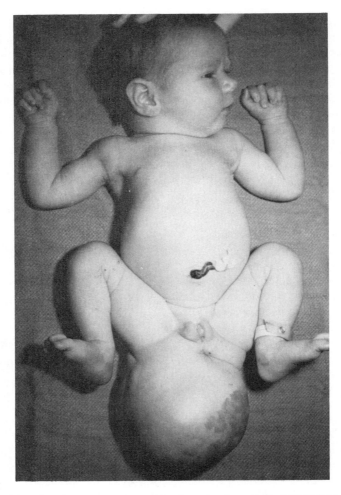

Fig. 15-16. Excision of such a sacrococcygeal teratoma involves marked blood loss as well as difficulty in positioning. (Courtesy Dr. Arnold Colodny, Boston, Mass.)

of genitourinary procedures performed during infancy. Congenital anomalies of kidneys, ureters, and bladder and correction of exstrophy of the bladder are being recognized shortly after birth, and early correction is essential in prevention of permanent damage. These procedures require careful preparation to recognize anemia, early renal failure, or signs of toxicity. Although the cardiorespiratory system should be unaffected, major problems may arise from the need of deep relaxation and prolonged duration of operation. These are described in Chapter 16. Wilms' tumors bear high incidence of metastasis, and removal is difficult, involving drastic manipulation and considerable blood loss. Cystic kidneys may be large (Fig. 15-17), but removal is easier and prognosis is good. Both types of tumor may cause intestinal obstruction. One of the more unusual lesions, that of abdominal muscular deficiency, or prune-belly syndrome, carries a high mortality in early life because of a multitude of associated anomalies, chiefly related to the urinary tract but also to the gastrointestinal and other systems. As the name implies, the

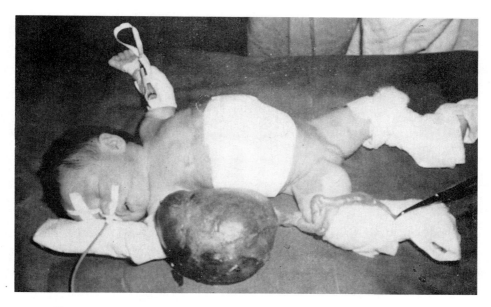

Fig. 15-17. Cystic kidneys often are large enough to cause intestinal obstruction.

abdomen has very weak but not absent musculature, and relaxation is complete at all times. This has widespread effect, especially in relation to expiratory effort, cough, digestion, and excretion (Welch, 1969) (p. 402).

BIBLIOGRAPHY

Adelman, S., and Benson, C. D.: Bochdalek hernias in infants; factors determining mortality, J. Pediatr. Surg. **11**:569, 1976.

Albert, M. S., and Winters, R. W.: Acid-base equilibrium of blood in normal infants, Pediatrics **37**:728, 1966.

Allen, M. S., and Thomson, S. A.: Congenital diaphragmatic hernias in children under one year of age; a 24-year review, J. Pediatr. Surg. **1**:157, 1966.

Aranda, J. V., Saheb, N., Stern, L., and Avery, M. E.: Arterial oxygen tension and retinal vasoconstriction in newborn infants, Am. J. Dis. Child. **122**:189, 1971.

Areechon, W., and Reid, L.: Hypoplasia of lung with congenital diaphragmatic hernia, Br. Med. J. **1**:230, 1963.

Avery, M. E.: The lung and its disorders in the newborn infant, Philadelphia, 1964, W. B. Saunders Co.

Ayre, P.: Anaesthesia for harelip and cleft palate in babies, Br. J. Surg. **25**:131, 1937.

Baffes, T. G.: Diaphragmatic hernia. In Mustard, W. T., Ravitch, M. M., Snyder, W. H., and others, editors: Pediatric surgery, ed. 2, Chicago, 1969, Year Book Medical Publishers.

Ballantine, T. V. N., Tapper, D., Mueller, H. L., and others: Pyloromyotomy; does surgery in infancy increase allergy? Pediatrics **56**:3, 1975.

Bell, M. J.: Congenital diaphragmatic hernia, J. Maine Med. Assoc. **211**:884, 1973.

Bennett, E. J.: Fluids for anesthesia and surgery in the newborn and the infant, Springfield, Ill., 1975, Charles C Thomas, Publisher.

Bennett, E. J., Auger, H. L., and Jenkins, M. T.: Pyloric stenosis. In Jenkins, M. T., editor: Common and uncommon problems in anesthesia, Boston, 1968, Little, Brown & Co.

Bennett, E. J., Bowyer, D. E., Gieseke, A. H., Jr., and Stephen, C. R.: Pancuronium bromide; a double blind study in children, Anesth. Analg. (Cleve.) **52**:17, 1973.

Benson, C. D.: Prepyloric and pyloric obstruction. In Mustard, W. T., Ravitch, M. M., Snyder, W. H., and others, editors: Pediatric surgery, ed. 2, Chicago, 1969, Year Book Medical Publishers, Inc.

Benson, C. D.: Swenson's procedure. In Ravitch, M. M., Welch, K. J., Benson, C. D., and others, editors: Pediatric surgery, ed. 3, Chicago, 1979, Year Book Medical Publishers, Inc.

Beven, J., and Burn, M.: Acid-base changes and anaesthesia; the influence of preoperative starvation and feeding in paediatric surgical patients, Anaesthesia **28**:415, 1973.

Bidwai, A. V., Stanley, T. H., Graves, C. L., and others: The effects of ketamine on cardiovascular dynamics during halothane and enflurane anesthesia, Anesth. Analg. (Cleve.) **54**:588, 1975.

Bill, A. H.: Hernias other than inguinal. In Mustard, W. T., Ravitch, M. M., Snyder, W. H., Jr., and others, editors: Pediatric surgery, ed. 2, Chicago, 1969, Year Book Medical Publishers, Inc.

331

Bock, H. B., and Zimmerman, J. G.: Study of selected congenital anomalies in Pennsylvania, Public Health Rep. **82**:446, 1967.

Boix-Ochoa, J., Geguero, G., Seijo, G., and others: Acid-base balance and blood gases in prognosis and therapy of congenital diaphragmatic hernia, J. Pediatr. Surg. **9**:49, 1974.

Boles, E. T., Jr., Schiller, M., and Weinburg, M.: Improved management of neonates with congenital diaphragmatic hernias, Arch. Surg. **103**:344, 1971.

Bower, B. D., Jones, L. F., and Weeks, M. M.: Cold injury in newborn; study of 70 cases, Br. Med. J. **1**:303, 1960.

Bunker, J. P., Brewster, W. R., Smith, R. M., and Beecher, H. K.: Metabolic effects of anesthesia in man. III. Acid-base balance in infants and children during anesthesia, J. Appl. Physiol. **5**:233, 1952.

Buntain, W. L., Lynn, H. B., Cloutier, M. D., and Dawson, B.: Management of the pediatric surgical patient, Mayo Clin. Proc. **47**:654, 1972.

Calverley, R. K., and Johnston, A. E.: The anaesthetic management of tracheo-oesophageal fistula; a review of ten years' experience, Can. Anaesth. Soc. J. **19**:270, 1972.

Chatrath, R. R., El Shafie, M., and Jones, R. S. L.: Fate of hypoplastic lung after repair of congenital diaphragmatic hernia, Arch. Dis. Child. **46**:633, 1971.

Clatworthy, H. W., Jr.: Special problems in surgery of newborn infants, Surg. Clin. North Am. **50**:771, 1970.

Collins, D. L., Pomerance, J. J., Travis, K. W., and others: A new approach to congenital posterolateral diaphragmatic hernia, J. Pediatr. Surg. **12**:149, 1977.

Collins, H. A., Stahlman, M., and Scott, H. W.: Occurrence of subcutaneous fat necrosis in infants following induced hypothermia used as adjuvant in cardiac surgery, Ann. Surg. **138**:880, 1953.

Conn, A. W.: Anaesthesia for pyloromyotomy in infancy, Can. Anaesth. Soc. J. **10**:18, 1963.

Coran, A. G., Das, J. B., and Eraklis, A. J.: Use of osmometry in the preoperative and postoperative management of the newborn, J. Pediatr. Surg. **6**:529, 1971.

Creighton, R. E., Whalen, J. S., and Conn, A. W.: The management of congenital diaphragmatic hernia, Can. Anaesth. Soc. J. **13**:124, 1966.

Creling, E. W.: Anatomy of the newborn, Philadelphia, 1969, Lea & Febiger.

Crino, M. H., and Nagel, E. L.: Thermal burns caused by warming blankets in the operating room, Anesthesiology **29**:149, 1968.

Daly, A. M., and Conn, A. W.: Anaesthesia for pyloromyotomy; a review, Can. Anaesth. Soc. J. **16**:316, 1969.

Davenport, H. T., and Barr, M. N.: Blood loss during pediatric operations, Can. Med. Assoc. J. **89**:1309, 1963.

Dibbins, A. W.: Neonatal diaphragmatic hernia; a physiologic challenge, Am. J. Surg. **131**:408, 1976.

Dibbins, A. W., and Kiesewetter, W. B.: Preoperative and postoperative care in infants and children. In

Mustard, W. T., Snyder, W. H., Ravitch, M. M., and others, editors: Pediatric surgery, ed. 2, Chicago, 1969, Year Book Medical Publishers, Inc.

Dibbins, A. W., and Weiner, E. S.: Mortality from neonatal diaphragmatic hernia, J. Pediatr. Surg. **9**:653, 1974.

Downes, J. J.: CPAP and PEEP—a perspective, Anesthesiology **44**:1, 1976.

Drop, L. J., and Laver, M. B.: Low plasma ionized calcium and response to calcium therapy in critically ill man, Anesthesiology **43**:292, 1975.

Dudrick, S. J., Wilmore, D. W., Vars, H. M., and Rhoads, J. E.: Long-term total parenteral nutrition with growth development and positive nitrogen balance, Surgery **64**:134, 1968.

Eckstein, H. B., and Glover, W. J.: Transport of neonatal emergencies, Lancet **1**:1272, 1974.

Eger, E. I. II: Anesthetic uptake and action, Baltimore, 1974, The Williams & Wilkins Co.

Eraklis, A. J., and Gross, R. E.: Oesophageal atresia; management following an anastomotic leak, Surgery **60**:4, 1966.

Exelby, P. R.: Sacrococcygeal teratomas in children, C.A. **22**:202, 1972.

Fanaroff, A. A., and Klaus, M. H.: Neonatal infections. In Klaus, M. H., and Fanaroff, A. A., editors: Care of the high-risk neonate, Philadelphia, 1973, W. B. Saunders Co.

Farman, J. V.: Heat losses in infants undergoing surgery in air conditioned theatres, Br. J. Anaesth. **34**:543, 1962.

Filler, R. M., Das, J. B., Haase, G. M., and Donahoe, P. K.: Muscle surface pH as a monitor of tissue perfusion and acid-base status, J. Pediatr. Surg. **6**:535, 1971.

Filler, R. M., Eraklis, A. J., Rubin, V. G., and Das, J. B.: Long-term total parenteral nutrition in infants, N. Engl. J. Med. **281**:589, 1969.

Finberg, L.: Dangers to infants caused by changes in osmolar concentrations, Pediatrics **40**:1031, 1967.

Fonkalsrud, E. W.: Phlebitis in infants, Anesthesiology **33**:652, 1970.

Fonkalsrud, E. W., Ogawa, H., and Clatworthy, H. W., Jr.: The surgery of premature infants, Surgery **58**:550, 1965.

Furman, E. B., Romas, D. E., Lemmer, L. A. S., and others: Specific therapy in water, electrolyte and blood-volume replacement during pediatric surgery, Anesthesiology **42**:187, 1975.

Gilbert, M. G., Mencia, L. F., Brown, W. T., and Linn, B. S.: Staged repair of large omphaloceles and gastroschisis, J. Pediatr. Surg. **3**:702, 1968.

Gordon-Jones, R. G.: A short history of anaesthesia for harelip and cleft palate repair, Br. J. Anaesth. **42**:548, 1970.

Goudsouzian, N. G., Morris, R. H., and Ryan, J. F.: The effects of a warming blanket on the maintenance of body temperature in anesthetized infants and children, Anesthesiology **39**:351, 1973.

Graff, T. D., Sewall, K., Lim, T. S., and others: Acid-base balance in infants during halothane anesthesia with use of an adult circle absorption system, Anesth. Analg. (Cleve.) **43**:583, 1964.

Graff, T. D., Sewall, K., Lim, T. S., and others: The ventilatory response of infants to airway resistance, Anesthesiology **27**:168, 1966.

Gravier, I., Dorman, G. W., and Votteler, T.: Congenital diaphragmatic hernia in children, Surg. Gynecol. Obstet. **132**:408, 1971.

Gray, S. W., and Skandalakis, J. E.: Embryology for surgeons, Philadelphia, 1972, W. B. Saunders Co.

Greenwood, R. D., and Rosenthal, A.: Cardiovascular malformations and tracheoesophageal fistula and esophageal atresia, Pediatrics **57**:87, 1976.

Greenwood, R. D., Rosenthal, A., and Nadas, A. S.: Cardiovascular anomalies associated with congenital diaphragmatic hernia, Pediatrics **57**:92, 1976.

Gregory, G. A.: Resuscitation of the newborn, Anesthesiology **43**:225, 1975.

Grob, M.: Conservative treatment of exomphaloceles, Arch. Dis. Child. **38**:148, 1963.

Gross, R. E.: A new method for surgical treatment of large omphaloceles, Surgery **24**:277, 1948.

Gross, R. E.: The surgery of infancy and childhood, Philadelphia, 1953, W. B. Saunders Co.

Gross, R. E., Clatworthy, H. W., Jr., and Meeker, I. A., Jr.: Sacrococcygeal teratomas in infants and children; a report of 40 cases, Surg. Gynecol. Obstet. **92**:341, 1951.

Gross, R. E., and Ferguson, C. C.: Surgery in premature babies, Surg. Gynecol. Obstet. **95**:168, 1966.

Hackel, A.: A medical transport system for the neonate, Anesthesiology **43**:258, 1975.

Haight, C.: Congenital esophageal atresia and tracheoesophageal fistula. In Mustard, W. T., Ravitch, M. M., Snyder, W. H., Jr., and others, editors: Pediatric surgery, ed. 2, Chicago, 1969, Year Book Medical Publishers, Inc.

Haller, J. A., and Talbert, J. L.: Surgical emergencies in the newborn, Philadelphia, 1972, Lea & Febiger.

Hampton, L. J., White, M. L., and Little, D. L.: Anesthesia for surgical correction of cardiorespiratory anomalies, Anesth. Analg. (Cleve.) **31**:105, 1962.

Hendren, W. H.: Pediatric surgery, N. Engl. J. Med. **289**:456, 1973.

Holder, T. M., McDonald, V. G., Jr., and Woolley, M. M.: The premature or critically ill infant with esophageal atresia; increased success with a staged approach, J. Thorac. Cardiovasc. Surg. **44**:344, 1962.

Johnston, A. E., and Conn, A. W.: The anesthetic management of tracheooesophageal fistula; a review of five years' experience, Can. Anaesth. Soc. J. **13**:28, 1966.

Johnstone, D., Rogimann, K., and Pless, G.: Factors contributing to the development of childhood respiratory allergy; roles of surgery, hospitalization and anesthesia, American Academy of Allergy, Bal Harbour, Fla., January 1974.

Jones, A., Steward, D. J., Donsky, G. J., and others: Incidence of respiratory allergy not increased after

anesthesia in infancy, Anesthesiology **45**:29, 1976.

Kasai, M.: Treatment of biliary atresia with special reference to hepatic portoenterostomy and its modifications, Prog. Pediatr. Surg. **6**:5, 1974.

Kay, B.: Neurolept-anesthesia for neonates and infants, Anesth. Analg. (Cleve.) **52**:970, 1973.

Kennedy, R. L., and Stoelting, V. K.: Anaesthesia for surgical repair of oesophageal atresia and tracheoesophageal fistula, Can. Anaesth. Soc. J. **5**:132, 1958.

Kissane, J. M.: Pathology of infancy and childhood, ed. 2, St. Louis, 1975, The C. V. Mosby Co.

Kitagawa, M., Hislop, A., Boyden, E. A., and Reid, L.: Lung hypoplasia in congenital diaphragmatic hernia; a quantitative study of airway, artery and alveolar development, Br. J. Surg. **58**:342, 1971.

Klaus, M. H., and Fanaroff, A. A.: Respiratory problems. In Klaus, M. H., and Fanaroff, A. A., editors: Care of the high-risk neonate, Philadelphia, 1973, W. B. Saunders Co.

Koop, C. W.: Biliary obstruction in the newborn, Surg. Clin. North Am. **56**:373, 1976.

Koop, C. E., Schnaufer, L., and Broennle, A. M.: Esophageal atresia and tracheoesophageal fistula; supportive measures that affect survival, Pediatrics **54**:558, 1974.

Korsch, B. M.: The child in the operating room, Anesthesiology **43**:251, 1975.

Krueger, C., Mostafo, S., and Regan, L. B.: Spontaneous pneumothorax in newborn infants, Surgery **2**:498, 1968.

Lank, B.: Anesthesia for premature babies, J. Am. Assoc. Nurse Anesth. **21**:238, 1953.

Lewis, M. A. H., and Young, D. E.: Ventilatory problems with congenital diaphragmatic hernia, Anaesthesia **24**:571, 1969.

Liebman, J., and Whitman, V.: The heart. In Klaus, M. H., and Fanaroff, A. A., editors: Care of the high-risk neonate, Philadelphia, 1973, W. B. Saunders Co.

Lynn, H. B.: Optimal ages for elective surgical procedures in infants, J.A.M.A. Georgia **52**:55, 1963.

MacDonald, D. J. F.: Cystic hygroma; an anaesthetic and surgical problem, Anaesthesia **21**:66, 1967.

Madding, G. F., and Kennedy, P. A.: Trauma to the liver, Philadelphia, 1971, W. B. Saunders Co.

Maisels, M., Li, T-K., Piechocki, J., and others: Effect of exchange transfusion on serum ionized calcium, Pediatrics **53**:683, 1974.

Martin, L. W.: Pediatric surgery—general. In Shirkey, H. L., editor: Pediatric therapy, St. Louis, 1975, The C. V. Mosby Co.

McNamara, J. J., Eraklis, A. J., and Gross, R. E.: Congenital posterolateral diaphragmatic hernia in the newborn, J. Thorac. Cardiovasc. Surg. **55**:55, 1968.

Merin, R. G.: Congenital diaphragmatic hernia from the anesthesiologist's viewpoint, Anesth. Analg. (Cleve.) **45**:44, 1966.

Moore, T. C., and Stokes, G. E.: Gastroschisis, Surgery **33**:112, 1953.

Morse, T. S.: Pediatric outpatient surgery, J. Pediatr. Surg. **7**:283, 1972.

Morse, T. S.: Transportation of sick and injured children. In Gans, S. L., editor: Surgical pediatrics, New York, 1973, Grune & Stratton, Inc.

Murdock, A. I., Burrington, J. B., and Swyer, P. R.: Alveolar to arterial oxygen tension difference and venous admixture in newly born infants with congenital diaphragmatic herniation through the foramen of Bochdalek, Biol. Neonate 17:161, 1971.

Mustard, W. T., Ravitch, M. M., Snyder, W. H., Jr., and others: Pediatric surgery, ed. 2, Chicago, 1969, Year Book Medical Publishers, Inc.

Nadas, A. S., and Fyler, D. C.: Pediatric cardiology, ed. 3, Philadelphia, 1972, W. B. Saunders Co.

Norman, A. P.: Congenital anomalies in infancy, ed. 2, Oxford, 1971, Blackwell Scientific Publications, Ltd.

Odell, G. B., Poland, R. L., and Ostrea, E. M.: Neonatal hyperbilirubinemia. In Klaus, M. H., and Fanaroff, A. A., editors: Care of the high-risk neonate, Philadelphia, 1973, W. B. Saunders Co.

Orringer, M. B., Kirsch, M. M., and Sloan, H.: Congenital and traumatic diaphragmatic hernias exclusive of the hiatus, Curr. Probl. Surg. 3:64, 1975.

Oski, F. A.: Designation of anemia on a functional basis, J. Pediatr. 83:383, 1973.

Pang, L. M., and Mellins, R. B.: Neonatal cardiorespiratory physiology, Anesthesiology 43:171, 1975.

Patz, A.: Retrolental fibroplasia, Surv. Ophthalmol. 14:1, 1969.

Podlesch, I., Dudziak, R., and Zinganell, K.: Inspiratory and expiratory carbon dioxide concentrations during halothane anesthesia in infants, Anesthesiology 27:823, 1966.

Potter, E. L., and Craig, J. M.: Pathology of the fetus and the infant, ed. 3, Chicago, 1976, Year Book Medical Publishers, Inc.

Psaltopoulo-Mehrez, M.: Anesthetic management of infants, Int. Anesthesiol. Clin. 1:169, 1962.

Raphaely, R. C., and Downes, J. J., Jr.: Congenital diaphragmatic hernia; prediction of survival, J. Pediatr. Surg. 8:815, 1973.

Ravitch, M. M.: Omphalocele; secondary repair with the aid of pneumoperitoneum, Arch. Surg. 99:166, 1969.

Ravitch, M. M., and Barton, B. A.: The need for pediatric surgeons as determined by volume of work and mode of delivery of surgical care, Surgery 76:754, 1974.

Real, F. R., and Esterly, J. R.: Pulmonary hypoplasia; a morphometric study of the lungs of infants with diaphragmatic hernia, anencephaly and renal malformation, Pediatrics 51:91, 1973.

Reid, L.: Embryology of the lung. In DeReuck, A. V. S., and Porter, R., editors: Development of the lung, Boston, 1967, Little, Brown & Co.

Replogle, R. L., and Reyes, H. M.: Management of trauma and shock in the pediatric patient. In Smith, C. A., editor: The critically ill child, ed. 2, Philadelphia, 1972, W. B. Saunders Co.

Reynolds, R. N.: Acid-base equilibrium during cyclopropane anesthesia and operation in infants, Anesthesiology 27:127, 1966.

Rickham, P. P.: Preoperative and postoperative care. In Mustard, W. T., Ravitch, M. M., Snyder, W. H., Jr., and others, editors: Pediatric surgery, ed. 2, Chicago, 1969, Year Book Medical Publishers, Inc.

Rickham, P. P.: Surgery for congenital defects, Anesthesiology 32:474, 1970.

Rickham, P. P., and Johnston, J. H.: Neonatal surgery, New York, 1969, Appleton-Century-Crofts.

Roe, B., and Stephens, H. B.: Congenital diaphragmatic hernia and hypoplastic lung, J. Thorac. Surg. 32:279, 1956.

Roe, C. F., Santulli, T. V., and Blair, C. S.: Heat loss in infants during general anesthesia and operations, J. Pediatr. Surg. 1:266, 1966.

Rowe, M. I.: Physiologic monitoring. In Gans, S. L., editor: Surgical pediatrics, New York, 1973, Grune & Stratton, Inc.

Rowe, M. I., and Uribe, F. L.: Diaphragmatic hernia in the newborn infant; blood gas and pH considerations, Surgery 70:758, 1971.

Rowe, M. I., and Uribe, F. L.: Hypoxia and the neonatal response to trauma, J. Pediatr. Surg. 7:482, 1972.

Rudolph, A. J.: Anticipation, recognition, and transitional care of the high-risk infant. In Klaus, M. H., and Fanaroff, A. A., editors: Care of the high-risk infant, Philadelphia, 1973, W. B. Saunders Co.

Ryan, D. W.: Anaesthesia for repair of exomphalocele; problems associated with immediate repair in the neonate, Anaesthesia 28:407, 1973.

Schulte, F. J.: Nerve conduction in newborns, Pediatrics 42:17, 1968.

Schuster, S. S.: A new method for staged repair of large omphaloceles, Surg. Gynecol. Obstet. 125:837, 1967.

Seashore, J. H., MacNaughton, R. J., and Talbert, J. L.: Treatment of gastroschisis and omphalocele with biological dressing, J. Pediatr. Surg. 10:9, 1975.

Segal, S.: editor: Manual for the transport of high-risk newborn infants, Vancouver, 1972, Canadian Paediatric Society.

Shaw, W.: The myth of gastroschisis, J. Pediatr. Surg. 10:235, 1975.

Shepard, F. M.: Arango, L. M., and Berry, F. A.: Acid-base response of the newborn to major surgery, Anesth. Analg. (Cleve.) 50:31, 1971.

Silverman, W. A., Sinclair, J. C., and Scopes, J. W.: Regulation of body temperature in pediatric surgery, J. Pediatr. Surg. 1:321, 1966.

Simmons, M. A., Adcock, E. W., Bard, H., and Battaglia, F. C.: Hypernatremia and intracranial hemorrhage in infants, N. Engl. J. Med. 291:5, 1974.

Smith, P. C., and Smith, N. T.: Anaesthetic management of a very premature infant, Br. J. Anaesth. 44:736, 1972.

Smith, R. M.: Temperature monitoring and regulation, Pediatr. Clin. North Am. 16:643, 1969.

Smith, R. M., Crocker, D., and Adams, J. C., Jr.: Anesthetic management of patients during surgery under hyperbaric oxygenation, Anesth. Analg. (Cleve.) 43:766, 1964.

Snyder, W. H., Jr., and Greaney, E. M., Jr.: Congenital diaphragmatic hernia; 77 consecutive cases, Surgery 57:576, 1965.

Soave, F.: Intrathoracic transposition of the transverse colon in complicated oesophageal atresia, Prog. Pediatr. Surg. 4:91, 1972.

Srouji, M. N.: The acid-base status of the surgical neonate on admission to hospital, Surgery 6:958, 1967.

Steward, D. J.: Panel discussion on problems in pediatric anesthesia, Annual Convention American Society of Anesthesiologists, San Francisco, 1977.

Stockman, J. A., Garcia, J. F., and Oski, F. A.: The anemia of prematurity, N. Engl. J. Med. 296:647, 1977.

Stogsdill, W. W., Miller, J. R., and Stoelting, V. K.: Review of anesthesia for tracheoesophageal fistula and anomalies, Anesth. Analg. (Cleve.) 46:1, 1967.

Strauss, J., Adamsons, K., Jr., and James, L. W.: Renal function of normal full-term infants in the first hours of extra-uterine life, Am. J. Obstet. Gynecol. 91:286, 1965.

Strong, M. J.: Anesthetic management of infants under one year of age with congenital heart disease. In Eckenhoff, J. E., editor: Science and practice in anesthesia, Philadelphia, 1965, J. B. Lippincott Co.

Strong, M. J., Keats, A. S., and Cooley, D. A.: Anesthesia for cardiovascular surgery in infancy, Anesthesiology 27:257, 1967.

Sunshine, P., and Lewis, G. B.: Disease of infants. In Katz, J., and Kadis, L. B., editors: Anesthesia and uncommon diseases, Philadelphia, 1973, W. B. Saunders Co.

Swenson, O.: A new surgical procedure for Hirschsprung's disease, Surgery 28:371, 1950.

Swyer, P.: An assessment of artificial respiration in the newborn, report of Fifty-ninth Ross Conference on Pediatric Research, 1969, p. 75.

Talbert, J. L., Karmen, A., Graystone, J. E., and others: Assessment of infant's response to stress, Surgery 61:626, 1967.

Tandon, G. C., Gode, G. R., Kalle, N. R., and others: Anesthetic management for surgical separation of thoracopagus twins, Anesthesiology 33:116, 1970.

Terry, T. L.: Extreme prematurity and fibroblastic overgrowth of persistent vascular sheath behind each crystalline lens. I. Preliminary report, Am. J. Ophthalmol. 25:203, 1942.

Vivori, E., Bush, G. H., and Ireland, J. T.: Tubocurarine requirements and plasma protein concentrations in the newborn infant, Br. J. Anaesth. 46:93, 1974.

Waterston, D. J., Carter, R. E., and Aberdeen, E.: Oesophageal atresia; tracheo-oesophageal fistula; a study of survival of 218 infants, Lancet 1:819, 1962.

Weiss, C.: Does circumcision in the newborn require an anesthetic? Clin. Pediatr. 7:128, 1968.

Welch, K. J.: Abdominal musculature deficiency syndrome. In Ravitch, M. M., Welch, K. J., Benson, C. D., and others, editors: Pediatric surgery, ed. 3, Chicago, 1979, Year Book Medical Publishers, Inc.

Weller, R. M.: Anaesthesia for cystic hygroma in a neonate, Anaesthesia 29:688, 1974.

Whittaker, L. D., Jr., Lynn, H. B., Dawson, B., and Cahves, F.: Hernias of the foramen of Bochdalek in children, Mayo Clin. Proc. 43:580, 1968.

Williams, P. R., and Oh, W.: Effects of radiant warmer on insensible water loss in newborn infants, Am. J. Dis. Child 128:511, 1974.

Wilton, T. N. P.: Anaesthesia for oesophageal surgery in infants and children, Anesth. Analg. (Cleve.) 31:267, 1952.

Wilton, T. N. P., and Wilson, F.: Neonatal anaesthesia, Philadelphia, 1965, F. A. Davis Co.

Wohl, M. E. B., Griscom, N. T., Strieder, D. J., and others: The lung following repair of congenital diaphragmatic hernia, J. Pediatr. 90:405, 1977.

Woolley, M. M.: Comments on symposium; management of the pediatric surgical patient; subject review, Mayo Clin. Proc. 47:654, 1972.

Woolley, M. M.: Congenital posterolateral diaphragmatic hernia, Surg. Clin. North Am. 56:317, 1976.

Yamazaki, T., Naito, H., Nakamura, K., and others: Lactate, pyruvate and excess lactate during ether and halothane anesthesia in infants and children, Anesthesiology 43:410, 1975.

Young, D. G.: Contralateral pneumothorax with congenital diaphragmatic hernia, Br. Med. J. 4:433, 1968.

Zindler, M., and Deming, M. V.: The anesthetic management of infants for the surgical repair of congenital atresia of the esophagus with tracheoesophageal fistula, Anesth. Analg. (Cleve.) 32:180, 1953.

CHAPTER 16

Anesthesia for intrathoracic and cardiac surgery

MARK C. ROGERS and ROBERT M. SMITH

GENERAL PROBLEMS

Infants and children who require thoracic surgery differ in many respects, but certain anesthetic fundamentals are common to all. Any infant, child, or adult whose chest is to be opened deserves scrupulous preoperative preparation with respect to history and physical examination, including chest x-ray films and indicated definitive tests. In addition, it is especially important that they be cleared of all possible foci of infection and be in the best possible state of health. Obstructing tonsils, carious teeth, and recent respiratory infections should be definite contraindications to elective thoracic surgery, as should such underlying conditions as urinary infection and mild anemia.

Special care also must be taken to prepare children emotionally. This means that children definitely should not be rushed through a series of upsetting tests the day before a critical operation but should be admitted to the hospital several days before operation so that they will not be confused, terrified, and exhausted on the morning of surgery.

It may be necessary for the anesthesiologist to make more than one preoperative visit to coax such children into receptive attitudes, to find the most appropriate type of medication to ease their anxiety, and to help reduce parental fears. Children who are to wake up in an oxygen tent or under continued support of a ventilator with assorted nasogastric, endotracheal, chest, and urinary catheters should be gently forewarned and also should be instructed as to the physiotherapy that they will receive. All this should be done without being too explicit, lest a child's preoperative night of rest be strewn with nightmares.

The anesthetic management of these children obviously will demand endotracheal intubation and usually a quiet chest, sometimes absolutely immobile for many minutes. Blood loss may not always require replacement, but any thoracic operation carries enough risk of sudden bleeding to call for routine preparation for transfusion. This means that at least one absolutely reliable infusion must be established. Additional cannulae for infusions, CVP, and arterial blood gas determination are used as indicated for special procedures. Only the stethoscope,

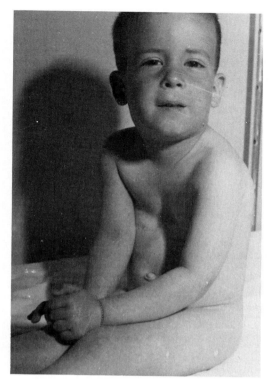

Fig. 16-1. Pectus excavatum deformity becomes most obvious when child is in sitting position.

blood pressure cuff, and thermistor are truly mandatory for all procedures.

In preparing for pediatric thoracic surgical procedures, the anesthesiologist must above all else prepare himself. Whether the child has cystic fibrosis, coarctation of the aorta, neuroblastoma, or endocardial cushion defect or is a 1-pound infant with patent ductus arteriosus (PDA) and respiratory distress syndrome, the variable aspects of respiratory and cardiovascular physiology must be understood if the child is to survive.

ANESTHESIA FOR OPERATIONS ON THE THORAX AND LUNGS

Although cardiovascular anomalies have attracted great interest, several surgical lesions also are seen in the rib cage and lungs of infants from birth onward.

Deformity of the thoracic cage

Pectus excavatum (funnel chest) and pectus carinatum (pigeon breast) consist respectively of concave and convex deformities of the sternum and adjoining ribs and costal cartilages. Sternal concavity that is of moderate degree when a child is lying down or standing appears greatly exaggerated in the sitting position (Fig. 16-1); in severe cases the sternum nearly touches the spine.

In spite of the occurrence of gross deformity of the chest, many years passed before evidence could be produced to show that either cardiac or respiratory function was significantly affected or that surgery was of measurable value. By application of technetium angiocardiography and xenon scans, however, studies of Beiser and associates (1972) and others have demonstrated that in the standing position, patients with relatively mild pectus deformities may have significant reduction of cardiac output and stroke volume and marked alteration of ventilation-perfusion patterns, especially in the left lung; the latter impairment shows definite improvement after surgery.

Early methods of surgical repair often were formidable undertakings involving bone grafts, extensive blood loss, and bilateral pneumothorax, but procedures have since become quite refined, requiring little or no blood replacement and causing only slight operative stress or postoperative discomfort. Three or more hours may be required while the surgeon excises the abnormal sternocostal cartilages and mobilizes the sternum. A series of 827 operations without a death (Welch, in press) attests to the safety of the procedure in experienced hands. Maintenance anesthesia in the first several hundred of these procedures consisted of ether or cyclopropane; the remainder were managed under halothane or intravenous-relaxant combinations. All of these agents evidently were satisfactory for patient and surgeon. In this series, the principal complications were left lower lobe collapse (7%) and pneumothorax (1%). A number of these patients also showed increased tendency to develop mild hyperpyrexia toward the end of operation, a phenomenon that may be related to the response of cartilage to surgical trauma (Folkman, 1978). Such complications have led us to take particular care to monitor both sides of the chest with individual stethoscopes and to pay strict attention to the child's temperature by using a water-circulating mattress and carefully calibrated thermistors with all patients. At termination of operation, the chest is reexamined for the presence of pneumothorax prior to extubation of the trachea. If pneumothorax is suspected, the anesthesiologist expands the lung while the surgeon attempts to close the chest more securely or inserts a chest drainage tube. A chest film is obtained immediately after the child's return to the recovery area and again after a 4- to 6-hour interval.

Diseases of the chest wall, mediastinum, and lungs

Developmental abnormalities of the trachea and bronchi, pulmonary infections, congenital cystic disease of the lungs, and primary or metastatic tumors of the chest wall, mediastinum, and lungs produce an interesting combination of problems. In most of the required operations there will be the expectation of considerable blood loss, interference with airways, alteration of ventilation-perfusion ratios, and the additional hazards of each particular disease.

Children with *congenital cystic disease of the lungs*, like those with diaphragmatic hernia, must not be subjected to increased airway pressure. In cystic disease, such pressure may overdistend the cysts, with resultant occlusion or collapse of remaining airways and alveoli (Ravitch, 1979). While a reasonable desire to retain spontaneous respiration might lead some anesthesiologists to choose the awake intubation technic, the patient's forceful struggling could easily produce more intrathoracic pressure than manual ventilation. On the basis of our experience at The Children's Hospital Medical Center, a quiet inhalation induction with limited ventilatory assistance or the use of relaxants with equally careful avoidance of increased airway pressure would be chosen

rather than the use of awake intubation. One must remember, of course, that following intubation, the danger of forceful inflation will continue until the cystic structures have been excluded from the airflow. During this phase, return to spontaneous respiration is advantageous but not mandatory.

A further consideration in management of children with lung cysts is the possible accumulation of nitrous oxide in the cystic areas, with resultant distension (Eger and Saidman, 1965). While this complication has not been a source of major concern, it can easily be avoided by replacing the nitrous oxide with morphine or other analgesics.

Lobectomy and pneumonectomy

Infants and children show quite remarkable tolerance to loss of functioning lung tissue. If the remaining pulmonary tissues are not diseased, excision of a single lobe will rarely cause any clinical or measurable ventilatory change. Children can often function well following pneumonectomy or excision of both lower lobes.

Investigation of compensatory adaptation to loss of pulmonary tissue by several workers, including Hislop and Reid (1974) and Wohl and associates (1977), has revealed that the remaining lung tissue expands to fill the space left following excision. Such expansion will consist of emphysematous enlargement of existing alveoli rather than any increase in the number of alveoli, as might be expected.

Lobectomy and pneumonectomy, formerly quite usual in the treatment of long-standing bronchiectasis in the presence of profuse suppuration, are rarely performed today. The occasional child undergoing lobectomy for bronchiectasis now is prepared with antibiotics and physiotherapy, and intraoperative secretions are of slight concern.

Excision of segments of lung and chest wall may be necessary in children having metastatic disease. Here the combination of repeated extensive operations, general debility, the effect of antineoplastic agents including the cardiotoxic doxorubicin (Adriamycin) (Rinehart and associates, 1974), and postoperative respiratory impairment through loss of several ribs may produce an extremely sorry picture. However, even these children may show unbelievable powers of endurance and survive.

Perhaps the most tragic cases are the children, often approaching adolescence, with advancing cystic fibrosis whose pulmonary involvement shows enough localization to justify lobectomy or pneumonectomy as a palliative measure.

In a series of 48 operations reported by Schuster and associates (1964), many children showed impressive improvement, but the overall picture still is most depressing. Despite prolonged medical therapy, most of these children, aged 6 months to 21 years, evinced continued loss of vitality, increasing cough and sputum, diffuse pneumonitis, and, as described in Chapter 3, significant reduction of ventilation. Several had undergone operations for other lesions associated with cystic fibrosis, such as nasal polyps and pansinusitis, and a few had developed cor pulmonale. Bronchoscopy had been performed on several patients to remove secretions or blood. Massive hemorrhage is not rare in patients with cystic fibrosis. Present treatment consists of bronchoscopy to locate the area of origin of bleeding followed by arteriography and embolization by injection of bits of Gelfoam (Fellows and associates, in press).

In the preparation of patients for lobectomy, a tracheostomy is established several days before operation to facilitate the clearing of blood and secretions during operation and the early postoperative period.

Preparation for tracheostomy includes full explanation to the patient of what is to be expected. One redeeming factor is that the tracheostomy will be needed for only 5 or 6 days after operation.

Medication for patients with cystic fibrosis should relieve anxiety without depressing the cough reflex or respiratory drive. Atropine should be eliminated, because the resultant thickened secretions and increased airway obstruction may cause severe respiratory distress.

Tracheostomy is performed under halothane-oxygen endotracheal anesthesia. The chief concern is to prevent irritation and coughing during induction and again as the child awakens, when continued violent coughing may produce extensive emphysema. Sedation and generous spraying of the throat with 4% lidocaine are helpful, but the situation is not easily controlled and may be extremely unpleasant for the patient.

Three to five days are allowed for the edges of the tracheostomy wound to heal, after which time lobectomy is performed.

Preparation for lobectomy includes antibiotic therapy (gentamycin and carbenicillin) plus an organized system of physiotherapy, coughing, and suctioning for maximum chest clearance. Adequate sedation without atropine again is in order. Anesthetic induction with the tracheostomy tube in place then is accomplished with thiopental or halothane; nitrous oxide is omitted if oxygenation is impaired.

Positioning a patient for lobectomy has always been a problem in patients with copious pulmonary secretions. Use of bronchial blocking technics or Carlen's double-lumen endotracheal tubes has never been satisfactory, especially in smaller patients. To overcome these difficulties, Schuster has employed the Overholt prone position with excellent success. Before the child is positioned, the tracheostomy tube is removed and replaced by a cuffed endotracheal tube, which will allow easier access and more reliable fixation during the operation. This tube should, above all else, have a straight adapter to allow optimal opportunity for suction throughout the procedure. The child is turned and positioned face down, the head held in neutral position in a posterior fossa headrest and the body tilted head downward at about 10°. This position naturally prevents cross-infection and promotes bilateral drainage into the endotracheal tube where secretions are easily accessible for suctioning. Surgeons who are familiar with this approach find it actually easier to use than the lateral approach, since it facilitates the exposure of hilar structures.

In most of these patients, arterial cannulation is performed following induction so that oxygen saturation can be followed during and after the procedure. Anesthesia has been maintained in our patients with either halothane or intravenous combinations using *d*-tubocurarine. Although both technics provide satisfactory conditions during operation, there is some question as to which promotes more prompt return of cough and spontaneous pulmonary protective responses. Inadequate elimination or reversal of either agent is possible, so the answer more probably relates to the manner of use rather than the agent itself. Since lobectomized patients usually need at least 24 hours of postoperative ventilatory support, the question has less relevance here than in other operations performed on patients with cystic fibrosis.

At the termination of surgery, the patient is placed in the supine position, all available air passages are thoroughly cleared, and the tracheostomy is reestablished for postoperative care. These children often remain in critical condition for several days and deserve the most talented personnel available.

In this period, during which children are unable to speak or communicate and are subjected to the extreme distress of incessant tracheal suctioning plus the pain of coughing and the misery of the disease, the emotional strain must be nearly unbearable. Caretaking personnel should be selected for their sensitivity as well as their knowledge. In particular, to avoid some of the distress of recurrent tracheal suctioning, most nurses and therapists need to be exhorted to hyperoxygenate the child more adequately before suctioning. Furthermore, they should be cautioned against pushing the suction catheter hastily into the trachea, jabbing it up and down forcefully, and then jerking it out. They should be encouraged instead to take 2 extra seconds to introduce it gently, move it up and down an inch, and withdraw it gradually, while the suction still acts to clear remnants left along the way.

Tracheoesophageal fistula and diaphragmatic hernia

Anesthesia for correction of these lesions has been described in Chapter 15.

ANESTHESIA FOR PEDIATRIC CARDIOVASCULAR SURGERY

For intelligent management of anesthesia in the field of pediatric cardiovascular surgery, the anesthesiologist should be aware of the diversity of cardiac defects found in infants and children, their hemodynamic effects and resultant symptoms, the indications for operation, the types of surgery involved, the anesthetic requirements, the specific problems most apt to be encountered, and methods of avoiding them as well as methods of treatment should they occur. Reference is recommended to texts on pediatric cardiology, such as Nadas and Fyler (1972), Rudolph (1974), Moss and associates (1977), and Keith and associates (1978), and information on pediatric cardiac surgery by Gross and associates (1940, 1950, 1970), Castaneda and associates (1974, 1977), and Sade and associates (1977) from this hospital as well as many other sources. The third edition of *Pediatric Surgery* by Ravitch and associates (1979) is especially valuable. Since all the nuances of diagnosis and surgery need not be mastered, an attempt will be made to sort out some of those believed to be of particular interest and importance to the anesthesiologist.

Background

To understand the current problems of anesthetic management in cardiovascular surgery of infants and children, it is helpful to trace the development of this field. An anesthesiology resident of today might find the prospect of anesthetizing a 7-year-old girl for repair of PDA considerably more interesting if he knew the historical background—that in 1938 the ligation of a PDA in a similar 7-year-old girl opened the door to the entire field of congenital cardiac surgery and that it was performed by a determined young surgical resident who was acting against the orders of the chief of surgery! The anesthetic was cyclopropane, administered without endotracheal intubation by a nurse anesthetist.*

*Surgeon: R. E. Gross; anesthetist: B. Lank.

The fortunate survival of this child and successive children after operations for PDA led to the rapid development of procedures for correction of other cardiovascular defects, several of which involved the great vessels rather than the heart itself. These included repair of vascular ring anomalies, also pioneered by Gross (1945), palliative shunts for tetralogy of Fallot (Blalock and Taussig, 1948; Potts and others, 1946), and repair of coarctation of the aorta (Gross, 1950). Two procedures devised at this time for correction of intracardiac defects were the Brock transventricular pulmonic valvotomy and Gross's repair of ostium secundum atrial septal defects (ASD) by means of his atrial well (1953).

At the time these operations were introduced, each one carried an appreciable risk: hemorrhage from a torn ductus arteriosus, hypotension following aortic repair, arrest during Blalock shunt, and many other problems related to the inability to control and monitor anesthesia and blood loss. It was reasonable in the 1930s and 1940s to limit such elective operations to children in relatively good condition. Repair of PDA was not considered advisable in children under 4 years old, while diagnosis of coarctation of the aorta was rarely made in children under 10 or 12 years of age. However, surgical relief of vascular ring was necessary in infants because of airway obstruction, and shunt procedures were performed on infants with tetralogy of Fallot who were critically hypoxemic but who, by present standards, were fairly durable. During the 1950s these procedures became standardized; mortality was virtually eliminated in PDA and coarctation operations and greatly reduced for palliative shunts.

During those first 10 years, little attempt had been made to increase the body's tolerance to hypoxia. Although problems of anesthesia were chiefly limited to maintenance of cardiorespiratory stability during open thoracotomy in the presence of hemodynamic and ventilatory stresses, they were challenging enough at the time, as documented by several early workers (Harmel and Lamont, 1946; McQuiston, 1949; Berger, 1948; Adelman, 1948; Harris, 1950).

The first step in altering body homeostasis was that of McQuiston, reported in 1950, which consisted of cooling children to 35° C while Potts performed his shunts. A wave of interest in surface cooling soon extended its application and led to the first open-heart operations by Lewis and Taufic in 1953. Immersion of patients in ice water and cooling them to 32° C allowed surgeons the 3 minutes necessary to perform pulmonic valvotomy under direct vision or to close ostium secundum ASDs.

Over the next 25 years there was a succession of developments. The anesthetic and physiologic considerations for the early procedures under hypothermia were described by Virtue (1955). After early application of surface cooling, it became evident that its use was restricted by the regular appearance of ventricular fibrillation at temperatures below 30° C. The pump-oxygenator, after years of development, came into clinical use at this time, extending to 30 minutes the 3-minute limitation allowed by surface cooling.

The fact that the heart continues to beat under both hypothermic and bypass technics was a major handicap in intracardiac surgery. Several methods of intentional cardiac arrest were devised, including anoxic arrest by cross-clamping of the aorta, arrest by intracardiac administration of potassium, and later, arrest by electrical induction of ventricular fibrillation.

Application of these methods made it possible to close the larger atrial ostium primum and ventricular septal defects (VSD) and perform total repair of tetralogy of Fallot (Kirklin and others, 1955).

For a brief period, interest in hypothermia receded. It was found, however, that more barriers could be broken down by combining hypothermia with extracorporeal perfusion. That was accomplished by the development of the so-called heat-exchanger (Sealey and others, 1958), the water-circulating device by which the patient's temperature is lowered and raised as desired during bypass.

The permissible time for intracardiac operations had been extended from 30 minutes to 2 hours and subsequently to more than 4 hours, thereby giving surgeons opportunity to correct most of the known cardiac anomalies, except those in young infants.

Despite the fact that the mortality in cardiac anomalies was known to be greatest during the first year of life, such surgery was rarely attempted. The greater risk of surgery and anesthesia were deterrents, but actual mechanical problems of operating inside such small hearts, further obscured by motion, cannulae, and blood, rendered such operations practically impossible. Total occlusion of cardiac inflow without the presence of cannulae was necessary.

Many advances were made under existing conditions, however. Skill and experience enabled Kirklin and DuShane (1961), Cooley and Hallman (1964), Mustard and associates (1964), McGoon and associates (1968), and others to make real progress in infant cardiac surgery in the 1960s and early 1970s. Use of the hyperbaric chamber gave Bernhard and associates (1963, 1966) an early advantage. Although the hyperbaric approach saved or prolonged the lives of many infants, the high cost of the facility and the poor return (3 minutes of operating time) were disappointing. More time and a more practical method were needed for total repair of major defects.

The Japanese team of Horiuchi and associates (1963) produced the key to the present solution. Using ether anesthesia, they were able to achieve profound hypothermia (20° C) by surface cooling, thereby demonstrating that the desired features of unimpeded access to an arrested heart were obtainable for periods of 30 to 45 minutes.

Later modification combining surface cooling and bypass perfusion was worked out by Barratt-Boyes and associates (1971) and was widely adopted (Mohri and others, 1972; Castaneda and others, 1974). Many lifesaving procedures have been devised for neonates, and total repair of tetralogy of Fallot is replacing the prolonged stress of two-stage management previously employed. Many problems remain unsolved, but infant cardiac surgery has gained solid footing and commands center stage.

CURRENT OVERALL APPROACH TO SURGERY FOR CONGENITAL CARDIAC DEFECTS

The general management of children with congenital cardiac defects has become a major institutional undertaking calling for experts in the fields of pediatric cardiology, radiology, anesthesiology, surgery, intensive care nursing, respiratory and physical therapy, and often psychotherapy. Operations for congenital cardiac defects should only be performed where such team organization is present and where several procedures are carried out each week.

Diagnosis is the first step. Accurate anatomic and hemodynamic evaluations are absolute essentials on which surgery must depend. For this it is necessary to have a team of astute cardiologists versed in all technics of electrocardiography, angiography, echocardiography, and all ramifications of cardiac catheterization. Personnel and facilities must be available at all times, for infants born at night frequently need immediate diagnostic investigation (often followed by predawn operation).

Diagnosis of some cardiac defects can be made without elaborate methods. Asymptomatic children with PDA or coarctation of the aorta seldom need cardiac catheterization. To make the delicate distinction between an inoperable hypoplastic left aortic arch and an operable aortic stenosis may be much more difficult, since it requires cardiac catheterization through the vena cava and foramen ovale.

The problem of diagnosis is understood more clearly when one finds that according to such authorities as Taussig (1960), Nadas and Fyler (1972), and Keith and associates (1978), there are over 100 different congenital cardiac anomalies. Table 16-1 shows a list of 29 major defects and their relative incidence as compiled by Nadas and Fyler (1972) at The Children's Hospital Medical Center.

In the subsequent investigation and treatment of these patients, it is helpful to classify

Table 16-1. Postmortem incidence of major congenital cardiac lesions at The Children's Hospital Medical Center, Boston, Mass. (1017 cases, mostly infants and children, in order of frequency)

	Number	Percentage
Tetralogy of Fallot	148	15
Transposition of the great arteries	93	9
Endocardial cushion defect	77	8
Hypoplastic left heart syndrome	64	6
Ventricular septal defect (simple)	61	6
Patent ductus arteriosus (complicated)	56	6
Total anomalous pulmonary venous drainage	52	5
Coarctation of the aorta	50	5
Ventricular septal defect (complicated)	38	4
Aortic stenosis	35	3
Levocardia	34	3
Pulmonary atresia	32	3
Patent ductus arteriosus (simple)	31	3
Tricuspid atresia	29	3
Dextrocardia	28	3
Mitral valve disease	27	3
Truncus arteriosus	25	2
Single ventricle	21	2
Ebstein's disease of the tricuspid valve	20	2
Corrected transposition of the great arteries	16	2
Ventricular septal defect and patent ductus	16	2
Coronary artery anomaly	15	1
Double outlet right ventricle	13	1
Atrial septal defect, secundum type	12	1
Pulmonary stenosis	11	1
Peripheral pulmonary stenosis	5	0.5
Cor triatriatum	4	0.4
Aortic regurgitation	2	0.2
Aorticopulmonary window	2	0.2
TOTAL	1017	100

From Nadas, A. S., and Fyler, D. M.: Pediatric cardiology, ed. 3, Philadelphia, 1972, W. B. Saunders Co.

them according to such features as operability, symptomatology, the presence or absence of cyanosis, or mortality. For the practical use of the anesthesiologist, it seems of advantage first to group the various lesions according to the type of *surgical approach currently employed* (without extracorporeal bypass perfusion [EBP], with EBP, or with EBP and profound hypothermia) and then to classify them further according to *hemodynamic effect* (whether acyanotic or cyanotic), whether the *lesion is extracardiac or intracardiac*, and whether the *operation is corrective or palliative*. Such a classification is attempted opposite.

ANESTHESIOLOGIST'S CLASSIFICATION OF OPERABLE CONGENITAL CARDIAC ANOMALIES
(Surgical approach, hemodynamic effect, extracardiac or intracardiac lesion, corrective or palliative repair)

Cardiac anomalies not requiring open-heart repair
1. Acyanotic patients
   Extracardiac lesions:
   Extracardiac corrective operation:
   Vascular ring anomalies (5)—repair
   Patent ductus arteriosus—division or ligation
   Coarctation of the aorta—excision and anastomosis
   Intracardiac lesions:
   Intracardiac corrective repair: inflow occlusion
   Pulmonic stenosis—Brock valvotomy, open valvotomy
   Aortic stenosis—aortic valvotomy

Extracardiac palliative operation:
  Ventricular septal defect—pulmonary banding
2. Cyanotic patients
  Intracardiac lesions:
    Extracardiac palliative operation:
      Tetralogy of Fallot—Blalock-Taussig, Potts, Waterston (Cooley) shunts

Cardiac anomalies corrected with use of extracorporeal perfusion (patients over 1 year old)

1. Acyanotic patients
  Intracardiac lesions:
    Intracardiac corrective operation:
      Pulmonic stenosis—valvotomy
      Aortic stenosis—valvotomy
      Atrial septal defect, ostium secundum—closure
      Atrial septal defect, ostium primum—closure
      Ventricular septal defect—closure
2. Cyanotic patients
  Intracardiac lesions:
    Intracardiac corrective operation:
      Tetralogy of Fallot—total repair

Defects corrected with use of extracorporeal perfusion and profound hypothermia (patients under 1 year old)

1. Acyanotic patients
  Intracardiac lesions:
    Intracardiac corrective operation:
      Aortic stenosis—valvotomy
      Ventricular septal defect—closure
2. Cyanotic patients
  Intracardiac lesions:
    Intracardiac corrective operation:
      Tetralogy of Fallot—total repair
      d-Transposition of great arteries—Mustard operation
      Total anomalous venous drainage—repair

It should be noted that there are faults in any of the classifications, and several are evident in the one above: (1) Many lesions differ in severity, size, the amount of shunt, or other factors and change the problem considerably. (2) The distinction between acyanotic and cyanotic patients is not always definite. Cyanosis in those having shunts between pulmonary and systemic circulations may vary with changes in pressure relationships. (3) There are many patients who have not only one of the defects listed but several different defects that occur together in complicating combinations, multiplying the difficulties of diagnosis, reducing one's ability to predict the hemodynamic and anesthetic responses, and increasing the risk of operation. In an infant operated on for VSD, the additional presence of a PDA may not be recognized until the VSD has been closed. The combined presence of coarctation of the aorta, bicuspid aortic valve, VSD, and PDA is relatively common, and that of five or six defects is not unusual. The variety of combinations defies classification and frustrates statisticians. (4) Still another problem in classification lies in the rapidly changing picture often presented in congenital cardiac defects, particularly the ductus arteriosus, which may be the only means of survival in newborns with pulmonary atresia but may close off rapidly at any time during the early neonatal period, with fatal results.

Indications and decisions for operation

The cardiologist arrives at his diagnosis by means of history, physical examination, and clinical signs. He also looks at the contours of the heart, vascularity of lung fields, size of shunts and form of the ejection streams, degree of pulmonary hypertension, signs of failure, and oxygen concentrations and pressure gradients in various heart chambers and should produce the correct diagnosis in 90% to 95% of cases. Based on his findings, three decisions may be necessary concerning operation: (1) is operation indicated, (2) what procedure should be used, and (3) when should it be performed?

Indications for operation stem from the physiologic consequences of the cardiac anomalies and, according to Nadas and Fyler (1972), include (1) overwork in terms of systolic or diastolic ventricular overloading, (2) inadequate systemic output, (3) pulmonary hypertension, and (4) arterial desaturation.

There are many instances where the need of operation is obvious and urgent, usually in neonates with congestive heart failure or extreme hypoxia. More frequently the indication is less obvious, and cardiologists present anatomic and hemodynamic findings in consultation with surgeons before decisions are made. While an increasing number of operations are being performed during infancy, many of these are preventive rather than mandatory, forestalling the probable effects of increasing heart strain and hypoxia. In a number of lesions, the defect is not apparent until early childhood. Secundum-type ASDs and coarctation of the aorta often are not diagnosed until the child is 6 or 8 years old, and operations for these defects and PDA serve prophylactic purposes to prevent gradual development of vascular obstruction, pulmonary hypertension, or infective endocarditis.

The bulk of the case load today probably consists of children 2 to 10 years old who have real signs of cardiac failure or hypoxia and are either in trouble or showing the signs of imminent danger. Many are seen who have already had operations and are nearing the end of their ability to function. In the near future, the greater part of cardiac surgery in young patients undoubtedly will consist of primary repair of lesions during infancy.

Anesthesiologist's evaluation of the patient

The anesthesiologist should participate in the preoperative deliberations and when the decision to operate has been made, reevaluate the patient from the standpoint of anesthesia, relating anatomic and hemodynamic data to the probable response to anesthetic management and operation. Although the cardiologist should be expected to know more about the heart, he should not be relied on to estimate the anesthetic risk involved.

Factors to be considered as potentially hazardous in these procedures include preoperative cardiorespiratory failure, patient anxiety, electrolyte disturbances, problems with airway maintenance, and sudden changes in blood pressure or heart rate during induction, followed by shifts in the degree of shunting, problems in output before and after bypass perfusion, blood loss, temperature change, acidosis, and clotting problems. One should know what complications are more apt to arise and which symptoms to look for as an indication of the severity of the situation.

At the outset, it is important to bear in mind that the two outstanding symptoms of congenital cardiac disease are *congestive heart failure* and *cyanosis*. Each congenital lesion has a predominant anatomicophysiologic tendency toward one or the other eventual development: cardiac failure or hypoxia. An understanding of the hemodynamics of different defects clarifies the progression toward either outcome and points to very different signs of increasing risk. It seems reasonable to review the underlying features of both derangements.

Congestive heart failure. The physiologic causes of congestive heart failure include two different categories. In the *first group*, failure is the result of *obstruction to left ventricular output*. A classic example of this is the infant with coarctation of the aorta, in which a congenitally narrowed aorta imposes an additional burden on the heart. Should the ventricle not be able to meet this increased work load, the diastolic pressure rises in the left ventricle and the left atrium. This increased pressure also is reflected in the pulmonary capillaries, where it causes transudation of fluid and pulmonary edema. With aortic stenosis, the same pattern may develop. If the mitral valve is stenotic (mitral stenosis), the increased pressure in the left atrium is transmitted directly to the pulmonary capillaries. When there is severe insufficiency of either the aortic or the mitral valve, there is no obstruction to blood flow, but the new effect may be similar, since the large volume of blood regurgitating to the left ventricle or left atrium results in a similar increase in diastolic pressure. Obstruction on the right side of either the pulmonary or tricuspid valve results in venous engorgement, hepatosplenomegaly, and edema.

The *second group* of congenital cardiac lesions that may lead to congestive failure are those in which there is a *pathologic communication between the pulmonary and systemic circuits* at the level of the atria (ASD), the ventricles (VSD), or the great vessels (PDA).

System-to-pulmonary communication allows blood from the higher pressure systemic circuit to enter the pulmonary circulation (left-to-right shunt). As a result, the pulmonary circuit has an increased blood volume and the left ventricle cannot meet the work demands of an adequate systemic flow plus the large extra pulmonary flow through a VSD or PDA. Here too, the result is congestive heart failure.

Cyanosis. When patients have cyanosis, the most common cause of the underlying systemic desaturation is obstruction of flow to the lungs and a right-to-left shunt. The obstruction to blood flow may be at the level of the pulmonary valve (pulmonic stenosis), in the muscle below the valve (tetralogy of Fallot), or at the tricuspid valve (tricuspid atresia). With the blood flow to the lungs obstructed, pressure increases in the right side of the heart and forces unoxygenated blood across either an ASD or VSD and into the systemic circuit, with resultant cyanosis. It should be pointed out that in the presence of any communication between the pulmonary and systemic circuits, it is actually possible to have right-to-left shunting without any valvular or muscular obstruction to blood flow, since the arterioles in the lungs may hypertrophy and develop an obstruction to pulmonary blood flow, as in pulmonary hypertension.

An alternative mechanism for the production of cyanosis is the situation in which the origin of the great vessels is reversed so that the pulmonary artery arises from the left ventricle and the aorta arises from the right ventricle (transposition of the great vessels). This results in the body having two parallel circulations instead of one continuous circulation. The pulmonary circuit (left atrium to left ventricle to pulmonary artery to pulmonary veins back to left atrium) does not mix with the systemic circuit (right atrium to right ventricle to aorta to systemic veins and back to right atrium). In this way, blood that flows to the lungs for oxygenation does not get to the aorta, and the patient is profoundly cyanotic and cannot survive without the development of some communication.

Specific features in patient evaluation. In addition to having a working understanding of the anatomy and hemodynamics of cardiac defects, the anesthesiologist should know which particular signs provide the most reliable information.

In the patient's history, his *exercise tolerance* often is the best single measure of his ability to tolerate the strain of operation. Before inducing anesthesia, the anesthesiologist should be well informed about whether the patient has the ability, suitable for his age, to sit up, feed himself, walk, attend school regularly, ride a bicycle, and compete physically or whether he is confined to bed. This information is equally valuable whether the child is threatened by heart failure or hypoxemia.

History of previous cardiac operation should be examined thoroughly, concerning both the procedure performed and the child's reaction to it. A second thoracotomy may be expected to involve greater blood loss. Reentering the chest through a median sternotomy has additional danger, for the aorta may have become bound to the sternum and may be torn open as the chest is entered. A Blalock-Taussig shunt will leave the patient without a functioning brachial artery on the side operated on, making that arm useless for blood pressure determination. Total repair of tetralogy following a Potts anastomosis will require total cardiac arrest to take the pulmonary-aortic anastomosis apart without exsanguinating the patient.

As shown on p. 347, other informative items are divided into those pertaining to the degree of cardiac failure or the degree of hypoxic involvement. Among those suggesting increased risk of heart failure, *cardiac enlargement* has been the most to be feared, because the large, flaccid heart is extremely difficult to start after a long period of perfusion. All signs and clues as to digitalis or other therapy for failure, as well as shortness of breath (tachypnea and sweating in infants), hypertension, arrhythmias, and abnormal concentrations of potassium and other electrolytes, should be noted. Infants and children with cyanotic anomalies are judged by their hypoxic "spells," squatting, hypotension, digital clubbing, hemoconcentration, and desaturation of arterial blood. The anesthesiologist should train himself to review the cardiac catheterization data with special regard to measurements of cardiac output and pressures in the various chambers as well as calculation of pulmonary and systemic resistance (Keown, 1966; Nadas and Fyler, 1972; Rudolph, 1974).

FACTORS DETERMINING RELATIVE RISK IN CARDIAC PATIENTS

All patients
Reduction of exercise tolerance

Acyanotic patients
History:
  Heart failure
  Hypertension
  Arrhythmias
Physical examination:
  Retarded growth
  Murmurs
  Cardiac enlargement
  Hypertension
X-ray:
  Heart size and shape
  Increased lung markings
Laboratory:
  Metabolic acidosis
  Serum sodium, potassium elevation or depletion
Cardiac catheterization:
  Increased pulmonary blood flow
  Pulmonary artery hypertension
  Pulmonary vascular obstruction
  Left-to-right shunt (size)
  Outflow obstruction (gradient)
Electrocardiogram
Phonocardiogram
Echocardiogram
Radionuclide

Cyanotic patients
History:
  Squatting
  Spells
  Hypotension
  Previous operations
Physical examination:
  Cyanosis
  Digital clubbing
  Hypotension
  Murmurs
X-ray:
  Heart shape
  Right ventricular enlargement
  Decreased lung markings
Laboratory:
  Reduced Po_2, O_2 saturation; O_2 content $\pm$

Elevated hematocrit
Increased platelets
Cardiac catheterization:
  Right ventricular hypertrophy
  Decreased lung markings
  Right-to-left shunt (size)

ANESTHESIA FOR CARDIOVASCULAR PROCEDURES NOT REQUIRING CARDIOPULMONARY BYPASS TECHNICS

As shown in the classification on p. 343, those anomalies regularly corrected without the use of bypass perfusion are vascular ring, PDA, and coarctation of the aorta.

Pulmonic stenosis and aortic stenosis are corrected under either inflow occlusion or bypass, depending on individual preferences. Prior to the development of the pump-oxygenator, closure of the ostium secundum ASD was performed without bypass, and attempts were made to correct total anomalous pulmonary venous connection (TAPVC) with some success. Palliative procedures include banding of the pulmonary artery for patients with pulmonary hypertension (large VSD, transposition of the great arteries, etc.) and shunt procedures for children with tetralogy of Fallot, pulmonic atresia, and other defects.

The hemodynamic problems presented by these patients differ considerably, but in general, anesthetic management of this group is less complicated than that for patients undergoing bypass perfusion. Those with vascular ring defects, and many with PDA and coarctation, come to operation with little or no cardiovascular symptomatology; the principal problems are thoracotomy and potential blood loss.

Children requiring pulmonary artery banding may be in moderate or marked distress, but the procedure is relatively simple and brief, while valvotomy for either pulmonic or aortic stenosis usually imposes only momentary strain on the patient.

Management includes premedication with individual consideration of each child's state of anxiety as well as his requirement for cardiovascular stability. The combination of pentobarbital, morphine, and atropine has been accepted for years. Morphine appears to be an excellent agent in respect to both the child's psychic response and the lack of effect on the heart, and its use has been extended to infants as young as 6 months of age, with dosages in the range of 0.1 mg/kg. Excitement following pentobarbital and the tachycardia and dry mouth caused by atropine make these agents less than ideal and invite the use of alternatives.

Induction of anesthesia should be carefully managed to avoid excitement, airway obstruction, or rapid changes in cardiac output, especially in children with preexisting failure or hypoxia. For a sleeping child, an inhalation "steal" is optimal. For a fearful child, a 25-gauge needle with a sleep dose of thiopental (2 mg/kg) may be least disturbing. If an intravenous infusion is already in place, it definitely should be used for induction.

The routine of preinduction oxygenation often alarms a child. We prefer to have the child take a few deep breaths to aerate his lungs and then give the thiopental and accomplish denitrogenation after loss of the lid reflex.

There is relatively free choice of agent in most of these cases. Induction with thiopental or nitrous oxide and halothane is usually tolerated if used with caution, and maintenance under 50% N_2O-O_2 mixture with halothane or relaxant should suffice. For cyanotic patients, halothane is avoided to prevent increase in right-to-left shunt. For patients with aortic stenosis, ketamine and pancuronium are avoided to prevent left ventricular strain. The use of morphine during these less severe cases is restricted because they are expected to be extubated at the end of operation and respiration should not be depressed.

Monitors consist of precordial or esophageal stethoscope, blood pressure apparatus (without arterial cannulation), and thermistor. Electrocardiography is of little real value in most of these procedures but is accepted as routine. Measurement of blood loss is indicated. With electrocautery one expects little blood loss, but the anesthesiologist must watch the field, for the danger of sudden, profuse bleeding is always present and if it

should occur, the surgeon might be too engrossed to pass the word on to an inattentive anesthesiologist. One reliable infusion is essential, with an immediately available supply of replacement fluid.

Following induction, the first potential problem comes with the opening of the chest. If the anesthesia is too light, the child may strain and react. If deep enough to tolerate rib spreaders and retraction of the lung, no greater depth will be needed at any time.

The reduction in cardiac output known to occur immediately after opening of the pleura in normal patients (Modell and Milhorn, 1972) has been especially striking in patients with cyanotic heart lesions. To prevent this response one should be sure of adequate blood volume and arterial pressure prior to thoracotomy. Treatment with calcium chloride (10 to 15 mg/kg) has been effective in restoring effective output.

Although mechanical ventilators may be used throughout most of these procedures, expansion of the lung should be controlled by hand as the pleura is opened and again while it is being closed. In addition, when the surgeon is attempting to place sutures in easily torn blood vessels, manual control enables the anesthesiologist to help greatly by immobilizing the entire chest for 3 or 4 seconds with each suture.

In operations where halothane has been used as the principal agent, it is important to reduce or discontinue the agent as soon as closure has begun; otherwise, awakening may be considerably delayed. Relaxants are reversed at the end of the procedure, and as previously noted, patients usually may be extubated on the operating table. Exceptional cases, such as premature infants undergoing PDA ligation and other patients in critical condition, require additional supportive care, as will be described.

Correction of vascular compression of trachea and esophagus (vascular ring)

Anomalies of the aortic arch that may act to compress the trachea and/or the esophagus have been grouped together under the term *vascular ring* (Fig. 16-2). The first five

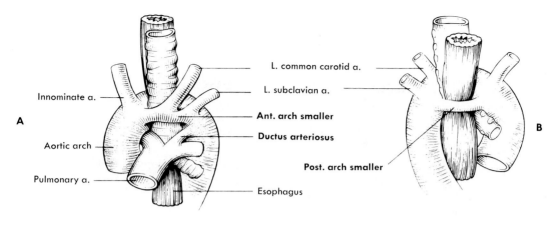

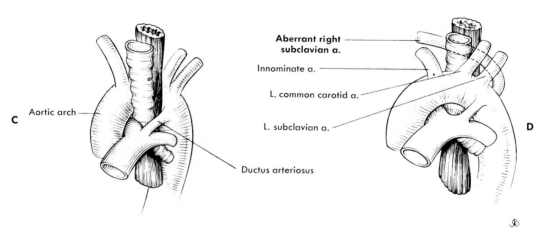

Fig. 16-2. Anomalies of the aortic arch. **A,** Double aortic arch, anterior view, posterior arch larger. **B,** Double aortic arch, posterior view, posterior arch smaller. **C,** Right aortic arch (going behind trachea and esophagus) with left ligamentum arteriosum or ductus arteriosus. **D,** Aberrant right subclavian artery.

types described by Gross in 1945 consisted of double aortic arch, right aortic arch with left ligamentum arteriosum, anomalous right subclavian artery, anomalous innominate artery, and anomalous left common carotid artery. Somewhat more recently, Edwards (1957) compiled over 100 different aortic arch anomalies.

These are vascular anomalies and do not involve any cardiac abnormality, nor do they impede vascular function. Obstruction of trachea or esophagus constitutes the entire clinical problem. Double aortic arch is seen most often; it is a true ring that causes compression of both trachea and esophagus and

consequently is more difficult to repair surgically than other forms (Gross, 1945).

The symptoms of these anomalies usually do not appear until several weeks or months after birth and will vary with the degree of tracheal or esophageal compression. Infants with tracheal compression have stridor, recurrent respiratory infection, and cough, and with severe obstruction they lie in opisthotonus in an attempt to stretch and distend the trachea. Esophageal compression causes difficulty in swallowing as well as postprandial vomiting. Diagnosis is made by demonstration of pulsating constriction by means of tracheoscopy and/or esophagoscopy and con-

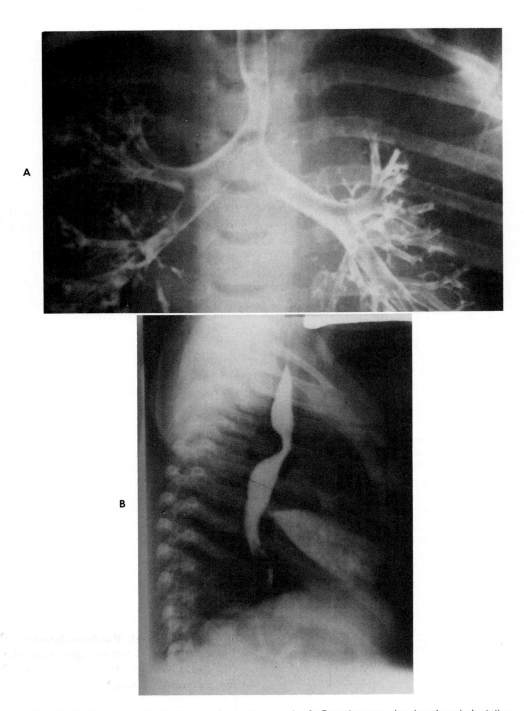

Fig. 16-3. X-rays of patient with vascular arch anomaly. **A,** Bronchogram showing deep indentation in trachea. **B,** Barium swallow showing filling defect of esophagus.

firmed by x-ray evidence of the indentation of the trachea and/or esophagus. Tracheal compression usually occurs just above the carina as shown in Fig. 16-3.

For the anesthesiologist, airway obstruction is the chief problem before, during, and *after* the operation. In addition, sudden hemorrhage can be disastrous during dissection of the great vessels.

For induction of anesthesia, either inhalation or relaxant technics may be used, since the airway obstruction is in the lower trachea and there is no increased danger of glottic spasm or reflex. After the chest is open, surgical manipulation may angulate the trachea and suddenly block ventilation. It is possible to prevent this by inserting the endotracheal tube beyond the area of tracheal constriction. In so doing, however, one is apt to pass the tip of the tube beyond the carina, thereby shutting off exchange to the left lung. To avoid this situation, it is advisable to cut an extra hole 1.5 to 2 cm above the tip of the endotracheal tube on the left-hand side, so that gases can reach the left main bronchus. However, one should avoid, if at all possible, passing the tube beyond the constriction, since, as reported by Wetchler and McQuiston (1956), this narrowed area may become irritated and edematous and lead to fatal postoperative edema, the constriction being too low to be relieved by tracheostomy.

During the course of the operation, the anesthesiologist must watch the surgical field continuously. Pressure of retractors and instruments may compress the heart, lungs, or trachea, and it is frequently necessary to have the surgeon back away quickly, simply to keep the infant alive. In the dissection of major vessels there is the ever present danger of sudden hemorrhage. The anesthesiologist should be in a position to see this the moment it occurs and also should watch the field in order to estimate the loss from incidental bleeding.

At the end of the operation, extubation may be accompanied by serious respiratory obstruction. It is to be remembered that the trachea does not resume a normal shape as soon as the compression is relieved, for the tracheal rings have become deformed and will require time to regain their normal shape. The airway is improved at operation, but obstruction may continue to be critical.

Extubation should be delayed until full respiratory power has returned but not so long that the child irritates the trachea further by forceful coughing and bucking. After the operation the child is treated with oxygen and humidity to minimize the danger of tracheitis. Steroids, in the form of dexamethasone (Decadron), 0.5 mg/kg, may be advisable if additional treatment is needed.

Patent ductus arteriosus

Management of the child undergoing division of an asymptomatic PDA offers very few problems to the anesthesiologist. However, the patent ductus stands historically and physiologically as the starting point in the understanding of correctable cardiac anomalies. Furthermore, its management in certain complicated situations, especially in the premature infant, presents problems of major concern that are being encountered with increasing frequency. Ongoing investigation of the physiology of spontaneous and induced closure of the ductus, especially that of Rudolph (1970, 1974), adds further to the interest of the lesion.

The ductus arteriosus is a normal fetal shunt from the pulmonary artery to the aorta (Fig. 16-4). Anatomic closure normally occurs in the first few hours of extrauterine life, followed by histologic closure in the second or third week (Cassels, 1966; Rudolph, 1974). Failure of the normal obliterative process allows blood to flow between systemic and pulmonary circulations. With increasing left ventricular preponderance, a continuous flow from aorta to pulmonary artery is established, producing the characteristic "machinery" murmur.

In the young child, the *hemodynamic effect* of the PDA is a left-to-right shunt that acts as continous run-off from the systemic to the pulmonic system (Nadas and Fyler, 1972). During systole a forceful contraction maintains normal arterial pressure, but during diastole the free escape of blood through

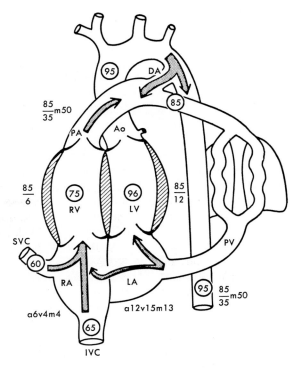

Fig. 16-4. Large patent ductus arteriosus. Course of the circulation, oxygen saturation data *(in circles)*, and pressures in the heart and great vessels in an infant 3 months old. (Reproduced with permission from Rudolph, A. M.: Congenital diseases of the heart. Copyright © 1974 by Year Book Medical Publishers, Inc., Chicago.)

the ductus causes sudden reduction of resistance and consequently an abnormally low diastolic pressure.

The shunt produces important effects on the lungs as well as the heart. An abnormal pattern of flow is established whereby arterial blood is pumped out of the left ventricle into the aortic arch and then much of it is shunted through the ductus back into the pulmonary artery and to the lungs and left heart again, thus being recirculated through the lungs without having reached the tissues. Not only is this obviously inefficient, but the amount of blood flowing through the lungs is significantly increased, pulmonic flow occasionally being three times the systemic flow.

The ratio of pulmonary flow to systemic flow may be estimated by cardiac catheterization. Ratios of less than 2:1 are considered small, those between 2:1 and 3:1 moderate, and those over 3:1 large. Pulmonary engorgement and the pulsation of enlarged pulmonary arteries known as "hilar dance" can be seen by fluoroscopy and usually give sufficient information without recourse to cardiac catheterization.

The effect of PDA on the heart is to place increased strain on the left ventricle, often initiating cardiac failure and death in early infancy and seriously overworking the hearts of females during pregnancy.

While some children show no obvious symptoms, operation is generally believed to be indicated in every patient found to have PDA. In addition to retarded bodily development, more serious effects consist of pulmonary hypertension, which often recedes after operation, and pulmonary vascular obstructive disease (PVOD). Although less frequently encountered, this is a more serious development that is not usually affected by operative closure of the ductus (Edwards, 1957). As shown on p. 353, these complications, as well as infective endocarditis and aneurysm formation, are all considered to be indications for surgery.

INDICATIONS FOR LIGATION OR DIVISION OF PDA

Urgent

Congestive heart failure in infancy, with respiratory distress syndrome, or with pregnancy in later life

Therapeutic

Retarded growth
Pulmonary artery hypertension

Prophylactic

Presence of the lesion
Pulmonary vascular obstructive disease
Infective endocarditis
Aneurysm formation

Diagnosis of PDA can usually be made by auscultation of the murmur and by observation of the wide pulse pressure. Added confirmation is made by x-ray film and fluoroscopy of lung fields. One should remember that the loudest murmur is caused by a medium-sized shunt. When the shunt is very large and allows free flow of blood, the decreased intensity of the murmur can be dangerously misleading. Cyanosis, of course, is not seen in PDA unless excessive pulmonary artery pressure causes reversal of flow through the ductus, in which case cyanosis will be seen only in the lower trunk and legs.

Surgical treatment of PDA involves division of the ductus and suturing of the divided ends, thereby producing normal vascular anatomy. When there are major hazards, as when one is treating sick premature infants, it may be preferable to ligate the ductus rather than take the time to divide and suture it. This situation is described later.

Unless there are such complicating factors, children should tolerate the procedure extremely well and show no side effects. Mortality has been reduced to less than 1%.

Anesthetic management. The anesthesiologist's preoperative evaluation of the child with PDA should focus on the child's general physical and emotional readiness for the procedure and on the extent of the lesion itself. Having in mind that its major hazards are related to increased pulmonary flow and left ventricular failure, one first notes the child's

overall activity capacity and then goes on to growth, heart size, character and intensity of murmur, pulse pressure, heart rate, and history of cardiac failure or digitalis therapy. An estimation of the shunt, including x-ray and fluoroscopic examination for evaluation of pulmonary hypertension in questionable or complicated cases, should be part of the cardiologist's workup.

Left-to-right pulmonary shunts approaching a 3:1 pulmonary-systemic flow ratio may produce pulmonary artery hypertension (PAH). In situations involving sudden increase of PAH, clamping the ductus may be followed by rapid development of right-heart failure and death.

Under normal conditions, the child is given average amounts of barbiturate and morphine for premedication, because these children rarely have been sick enough to develop the emotional sensitivity often seen in those with more restrictive lesions. Atropine is used also but preferably delayed until after induction of anesthesia.

There are few restrictions on technic or agent. Circle or adapted T-systems, anesthetic induction with nitrous oxide or intravenous agents, oral endotracheal intubation, and maintenance with halothane or nitrous oxide–relaxant combination are all acceptable. The surgeon's chief requisites are a moderately quiet diaphragm at all times and complete apnea when sutures are placed in the divided ductus.

The anesthesiologist may notice that a loud murmur heard before anesthesia has completely disappeared following induction and intubation. This probably is because of increased pulmonary artery pressure and reduction of systemic/pulmonic gradient. Monitors required are stethoscope, blood pressure cuff, and thermometer. ECG adds little, but failure to use it draws criticism from inexperienced bystanders. One reliable intravenous line is mandatory. A central venous line is unnecessary unless the child has shown signs of cardiac failure, and arterial cannulation is rarely justified. Intubation may be performed with halothane or relaxant, because the attendant reduction of blood

353

pressure is easily tolerated by these children.

Following induction, intubation, and placement of monitors, the child is positioned on his right side, lying at a 45° tilt or in a true lateral position, for anterolateral or lateral thoracotomy. Before any thoracotomy, blood should be immediately available. The first upsetting incident during thoracotomy is apt to occur when the surgeon opens the chest, spreads the ribs, and retracts the lungs. Any or all of these maneuvers may provoke active bucking unless the child is comparatively well relaxed. For this reason, the anesthesiologist should be fully aware when the chest is about to be opened and should warn the surgeon if the child is not ready. If the child tolerates this stimulation without reacting, the anesthesiologist may be reassured, for the child will need no greater depth of anesthesia throughout the remainder of the operation.

The retraction of the lung necessary for performance of the operation usually involves appreciable restriction of ventilation. To ensure adequate exchange, the anesthesiologist must be able to hear satisfactory breath sounds in the contralateral lung and to visualize the degree of expansion in the exposed lung. In spite of surgical retraction, the exposed lung should be inflated to at least 30% of capacity with each breath and to full expansion every 15 minutes or as indicated.

To expose the ductus arteriosus, the vagus nerve is followed to the origin of the recurrent laryngeal nerve, which loops underneath the ductus. Although manipulation of the vagus nerve rarely causes any response during this operation, the laryngeal nerve is easily damaged, causing prolonged hoarseness.

During dissection of the ductus, and especially during its division and suturing, a quiet field is mandatory. Total control of respiration, whether by use of halothane or relaxant, and manual bag compression allow one to keep the chest motionless during the placement of each suture and to ventilate before placement of the next.

Prior to clamping of the ductus, pulse and blood pressure usually remain stable. When the ductus is occluded, there often is an abrupt elevation of diastolic pressure (Fig. 16-5), although this does not always occur.

The anesthesiologist can be of additional value at the time the ductus is ligated or clamped. The murmur of the ductus should be clearly audible prior to its occlusion. If a murmur is still audible after placement of the clamps, it suggests that the wrong vessel has been occluded. This could be a grave mistake but is understandable with many of the complicated anomalies. If noticed promptly, it should be easily corrected.

Suturing of the divided ends of the ductus may require 8 or 10 minutes. Immediately thereafter comes the moment of truth when the clamps are removed, exposing the adequacy of the sutures. Any bleeding will require more suturing, continued absolute diaphragmatic control, and occasionally the rapid administration of blood.

As previously mentioned, prompt awakening at termination of operation is desirable after simpler procedures, and halothane should be reduced at the time of pleural closure. It is preferable to wait until the last suture is placed before reversing muscle relaxants, however, since premature arousal is upsetting to all concerned.

Following careful tracheal toilet, the chest tube is clamped and the child is moved to the recovery area. He is routinely placed in an oxygen tent with FI_{O_2} of 0.4 or 0.5, though it is seldom actually necessary.

There are two dangers characteristic of this operation. Sudden hemorrhage, especially from tearing of the ductus, is always possible. Though a rare occurrence, it may be extremely difficult to control and then will require rapid infusion of large quantities of blood.

The danger of overinfusion is more subtle and more frequently experienced. Since the pulmonary circulation of patients with PDA is considerably increased, clamping of the ductus and subsequent equalization of the systemic and pulmonary volumes results in an appreciable shift of blood to the systemic side, thereby actually simulating a transfu-

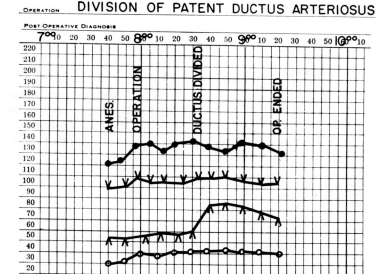

Fig. 16-5. Anesthesia chart of a 4-year-old child during division of patent ductus arteriosus. Sharp rise in diastolic pressure is a characteristic response to occlusion of ductus shunt.

sion. Thus, one should administer all fluids sparingly, preferably not more than 2 or 3 ml/kg/hr. Although blood should be prepared and ready for emergency use, none should be required in uncomplicated procedures. (One should bear in mind the study of Barr and Davenport [1963] that showed greater blood loss in closure of colostomy than in ductus arteriosus repair.)

Patent ductus arteriosus in full-term and premature infants

If a full-term infant has a ductus arteriosus of normal size that remains open, it should be tolerated well, the only sign being the characteristic murmur (Nadas, 1976).

If a full-term infant has a large ductus that remains open, the increased flow to pulmonary vessels may cause pulmonary hypertension and right heart failure. Surgical ligation of the ductus is now advised for these infants, since excellent results have been reported by several groups (Edmunds and others, 1973; Zachman and others, 1974; Sade and Castaneda, 1976).

The situation that we now see with increasing frequency is that of an 800- to 1200-gram premature infant who has a patent ductus plus idiopathic respiratory distress syndrome (IRDS) (Fig. 16-6). Ligation of the ductus is indicated to shorten the course of the IRDS and reduce complications. According to Sade and associates (1977), however, recovery of these infants is often marked by initial improvement while the right-to-left shunt is still predominant, but as systemic pressure exceeds pulmonic pressure and reverses the direction of the shunt, blood gas levels deteriorate for a period before showing recovery, and mortality still is appreciable. Optimum time for operation is believed to be before IRDS reaches a critical stage, but the problem remains unsettled.

The operation involved in any of these situations is relatively simple, requiring only 15 to 20 minutes to perform. The complicated business of detaching monitors and transporting these sick infants from nursery to operating room and back can be more of an undertaking than the operation and has

355

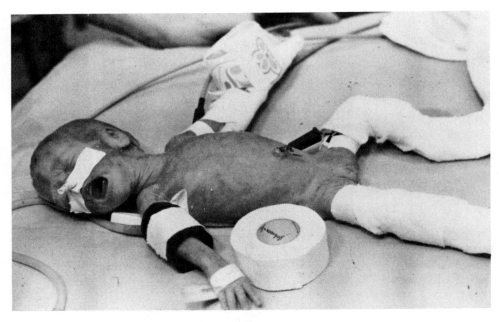

Fig. 16-6. A 900-gram premature infant with respiratory distress syndrome and patent ductus arteriosus (lying beside a 1-inch roll of tape).

been avoided by some who perform the procedure in the nursery (Edmunds and associates, 1973).

Anesthetic management of full-term infants has much in common with that of premature infants. Preparation may require digitalization, correction of fluid and electrolyte imbalances, chest and abdominal x-ray films, vitamin K, and warming, in addition to preliminary cardiac catheterization. Stethoscope, blood pressure cuff and Doppler monitor, thermometer, ECG, and one intravenous cannula are applied, after which intubation is performed without anesthesia. Oxygen is administered with dual concern for sufficient oxygen and avoidance of damage to lungs and eyes.

For the operation, a 50% nitrous oxide–oxygen mixture with atropine (0.1 mg) and *d*-tubocurarine or metocurine should suffice. Humidified gases, a small stockinette hat, and maximal covering of limbs and other exposed parts contribute to the infant's warmth and viability. An arterial line may have been established prior to operation. If so, samples may be taken for determination of blood gases, but care must be taken to replace withdrawn blood with accuracy.

The full-term infant will suffer primarily from congestive failure, and the premature infant from IRDS, but both will show definite reduction of pulmonary compliance. Although excessive ventilatory assistance will cause increased pulmonary pressure, some assistance may be necessary to provide adequate exchange.

Adequacy of ventilation during recovery may be as difficult to provide as adequacy of circulation following cardiac surgery in infants. Hatch and associates (1973), Stewart and associates (1973), Downes and associates (1970), and Gregory and associates (1975) agree on the value of positive pressure respiration in these patients. While one must individualize therapy, Gregory and associates recommend the use of continuous positive airway pressure (CPAP), or spontaneous breathing against a positive end-expiratory pressure, citing evidence of increasing FRC by 35% in cyanotic and 33% in acyanotic infants. In the very small premature infant this becomes particularly important.

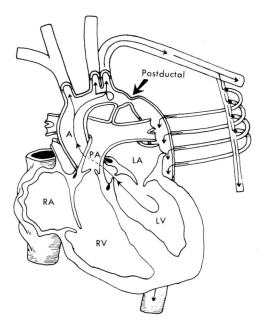

Fig. 16-7. Coarctation of the aorta (postductal type). Obstruction of the descending aorta sends collateral circulation through subclavian, internal mammary, and intercostal arteries to regain distal aortic segment.

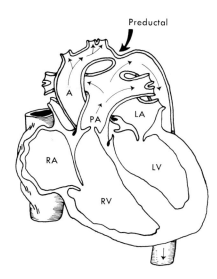

Fig. 16-8. Preductal coarctation with a patent ductus arteriosus entering the aorta distal to the coarctation.

The ductus arteriosus continues to be a center of interest. The demonstration of pharmacologic control of the ductus has been an important new development. The use of prostaglandin E to maintain patency of the ductus, as noted by Coceani and Olley (1973), and the use of indomethacin to close the ductus, as reported by Heymann and Rudolph (1976), Friedman and associates (1976), and Rudolph and Heymann (1977) have already been put into clinical practice with good results.

Still another modification has been the injection of the ductus with formalin to prevent it from closing when the survival of an infant with pulmonary atresia depends on its' remaining open.

Coarctation of the aorta

Although several forms of coarctation of the aorta exist, that termed simple, postductal, or "adult" type is most frequently seen. It consists of a constriction of the aorta that may occur at any level but in 98% of cases oc-

curs in the first part of the descending aorta. Since the coarctation or constriction usually causes almost total obliteration of the aortic lumen, survival depends on collateral circulation. In the simple postductal coarctation, the ductus arteriosus is occluded and arterial blood of the entire body is pumped by the left ventricle to the aortic arch, where it supplies head and arms, and then, meeting the obstructing coarctation, detours via subclavian and internal mammary arteries to be shunted through intercostal arteries back into the peripheral aorta and thence to the lower trunk and legs (Fig. 16-7).

In contrast to this, the circulation in patients with preductal coarctation has dual origin; the left ventricle supplies only the aortic arch, head, and upper limbs, while the right ventricle pumps blood via the ductus arteriosus, which has remained open, into the descending aorta, lower body, and legs (Fig. 16-8). Although the latter form is termed the "infant" type, it does not preclude survival.

Simple coarctation may cause congestive heart failure in early infancy but rarely produces any overt signs between 2 and 12 or more years of age. The obstruction of aortic

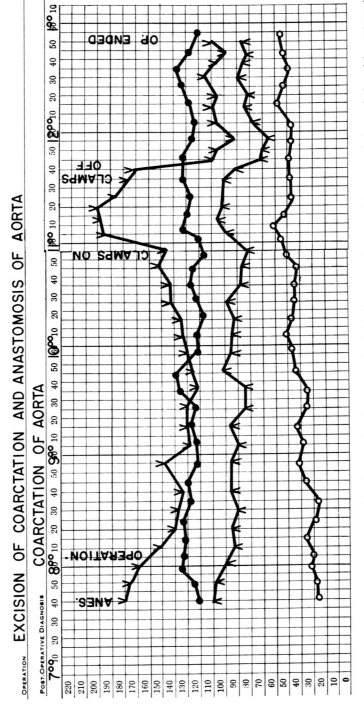

Fig. 16-9. Anesthesia chart during correction of coarctation of the aorta, showing typical sharp rise in arterial pressure during occlusion of the aorta and subclavian artery.

heart failure during the first weeks of life. This is a common cause of death in infancy. Cardiac catheterization is carried out to determine whether the lesion is the simple postductal or the complicated preductal form. Infants with simple coarctation are first given digitalis for control of cardiac failure, and they are only operated on if unresponsive to medical therapy. For these infants, nitrous oxide–relaxant technics have provided more cardiac stability than halogenated agents, and we should consider ketamine to be contraindicated in the presence of outflow obstruction. Operation requires finesse, but there is little blood loss, and cross-clamping of the aorta seldom causes obvious pressure change as in older patients, possibly because of greater expansibility of the vasculature.

Postductal coarctation often appears in association with aortic or mitral obstructive lesions, which do not add excessive morbidity.

The preductal, or infant, type of coarctation has been more difficult to correct, in part because of the high incidence of major defects accompanying it, including hypoplastic left heart, hypoplastic aortic arch, and VSD (Keith and others, 1978). Preoperative reduction of ductal flow by use of indomethacin has been helpful, and bypass perfusion with hypothermic arrest has been necessary in some cases where the situation was complicated by the additional presence of VSD.

Aortic stenosis

Congenital aortic stenosis may be due to obstruction above, below, or at the aortic valve, producing congestive failure in infants and chest pain, fainting, left ventricular hypertrophy, and occasionally sudden unexpected death in older children. Indications for operation are cardiac enlargement and a pressure gradient of 100 mm Hg or more, regardless of symptoms, which may not be indicative of the patient's condition (Bahnson, 1979).

For incision and dilation of valvar stenosis, 1 to 2 minutes may suffice, but subvalvar and supravalvar stenosis may require more time for patching of a stenotic area or for resection of a subaortic membrane.

Because of aortic obstruction, anesthesia is planned to avoid tachycardia, hypertension, and inotropic responses; thus, the use of atropine, ketamine, and pancuronium is reduced or omitted. As noted by Hansen (1977), these patients have increased tendency to develop arrhythmias and more frequently become hypotensive under halothane. Consequently, our approach has been to begin anesthesia with small doses of morphine (0.1 mg/kg) and thiopental (1 to 2 mg/kg) and follow with nitrous oxide, oxygen, and curare for maintenance.

Aortic valvotomy calls for more precision than does pulmonic valvotomy, and there is greater tendency to use bypass perfusion. However, as noted by Sade and associates (1977), inflow occlusion is adequate in many situations.

Pulmonic stenosis

In its pure form with intact ventricular septum, pulmonic stenosis (PS) can be critical in small infants, with great right ventricular enlargement (Fig. 16-10) and rapidly progressing failure. PS has many variants, however, and strictures not precisely at the valvar level offer more difficulty. Hence, catheterization may be necessary to delineate the exact lesion and to measure pressures.

Right ventricular pressures of 150 to 200 mm Hg obviously will equal or exceed systemic pressures, with corresponding effects. Operation is considered to be indicated when right ventricular pressures exceed 75 to 80 mm Hg and mandatory when they exceed 150 mm Hg (Mustard, 1969).

Cyanosis seldom is evident in milder cases, and right ventricular hypertrophy without cyanosis is practically pathognomonic of PS. Peripheral cyanosis can occur as a result of prolonged circulation time and oxygen depletion. Generalized cyanosis does not occur unless there is a septal defect or the infant develops failure, with right-to-left shunt through a patent foramen ovale.

In the infant with marked cardiac enlargement, valvotomy is considered imperative to

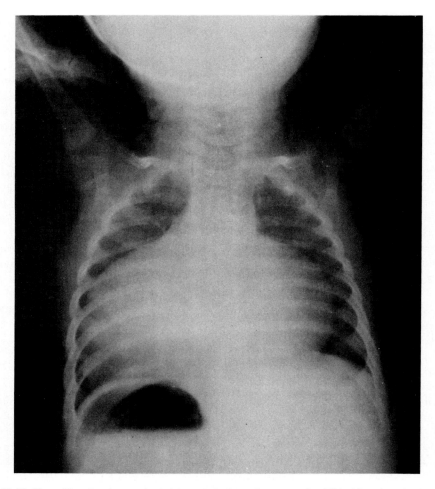

Fig. 16-10. X-ray film showing marked right ventricular enlargement in child with pulmonic stenosis.

prevent rapid succession of failure and death. In older children, progression of right ventricular overload is more gradual, hypertrophy less marked, and cyanosis rarely seen; these children come to operation in near normal condition.

Although operation may be performed as an emergency procedure in infants, pulmonic valvotomy at any age is one of the simplest of the cardiac operations and one of the most successful. Several operative approaches have been used, each requiring very little time (½ to 2 minutes) for actual valvotomy. The Brock transventricular valvotomy was quick but inaccurate and often

brought sudden bursts of blood loss. At present, bypass perfusion is chosen by those preferring more time, but PS is the single cardiac defect for which inflow occlusion seems particularly suited, combining adequate conditions with minimal hazard.

Anesthetic management for both infant and child should not add to the work of the right ventricle, whether by excitement, pharmacologic stimulation, or hypoxia. Thus, moderate premedication and use of agents that avoid excessive inotropism are indicated. When inflow occlusion is employed, air embolism may be a threat, but the near-zero mortality is evidence of the overall safety of the procedure. These patients should react promptly after operation and tolerate extubation on the operating table.

Pulmonary atresia

Pulmonary atresia is quite different from PS. Fortunately it is less common, its incidence being approximately one-tenth that of PS. Pulmonary atresia may occur with intact ventricular septum or with VSD. Infants born with *pulmonary atresia with intact ventricular septum* depend on the patency of the ductus arteriosus for survival; consequently, most die soon after birth unless operated on, and even then, mortality is high, for operation requires either difficult patch graft of the pulmonary artery or construction of a bifurcated tubular graft from right ventricle to distal pulmonary artery.

These infants are severely cyanotic and hypoxic and obviously require prolonged bypass perfusion or deep hypothermia. While tachycardia is to be avoided, cardiovascular support and adequate ventricular action must be maintained. We have used small increments of morphine, with nondepolarizing muscle relaxants, with minimal problems. Monitoring atrial pressures postoperatively has been valuable, and patients are supported on ventilatory assist until stable.

Pulmonary atresia with VSD includes several malformations having no direct connection between right ventricle and pulmonary circulation. Shunts allow survival of these infants, but intricate repairs are necessary to achieve a reasonable end product. This area is in a developmental stage, neither surgery nor anesthesia having become well established. The patients are cyanotic, the operation is complex, and bypass perfusion is definitely necessary for those thus far attempted.

Tetralogy of Fallot

Tetralogy of Fallot (TOF) was classified as the most common type of cyanotic heart disease by Taussig (1960). Although it is only one of several varieties of PS, the remarkable frequency of incidence makes it stand out as one of the best known of congenital anomalies.

The defects that make up the tetrad are PS, dextroposition of the aorta or overriding aorta, VSD, and right ventricular hypertrophy (Fig. 16-11). The right ventricular hypertrophy would appear to be a result of the other lesions rather than an independent defect.

The hemodynamic effect of these defects is reduction of pulmonary flow and a right-to-left shunt, which varies with the anatomic degree of aortic overriding and with the pressure variations in pulmonic and systemic circulations. The course of circulating blood is altered in that much of the blood returning to the right atrium and right ventricle is denied entrance to the pulmonary artery and passes through the VSD into the aorta and out to the tissues again, without passing through the lungs. The obvious result is hypoxemia, which is manifested in relation to the severity of the derangement.

With marked pulmonary stenosis, aortic overriding, and a large right-to-left shunt, Pa_{O_2} may fall as low as 15 mm Hg, with O_2 saturation at 25%. To compensate for this hypoxia, there is increased red blood cell production, the hematocrit often rising to 60% or 70% and occasionally as high as 90%. With this polycythemia there is a corresponding increase in total O_2 content. Of greater value to the patient is a shift of the O_2 dissociation curve to the right and an increase in 2,3-DPG, which facilitates O_2 dissociation at the tissue level. Although the bone marrow is stimulated to produce more red cells, platelets are significantly reduced, resulting in some tendency toward increased bleeding. The hemoconcentration produces greater difficulty, however, causing thrombosis and abscess formation, particularly in cerebral tissues.

Cyanosis is the most prominent sign in many patients, but with milder degrees of PS and aortic overriding, cyanosis may be mild or absent. These children are often labeled "pink tets," while those having severe PS and aortic overriding are the more

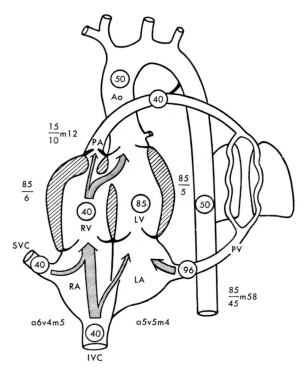

Fig. 16-11. Ventricular septal defect with severe obstruction to right ventricular outflow (tetralogy of Fallot). Course of the circulation, oxygen saturations *(in circles)*, and pressures are shown in an infant after the ductus arteriosus had closed. (Reproduced with permission from Rudolph, A. M.: Congenital diseases of the heart. Copyright © 1974 by Year Book Medical Publishers, Inc., Chicago.)

common "blue tets." Other clinical findings vary in similar fashion.

Clinical signs of TOF may not appear for several weeks after birth but become well developed in the first year, with increasing cyanosis, slow weight gain, and exercise intolerance. The typical squatting of children with TOF occurs mostly between the ages of 2 and 4 or 5 years. During infancy the outstanding sign of this syndrome consists of "spells," or periods of acute hypoxia with fainting, believed to be due to infundibular spasm.* Digital clubbing appears more gradually but may become marked during adolescence. A child's exercise tolerance is poor, because right ventricular output is fixed by the narrowed orifice of the pulmonary artery.

*The infundibulum, or conus, forms a funnel below the pulmonic valve, through which blood must pass to enter the pulmonary artery. Spasm or contraction is believed to be stimulated by effort, excitement, stress, or hypoxia and to be relieved by propranolol or morphine.

Cardiac output can be increased to some extent by speeding the heart, but the usual ability to increase stroke volume in response to increased oxygen demands is lost, and exercise usually produces further reduction of Pa_{O_2}.

X-ray films of the lungs of children with TOF show underperfused tissue and the characteristic sabot-shaped heart; lack of pulmonary artery shadow and upward tilting of the apex by the large right ventricle give it the shape of the wooden peasant shoe.

Several operations may be performed for TOF. Palliative procedures first developed consisted of the Blalock-Taussig anastomosis, whereby one subclavian artery was dissected out nearly to the axilla, transected, and brought down to form an end-to-side anastomosis with the ipsilateral pulmonary artery, as described in 1948, and the Potts side-to-side anastomosis of pulmonary artery to descending aorta (1946). With improved open-heart technics, primary repair is now preferred in most cases. The Blalock shunt frequently became thrombosed, while the Potts shunt, if 2 mm too large, could cause cardiac failure, and both types of shunt caused unequal flow rates in the two lungs, with consequent problems. Since patients frequently are encountered who have had these repairs, it is important to know that the Potts procedure, although considerably easier to perform, offers far greater risk if the patient returns for complete repair. To close the pulmonary artery–aortic shunt, circulatory flow must be totally arrested.

Since both operations are difficult in small infants, a central shunt (Waterston or Cooley procedure) is preferable as a palliative procedure. In this operation the right pulmonary artery is anastomosed to the ascending aorta.

Following any temporizing procedure, the child usually faces continued physiologic restrictions and generally may expect eventual total repair. Consequently, there is increasing preference for total repair during infancy. These procedures obviously require the application of bypass technics.

Anesthetic management. Anesthetic management is of particular importance for patients undergoing shunt procedures. Hypotension, hypoxia, and hemoconcentration constitute major threats at several different stages of the operation.

The necessity for maintaining fluid intake before operation has been mentioned. Premedication is also more of a problem than usual, for these children are both apprehensive and delicate. Because oxygen saturation is 20% to 30%, either excitement or respiratory depression may initiate extreme hypoxia at the outset. Barbiturates must be used with caution in patients with TOF, but morphine is well tolerated and helps prevent infundibular spasm and right-to-left shunting.

Since these infants should have infusions previously established, premedication can be managed by small intravenous increments of morphine (0.05 mg/kg) after they are 6 months old. Medication for younger infants should be highly individualized, if given at all.

Blood pressure should be measured carefully prior to induction, for this must be followed with accuracy at all times. Pressure cuff and Doppler sensor may be all that is necessary. Before a Blalock shunt, one naturally should place the cuff on the arm that will not be affected by interruption of the subclavian artery. If previous shunts have been performed, it may be necessary to use a leg for blood pressure measurement.

Other monitors for these procedures include precordial or esophageal stethoscope, thermometer, ECG, and frequently CVP measurement. Blood loss rarely is a problem, and replacement with plasma usually serves as the principal supportive measure.

Anesthetic induction of hypoxic, hypotensive patients with right-to-left shunts holds several hazards. Any reduction of left ventricular pressure or decrease in peripheral resistance will increase the right-to-left shunt. Reduction of cardiac output will reduce both systemic and pulmonary arterial pressures, and all factors will act to decrease oxygenation. In addition, presence of the shunt alters the action of the drugs used. Inhalation agents, especially those of low solubility, require more time to act. Intravenous agents, on the other hand, cross the ventricular defect and reach the brain more quickly than in normal patients.

Because of its cardiovascular supportive action, cyclopropane was popular among such early workers as Lank, Berger (1948), Harmel and Lamont (1946), and McQuiston (1949). The prolonged induction time was evident but was not a major problem. Ketamine recently has been used for induction and has the double advantage of supporting cardiac output and systemic resistance while being an intravenous agent. Its superiority for shunt procedures has been attested to by Radnay and associates (1974) but questioned by Levin and associates (1975), who found it of little advantage over halothane-relaxant combinations. When possible, we prefer induction with intravenous agents, intubation with succinylcholine, and maintenance with

N_2O and d-tubocurarine or metocurine.

A sharp fall in blood pressure following opening of the chest has been a frequent occurrence, especially when plasma was given at the start. Reducing the rate of plasma administration, or treating the hypotension with calcium chloride (10 to 15 mg/kg), and correcting anesthetic overdosage or excessive ventilatory pressure have been effective steps in minimizing this response.

Systolic pressure of 80 mm Hg has been considered adequate for these patients, but below that level oxygenation may be compromised, and the operation is halted until the patient's condition has stabilized.

Undoubtedly the period of greatest stress during shunt procedures occurs when one branch of the pulmonary artery is occluded for anastomosis to the subclavian artery or aorta and the reduced pulmonary blood flow existing beforehand is approximately halved. It is important for the surgeon to perform the anastomosis with dispatch. To provide maximum oxygenation under the circumstances, the anesthesiologist can increase the heart rate (and cardiac output) by repeating atropine prior to pulmonary artery occlusion, use 100% oxygen, relaxant, and narcotic during occlusion, and at signs of bradycardia, hypotension, or T-wave ECG changes, support the heart with calcium chloride and isoproterenol infusion. Sodium bicarbonate also may be indicated.

Following Blalock shunts there is danger of thrombosis in the presence of hypotension and/or hemoconcentration. Consequently, special care must be taken to prevent these situations at all times, particularly in the early postoperative period.

Prompt awakening is expected after shunt procedures, and extubation usually is performed in the operating room. Hypoxia must be avoided, however. Since children who are cold enough to shiver increase their oxygen requirement by three or four times, warmth on awakening is of major importance.

Inflow occlusion

During the past 20 years, inflow occlusion has been used for correction of several car-

diac defects, including PS, aortic stenosis, atrial septostomy, and repair of small ASDs. At present its use is limited primarily to pulmonic valvotomy and atrial septostomy. The maneuver consists of occluding superior and inferior venae cavae by tourniquets (and cross-clamping the aorta for aortic valvotomy), thereby allowing the surgeon 2 minutes of unencumbered access to the interior of the heart and major valves.

Prior to inflow occlusion, patients are stabilized in light planes of anesthesia and preferably completely immobilized by muscle relaxants. Vagal reflexes are blocked by adequate atropinization, and 100% O_2 is administered as occlusion is initiated. If more than 2 minutes of occlusion are needed, or if arrhythmias or other signs of stress appear, tourniquets are released to allow reoxygenation and then may be reapplied as needed.

The principal danger associated with inflow occlusion is that of air embolism. To avoid this, the anesthesiologist should prevent all respiratory action while the heart is open; then, as the heart is being closed, he should inflate the lungs in order to compress the pulmonary vessels and fill the heart with blood, thereby displacing any air from pulmonary veins and heart.

Upon release of the tourniquets, return of normal cardiac activity is expected, and healthy infants may show sympathetic rebound and hypertension for 20 to 30 minutes. In others, delayed recovery may call for use of calcium chloride (10 to 15 mg/kg), digital cardiac compression, or limited use of sodium bicarbonate (1 mEq/kg).

Inflow occlusion with moderate hypothermia. The addition of local and general hypothermia to inflow occlusion has been employed to prolong the duration of operating time within the heart. Surface cooling by immersion in ice water to 30° C was used by Lewis in 1953 to perform the first open-heart procedures. The anesthetic and physiologic responses of patients undergoing these procedures was described by Virtue (1955).

Local application of sterile ice chips around the heart has also been used to reduce oxygen consumption and facilitate inflow occlusion. Development of reliable bypass technics and profound hypothermia have supplanted these methods almost completely.

Inflow occlusion with hyperbaric oxygenation. The survival rate for infant cardiac surgery was improved by the combining of inflow occlusion with hyperbaric oxygenation (Bernhard and others, 1963, 1966). When operation was performed in chambers pressurized to 3 atmospheres, the greater amount of oxygen dissolved in the infant's blood appeared to increase his tolerance to anesthesia and thoracotomy as well as to prolong the allowable inflow occlusion. Anesthesia for these procedures was carried out in approximately the same manner as for those at atmospheric pressure, except that the nitrous oxide became three times as potent and had to be reduced accordingly (Smith and associates, 1964). The development of deep hypothermic technics, which allow 60 minutes or more of operating time and require much less extensive outlay, ended our use of the hyperbaric approach.

ANESTHESIA FOR PROCEDURES REQUIRING BYPASS PERFUSION
Technical aspects of the pump-oxygenator

In spite of the anatomic and physiologic differences in the cardiac defects involved, the management of patients who are operated on under bypass perfusion involves many steps that are used for all. For this reason, it seems practical to describe the technical aspects of extracorporeal perfusion at the outset.

Anesthesiologists played a part in the development of pump-oxygenators and in many instances have been responsible for their management. The contributions of Patrick, Moffitt, and Theye of Mayo Clinic have been particularly valuable.

While total care of these devices now more frequently rests in the hands of trained technicians, it is to the advantage of all concerned for the anesthesiologist to be familiar with the fundamentals of extracorporeal circulation and to know something of the develop-

ment and mechanics of pump-oxygenators. For details and references one may refer to Gibbon (1954), Gollan (1959), Norman (1972), Arens (1975), and Sade and associates (1977).

For many years before the clinical application of bypass perfusion, surgeons had recognized the need for some method that would enable them to operate inside the heart, but its development, like that of the automobile and airplane, was a gradual advance of theories, obstacles, and problems through which investigating teams struggled, often with discouraging results. During the first 20 years, between 1930 and 1950, Dr. John Gibbon worked virtually alone on what began as an impossible dream and finally was recognized as a matter of urgent need, and investigation pushed ahead with vigor on many fronts. For several years there seemed to be daily progression of new advances and new obstacles. Problems met along the way included attempts to reproduce a pulsatile flow, the clotting of blood on contact with glass surfaces, determination of correct rate of perfusion, hemolysis due to excessive bubbling or suction devices, the balancing of inflow to outflow, production of intentional cardiac standstill, combination of moderate hypothermia (30° C) with bypass methods, and finally use of bypass plus deep hypothermia (20° C) to prepare for reversible cardiac arrest. Gollan's *Physiology of Cardiac Surgery* (1959) gives an interesting and enjoyable account of the development of deep hypothermia for cardiac surgery.

After 20 years there has been some standardization, but changes are still going on. The disk oxygenator, for many years more widely employed, has now been displaced by bubble oxygenators that have disposable components. The membrane oxygenator, theoretically less traumatic, has been more difficult to adapt to clinical use but promises to be particularly valuable for postoperative or nonsurgical support of patients over a course of several days (Drinker, 1972). There are at present two chief limitations to the use of heart-lung bypass devices: (1) the duration of use, this being limited to 4 to 5 hours,* and (2) the size of the patient, since the heart of an infant weighing less than 15 kg is so small that the presence of necessary cannulae and the blood coming through the coronary sinus render operation virtually impossible.

Side effects of cardiopulmonary perfusion

Early experience with bypass perfusion was filled with complications believed to be caused by the pump-oxygenator. The presence of pulmonary edema and severe pulmonary congestion, often termed "pump lung," was one of the most troublesome. The chief cause of this was found to be failure to drain the left atrium during bypass. This and many other problems have been overcome, and Laver and Bland (1975) have refuted the existence of any pulmonary dysfunction due purely to extracorporeal circulation.

Hyperglycemia during bypass was reported by Moffitt and associates (1970) and Mills and associates (1973). Moffitt and associates also reported elevation of lactic and pyruvic acid. Castaneda and associates (1974) found significant lactic acid elevation only in patients developing terminal acidosis.

Coagulopathy remains the cause of some difficulty and is best treated by fresh whole blood. Platelet reduction has been a constant finding during bypass. Although some of this may be due to filters in the pump-oxygenator, and there has been reference to "platelet destruction," there is usually a rapid replenishment shortly after return of normal circulation.

The higher mortality associated with longer bypass perfusion procedures has been cited as direct evidence of the harmful effect of perfusion. This may be a factor in the case of microemboli, whose occurrence has been an increased danger in longer operations; however, the higher mortality of longer bypass is also related to greater complexity of the lesion being repaired and the reduced strength of the patient bearing the lesion.

*Survival after 9 hours of bypass perfusion has been reported (Moffitt and others, 1970).

Acidosis has been associated with decreased tissue perfusion, especially during hypothermia. This has been controlled by hyperventilation, alkalinization, and maintenance of tissue perfusion by use of steroids.

Hemoconcentration and cooling, particularly in cyanotic patients, leads to thrombosis, for which hemodilution has been an effective measure (Laver and Bland, 1975; Sade and others, 1977). This may be accomplished by use of Ringer's lactate solution and heparinized whole blood in proportions calculated to produce a hematocrit of 30% during bypass (or 20% during hypothermia), determined by the following formula (Sade and others, 1977):

$$RL = \left(\frac{Hct\ I}{Hct\ D} \times BV \right) - BV$$

where

RL = volume of Ringer's lactate solution
$Hct\ I$ = initial hematocrit
$Hct\ D$ = desired hematocrit
BV = patient's blood volume

Procedural steps in extracorporeal circulation

The use of bypass perfusion requires several additional steps in anesthetic, surgical, and pharmacologic control. In our hospital such procedures include the following:

1. Induction of anesthesia is performed, and at least one peripheral intravenous infusion and one central venous infusion are established. Arterial cannulation is used for determination of blood gas levels and arterial pressure in all but such simple procedures as repair of ostium secundum defects and pulmonic valvotomy.
2. A Foley catheter is inserted.
3. The patient is placed in supine position, and a midline sternal-splitting incision is made.
4. An arterial inflow cannula is inserted into the ascending aorta (rarely, into the femoral artery).
5. Venous drainage lines are established by passing catheters through the right atrium into the inferior and superior venae cavae.
6. Heparin anticoagulant (2 mg/kg) is administered.

7. The pump-oxygenator is readied with suitable prime. Whole blood and a balanced electrolyte solution, buffered to pH 7.4 (Normosol-R, pH 7.4), are used in our institution. Ringer's lactate solution is used by some groups. Blood may be omitted with polycythemic patients.

8. When pump connections are completed, the surgeon gives the word and releases clamps on venous and arterial lines; then the pump is switched on and regulated to a flow rate suited to the child's size.

9. Suction sumps are fixed in the atria.

10. The surgeon proceeds to repair the lesion, often beginning by arresting the heart by electric fibrillation or by injection of a cardioplegic solution of potassium chloride.

11. During cardiac repair, the anesthesiologist keeps the lungs immobilized in partial expansion, maintaining a 50-50 mix of N_2O and O_2, with addition of 0.5% halothane. Arterial pressure now is nonpulsatile, showing mean pressure, and is maintained between 50 and 100 mm Hg. Hypotension is corrected by adding volume, hypertension by reducing volume or increasing halothane. The anesthesiologist watches for suffusion of the head, denoting obstruction of the superior vena cava. A technician monitors the rate of bypass flow and suction lines, maintains volume, and draws blood for pH, gases, electrolytes, and hematocrit, usually reducing hematocrit to 25% for normothermic bypass and to 20% for hypothermic bypass. Halothane and 3% CO_2 are added via pump.

12. On completion of repair, as the heart is closed the anesthesiologist inflates the lungs, filling the pulmonary vessels and heart with blood in order to drive out any air. The heart is defibrillated or allowed to start by washout of the potassium solution.

13. The patient remains on total bypass until the heart has regained normal activity; then caval ligatures are released, allowing the heart to accept more of the burden.

14. With adequate return of blood pressure, "coming off the pump" is accomplished by initial clamping of the venous line. The arterial line is clamped if the patient appears to be in proper fluid balance as shown by satisfactory arterial pressure (80 to 100 mm Hg) and left atrial pressure (10 to 20 mm Hg). More frequently the pump is allowed to continue to return blood into the patient for a few moments after occlusion of the venous line in order to make up volume deficit, after which the pump is stopped and the arterial line is clamped. Should more blood be needed, the process is repeated.

15. Inflow and outflow cannulae are removed, and protamine is administered (1.5 mg of protamine for each 1.0 mg of heparin previously given). Protamine is given slowly or in divided doses to prevent hypotension.

16. Bleeding is controlled, chest tubes are inserted, pacing wires and atrial cannulae are often placed, and the wound is closed.

17. Following less extensive procedures, the patient is awakened and the endotracheal tube removed in the operating room. Others are maintained on ventilatory support until their condition warrants its discontinuation.

Additional drugs are not routinely given and are not required under usual circumstances. The use of ϵ-aminocaproic acid to prevent fibrinolysis is not believed to be a reasonable practice. Routine use of inotropic agents masks the actual strength of cardiac function and also confuses the signs of fluid imbalance.

Hypopotassemia commonly occurs during bypass, and aliquots of potassium chloride, 2 to 5 mEq, are given if serum potassium falls below 2 mEq/L. Similarly, calcium chloride is added (10 to 15 mg/kg) if ionized calcium falls below 2 mM/L.

Urine output should continue at 1 ml/kg/hr. If, in the presence of adequate fluid intake, urinary output falls below that amount, diuretics are used.

The pump-oxygenator

Having passed through innumerable mutations, the pump-oxygenators currently used vary in minor details, but many are basically similar in function and design. As stated by Sade and associates (1977), the requirements of the pump-oxygenator are to provide (1) sufficient blood flow to perfuse vital organs, (2) required concentrations of dissolved oxygen and carbon dioxide, (3) appropriate acid-base control, and (4) desired body temperature.

At present, most pump-oxygenators consist of a heavy chassis constructed with four or five roller pumps, with individual speed control, pipes for O_2, CO_2, and hot and cold water, a halothane vaporizer, and apparatus for holding the disposable plastic blood-carrying components. These include tubing, collecting, oxygenating, and debubbling chambers, heat exchanger, and filters. Some of the more sophisticated oxygenators also carry built-in tape decks.

Collecting tubes carry blood from the heart to the collecting chamber by gravity. Blood or priming solution mixes with venous blood and blood suctioned from the wound and passes into the oxygenating chamber. In addition to blood and Normosol, the following ingredients have been included in our priming solution:

1. Heparin, 1000 units/L
2. Calcium chloride, 1 g/500 ml blood
3. Sodium bicarbonate, 15 mEq/500 ml blood
4. Oxacillin, 50 mg/kg (maximum 1 g)
5. Mannitol, 0.5 mg/kg
6. Methylprednisolone, 30 mg/kg for prolonged cases or hypothermia

To provide adequate oxygenation at normal temperature, the flow rate is adapted to the size of the patient as follows:

Weight	Flow rate
Under 35 kg	100 ml/kg/min
35 to 60 kg	75 ml/kg/min
Over 60 kg	50 ml/kg/min

Open-heart procedures

Fundamental considerations. Three major hemodynamic factors concerned with congenital cardiac defects are *blood flow, pressure,* and *resistance* in systemic and pulmonary circuits. As previously mentioned, the defects include left and right ventricular outflow obstruction, shunts, and abnormal anatomic structures interfering with the usual flow of blood, with eventual tendency to cause either cardiac failure or hypoxemia, or both. To reduce a very large problem to a few words, anesthesia should be planned with the appreciation of these hemodynamic factors in mind, and one should follow three

simple rules: (1) avoid addition of stress to hearts working against increased obstruction, (2) avoid increasing systemic (left-heart) stimulation in defects causing left-to-right shunting and increased pulmonary artery pressure, and (3) with cyanotic patients, avoid further reduction of pulmonary flow (hypoxia, hypotension, acidosis, hyperventilation).

As previously stated, technical management of anesthesia varies with the child's condition and the defect involved, in general depending on whether the child is in relatively good condition, as would be a 3-year-old with ostium secundum ASD, an 8-year-old with a large endocardial cushion defect in danger of congestive heart failure, or a 1-year-old with TOF and severe pulmonary hypoperfusion.

For children in good condition, induction may depend chiefly on their choice of either mask or needle. Nitrous oxide, oxygen, and halothane are acceptable, as would be thiopental or ketamine, and maintenance may consist of a variety of popular intravenous or inhalation agents suitably administered. Intravenous narcotics and other long-acting depressants are to be avoided, since these patients are usually extubated at the end of operation.

Acyanotic cardiac lesions call for a delicate balance between drugs that will sustain the action of the heart without adding to its burden. In aortic or mitral valvular stenosis, agents that increase the heart rate or systolic pressure may induce failure. On the other hand, if failure is already present, these drugs may be needed to stimulate the heart. Thus, there is greater need to know the exact state of myocardial efficiency before and during operation and greater need to use agents that are controllable. Here the use of measurement of cardiac output and atrial pressures will be of considerable value. They can be measured during operation by direct cannulation of the heart, but Swan-Ganz catheters may be needed in the postoperative period.

When the greatest danger appears to involve excessive pressure or increased resistance, induction with thiopental and maintenance with halothane have been our usual approach, with either succinylcholine or d-tubocurarine used for intubation. When cardiac failure is present or seems imminent, a more rational approach would be to use ketamine for induction and pancuronium for intubation and maintenance, with morphine and nitrous oxide for analgesia. We have found the tachycardia of both ketamine and pancuronium to be difficult to control. While Laver and Bland (1975) might use morphine as the principal agent here, our approach would consist of generous atropinization, ketamine induction for small infants and thiopental or nitrous oxide induction for larger children, followed by succinylcholine for intubation and morphine, nitrous oxide, and d-tubocurarine or metocurine for maintenance.

For children who are cyanotic and hypotensive, the chief danger is reduction of cardiac output. Hence, all agents that reduce the activity or efficiency of the heart must be avoided or used with extreme caution.

Several phases of open-heart operations may prove to be particularly upsetting. Induction is the first and as usual may involve either physical or physiologic stress. As previously noted, opening the chest often evokes responses in normal patients as well as in some of those previously operated on, and forceful separation of the ribs followed by retraction of the lung can cause either stimulation or depression.

Upon first touching the heart, the surgeon often initiates arrhythmias of brief duration and slight apparent harm. When the surgeon proceeds to the insertion of caval cannulae, more serious problems may arise in the form of definite bradycardia and hypotension. While this may be due primarily to the more active manipulation of the heart, the sudden jets of blood that may occur at the time of insertion of cannulae may play a part. This situation calls for prompt replacement of blood and reduction of anesthetic concentration. Heparin should be administered, and the surgeons should attempt to "get on the pump" as soon as possible. To support the patient during the intervening minutes, fur-

ther assistance in the way of atropine or calcium may be given while the child is ventilated with pure oxygen.

Since the pump-oxygenator is primed with fluid containing no anesthetic, infusion of this fluid at initiation of the pump may tend to arouse a patient who is lightly anesthetized. To control a patient who appears on the verge of awakening, thiopental, administered via the pump-oxygenator, has the most rapid effect.

Particular care must be taken at all times when one is dealing with patients who have intracardiac shunts in order to prevent air from entering either arteries or veins. The anesthesiologist should also help by watching for the appearance of air bubbles in the coronary vessels during perfusion.

Ostium secundum atrial septal defect. This defect is situated high in the atrial septum and may consist of a single opening or several small perforations. Flow through the shunt is from left to right, causing some increase in pulmonary flow but seldom enough to cause symptoms during childhood. The lesion is usually noticed by auscultation when the child is 6 to 8 years old. The child may appear frail and occasionally has protrusion of the left chest, but most of those coming to operation appear to be normal and healthy. Partial anomalous pulmonary venous return is commonly associated with ostium secundum defects, the two right pulmonary veins entering the right atrium instead of the left.

Operation for ostium secundum defects is one of the least difficult of the cardiac procedures and is one of those that were initially performed under inflow occlusion and hypothermia without bypass. Sewing over the atrial defect usually is quite simple. The additional presence of anomalous pulmonary veins does not add appreciably to the risk of the operation, but the required patch repair takes an added 10 to 20 minutes, thereby making bypass perfusion necessary.

Anesthetic preparation and management seldom require special technics. These children tolerate inhalation and intravenous agents and should awaken and be extubated on the operating table.

Endocardial cushion defects (including ostium primum atrial septal defects). The endocardial cushions, or atrioventricular cushions, are derived from mesenchymelike connective tissue and make up the central part of the heart, including the lower part of the atrial septum, the mitral and tricuspid valves, and the upper part of the ventricular septum. The valves and septa are formed by approximation and fusion of four segments of the embryologic endocardial cushions (Rudolph, 1974; Skidmore, 1975). Abnormal fusion of these components results in the various defects described below.

The partial endocardial cushion defect, also called the ostium primum ASD, is a lesion of the lower part of the atrial septum that is larger than most secundum defects, usually involving mitral and tricuspid valves but retaining two separate valve rings and the ventricular septum.

In the complete endocardial cushion defect, or common atrioventricular canal, the two valves are confluent and the atrial defect is continuous with a large VSD. This is the cardiac defect most commonly seen in Down's syndrome (Fig. 16-12).

The clinical effect of these lesions varies greatly with the extent of the lesion. Small primum defects simulate the secundum defect, but larger lesions, especially with the addition of mitral regurgitation, cause increasing left-to-right shunting, pulmonary vascular obstructive disease, and great en-

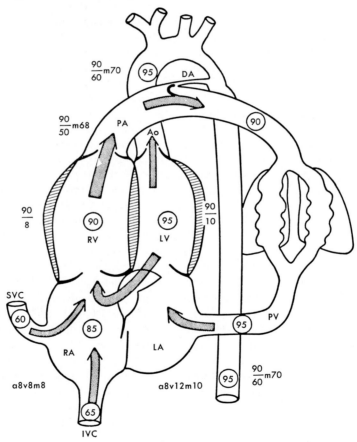

Fig. 16-12. Endocardial cushion defect with obligatory left-to-right shunt. Course of the circulation, oxygen saturations *(in circles)*, and pressures in the heart and great vessels are shown. (Reproduced with permission from Rudolph, A. M.: Congenital diseases of the heart. Copyright © 1974 by Year Book Medical Publishers, Inc., Chicago.)

largement of the heart. Thorough evaluation of all ASD primum patients is essential, with special attention to heart size, presence of failure, rate of progress of the signs, and exercise tolerance (see list of factors on p. 347). The anesthesiologist does well to view the chest film himself to get a clear idea of the heart size, and he should also scan the catheterization report for data on shunting, blood flow, or pulmonary vascular disease. In our experience, a grossly enlarged heart has been one of the most valuable indications of impending danger. Typical catheterization data of patients with endocardial cushion defects (Fig. 16-12) show O_2 content increasing at right atrial and right ventricular levels, right and left atrial pressures nearly equal, and pulmonary resistance increasing with developing mitral stenosis. The risk of operation is largely dependent on the degree of pulmonary vascular obstruction and cardiac enlargement. Children with an incomplete form of endocardial cushion defect often get along fairly well until reaching school age, but during the next 10 years they may suddenly develop severe failure. The repair may involve application of an atrial patch and mitral reconstruction in moderately severe lesions, while pulmonary artery banding may be the safest procedure in small infants.

The degree of cardiac impairment varies greatly in ASD primum, and anesthesia requirements vary accordingly. Patients with major defects need expert application of technics directed toward maintenance of stable cardiac output and avoidance of added work. Halothane may be used for induction but must be strictly controlled to avoid excess dosage. Divided doses of morphine seem safest when the heart is distended, to be followed by nasal intubation with d-tubocurarine and topical anesthesia. Full use is made of monitors, including arterial and central venous cannulation with continuous display, ECG, and urinary catheter established at the start and pacemaker wires and atrial pressure cannulae placed during operation.

Repair of complete endocardial cushion defect may require 3 hours of bypass perfusion, after which an enlarged heart may be difficult to restart. Brief manual massage may stimulate action, but knowledge of potassium and ionized calcium levels and blood gases, as well as the ability to correct abnormal findings, is essential here. If ionized calcium (Ca^{++}) falls below 2 mM/L, it is corrected by addition of calcium chloride, 5 to 10 mg/kg. Drop and Laver (1975) have found that isoproterenol given with calcium hastens return to normal levels. Warmth, adequate volume, and dopamine are additional aids. Heart block due to injury of the conductive system has been a source of trouble in the past but has been reduced by mapping of the course of the bundle of His and by pacemaker control. The mortality of repair of partial endocardial cushion defects should be less than 10% and results are equally good. The complete defect bears a much higher mortality, and results often are unsatisfactory.

Ventricular septal defect. VSD is the most common of all congenital cardiac anomalies (Nadas and others, 1973). Depending on the age of the child and the size of the lesion, VSD tends to cause left-to-right shunting, pulmonary artery hypertension, and congestive heart failure. The smallest defects cause no clinical symptoms and usually close spontaneously early in infancy, while those of moderate size decrease gradually and rarely require medical or surgical therapy.

Infants born with large VSDs show signs of congestive heart failure most often manifested by tachypnea, tachycardia, and dyspnea. Sweating and hepatomegaly are also seen, but less frequently. The present approach is to attempt to control these infants with digitalis and diuretics over a period of 3 to 4 weeks, following which, if failure and pulmonary artery hypertension persist, operation is indicated. While pulmonary artery banding formerly was the accepted procedure for small infants, unsatisfactory results have led many surgeons to abandon this approach in favor of total repair.

In older infants and children, acute congestive failure is less common. Large VSDs are more frequently recognized by loud systolic murmur and subsequent cardiac catheterization. Operation is indicated when pulmonary artery systolic pressure is greater than half systemic, when pulmonary artery/systemic blood flow ratio is 2:1 or more (large VSDs may reach 5:1 ratios), and in the presence of increasing pulmonary vascular resistance.

Operation for all older children consists of closure of the defect or defects, usually by Teflon patch, under bypass perfusion. When VSD is not associated with other lesions, the management is not complicated. In many of the milder cases, a wide variety of anesthetic agents may be used. In the presence of large left-to-right shunts, agents that raise systemic pressure or cardiac output are avoided to prevent increase of the shunt.

VSD occurs in association with a host of other defects, including PDA, mitral stenosis, coarctation of the aorta, and TOF. Management of anesthesia in these situations will vary with the total effect of the combined lesions.

Complete transposition of the great arteries. The morphologic classification of transposition includes lesions such as double-outlet right ventricle (Taussig-Bing) and double-outlet left ventricle. In addition, transpositions may be complete or corrected, depending on the atrial situs as well as the ventricular loop. Dextrotransposition of the great arteries (d-TGA) far outnumbers all other varieties, and this lesion is usually intended when the abbreviation TGA is used alone.

In TGA the complete transposition of the aorta and pulmonary artery results in two separate circuits. Systemic blood passes from right atrium to right ventricle to aorta, tissues, vena cava, right atrium, and back to right ventricle without going to the lungs. Pulmonary venous blood goes to the left atrium, left ventricle, pulmonary artery, lungs, pulmonary veins, and back to the left atrium without going to the tissues. Infants become cyanotic and hypoxic, and cannot survive unless some communication develops between the two circuits.

There are three important variants to d-TGA: one having no VSD (Fig. 16-13), another having VSD and severe PS, and a third having VSD but no PS. All develop cyanosis at birth, with arterial O_2 saturations of 20% to 40%. Those with intact VSD do not survive unless there is shunting via the foramen ovale. Those having a VSD alone may obtain enough oxygen to survive but develop severe pulmonary hypertension and congestive failure.

Current treatment combines several approaches. Treatment employed at The Children's Hospital Medical Center, as described by Sade and associates (1977), is to catheterize all infants with diagnosis of TGA at birth and perform balloon atrial septostomy on those with inadequate shunt. If this does not suffice, it is followed by a Blalock-Hanlon atrial septostomy under inflow occlusion. If infants develop severe failure, they undergo pulmonary artery banding in the early months of life or the total repair devised by Mustard and associates (1964) at 6 months. In those that remain in fair condition, the Mustard procedure is performed at 1 year. The Mustard operation consists of excision of the atrial septum and construction of a tunnel of pericardium that conducts blood from the venae cavae through the mitral valve into the left ventricle, leaving the blood from the pulmonary veins to pass through the right atrium and into the right ventricle (Fig. 16-14). Senning's repair also is used here.

The anesthesiologist caring for these infants is faced with the dual problem of hypoxia and threatened or actual congestive heart failure. The initial balloon atrial septostomy often is performed without anesthesia by the cardiac catheterization team, but Blalock-Hanlon, pulmonary artery banding, and Mustard procedures require general anesthesia adapted to each situation. Pulmonary artery banding is the simplest of the three, requiring only thoracotomy. The Blalock-Hanlon procedure requires inflow occlusion of 30 to 90 seconds in good hands, while the total (Mustard) repair takes 1 to 2 hours of bypass perfusion or hypothermic arrest.

Ketamine serves well to start any of the above procedures and may be followed by

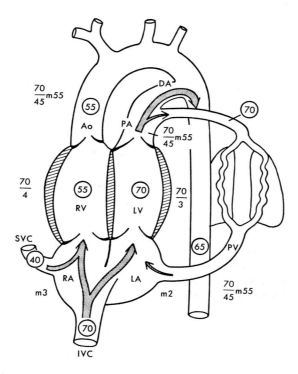

Fig. 16-13. Aortopulmonary transposition with no associated defects. Course of the circulation, oxygen saturations *(in circles)*, and pressures in the fetus are shown. (Reproduced with permission from Rudolph, A. M.: Congenital diseases of the heart. Copyright © 1974 by Year Book Medical Publishers, Inc., Chicago.)

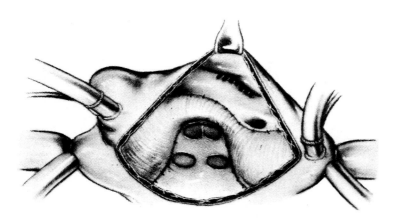

Fig. 16-14. The Mustard procedure for repair of transposition of great arteries. Pericardial baffle has been sewn into the right auricle so as to divert pulmonary venous and coronary sinus blood into the tricuspid valve, and SVC and IVC blood into the mitral valve. (From Stark, J., de Laval, M. R., Waterston, D. J., and others: J. Thorac. Cardiovasc. Surg. **65**:673, 1974.)

intubation under any of the muscle relaxants. One should consider the hazard of retrolental fibroplasia before using 100% O_2, but with severely hypoxic infants it may be necessary. If the infant will tolerate it, 30% to 50% N_2O may be used as a diluent and analgesic. In neonates, arterial blood gases may be measured by umbilical route. For older infants undergoing Mustard procedure, radial or dorsalis pedis arteries should be used. Following the two shorter operations, infants often get along without postoperative ventilatory support, but at least 24 hours of support is necessary following total repair.

Total anomalous pulmonary venous connection. There are several variations of total anomalous pulmonary venous connection (TAPVC). The basic defect is failure of the pulmonary veins to drain into the left atrium.

Instead, all four pulmonary veins converge to form a common vein or sinus. The different defects are classified according to the route by which this sinus carries blood to the heart. According to Gathman and Nadas (1970), the supracardiac type (45% of total) (Fig. 16-15) carries blood by way of the left innominate vein, superior vena cava, or azygos vein to the right atrium; the cardiac type (23%) routes blood via the coronary sinus; the subdiaphragmatic type (2%) routes blood via the portal vein; and the mixed type (11%) consists of combinations of the above routes.

The chief clinical features are cyanosis, pulmonary venous obstruction, pulmonary hypertension (pulmonary artery pressure often exceeding systemic), respiratory distress, cardiac failure, and pulmonary edema. In mild cases, patients may remain asymptom-

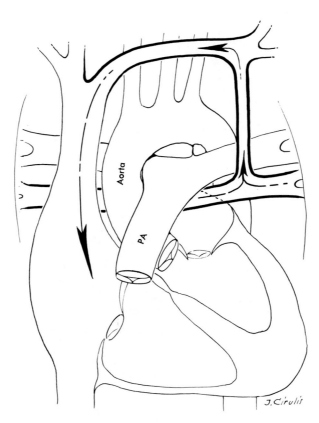

Fig. 16-15. Total anomalous pulmonary venous drainage. One of several variations, this one involving union of pulmonary veins and connection to the right heart via the superior vena cava.

atic for years, but the majority need operation in infancy, often in the first week of life.

Operation is performed under bypass perfusion (with the use of hypothermic arrest for neonates) and consists of anastomosing the common pulmonary sinus to the left atrium and then ligating the anomalous part of the system that had carried blood to the right atrium. Closure of the ASD is performed as the last step. When the operation is carried out as an emergency procedure on hypoxic infants with high pulmonary artery pressure, one must tread a narrow path between hypoxia on the one hand and hypervolemia and cardiac failure on the other. The underdeveloped left atrium and ventricle are faced with a sudden increase in work, and pulmonary edema has followed immediately after anastomosis in several instances.

Anesthetic agents are chosen to maintain myocardial contractility and avoid bradycardia. The threat of pulmonary edema is imminent during and after operation, and left atrial pressure measurement has definite value. To hold this at the desired level of 15 to 20 mm Hg, ventilation is supported, cardiac output is monitored, pacemaker wires are implanted in ventricles, and inotropic infusions of calcium plus isoproterenol or dopamine are held in readiness.

Truncus arteriosus. In this defect a single arterial trunk bridges the ventricular septum and carries blood from both ventricles. The pulmonary arteries branch off of the ascending trunk to carry blood to the lungs at systemic pressure. Pulmonary flow is greatly increased, causing severe congestive failure in infancy. The mixture of oxygenated and unoxygenated blood causes marked cyanosis. In infancy pulmonary artery banding may be helpful, but in older children a more complicated repair is more satisfactory. This consists of removing the pulmonary arteries from the trunk, connecting the right ventricle to the pulmonary arteries by a homograft conduit with Hancock valve, and closing the VSD (McGoon, 1979).

This is another case where anesthesia must be given to hypoxic infants in congestive failure. Simple banding and major correction are managed as previously described for these situations.

ANESTHESIA FOR PROCEDURES REQUIRING BYPASS PERFUSION AND CARDIAC ARREST UNDER PROFOUND HYPOTHERMIA

Early users of hypothermia were discouraged by the appearance of arrhythmias below 35° C and the more disturbing incidence of postoperative cerebral damage. Attempts to achieve deep hypothermia were abandoned for several years. In 1963, however, the Japanese team of Horiuchi and associates succeeded in cooling small infants to 20° C using ether as the general anesthetic. Subsequent work reported by Mohri and associates (1966), Hikasa and associates (1967), Barratt-Boyes and associates (1971), and Sade and Castaneda (1976) has established bypass perfusion with profound hypothermia as a highly advantageous method for intracardiac operations on infants under 1 year old and weighing less than 14 kg. The series reported by Sade and Castaneda, as shown in Table 16-2, included 153 operations with a mortality of only 11.1%. As is evident in the table, the lesions most frequently repaired under this technic have been VSD, d-TGA, TOF, and TAPVC. The ages of these infants varied between 1 and 90 days.

Technic of profound hypothermia

Infants are brought to the operating room in isolettes or covered cribs, some of them with endotracheal tubes already in place. If not previously intubated, an endotracheal tube is inserted under metocurine and oxygen, and one peripheral venous line, one central venous line, and an arterial cannula are established. The venous lines are placed in the best available sites in arms, legs, or neck using 20- or 22-gauge Teflon cannulae. The arterial cannula is inserted by open exposure of a radial artery using a 22-gauge Teflon needle under direct vision and is connected to a Harvard pump. The esophageal stethoscope and ECG are fixed in place, thermistor probes are inserted in nose,

Table 16-2. Deep hypothermic circulatory arrest in infancy (1/1/73 to 5/1/76)

Correctable lesion	No. patients	Age (D)	Weight (kg)	Hosp. mort.
VSD	50	20-340	2.0-7.5	3 (6.0%)
TOF	33	12-355	2.0-8.5	2 (6.0%)
DORV	2	362-400	6.0-7.5	0 —
d-TGA	40	4-365	3.5-9.0	6 (15.0%)
IVS	(30)	4-365	3.5-9.0	(4) (13.0%)
VSD	(10)	60-320	4.0-8.0	(2) (20.0%)
Taussig-Bing	1	210.0	5.0	0 —
TAPVC	13	1.5-180	2.2-5.0	2 (15.0%)
AS	3	20-270	3.5-8.0	0 —
A-V canal	10	5-270	2.0-8.0	4 (40.0%)
Dyspl. pulm. valve	1	360.0	7.5	0 —
	153	1.5-400	2.0-9.0	17 (11.1%)

From Sade, R. M., and Castaneda, A. R.: Recent advances in cardiac surgery in the young infant, Surg. Clin. North Am. **56:**451, 1976.

esophagus, and rectum, and nasogastric and urethral catheters are passed.

ANESTHETIC MANAGEMENT OF INFANTS UNDERGOING CARDIAC SURGERY UNDER DEEP HYPOTHERMIC ARREST

Premedication
Atropine (0.1 to 0.2 mg IM) 30 minutes before operation

Anesthetic management
Under 3 months old:
Induction: metocurine—O_2
Maintenance: nitrous oxide—O_2—curare (1.5-mg supplements), occasionally morphine (0.2 mg/kg)
3 months and over:
Induction: ketamine (1 to 2 mg/kg IV)—O_2—succinylcholine
Maintenance: nitrous oxide—O_2—curare—morphine (0.2 to 0.5 mg/kg)
Nasotracheal intubation from start; controlled ventilation for at least 24 hours after operation

In the series of Sade and Castaneda (1976) and others, cooling was initiated by placing the infant and assorted attachments into a large plastic sack and immersing all in a small plastic tub filled with ice and water. Cooling to a core temperature of 25° C was accomplished in this manner. The infant was then removed from the tub, dried, placed on the operating table, and prepared, thoracotomy performed, the pump-oxygenator connected, and final cooling to 20° C attained by the heat exchanger. External cooling by ice immersion has been abandoned, however, and the entire process now is accomplished by internal perfusion. When 20° C is reached, the pump-oxygenator is stopped and cannulae are removed from the heart, giving the surgeon 60 to 90 minutes of unimpeded access to a relaxed, immobile heart. Following satisfactory cardiac repair, bypass is restarted and rewarming continued until nasopharyngeal temperature reaches 32° C. Further rewarming to 37° C is performed by surface warming with a thermal blanket.

During the process of cooling, the infant is hyperventilated to counterbalance the expected metabolic acidosis. The heart slows gradually from initial rates of 140 to 180 down to 100, 80, and 60 beats/min. The starting blood pressure usually is maintained until the heart rate falls to 60 beats/min. By this time, the surgeons should be about to connect the pump. It is essential to start heparin while circulation is still sufficient to distribute it throughout the infant's body; consequently, the anesthesiologist must see that it is administered (2 mg/kg) before bypass is begun and well ahead of that time if arrhythmia or hypotension threatens.

The effects of profound hypothermia have been investigated extensively over the past 30 years. The reduction of oxygen requirement is obviously the principal object. Increased solubility of gases, shift of the dissociation curve to the left, and tendency to develop metabolic acidosis with spontaneous respiration are well known. The necessary amount of counteracting of hyperventilation, the ideal level of PCO_2 to prevent cerebral vasoconstriction, the effect of intercurrent hyper- and hypoglycemia, and the meaning of altered acid-base balance have not been determined. Johnston and associates (1974), after a careful study, found that 15% CO_2 was necessary during the procedure. Johnson and Hansen, in our work, have not found the addition of CO_2 to be of importance, in either the operative or the postoperative course. It is possible that the contents of the pump prime and other details might explain such differences, but as yet, each team appears to have individual differences. Certainly, all the supportive and monitoring methods needed for normothermic bypass are required during hypothermic bypass. Ionized calcium levels have frequently been found to be below the normal 2 mEq/L after hypothermia and call for prompt correction. Hemodilution and steroids are also more essential for prevention of thromboemboli and coagulation defects.

Psychologic and mental changes related to bypass perfusion and deep hypothermia

The question of brain damage related to bypass perfusion at normothermic levels and especially at deep hypothermic levels has raised some doubt. Heller and associates (1970) studied the incidence of delirium in patients following normothermic procedures and found that 37% had some evidence of delirium during recovery. They related it to severity of the underlying lesion, age of the patient (all were over 18 years old), and duration of the pump run. While it is impossible to determine such statistics in small children, studies by Perna and associates (1973) and experiences of Barratt-Boyes (1971), Sade and Castaneda (1976), and others attest to the

safety of 60 minutes of cardiac arrest in infants at 20° C.

ANESTHESIA FOR CARDIAC CATHETERIZATION, ANGIOCARDIOGRAPHY, AND CARDIOVERSION

Catheterization studies of the right and left heart may involve special problems for the anesthesiologist. Since the two procedures are distinctly different, they will be discussed individually.

Right-heart catheterization

Right-heart catheterization is used for the diagnosis of various types of cyanotic heart disease and of lesions involving shunts, the exact nature of which is uncertain. The studies require from 1 to 3 hours, and since measurement of oxygen saturation and pressure gradients constitutes the principal goal of the project, it is desirable to avoid the use of oxygen, whether mixed with an anesthetic or used purely for supportive therapy. The process of right-heart catheterization usually requires exposure of a vein in the antecubital space and passage of a catheter into this vein and thence into the chambers of the heart. The procedure does not cause excessive pain but is uncomfortable, and it is something one could hardly expect a small child to tolerate quietly. Sedation is indicated but must be of a type that has a prolonged, even action without peaking. This has been a difficult problem to solve, and most approaches have fallen short of expectations.

The variety of agents and technics thus far employed include most of the general anesthetics and sedation under tribromoethanol, rectal and intramuscular thiopental, ketamine, hydroxyzine, and diazepam. The combination of chlorpromazine, promethazine, and meperidine, suggested by Smith and associates (1958) of Toronto, has undoubtedly been used most extensively. It is made up as follows:

Promethazine	50 mg (2 ml)
Chlorpromazine	50 mg (2 ml)
Meperidine	200 mg (4 ml)
	8-ml solution

The suggested dose is 1 ml/20 lb in non-cyanotic children and 0.7 ml/20 lb in cyanotic or debilitated children, given intramuscularly 1 hour before catheterization.

The prolonged depression caused by chlorpromazine has been disturbing, and for this reason it seems preferable to use a combination of meperidine, 1 mg/lb, and pentobarbital, 2 mg/lb, by intramuscular route and supplemented as required by divided intravenous doses during the course of catheterization.

Left-heart catheterization

General anesthesia was often required for left-heart catheterization performed by passing a needle through the chest wall into the heart. The present method of femoral artery catheterization almost always can be managed under sedation, as with right-heart catheterization.

Angiocardiography

Whereas the injection of radiopaque solutions into veins and arteries once was so irritating that anesthesia was necessary, the development of Renovist* and similar contrast media has eliminated the need for anesthesia in these studies.

Cardioversion

The sharp, shaking impact of cardioversion calls for brief but appreciable sedation. Diazepam has been employed for older patients, but dosage sufficient to be effective for children may leave them depressed for some time. Our present preferred sedative for cardioversion is methohexital, prepared by adding 50 ml of water to the 500-mg bottle of powdered methohexital to make a 1% solution (10 mg/ml). A typical situation where methohexital might be used would be for cardioversion in a 12-year-old child with paroxysmal auricular tachycardia. If suction, an oxygen source with anesthesia bag and mask, and complete resuscitation equipment are available, this may be undertaken in an intensive care unit. Atropine and sedatives

*E. R. Squibb & Sons, Inc., Princeton, N.J.

are not mandatory, but oral intake should have been withheld as for any anesthetic.

Preoxygenation is advisable. If a child objects to application of a mask, 10 or 12 deep breaths should be of appreciable value. Methohexital is injected directly into a previously established infusion close to the patient for prompt effect. An initial dose of 1 mg/kg may suffice to induce light sleep, at least deep enough to abolish the eyelash response, but added doses of 0.5 mg/kg may be needed if the child is alert and apprehensive. There may be signs of conscious reaction at the moment of countershock, but it is rarely remembered. Thiopental may be used in similar fashion, but less prompt awakening after cardioversion must be expected. Dosage for thiopental would be two to three times that of methohexital. In either case, one should be prepared for initial failure of cardioversion and several repetitions, with the possibility of requiring added sedation.

BIBLIOGRAPHY

Adelman, M. H.: Anesthesia in surgery of patent ductus arteriosus, Anesthesiology 9:42, 1948.
Arens, J. F.: Extracorporeal circulation; practical considerations in use of the heart pump, refresher course, American Society of Anesthesiologists, 1975.
Bahnson, H. T.: Aortic stenosis. In Ravitch, M. M., Welch, C. D., Benson, C. D., and others, editors: Pediatric surgery, ed. 3, Chicago, 1979, Year Book Medical Publishers, Inc.
Barr, M. N., and Davenport, H. T.: Blood loss during pediatric operations, Can. Med. Assoc. J. 89:1309, 1963.
Barratt-Boyes, B. G.: Cardiac surgery in neonates and infants, Circulation 44:924, 1971.
Barratt-Boyes, B. G., and Neutze, J. M.: Primary repair of tetralogy of Fallot in infancy using profound hypothermia with circulatory arrest and limited cardiopulmonary bypass, Ann. Surg. 178:406, 1973.
Barratt-Boyes, B. G., Simpson, M., and Neutze, J. M.: Intracardiac surgery in neonates and infants using deep hypothermia with surface cooling and limited cardiopulmonary bypass, Circulation 43(1):25, 1971.
Beiser, G. D., Epstein, S. E., Stampfer, M., and others: Impairment of cardiac function in patients with pectus excavatum with improvement after operative correction, N. Engl. J. Med. 287:267, 1972.
Berger, O. L.: Anesthesia for surgical treatment of cyanotic heart disease. J. Am. Nurs. Anesth. 16:1948.
Bergner, R. P., and Schafer, G. W.: General anesthesia for pediatric thoracic surgery, Anesth. Analg. (Cleve.) 35:194, 1956.

Bernhard, W. F., Navarro, R. V., Yagi, H., and others: Cardiovascular surgery in infants performed under hyperbaric conditions, Vasc. Dis. 3:33, 1966.

Bernhard, W. F., Tank, E. S., Fritelli, G., and Gross, R. E.: The feasibility of hypothermic perfusion in surgical management of infants with cyanotic congenital heart disease, J. Thorac. Cardiovasc. Surg. 46:651, 1963.

Blalock, A., and Taussig, H. B.: Surgical treatment of malformations of the heart in which there is pulmonary stenosis or pulmonary atresia, J.A.M.A. 128:189, 1948.

Brewer, L. A. III, Fosburg, R. G., Mulder, G. A., and others: Spinal cord complications following surgery for coarctation of the aorta; a study of 69 cases, J. Thorac. Cardiovasc. Surg. 64:368, 1972.

Cassels, D. E., editor: The heart and circulation in the newborn and infant; an international symposium, New York, 1966, Grune & Stratton, Inc.

Castaneda, A. R., Freed, M. D., Williams, R. G., and Norwood, W. I.: Repair of tetralogy of Fallot in infancy; early and late results, J. Thorac. Cardiovasc. Surg. 74:372, 1977.

Castaneda, A. R., Lamberti, J., Sade, R. M., and others: Open heart surgery during the first three months of life, J. Thorac. Cardiovasc. Surg. 68:719, 1974.

Coceani, F., and Olley, P. M.: The response of the ductus arteriosus to prostaglandins, Can. J. Physiol. Pharmacol. 51:220, 1973.

Conn, A. W., and Millar, R. W.: Postocclusion hypertension and plasma catecholamine levels, Can. Anaesth. Soc. J. 7:443, 1960.

Cooley, D. A., Berman, S., and Santibaneg-Woolrich, A.: Surgery in the newborn for congenital cardiovascular lesions, J.A.M.A. 182:912, 1962.

Cooley, D. A., and Hallman, G. L.: Cardiovascular surgery during the first year of life, Am. J. Surg. 107:474, 1964.

Crafoord, C., and Nylin, G.: Congential coarctation of the aorta and its surgical treatment, J. Thorac. Surg. 14:347, 1945.

Davis, T. B., Morrow, D. H., Hebert, C. L., and Cooper, T.: An increased incidence of paradoxical hypertension following resection of aortic coarctation under halothane anesthesia, Anesthesiology 22:132, 1961.

Downes, J. J., Nicodemus, H. F., Pierce, W. S., and Waldhausen, J. A.: Acute respiratory failure in infants following cardiovascular surgery, J. Thorac. Cardiovasc. Surg. 59:21, 1970.

Drinker, P. A.: Progress in membrane oxygenator design, Anesthesiology 37:242, 1972.

Drop, L. G., and Laver, M. G.: Low plasma ionized calcium and response to calcium therapy in critically ill man, Anesthesiology 43:300, 1975.

Edmunds, L. H., Gregory, G. A., Heymann, M. A., and others: Surgical closure of the ductus arteriosus in premature infants, Circulation 48:856, 1973.

Edwards, J. E.: Functional pathology of the pulmonary vascular tree in congenital cardiac disease, Circulation 15:164, 1957.

Eger, E. E. II, and Saidman, L. J.: Hazards of nitrous oxide anesthesia in bowel obstruction and pneumothorax, Anesthesiology 26:61, 1965.

Fellows, K. E., Khaw, K. T., Schuster, S. S., and Shwachman, H.: Bronchial embolization; technique and results, J. Pediatr., in press.

Fermoso, J. D., Richardson, T. O., and Guyton, A. C.: Mechanism of decrease in cardiac output caused by opening the chest, Am. J. Physiol. 207:1112, 1964.

Folkman, J.: Personal communication, 1978.

Friedman, W. F., Hirschklan, M. J., Printz, M. P., and others: Pharmacologic closure of patent ductus arteriosus in the premature infant, N. Engl. J. Med. 295:526, 1976.

Gathman, G. E., and Nadas, A. S.: Total anomalous pulmonary venous connection—clinical and physiological observations of 75 pediatric patients, Circulation 42:143, 1970.

Gattiker, R. I.: Anesthesia during surgery for transposition of the great arteries, Int. Anesthesiol. Clin. 10:93, 1972.

Gibbon, J. H.: Application of a mechanical heart and lung apparatus to cardiac surgery, Minn. Med. 37:171, 1954.

Glenn, W. W., Ordway, N. K., Talner, N. S., and Call, E. P.: Circulatory bypass of the right side of the heart. VI. Shunt between superior vena cava and distal right pulmonary artery; report of clinical application in thirty-eight cases, Circulation 31:172, 1965.

Gollan, F.: Physiology of cardiac surgery, Springfield, Ill., 1959, Charles C Thomas, Publisher.

Gregory, G. A., Edmunds, L. H., Jr., Kitterman, J. A., and others: Continuous positive airway pressure and pulmonary and circulatory function after cardiac surgery in infants less than three months of age, Anesthesiology 43:426, 1975.

Gross, R. E.: Surgical relief for tracheal obstruction from a vascular ring, N. Engl. J. Med. 233:586, 1945.

Gross, R. E.: Coarctation of the aorta; surgical treatment in one hundred cases, Circulation 1:41, 1950.

Gross, R. E.: Surgery of infancy and childhood, Philadelphia, 1953, W. B. Saunders Co.

Gross, R. E.: An atlas of children's surgery, Philadelphia, 1970, W. B. Saunders Co.

Gross, R. E., Emerson, P., and Green, H.: Surgical obliteration of patent ductus arteriosus in 7-year-old girl, Am. J. Dis. Child. 59:554, 1940.

Guntheroth, W. C.: Medical emergency management; neonatal and pediatric cardiovascular cases, J.A.M.A. 232:168, 1975.

Gutierrez, J., Strong, M. J., and Keats, A. S.: Increase in cyanosis during controlled respiration in patients with tetralogy of Fallot; abstract, Anesthesiology 27:217, 1966.

Hansen, D. D.: Anesthesia. In Sade, R. M., Cosgrove, D. M., and Castaneda, A. R., editors: Infant and child care in heart surgery, Chicago, 1977, Year Book Medical Publishers, Inc.

Harmel, H. H., and Lamont, A.: Anesthesia in the surgical treatment of congenital pulmonary stenosis, Anesthesiology 7:477, 1946.

Harris, A. J.: Management of anesthesia for congenital heart operations in children, Anesthesiology 11:328, 1950.

Hatch, D. J., Taylor, B. W., Glover, W. J., and others: Continuous positive-airway pressure after open-heart operations in infancy, Lancet 2:469, 1973.

Heller, S. S., Frank, K. A., Malm, J. R., and others: Psychiatric complications of open-heart surgery; a re-examination, N. Engl. J. Med. 283:1015, 1970.

Heymann, M. A., Rudolph, A. M., and Silverman, N. M.: Closure of the ductus arteriosus in premature infants by inhibition of prostaglandin synthesis, N. Engl. J. Med. 295:530, 1976.

Hikasa, Y., Shirotani, H., Satomura, K., and others: Open-heart surgery in infants with an aid of hypothermic anesthesia, Arch. Jap. Chir. 36:595, 1967.

Hislop, A., and Reid, L.: Growth and development of the respiratory system; anatomical development. In Davis, J. A., and Dobbing, J., editors: Scientific foundations of paediatrics, Philadelphia, 1974, W. B. Saunders Co.

Ho, E. C., and Moss, A. J.: The syndrome of "mesenteric arteritis" following surgical repair of aortic coarctation; report of nine cases and review of the literature, Pediatrics 49:40, 1972.

Horiuchi, T., Koyamada, K., Matano, I., and others: Radical operation for ventricular septal defect in infancy, J. Thorac. Cardiovasc. Surg. 46:180, 1963.

Johnston, A. E., Raddle, I. C., Steward, D. J., and Taylor, J.: Acid-base and electrolyte changes in infants undergoing profound hypothermia for surgical correction of congenital heart defects, Can. Anaesth. Soc. J. 21:23, 1974.

Keith, J. D., Rowe, R. D., and Vlad, P.: Heart disease in infancy and childhood, ed. 3, New York, 1978, Macmillan, Inc.

Keown, K. K.: Anesthesia for surgery of the heart, ed. 2, Springfield, Ill., 1966, Charles C Thomas, Publisher.

Kirklin, J. W.: Advances in cardiovascular surgery, New York, 1973, Grune & Stratton, Inc.

Kirklin, J. W., and DuShane, J. W.: Repair of ventricular septal defect in infancy, Pediatrics 21:961, 1961.

Kirklin, J. W., DuShane, J. W., Patrick, R. T., and others: Intracardiac surgery with the aid of a mechanical pump-oxygenator system (Gibbon type), Proc. Staff Meet. Mayo Clin. 30:201, 1955.

Kirklin, J. W., and Karp, R. B.: The tetralogy of Fallot; from a surgical viewpoint, Philadelphia, 1970, W. B. Saunders Co.

Kitterman, J. A.: Patent ductus arteriosus in premature infants, Clin. Res. 18:209, 1970.

Kitterman, J. A., Edmunds, L. H., Jr., Gregory, G. A., and others: P.D.A. in premature infants; incidence relation to pulmonary disease and management, N. Engl. J. Med. 287:473, 1972.

Laver, M. B., and Austen, W. G.: Cardiorespiratory dy-namics. In Gibbon, J., editor: Surgery of the chest, Philadelphia, 1969, W. B. Saunders Co.

Laver, M. B., and Bland, J. H. L.: Anaesthetic management of the pediatric patient during open-heart surgery, Int. Anesthesiol. Clin. 13:149, 1975.

Levin, R. M., Seleny, F. L., and Streczyn, M. V.: Ketamine-pancuronium-narcotic technic for cardiovascular surgery in infants—a comparative study, Anesth. Analg. (Cleve.) 54:800, 1975.

Lewis, F. V., and Taufic, M.: Closure of atrial septal defects with the aid of hypothermia, Surgery 33:52, 1953.

Lowenstein, E., and Bland, J. H. L.: Anesthesia for cardiac surgery. In Norman, J. C., editor: Cardiac surgery, ed. 2, New York, 1972, Appleton-Century-Crofts.

Lowenstein, E., Hallowell, P., Levine, L. H., and others: Cardiovascular response to large doses of intravenous morphine in man, N. Engl. J. Med. 281:1389, 1969.

McClure, P. D., and Izsak, J.: The use of epsilonaminocaproic acid to reduce bleeding during cardiac bypass in children with congenital heart disease, Anesthesiology 40:604, 1974.

McGoon, D. C.: Truncus arteriosus and pulmonary atresia with ventricular septal defect. In Ravitch, M. M., Welch, K. J., Benson, C. D., and others, editors: Pediatric surgery, ed. 3, Chicago, 1979, Year Book Medical Publishers, Inc.

McGoon, D. C., Rastelli, G. C., and Ongley, P. A.: An operation for the correction of truncus arteriosus, J.A.M.A. 205:69, 1968.

McQuiston, W. O.: Anesthetic problems in cardiac surgery in children, Anesthesiology 10:590, 1949.

McQuiston, W. O.: Anesthesia in cardiac surgery; observations in 362 cases, Arch. Surg. 61:892, 1950.

Mills, N. L., Beaudet, R. L., Isom, W. O., and Spencer, F. C.: Hyperglycemia during cardiopulmonary bypass, Ann. Surg. 177:203, 1973.

Modell, H., and Milhorn, H. T., Jr.: Quantitation of factors affecting the alveolar-arterial PO_2 difference in thoracotomy, Anesthesiology 37:592, 1972.

Moffitt, E. A., Rosevear, J. W., and McGoon, D. C.: Myocardial metabolism in open-heart surgery; arterial levels of metabolites, electrolytes, oxygenation, and acid-base balance, Anesth. Analg. (Cleve.) 48:633, 1969.

Moffitt, E. A., Rosevear, J. W., and McGoon, D. C.: Myocardiac metabolism in children having open-heart surgery, J.A.M.A. 211:1518, 1970.

Mohri, H., Dillard, D. H., and Merendino, K. A.: Hypothermia; halothane anesthesia and the safe period of total circulatory arrest, Surgery 72:345, 1972.

Mohri, H., Hessel, E. A., Jr., Nelson, R. J., and others: Use of rheomacrodex and hyperventilation in prolonged circulatory arrest under deep hypothermia induced by surface cooling, Am. J. Surg. 112:241, 1966.

Moss, A. J., Adams, S. H., and Emmanouilides, G. G.:

Heart disease in infants, children, and adolescents, Baltimore, 1977, The Williams & Wilkins Co.

Mustard, W. T.: Bulbus cordis anomalies. In Mustard, W. T., Ravitch, M. M., Snyder, W. H., and others, editors: Pediatric surgery, ed. 2, Chicago, 1969, Year Book Medical Publishers, Inc.

Mustard, W. T., Keith, J. D., Trusler, G. A., and others: The surgical management of transposition of the great vessels, J. Thorac. Cardiovasc. Surg. **48:** 953, 1964.

Nadas, A. S.: Patent ductus revisited, N. Engl. J. Med. **295:**563, 1976.

Nadas, A. S., and Fyler, D. C.: Pediatric cardiology, ed. 3, Philadelphia, 1972, W. B. Saunders Co.

Nadas, A. S., Fyler, D. C., and Castaneda, A. R.: The critically ill infant with congenital heart disease, Mod. Concepts Cardiovasc. Dis. **42:**53, 1973.

Norman, J. C.: Cardiac surgery, ed. 2, New York, 1972, Appleton-Century-Crofts.

Patrick, R. T., Theye, R. A., and Moffitt, E. A.: Studies in extracorporeal circulation. V. Anesthesia and supportive care during intracardiac surgery with the Gibbon-type pump-oxygenator, Anesthesiology **18:** 673, 1957.

Perna, A. M., Gardner, T. J., Tabaddor, K., and others: Cerebral metabolism and blood flow after circulatory arrest during deep hypothermia, Ann. Surg. **178:**95, 1973.

Potts, W. J., Smith, S., and Gibson, S.: Anastomosis of aorta to pulmonary artery, J.A.M.A. **132:**627, 1946.

Radnay, P. A., Arai, T., and Nagashima, H.: Ketamine-gallamine anesthesia for great-vessel operations in infants, Anesth. Analg. (Cleve.) **53:**365, 1974.

Rashkind, W. J., and Miller, W. W.: Creation of an atrial defect without thoracotomy, a palliative approach to complete transposition of the great arteries, J.A.M.A. **196:**991, 1966.

Ravitch, M. M.: Congenital cystic disease of the lung. In Ravitch, M. M., Welch, K. J., Benson, C. D., and others, editors: Pediatric surgery, ed. 3, Chicago, 1979, Year Book Medical Publishers, Inc.

Reifenstein, G. H., Levine, S. A., and Gross, R. E.: Coarctation of the aorta; a review of 104 autopsied cases of the "adult type," 2 years of age or older, Am. Heart J. **33:**146, 1947.

Rinehart, J. J., Lewis, R. P., and Balcerzak, D. P.: Adriamycin cardiotoxicity in man, Ann. Int. Med. **81:** 475, 1974.

Rittenhouse, E. A., Mohri, H., Dillard, D. H., and Merendino, K. A.: Deep hypothermia in cardiovascular surgery, Ann. Thorac. Surg. **17:**63, 1974.

Rudolph, A. M.: The changes in the circulation after birth; their importance in congenital heart disease, Circulation **41:**343, 1970.

Rudolph, A. M.: Congenital diseases of the heart, Chicago, 1974, Year Book Medical Publishers, Inc.

Rudolph, A. M., and Heymann, M. A.: Medical treatment of the ductus arteriosus, Hosp. Prac. **12:**57, 1977.

Sade, R. M., and Castaneda, A. R.: Recent advances in cardiac surgery in the young infant, Surg. Clin. North Am. **56:**451, 1976.

Sade, R. M., Cosgrove, D. M., and Castaneda, A. R.: Infant and child care in heart surgery, Chicago, 1977, Year Book Medical Publishers, Inc.

Sade, R. M., Williams, R. G., and Castaneda, A. R.: Corrective surgery for congenital cardiovascular defects in early infancy, Am. Heart J. **90:**656, 1975.

Schuster, S. S., Shwachman, H., Harris, G. B., and others: Pulmonary surgery for cystic fibrosis, J. Thorac. Cardiovasc. Surg. **48:**750, 1964.

Sealey, W. C., Brown, I. W., Jr., and Young, W. G., Jr.: Report on the use of both extracorporeal circulation and hypothermia for open heart surgery, Ann. Surg. **147:**603, 1958.

Senning, A.: Correction of the transposition of the great arteries, Ann. Surg. **182:**287, 1975.

Skidmore, F. D.: The embryology of the heart. In Goor, D. A., and Lillihei, C. W., editors: Congenital malformations of the heart, New York, 1975, Grune & Stratton, Inc.

Smith, C., Rowe, R. D., and Vlad, P.: Sedation of children for cardiac catheterization with an ataractic mixture, Can. Anaesth. Soc. J. **5:**35, 1958.

Smith, R. M.: Circulatory factors affecting anesthesia in surgery for congenital heart disease, Anesthesiology **13:**38, 1952.

Smith, R. M., Crocker, D. C., and Adams, J. G., Jr.: Anesthetic management of patients during surgery under hyperbaric oxygenation, Anesth. Analg. (Cleve.) **43:**766, 1964.

Steward, D. J., Sloan, J. A., and Johnston, A. E.: Anaesthetic management of infants undergoing profound hypothermia for surgical correction of congenital heart defects, Can. Anaesth. Soc. J. **21:**15, 1974.

Stewart, S., Edmunds, L. H., Kirklin, J. W., and others: Spontaneous breathing with continuous positive airway pressure after open intracardiac operations in infants, J. Thorac. Cardiovasc. Surg. **65:**37, 1973.

Stoelting, R. K., and Gibbs, P. S.: Hemodynamic effects of morphine and morphine-nitrous oxide in valvular heart disease and coronary artery disease, Anesthesiology **38:**45, 1973.

Strong, M. J., Keats, A. S., and Cooley, D. A.: Anesthesia for cardiovascular surgery in infants, Anesthesiology **27:**257, 1966.

Strong, M. J., Keats, A. S., and Cooley, D. A.: Arterial gas tensions under anaesthesia in tetralogy of Fallot, Br. J. Anaesth. **39:**472, 1967.

Taussig, H. B.: Congenital malformations of the heart, Cambridge, Mass., 1960, The Commonwealth Fund, Harvard University Press.

Theye, R. A., Moffitt, E. A., and Kirklin, J. W.: Anesthetic management during open intracardiac surgery, Anesthesiology **23:**823, 1962.

Virtue, R. W.: Hypothermic anesthesia, Springfield, Ill., 1955, Charles C Thomas, Publisher.

Wakusawa, R., Shibata, S., and Kazutoshi, O.: Simple deep hypothermia for open-heart surgery in infancy, Can. Anaesth. Soc. J. **24:**491, 1977.

Welch, K. J.: Surgical repair of pectus excavatum. In Holder, T. M., and Ashcraft, K. W., editors: Surgery of infants and children, Philadelphia, W. B. Saunders Co., in press.

Wetchler, Z. V., and McQuiston, W. O.: Anesthetic management of infants and children with double aortic arch; paper presented before American Society of Anesthesiologists, Kansas City, Mo., October 1956.

Wilson, R. D., Traber, D. L., Priano, L. L., and others: Anesthetic management of the poor risk pediatric patient, South. Med. J. 62:767, 1969.

Wohl, M. E., Briscom, N. T., Strieder, D. J., and others: The lung following repair of diaphragmatic hernia, J. Pediatr. 90:405, 1977.

Zachman, R. D., Steinmetz, G. P., Botham, J. R., and others: Incidence and treatment of the patent ductus arteriosus in the ill premature infant, Ann. Heart J. 87:697, 1974.

CHAPTER 17

Anesthesia for general, urologic, and plastic surgery

ANESTHESIA FOR OPERATIONS ABOUT THE HEAD AND NECK

There is considerable contention between general, plastic, and otolaryngologic surgeons for operations about the head and neck. For the sake of simplicity, most of these procedures will be discussed together without dividing them among specific fields of surgery. Hemangiomas, lymphagiomas, thyroglossal, branchiogenic, and preauricular cysts and sinuses, cystic hygromas, cervical nodes, and malignant tumors are seen in varying frequency during childhood. Surgical requirements are a clear airway, free access to the child's head, analgesia, and very little relaxation.

Endotracheal intubation will be indicated in most of these operations. If the airway is not occluded in any way, there will be relatively free choice of anesthetic agent and technic. Probably the most important consideration in uncomplicated situations is to be sure that the vagus nerve is adequately blocked by an effective dose of atropine (0.03 mg/kg) within 30 minutes prior to anesthesia, for vagal responses may be hyperactive during operations in this general area.

When there is either inflammation or obstruction of the airway, management becomes more exacting. Preoperative sedation is reduced in proportion to the degree of obstruction. Induction of anesthesia providing maximal oxygenation with minimal irritation probably consists of halothane and oxygen. Nitrous oxide may be used initially if the obstruction is not severe.

Among the lesions offering greatest difficulty are lymphangiomas and hemangiomas of the tongue and oral tissues. These are not uncommon and occasionally reach considerable size (Fig. 17-1). Preoperative tracheostomy may be advisable to provide an airway during and after operation. Excessive bleeding may complicate removal of such tumors, and pharyngeal packing will be necessary in addition to endotracheal intubation or tracheostomy. Cystic hygromas also occur frequently, usually in the anterior cervical region, but they may be found extending into the floor of the mouth, the axilla, and substernally into the chest (MacDonald, 1967).

Operations involving cervical masses appear to present increased danger. Four different instances of cardiac arrest are known to have occurred during relatively simple procedures in the cervical region, each time seemingly caused by excessive vagal stimulation, inadequate atropinization, and the use of cardiac sensitizing agents. In each case the head was turned sharply to the side, and there probably was appreciable manual pressure on the carotid sinus.

At termination of operations about the neck, it is best to keep the child asleep until

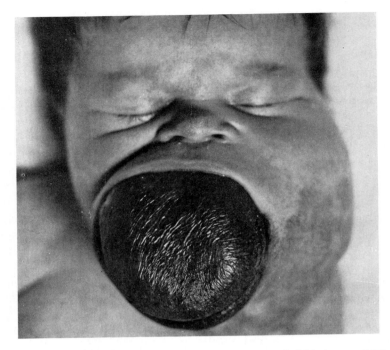

Fig. 17-1. Obstructive lesions about the mouth are not uncommon, but this hemangioma offered exceptional difficulties.

the wound is closed and the dressing has been applied. Premature awakening, bucking, and coughing may cause renewed bleeding into the tissues adjacent to the trachea.

Esophagoscopy and esophageal dilation may be included in the sphere of the general surgeon. Patients with congenital, traumatic, or postoperative stricture may require repeated dilation. At the Children's Hospital Medical Center, one of our patients underwent 99 general anesthetics for dilation following lye ingestion. Esophagoplasty was performed on the one-hundredth admission.

Anesthesia for fiberoptic esophagoscopy has been added to this general category. For all of these procedures, deep relaxation and the use of a relatively small endotracheal tube make it easier for the surgeon and less traumatic for the child. We prefer muscle relaxants and controlled respiration. One should be sure to clean the mouth and hypopharynx after the surgeons have completed their work and then extubate.

ANESTHESIA FOR OPERATIONS ON THE TRUNK AND LIMBS

The general surgeon performs relatively few challenging procedures on the trunk and limbs, with the possible exception of trauma and occasional severe infections. Plastic and orthopedic surgeons manage most of the burns, crushing trauma, and reconstructive work. Lacerations, removal of superficial tumors, mastectomy, and excision of pilonidal sinuses are managed according to standard anesthetic principles. We do not feel that endotracheal intubation is necessary when these patients are supine unless there are extenuating circumstances.

ANESTHESIA FOR ABDOMINAL OPERATIONS
Surgical lesions

Abdominal conditions requiring surgery during the pediatric period may be due to the presence of congenital anomalies, metabolic disorders, or hormonal disturbances and thus may be charactistic of this age group, but they also include the inflammatory lesions, tumors, and traumatic states seen in older patients. The following indications for abdominal surgery may be encountered in infants and children:

Intestinal obstruction
  Atresia
  Stenosis
  Duplication
  Volvulus
  Meconium ileus
  Tumor
Pyloric stenosis
Appendicitis
Meckel's diverticulum
Regional enteritis
Acute necrotizing enteritis
Inguinal, umbilical hernia
Biliary atresia
Liver cysts, tumors
Neuroblastoma
Wilms' tumor
Hirschsprung's disease
Portal hypertension
Splenomegaly
Ruptured viscus
Exstrophy of bladder
Tumors of bladder
Adrenogenital syndrome
Ovarian cyst, tumors
Glycogen storage disease

Anesthetic problems

Some of the anesthetic problems of infants have been mentioned. For the most part, the anesthetic requirements for abdominal surgery in children are similar to those for adults. In addition to analgesia, full relaxation is usually needed, and the use of a potent general anesthetic, muscle relaxant, or regional block will be necessary. In exceptional situations, very weak patients may require only analgesic concentrations of anesthetic agents.

For most infants and children, halothane affords easy induction and adequate relaxation for abdominal procedures, but enflurane may be preferred for better relaxation in larger children or for procedures that require an unusual degree of relaxation, such as esophageal reconstruction.

Nitrous oxide should be avoided in the presence of bowel obstruction but may be replaced by morphine, fentanyl, or meperidine in small doses and reversed later if indicated. Spinal and epidural anesthesia have some place in abdominal surgery, but regional anesthesia of this type usually is reserved for particular indications, such as for a child who has also sustained a head injury.

Although the first two requirements for abdominal surgery are analgesia and relaxation, a number of other problems confront the anesthesiologist. The aspiration of regurgitated intestinal contents is always to be feared but is of greatest danger in patients with intestinal obstruction. Gastric suction must be established in such patients prior to anesthesia.

Awake intubation is useful in small infants but is not tolerated well in children more than 6 months old unless they are quite ill. Induction of general anesthesia prior to intubation is justifiable in older children by either inhalation or intravenous technic if the stomach has been relieved of most of its contents and effective suction equipment is at hand. After operation the endotracheal tube is left in place until the child has awakened.

Children facing abdominal surgery may be in an extremely toxic condition because of peritonitis, prolonged vomiting, uremia, or cachexia. In fact, of all types of pediatric patients, the sickest may be found among those requiring abdominal operation. Time must be allowed for adequate preparation of these children by correction of dehydration, hypovolemia, anemia, and metabolic imbalances.

In prolonged intra-abdominal procedures such as abdominoperineal resection for Hirschsprung's disease, additional fluid and electrolyte replacement are needed, and allowance of 8 to 12 ml/kg is reasonable. Blood replacement may not be required, but either blood or colloid probably will be advisable.

Excision of neuroblastoma, Wilms' tumor, and hepatic tumors and repair of ruptured liver, in that order, carry increasing danger of massive blood loss. In past years, exsanguinating hemorrhage was the principal cause of death in our operating rooms. Reliable infusions, ample blood stores carefully prepared, and deliberate surgical technic have practically eliminated this problem.

Traumatic lesions of the abdomen are most frequently caused by automobiles, but bicycles and sleds take an appreciable toll when in season. Ruptured spleen can cause considerable blood loss, but less rapidly than the liver. If the liver has been badly torn, the edges may be held together so tightly within the peritoneum that hemorrhage is held to a minimum. When the surgeon opens the peritoneum, however, the edges may fall apart, with immediate exsanguination.

In addition to the rather general problems referred to, other hazards are associated with certain specific lesions or organs.

Inguinal and umbilical herniorrhaphy

Beyond infancy, inguinal herniorrhaphy is one of the least complicated pediatric operations. The hernia rarely is either large or strangulated, and the surgeon requires only 20 to 30 minutes of moderate relaxation to perform a bilateral repair. Nitrous oxide and halothane seem ideal for the procedure, and intubation is optional. Our preference usually is to intubate older children but to use only a mask for those under 8 years old. There seems to be some discomfort after these operations, possibly noticed more because the child had no sense of being sick before operation and does not understand why he should wake up hurting. An intravenous infusion is not necessary for fluid therapy in early morning cases, but it serves as an excellent means of painless sedation on awakening and may be removed shortly after the child is made comfortable.

Umbilical herniorrhaphy is even less exacting than inguinal herniorrhaphy, but general anesthesia always demands careful attention. In both types of hernia, awakening may be accompanied by glottic spasm, bradycardia, and severe hypoxia. Any procedure performed as frequently as hernia repair will produce a certain number of catastrophes, as the courts of law easily bear proof, and the concept that an operation is uncomplicated is an invitation to negligence and inadequate attention.

Orchidopexy

Although belonging more strictly to genitourinary surgery, orchidopexy and inguinal herniorrhaphy usually are treated together and should be discussed together. Two points differentiate anesthetic management of children for orchidopexy. First, there is more stimulus because of traction on the spermatic cord, and there will be more reflex responses and greater need for relaxation. Halothane and nitrous oxide remain adequate for small children, without tracheal intubation, but beyond 6 or 8 years of age intubation becomes distinctly desirable, and relaxant technics have increasing advantage.

The second point of difference is the increased amount of postoperative discomfort following orchidopexy. After herniorrhaphy a child may be restless and upset, but there is often enough evidence of real pain following orchidopexy to call for at least one dose of morphine. With an infusion running, our preference is to use divided intravenous doses of morphine, starting with a maximum of 1 mg for children under 25 kg and 2 mg for those between 25 and 50 kg.

Intestinal obstruction

The anesthetic handling of newborns with intestinal obstruction has been described and usually consists of local infiltration or awake intubation followed by halothane. The greatest problem with these infants often lies in postoperative support.

Some forms of intestinal obstruction are relatively benign. Intussusception may be serious if it has progressed far, but the condition usually occurs in relatively healthy 1- or 2-year-old children and generally is diagnosed before the child becomes acutely ill (Evrard, 1973).

In our practice, gastric suction is established, and anesthesia is induced with halothane and oxygen, after which the trachea is intubated and anesthesia continued with halothane supplemented by relaxants as necessary. Fluid therapy is suited to the degree of dehydration, as described in Chapter 25.

More seriously disturbed fluid and electrolyte balance may be seen in children in late stages of regional enteritis or in those with acute distension due to peritonitis or intestinal tumors. Operation should be delayed until safe levels of blood volume, electrolytes, and blood gases have been restored and the upper gastrointestinal tract has been at least partially relieved of its contents by means of a relatively large sump tube with numerous holes. After such a tube has been in place for 2 or 3 hours and fluids have been properly initiated, it may be reasonable to proceed with the operation. Endotracheal intubation will be an important step, but if the patient is no longer distended, one should be able to use either inhalation or intravenous induction with success. As noted earlier, nitrous oxide is best avoided when distension is present. The point of chief concern will be to leave the endotracheal tube in place after the operation until one is sure that the child's gag reflex is completely restored.

Incarcerated hernia falls into much the same category as intussusception. These infants seldom are very ill and tolerate most anesthetics well. Occasionally this condition is seen in weak, premature infants, or it may progress sufficiently to cause dehydration and electrolyte imbalance, in which case time must be taken to restore essential conditions.

Appendicitis

The declining rate of tonsillectomy probably leaves appendectomy as the operation most frequently performed in childhood. Appendicitis can occur during infancy but is uncommon in children under 3 or 4 years of age.

Children who are brought to the operating room with diagnosis of acute appendicitis differ greatly in the duration and degree of illness, and anesthetic management should be adapted to the particular situation.

The anesthesiologist frequently is called to the hospital to find his young patient about to be placed on the operating table. This operation is never so urgent that time cannot be allowed for standard review of the child's history and evaluation of his physical condition. In addition, there are several essential pieces of information relating to patients with appendicitis that one should obtain in order to determine the risk and decide on the management. These include the following:

1. The child's present temperature. If over 102° F, we prefer to delay operation until it can be corrected.
2. The previous course of the temperature. If less than 102° F, this temperature could merely be the low point in the course of a spiking fever. One should know how long there has been a fever and how high it has been in order to assess the child's illness.
3. When and what the child has eaten. Appendicitis usually causes anorexia, and patients seldom will have undigested stomach contents. However, precautions must be taken in case one encounters a child who has just eaten corn and a hamburger.
4. If the child has vomited. If so, the duration and frequency are of much concern, since they suggest more severe illness, the degree of dehydration, and possible presence of peritonitis.
5. The time of last voiding. This is a valuable clue to the state of hydration.
6. What therapeutic steps have been initiated, including the type and amount of intravenous fluids, antibiotic therapy, and whether antipyretic drugs have been given.
7. The white cell count is often misleading and of little value. Of laboratory data, urine specific gravity may be of assistance in judging hydration.

After gathering this information, one proceeds with two additional considerations in mind:

1. The actual pathology often is more advanced than a child's symptoms suggest, and perforation is found in many small children when not suspected.
2. Although fever and toxicity might not be present at the start, overwhelming sepsis can occur during operation, with mounting fever, convulsions, and death. As with all patients having real or threatened sepsis, preparations must be made to monitor and control body temperature throughout the entire operation.

Anesthetic management of acute appendicitis varies with the child's condition. The child who has minimal signs of short duration, is hydrated, and has not eaten presents minimal difficulty. Premedication with narcotic and atropine is acceptable, and preliminary barbiturate may be given if time permits. In many instances, an infusion is started at the time of admission and enough morphine added to relieve anxiety. If an infusion is already running, induction by this route is more pleasant than by inhalation. If veins are difficult to find, inhalation technics are used. Tracheal intubation is not an absolute necessity but is definitely indicated.

In early unruptured appendicitis a nasogastric tube is not required and if used is rarely left in place after the operation. Should the appendix be perforated, however, a nasogastric tube is inserted and left in place for 24 to 48 hours.

At the end of any operation of this type, the endotracheal tube is not removed until the child is awake and there is complete return of the gag reflex.

Appendicitis with fever and moderate dehydration. If the child's temperature is 102° F or higher and there are obvious signs of dehydration, the operation is delayed to allow for partial correction of dehydration and initiation of antibiotic effect. An infusion of 5% dextrose in 0.2N saline solution is given (10 ml/kg). A nasogastric tube is passed before anesthetic induction if there has been vomiting. No attempt at surface cooling is made for fear of causing shivering and increasing oxygen demands.

Within 30 to 60 minutes enough fluid can usually be given to improve tissue turgor, induce voiding, and justify induction of anesthesia even if the temperature is still elevated. Atropine is added via the infusion, to be followed by thiopental and succinylcholine or halothane for tracheal intubation. If by this time the temperature is not well below 102° F, operation is delayed further while ice bags are applied to neck, axillae, and other exposed areas, and hydration is continued.

These measures should be effective within 10 to 15 minutes and should be discontinued when the temperature has reached 100° F to prevent excess cooling. Since it is also possible for the temperature to rebound, it must be watched closely throughout the entire operation. Subsequent temperature elevation is best treated by rinsing the stomach with iced saline solution or pouring ice water under the child's neck and back rather than relying on a cooling mattress.

Following operation, these sick children are more apt to vomit during awakening, and tracheal extubation must be delayed until they are actually conscious.

Appendiceal perforation and peritonitis. When children are severely sick with peritonitis, toxic signs of high spiking fever, abdominal distension, and mental disorientation may be present. The duration of illness is important here, since prolonged vomiting and peritoneal irritation may have produced marked depletion of plasma protein. Nasogastric suction, antibiotics, and replacement of fluid, electrolytes, and colloid will be necessary before operative intervention. X-ray films of chest and abdomen should be obtained to determine presence of complicating atelectasis, pneumonia, or loculation of infection, while measurement of arterial blood gases, total serum proteins, and electrolytes is also in order.

After some stability has been established, operation may be undertaken to drain the site of perforation or to remove the appendix. Temperature must be controlled as before; nitrous oxide should be avoided if there is distension. Requirement for anesthetic agents may be considerably reduced, and small amounts of controllable agents are preferable. Morphine, topical spray for intubation, and 0.5% halothane might be adequate for a child of this type, with use of oxygen and assisted respiration throughout. These children will be critically ill for some time, and recovery will depend on the excellence of postoperative attention.

Operations on the liver

There is general agreement that operations on the liver rank among the most dangerous in pediatric surgery (Martin and Woodman, 1969; Ein and Stephens, 1974, 1974a; Head and Smyth, 1974). Factors contributing to this picture are the high incidence of hepatic tumors in early infancy, the difficulty in dealing with hepatic injury, the numerous essential functions of the liver that may be disrupted by surgical lesions, and the susceptibility of the liver to total failure.

Operations involving the liver include biopsy, biliary tract exploration, excision of cysts and benign and malignant tumors, repair of traumatic lesions, and transplantation. With the exception of liver biopsy, these procedures are of major proportion. Varieties of benign cysts and hamartomas are among the less challenging procedures but still require a high degree of skill to remove safely, while hemangiomas, primary-cell carcinomas, and hepatomas usually involve partial hepatectomy and maximal risk.

The principal anesthetic requirements for hepatic surgery are the avoidance of toxicity, provision of full relaxation, and replacement of large amounts of blood. The danger of toxicity, as discussed in Chapters 5 and 26, probably has been exaggerated, for children tolerate fluorinated anesthetics remarkably well. Except for occasional liver biopsy and the rare transplant, serious hepatic dysfunction seldom is involved in pediatric surgical lesions. Infants explored for biliary atresia may have marked jaundice, but this is related more to obstruction or absence of biliary ducts than to cellular pathology. This type of liver disease should not contraindicate use of halogenated agents on scientific grounds. However, nonhalogenated agents may reasonably be chosen to avoid the nuisance of uninformed criticism. In choice of the agent, it still might be borne in mind that halothane has been shown to reduce hepatic perfusion (Berger and others, 1976). Furthermore, when large amounts of blood are needed, there will be increased risk of an incompatibility that could cause jaundice. If no halothane has been used, the usual accusation of "halothane hepatitis" can be tossed out at once.

The choice of agents varies slightly with the type of surgery. Agents metabolized by the liver are not contraindicated but may be expected to have more prolonged effect. Succinylcholine and thiopental are used in slightly reduced amounts. Relaxation is obtained with d-tubocurarine, and analgesia is obtained with nitrous oxide and morphine, but other combinations would be quite acceptable.

Liver biopsy. Although liver biopsy can be performed on adults under local anesthesia, the danger of hemorrhage is increased in children who are unable to remain still; thus, general anesthesia is indicated. The child must be prone, and respiration may be impeded by placement of a pad under the upper abdomen. Since the diagnosis of active liver disease usually is in question, halogenated agents are avoided. The chief hazard is bleeding. Consequently, these patients must be watched carefully for several hours after the procedure. While the operation should require only 10 or 15 minutes and anesthesia little more, the child should be kept in bed, supine, for several hours.

Major hepatic surgery. Partial hepatectomy for tumor, repair of lacerated liver, and liver transplantation all involve extensive surgery with danger of massive blood loss and possible disturbance of liver function following operation. All three types of surgery require increased monitoring facilities and additional personnel to assist with administration of blood and to help in the maintenance of other supportive measures.

Preoperative studies seldom will be possible for children with ruptured liver but definitely are in order for those scheduled for partial or total hepatectomy. Patients with benign or metastatic tumors should have near-normal metabolic liver function, but as noted by Turmel and associates (1973), preoperative findings are useful in evaluating postoperative recovery. Children facing liver transplantation may show a wide range of dysfunction, which should be evaluated as thoroughly as possible. Studies recommended by Turmel and associates include transaminase, lactic dehydrogenase, alkaline phosphatase, serum electrophoresis, and

391

others. In addition, elevation of urinary catecholamines, particularly vanillylmandelic acid (VMA), may be found in patients having metastatic neuroblastoma, and cystothionuria may be found in those with hepatoblastoma.

All of these patients should be thoroughly screened for bleeding disorders, with complete coagulograms as well as serum albumin, total protein, and bilirubin concentration. Although several of these factors are not easily corrected, time should be taken when possible to treat hypovolemia and anemia.

Other studies of importance include blood glucose metabolism and x-ray evaluation by liver scan, inferior vena cavogram, and aortography.

A competent blood bank is essential for this type of surgery. At least 50 ml of blood per kg, preferably fresh, should be prepared at the start, with more available.

Standard premedicant drugs should be tolerated by patients scheduled for tumor excision but rarely would be given to patients in shock or in a toxic condition. Preoperative preparation would include warming the operating room to 75° F and providing a warming blanket as well as a heating lamp for smaller children. When children are alert and not in critical condition, induction of anesthesia may be started with the simple stethoscope and blood pressure apparatus and one intravenous infusion. If a large vein is not obvious, a 25-gauge needle may be used for induction. To avoid all use of halogens, one starts with either N_2O-O_2 or a small amount of thiopental, establishing a standard "balanced anesthesia" thereafter. While thiopental and muscle relaxants may be metabolized more slowly by affected livers, these agents should not aggravate any existing toxicity or dysfunction.

As soon as the child is asleep, at least two large-bore infusions are started using arms or neck so that their course to the heart and head cannot be obstructed during the operation. One of the infusions can be adapted for use as a CVP monitor. An arterial line is set up for blood gas and pressure determination, and nasogastric tube, urethral catheter,

and ECG, as well as the usual stethoscope, thermistor, and blood replacement record, are installed. Furman (1971), who reported a partial hepatectomy in an 18-month-old child, also measured serial osmolality, serum protein, and hematocrit, which proved invaluable in detecting the presence of metabolic acidosis during the procedure. We now monitor ionized calcium and potassium in such cases for guidance in their replacement and sodium for estimation of osmolality.

Massive blood replacement is discussed in greater detail in Chapter 25, but it should be emphasized here that when the neck or arm is used as the intravenous site and a catheter is threaded nearly to the right atrium, infused fluids enter the heart practically as a bolus, and cold or acidotic blood will have much greater effect than when infused via the internal saphenous vein. Consequently, it is particularly important to use fresh blood that is warm and chemically suitable for administration to a hypovolemic patient.

During the course of these operations there are distinct differences in the problems encountered. Surgical and anesthetic management of children for *excision of large hepatic tumors* has been described by Martin and Woodman (1969), Ein and Stephens (1974, 1974a), Turmel and associates (1973), and Steward and Creighton (1975). Mortality has varied between 18% and 80%, and the chief problem has been blood loss. Taylor and associates (1969) described 22 hepatic resections performed at our hospital between 1953 and 1968 with four deaths (one child moribund on admission, one death due to air embolus, one due to malposition of CVP line, and one due to hemorrhage).

Children with hepatic tumors often come to operation in reasonably good general condition. As the operation proceeds, a moderate degree of anesthesia, full relaxation, and control of blood loss can preserve the initial homeostasis, although there may be moments of considerable stress.

It is of primary importance throughout all such operations for anesthesiologist and surgeon to work in close cooperation. Rapid surgery, exposing extensive cut surfaces of the liver, and lifting the liver out of its normal position can precipitate sudden hemorrhage or angulate and occlude the vena cava. The anesthesiologist must watch the operation continuously to be aware as soon as such complications take place. A continuously visible readout of arterial and central venous blood pressure is particularly valuable here to show the sudden complete drop in pressures that occur after caval obstruction.

Proper steps must be taken at once to correct such major complications. Replacement of the liver in its natural bed should restore blood pressures promptly. Replacement of massive hemorrhage is only possible when there is adequate equipment and skilled personnel. A pumping device capable of infusing 500 ml in 1 minute is needed. For this, a rotary pump similar to those used in pump-oxygenators is best suited.

Prior to beginning such operations, we impress upon the surgeon the need of proceeding slowly to allow us to keep up with the blood loss and of stopping the operation if blood loss or manipulation of the liver appears excessive. It has been our practice to keep arterial pressure at or above 80 mm Hg. In addition to fresh whole blood, these patients need albumin and glucose (Steward and Creighton, 1975).

Turmel and associates (1973) point out the importance of temperature control in these patients. While moderate hypothermia (32° to 36° C) may reduce anesthetic requirement and also protect the liver during emergency occlusion of the hepatic artery, extreme hypothermia, easily caused by rapid transfusion, can cause serious arrhythmias and arrest during operation and cardiorespiratory depression during recovery.

Air embolism is another danger during hepatic surgery, as we have learned by experience. Experience has also taught us not to assume that bleeding will stop as soon as a large tumor has been removed. There usually are open vessels in the tumor bed that can continue to flow freely, with rapid progression to hypovolemia and shock. It is also important to realize that catastrophe is apt to occur while blood is being replaced if it is cold or acidotic.

Traumatic lesions of the liver, whether caused by blunt forces or penetrating injuries, may present overwhelming problems, primarily related to hemorrhage. Any child who is bleeding from a large abdominal wound should be explored at once. If the wound involves the liver, the child is not apt to reach the hospital alive, but should this occur, his life will depend on the efficiency with which replacement therapy and immediate surgery can be carried out.

Following blunt trauma, as mentioned earlier, a child may at first show minimal signs of blood loss because the segments of liver are compressed firmly within the intact peritoneum. Gradual distension of the abdomen, hypotension, and needle aspiration of intraperitoneal blood should alert one to the true situation. Unfortunately, we can recall several instances in which operation was attempted and, when the peritoneum was opened, the liver simply fell apart, with immediate and final exsanguination.

To save the life of a patient with a major tear of the liver requires preparation, experience, and speed. These accidents do not occur often enough to provide most children's hospitals with such facilities, and we must rely on occasional cases and the experience of others (Kaufman and Burrington, 1971; Ein, 1975; Steward and Creighton, 1975). As soon as the diagnosis of lacerated liver is made, shock therapy is started, and at least two maximum-sized catheters are placed in arm or neck veins. Volume expanders are started immediately, followed by plasma and blood as soon as they can be obtained. Oxygen is administered. If the child has lost consciousness, the trachea is intubated; otherwise the child is transported to the operating room and intubated under 50% nitrous oxide–oxygen, topical spray, and morphine.

Several approaches have been attempted to attain exposure of the torn liver without allowing free escape of volumes of blood. Hypothermia was used in cases reported by Bernhard (1955) and Welch (1979), and others have used the pump-oxygenator. More recently surgeons have tried to gain early control of hepatic vessels and inferior vena cava but disagree on whether to enter the chest first and place a ligature around the inferior vena cava or go directly into the abdomen and ligate the hepatic artery and vena cava. Flint and associates (1977), reporting 178 cases of hepatic trauma with 20% mortality, support the latter. Control of caval bleeding can be gained by passing a cuffed endotracheal tube into the inferior vena cava, starting either at the right atrium and passing it caudally or at the abdominal cava and passing it upward, and then inflating the cuff, thus bridging that part of the cava that most frequently is the site of fatal bleeding (Welch, 1979). It may be necessary to clamp the aorta for brief periods as well. With some control of the bleeding, and aided by rapid blood replacement and all supportive assistance, it should be possible to improve the salvage rate of these children.

The sickest patients facing operations on the liver are those undergoing *liver transplantation*. Although it is possible that interest may be rekindled in this procedure, results of most workers have been so discouraging that few are being performed at this time, and it does not seem practical to attempt a detailed discussion of the problem. The surgical success of Starzl and associates (1968) has been almost unique in this field, and the anesthetic management of the cases by Aldrete and associates (1969) should be examined by those interested in this area. Points of particular interest in the latter report bear repetition. A group of 25 patients (1 to 68 years of age) underwent orthotopic liver homotransplantation, and four more (1 to 50 years of age) had auxiliary hepatic homotransplants. Most notable in the care of these patients is the anhepatic state during which the portal vein is occluded and severe derangements occur, particularly in blood glucose and acid-base imbalance. The problems introduced by use of immunosuppressants resemble those related to kidney transplants. Hypothermia is difficult to control because of the tremendous amounts of blood

required (50 to 350 ml/kg) and the extensive exposure of abdominal viscera.

Other extensive abdominal procedures

A variety of extensive abdominal operations can be listed that involve either danger of hemorrhage, as in excision of Wilms' tumors and neuroblastomas, or prolonged manipulation of the viscera plus less marked blood loss, as in abdominoperineal procedures for Hirschsprung's disease, colectomy, and excision of intestinal duplications. The anesthetic management of children undergoing excision of large abdominal tumors has been a battleground of bitter experience from which most of our understanding of massive blood replacement has been gained (Figs. 17-2 and 17-3). This is discussed in Chapter 25.

Since the advent of electrodissection, blood loss has been approximately halved, but it remains the chief source of danger during the removal of large tumors. Crossmatching large amounts of blood is the first prerequisite in preparation; 50 to 100 ml/kg is a reasonable figure to start with, if more is available. This blood should be fairly fresh and should be warmed to room temperature before use.

As with hepatic operations, anesthesia is chosen to provide relaxation without depression of cardiovascular function, and our choice again is nitrous oxide, oxygen, and *d*-tubocurarine, but halothane now is added if so desired for analgesia and succinylcholine may be used for intubation. A gastric sump suction is kept in place throughout the operation to allow optimal working conditions for the surgeon.

At the start of these operations, two reliable infusions are established using the arms in operations in which the inferior vena cava may be cut or occluded and in Duhamel or other operations in which the legs may be supported in stirrups.

For most of these operations, patients will be supine or possibly in the Trendelenburg position. If a thoracoabdominal wound is necessary, greater blood loss should be ex-

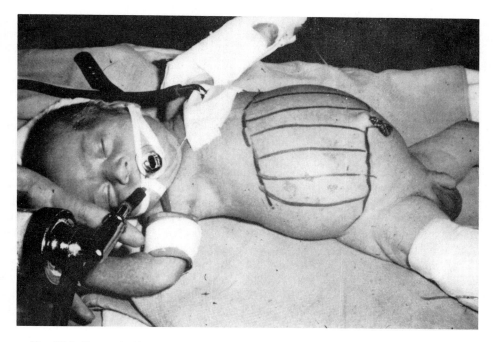

Fig. 17-2. Removal of large tumors from upper abdomen may involve copious blood loss.

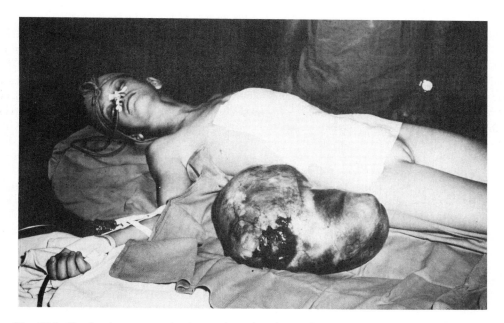

Fig. 17-3. Ovarian tumors may be tremendous, but danger lies in change in abdominal pressure rather than in blood loss.

pected, but the extent may be concealed if blood is allowed to accumulate in the thorax and abdomen. It is important for the anesthesiologist to watch the progress of the operation in order to estimate the rate of blood loss. A urethral catheter is used in such procedures, and an hourly output of 1 ml/kg is considered evidence of satisfactory renal perfusion. CVP measurement may be helpful but is less reliable in children and is not considered by us to be mandatory for children with normal cardiovascular function.

When one is dealing with children with Wilms' tumors, the tumor may be so large and unusual in appearance that one immediately has the urge to palpate it. The anesthesiologist should refrain from this during preoperative preparations and keep others away from the child as he lies unprotected on the operating table during anesthetic induction, for such palpation is believed to increase the risk of metastasis.

As noted with hepatic tumors, following removal of a large Wilms' tumor or neuroblastoma there may be active bleeding from the tumor bed, and one should continue to monitor blood loss closely during closure of the abdomen, expecting to continue replacement of appreciable amounts of blood.

Abdominal operations not involving tumors introduce other problems. Esophageal varices secondary to portal hypertension may bleed copiously, and patients requiring shunt procedures often have cystic fibrosis as underlying pathology. One avoids use of the esophageal stethoscope and gastric sump in these children. Pulmonary complications and general debility are to be expected.

The fluid replacement is especially important in patients undergoing prolonged intraabdominal operations in which there is continued handling of intestine, particularly Swenson or other procedures for Hirschsprung's disease. In such operations there may be relatively small blood replacement, but the loss of fluid by evaporation and third-space loss will far exceed that of most extra-abdominal operations, and there will be increased need of protein and electrolyte. It seems advisable to figure on a basic allowance of 8 ml/kg/hr of Ringer's lactate solution alternated with 5% dextrose in 0.5% saline solution, plus albumin as indicated by the clinical situation and measured serum protein. Urinary output is of major significance in such situations, and reduced output should be considered an indication for increased fluid intake rather than immediate recourse to a diuretic.

Splenectomy. Splenectomy, once a relatively common operation, now is reserved for definite therapeutic measures in treatment of selected anemia patients and as a diagnostic method in Hodgkin's disease. The observations of King and Shumacker (1952), Eraklis and associates (1967, 1972), and Welch (1979) that splenectomized children become highly susceptible to infections brought a sudden reduction in the removal of traumatized spleens and considerable reluctance to perform splenectomy for treatment of anemia in children under 2 years old. The child with a diagnosis of ruptured spleen is now given a trial on bed rest, or, if laparotomy is indicated, the spleen may be sutured together. Appropriate blood replacement is carried out in either situation.

Removal of the spleen is effective in treatment of both familial hemolytic anemia (spherocytosis) and thalassemia, and it is approximately 20% effective in curing idiopathic thrombocytopenic purpura (ITP). In spite of its value in these situations, the operation is withheld until children are out of infancy if possible, since the danger of infection is greatly increased in this age group. Only if transfusions are needed with unusual frequency is splenectomy performed in very young children.

Children with familial hemolytic anemia may have reduced red cell count. The destruction of the red cells is gradual, however, and the circulating blood volume is not reduced. The use of transfusions to restore the normal red cell count may result in bursts of hemolysis, leaving the child unimproved. For this reason, children frequently are accepted for operation with depleted red cells. An infusion is started at the beginning of operation, but blood is not given until the splenic pedicle has been clamped. From that point on, blood transfusion is tolerated normally.

ITP involves a different problem. Children with this disease usually have received cortisone to stimulate platelet formation. Consequently, an adequate steroid level should be established and maintained before, during, and after operation. Administration of 50 mg of hydrocortisone to children under 4 years and 100 mg to older patients is a reasonable measure.

Choice of an anesthetic agent for splenectomy once aroused controversy over whether one should use ether or cyclopropane. Those favoring ether believed that the sympathomimetic effect helped to contract the spleen, thereby releasing useful amounts of blood and shrinking the spleen to facilitate surgery. Now we use muscle relaxants, with halothane added as needed. The operation is not challenging unless the spleen is grossly enlarged. The patient usually is positioned right-side down for left subcostal incision. The surgeon's preference for head-down position with punishing tablebreak and kidney lift under the child should be moderated considerably. It should be possible to start the procedure with a rather mild break in the table, allowing the surgeon more angulation as it becomes necessary. An empty stomach is definitely required here, and no self-respecting anesthesiologist should need to be reminded to insert a sump after the operation has begun.

Splenectomy is now performed on all patients suspected of Hodgkin's disease. The accepted method of evaluating these patients consists of staging procedures that include x-rays, lymphangiograms, laparotomy, and splenectomy. Removal of the spleen is necessary because the entire organ must be examined for histologic changes. Ultimate therapy and decision on radiotherapy and antineoplastic drugs will depend on whether the child is categorized as stage 1, with a single node above the diaphragm, stage 2, with more than one node above the diaphragm, stage 3, with subdiaphragmatic spread, or stage 4, with systemic disease

(Rubin, 1972; Rosenberg, 1972; Aisenberg, 1978).

ANESTHESIA FOR GENITOURINARY SURGERY

The volume of pediatric genitourinary surgery has expanded tremendously during the past 10 years. Because of more perceptive diagnosis of congenital defects in early infancy, a more aggressive approach to their correction, and many operative procedures associated with renal failure, operations on the genitourinary tract occupy 20% to 30% of the pediatric surgical schedule, and the proportion is still increasing. This is fortunate, for success in these operations is relatively high, and the benefit gained in relief of urinary cripples is doubly appreciated by the patients and by others around them.

Surgical procedures and requirements

The variety of pediatric genitourinary operations presently being performed is suggested in the list on p. 398. The anesthetic requirements naturally vary—circumcision in a neonate bears little resemblance to renal transplant in a 12-year-old. For operations on external genitalia, there is definite need of analgesia. We still have not solved the age-old problem of anesthesia for neonatal circumcision. Our continued acceptance of circumcision without analgesia does not seem humane. It is excusable in many instances on the grounds that it is considerably safer than fumbling attempts at anesthesia. However, one is repeatedly reminded that the problem has been overlooked for too long (Weiss, 1968). It is our custom to use general (halothane) anesthesia for these infants and apply an analgesic ointment (Obtundia, Otis Clapp) and dressing for postoperative relief. Where suitable anesthetic facilities are not available, local anesthesia may be used, or the operation might well be omitted.

Relatively few of the urologic procedures may be considered as minor undertakings or suitable for ambulatory surgical approach. Paraphimosis, usually present in a slightly older age group than circumcision, requires general anesthesia but is appropriate for outpatient management, as are cystoscopy and urethral dilation. Girls tolerate cystoscopy rather easily, but boys need both analgesia and relaxation. Our choice for all is light general anesthesia with N_2O, oxygen, and halothane and occasionally with thiopental for induction in larger children. The use of topical anesthetic with instrumentation allays some of the postoperative discomfort.

Several widely divergent urologic conditions are reasonably considered urgent. These include impacted renal calculus, traumatic rupture of kidney or bladder, and emergencies of acute renal failure that are seen in all age groups. They also include others seen primarily in the pediatric age group. The small child with paraphimosis should be relieved within a few hours, but one may wait for his food to digest. A small child with a large, recently diagnosed Wilms' tumor should have a prompt workup and be operated on within 24 hours to reduce the chance of metastasis. The boy with painful torsion of the testicle is taken directly to the operating room, routine tests are cleared as efficiently as possible, and the operation is performed without delaying for digestion of food. In skilled hands, the danger of aspiration should be small compared with the probable loss of a testicle during a 4-hour postponement of surgery.

As may be seen below, the greater part of pediatric urologic survey is made up of fairly extensive procedures, often invading the deeper areas of the body and consuming considerable time. Such is the enthusiasm of current surgeons that one is known to have spent 20 hours in an attempt to reconstruct the kidneys, ureters, and bladder of a small child in a single operation. Obviously any procedure of this nature demands all available refinements in anesthetic care. Under more usual circumstances, where several shorter operations would be used, it would still call for full relaxation, light analgesia, meticulous fluid and metabolic control, and administration of anesthesia with a clear understanding of the underlying pathology of the specific condition. There are similar features in each of the groups categorized below. Many of the procedures to correct anomalies are relatively long, usually performed on young children in fair-to-good condition. Blood loss should be less of a problem than maintainance of metabolic equilibrium. The tumor group carries the potential for massive blood loss, with additional complications in several varieties of tumor. Trauma brings the problems of shock and unassessed hidden bleeding. Complex syndromes involving renal pathology introduce problems of muscle weakness and related disability, while chronic renal failure opens up a multitude of questions concerning renal dysfunction, tissue response, and immunology.

MORE COMMONLY ENCOUNTERED GENITOURINARY CONDITIONS REQUIRING SURGERY DURING INFANCY AND CHILDHOOD

Congenital anomalies
Double renal pelvis and ureters
Ectopic ureter
Megaureter
Ureterocele
Neurogenic bladder
Exstrophy of bladder
Undescended testes
Hypospadias, epispadias
Phimosis
Vaginal anomalies

Cysts and tumors
Wilms' tumor
Cystic kidney
Neuroblastoma
Ganglioneuroma
Adrenogenital tumors
Pheochromocytoma
Retroperitoneal teratoma
Ovarian tumor

Trauma
Ruptured kidney
Ruptured bladder
Urethral injuries

Renal failure (operative procedures)
Renal biopsy
Nephrectomy
Shunt and fistula creation
Parathyroidectomy
Renal transplantation

Infections
Cystitis
Urethritis
Paraphimosis

Anesthetic evaluation and management of urologic patients

Some degree of similarity among urologic patients may lull one into the idea that they are all alike. They are not, and one must know when to look for trouble.

The loss of renal function is only one of the defects seen in urologic patients. Urinary infection and obstruction are present in a great many urologic lesions, and their presence and degree of development are primary considerations in patient evaluation. History of fever is of importance, as are weight loss (or gain), change in voiding habits, and fluid intake. Fatigue, anorexia, bed-wetting, vomiting, anuria, pain, anemia, acidosis, urgency, and pyuria all may be associated with developing renal infection.

Laboratory evidence of renal disease may include leucocytosis, bacterial growths in urine culture, proteinuria, and hematuria. The most informative test of overall renal function, according to Welch (1979b), is the creatinine clearance test. The normal values range from 45 to 60 ml/m^2/min, based on 24-hour collection. For immediate information, serum creatinine (normal values 0.4 to 0.8 mg/dl) and blood urea nitrogen (normal, 8 to 20 mg/dl) give reliable guidance. Intravenous pyelography and other filming technics aid in diagnosis and in prediction of the magnitude of the coming operation.

Psychologic and emotional considerations. It should be remembered that many children with urologic problems have deeply seated emotional involvement. This may be due to the chronicity of several defects and the need of repeated operations, it may be due to embarrassment caused by urinary leakage, or it may be due to sensitivity related to abnormal genitalia. This is frequently found in young boys with hypospadias, many of whom have taken muscle-building courses to restore their self-confidence. Special encouragement and consideration are due such individuals, and physicians should avoid unnecessary exposure or discussion of their patients' defects.

Positioning and anesthetic technics. Position during operation is of some importance.

While cystoscopy in lithotomy position is relatively harmless, and the majority of procedures performed through the abdomen are acceptable, those requiring the lateral, angulated kidney position can be quite punishing if carried to the extent desired by the surgeon. As with the position for splenectomy, the patient may be placed over the break in the table and flexed mildly until more angulation actually is necessary; then enough angulation is allowed to facilitate the operation without compromising cardiorespiratory function.

General principles of anesthetic management for urologic patients in this age group call for mild preoperative sedation, relatively full relaxation under controlled ventilation, and moderate degrees of analgesia, all of which can be provided by one's favorite sedative plus a balanced type of anesthesia. Halothane or ethrane may be used as supplements in the presence of normal renal function, but for prolonged relaxation, excessive amounts of these agents might be required if relied on as primary agents. Standard monitoring apparatus should suffice for operations less than 3 hours long and not involving massive blood loss or unusual risks. Arterial cannulation would be indicated for any of the increased risks, such as those encountered in removal of large tumors, severe trauma, or pheochromocytoma.

Measurement of body temperature has special significance during most urologic operations because of the increased potential for infection. Most procedures on kidneys, ureters, bladder, or lower urinary tract may allow release of organisms into surrounding tissues, with resulting sudden temperature elevation to 104° to 105° F. Current interest in malignant hyperthermia will probably bring that rarity to mind at once, but sepsis will be a more likely diagnosis. Unfortunately, the urine is not collected during many of these cases, and diagnosis is less easily determined, but absence of tachycardia or arrhythmias, muscle spasm, and other signs of malignant hyperthermia should help to settle the question.

Inability to measure urine excretion or

content is a definite disadvantage in any procedure, but particularly in operations where kidneys are both diseased and stressed. If possible, at least one kidney should be monitored by urethral catheter. Fluid administration during renal operations usually will require moderate increase over standard minimal allowances, unless one is dealing with renal failure. This is discussed below. For children with near-normal kidneys who are undergoing relatively long urologic procedures, the manipulation of abdominal viscera should increase third-space accumulation appreciably, and the standard minimal fluid allowances of 4 to 6 ml/kg/hr could easily be increased to 6 to 8, with additional fluids to replace blood and protein losses. During such operations, children also will need fluid, glucose, sodium, chloride, and possibly potassium and magnesium.

Management of specific lesions

In each of the subgroups of urologic surgery, there are specific lesions that deserve additional consideration. Although many are of interest, there is space here for only a few. References for more complete information include texts by Kelalis and King (1976), Ravitch and associates (1979), and Holder and Ashcraft (in press) as well as other texts on the medical aspects of renal disease.

Megaureter stands as a typical major problem resulting from ureteral obstruction. Hendren (1979) has developed repair of this lesion to an advanced stage that offers excellent results but requires extensive operation and highly refined anesthetic care.

Exstrophy of the bladder in the past involved several operations in order to turn in the bladder, reconstruct the phallus, and pull together the divided pelvis. Gross reported a series of 80 such cases at our hospital in 1959. The procedure now often undertaken combines an orthopedic maneuver to separate sacroiliac joints, with the infant prone, and then the infant is turned over to allow the general or urologic surgeon to perform the extensive turn-in of the bladder. This in reality constitutes two extensive and bloody operations in one and rates with excision of tu-

mors for incidence of hypovolemic shock. Extensive preparation for support and massive blood replacement is necessary, and the combined procedure should only be attempted where optimal facilities and personnel are involved.

Wilms' tumor, neuroblastoma, and cystic kidney stand out among some 20 tumors of the region as being strikingly large, relatively common, and quite challenging. The first two have already been mentioned in this chapter. Considerable experience in dealing with these tumors has been gained in our hospital, and there has been keen interest in the coordination of surgical, radiation, and chemotherapeutic approaches (Gross and others, 1959; Farber, 1966).

All three of these tumors may reach remarkable size before being recognized, because parents may mistake the bulging abdomen for normal baby development until jolted to reality by palpation of an unyielding mass. There are innumerable differences in origin, diagnosis, therapy, and prognosis. For the anesthesiologist, Wilms' tumor and neuroblastoma represent major problems in relaxation, blood replacement, and critical care. Both are malignant, present the hazards of metastasis, and are treated with a variety of antineoplastic agents, among which doxorubicin (Adriamycin) must be identified and evaluated for possible cardiotoxic effects prior to anesthesia (Rinehart and others, 1974). Removal of both may involve enough manipulation to release catecholamines and initiate bursts of hypertension. However, the two differ in that the catechol released during excision of Wilms' tumors comes from handling of the adjacent adrenal gland, whereas the hypertension, tachycardia, and arrhythmias evoked during surgery of neuroblastoma, and the less malignant ganglioneuroma, come from the neurogenic tissues of which they are composed. None of these reactions is apt to be as upsetting as those seen in treatment of pheochromocytoma, where the continued release of catecholamines often brings the patient to the operating room with a history of continued hypertension and significant generalized vasoconstriction, and extremes of high and low blood pressure occur during the operation. Treatment directed against catechol excess has not been necessary in our experience with Wilms' or neurogenic tumors but is part of the standard management of pheochromocytoma, as mentioned below.

Adrenogenital disorders are rare but involve particular danger during anesthesia. Adrenal hyperplasia and adrenal tumors with virilizing effects bring girls to surgery for excision of an enlarged clitoris and boys for exploration for adrenal tumors. Therapy with hormones, steroids, and antihypertensive agents introduces a variety of complications. In our experience, acute sodium depletion has been the chief problem. On two occasions small girls have developed sudden cardiovascular collapse shortly after clitorectomy; both were later found to be severe "salt losers" who had been without their usual therapy for several hours. Though not present in all patients having adrenal hyperplasia, the salt-losing defect should be ruled out before operation or suitable therapy instituted to prevent complications.

Pheochromocytoma, although one of the more exotic pathologic lesions, is one of the least common, occurring in children less frequently than in adults. It has been seen in our operating rooms less than five times among the last 200,000 patients. The tumor causes headache, hypertension, nausea, and sweating in both young and old, and operation has been associated with mortality of 10% to 40% (Hume, 1960) due to hypertension, hypovolemia, and shock. Greater problems occur when the tumor had not been suspected and when it is multilocular. In children pheochromocytoma produces more norepinephrine than epinephrine, a difference that should cause fewer arrhythmias. In a majority of cases it occurs bilaterally (Schwartz and others, 1974).

Continuous production of sympathomimetic substances causes hypertension and peripheral vasoconstriction, with resultant reduction of circulating blood volume. Prior to operation it is important to lower blood pressure and expand blood volume. This may

be accomplished by administration of alpha adrenergic–blocking phenoxybenzamine (30 to 60 mg/day PO) for 7 to 10 days and beta-blocking propranolol (30 mg/day PO) for 2 to 3 days prior to operation (Kumar and Zsigmond, 1978; Pratilas and Pratila, 1979).

Few workers have had sufficient experience to speak with authority concerning management of children with pheochromocytoma. Consequently, there are brief reports favoring and condemning most of the major anesthetics. Recent preference has been shown for halothane, ethrane, and balanced anesthesia with sodium nitroprusside (Katz and Wolf, 1971). However, Innovar and droperidol both are known to induce marked hypotension in patients with pheochromocytoma and appear to be poorly suited to this use. If the patient is well prepared and one has a method of controlling the fluctuating pressure, it seems possible to use a variety of agents.

Several conditions characterized by defective abdominal muscle strength have important bearing on urologic function. Though rare (a total of 184 in world literature), that labelled *prune-belly syndrome* by Osler in 1901 is one of the most striking. Abdominal musculature is not absent, as often inferred, but is moderately to severely deficient. The abdominal wall hangs like a loose, wrinkled sac, with resultant lack of support of viscera (Fig. 17-4). Additional loss of bladder musculature underlies much of the urologic pathology caused by inability to void spontaneously. Bladder distension, ureteral reflux, hydronephrosis, and renal failure naturally follow.

Also known as abdominal musculature deficiency (AMD), it affects males in 95% of cases and varies widely in organs involved and degree of involvement. The typical combination is primary defect of the urologic system with malrotation of the gut, talipes equinus, and a congenital heart lesion. Welch (1979a), summarizing 45 patients treated at our hospital, listed a total of 276 urologic anomalies plus 37 orthopedic, 15 gastrointestinal, 10 cardiovascular, and 30 other defects identified in this group.

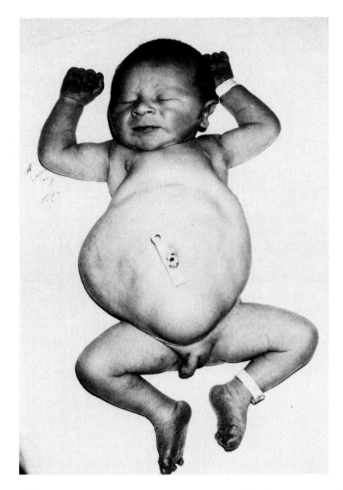

Fig. 17-4. Abdominal musculature deficiency, or prune-belly syndrome.

Urologic operations most frequently required for these infants include ureterostomy, bladder neck resection, and ureteral reimplantation. As pointed out by Hannington-Kiff (1970), these infants present severe anesthetic problems. The presence of an enlarged, atonic bladder and associated urologic pathology means that the infant may have renal infection, anemia, and uremia, while cardiac and other defects add further problems. Of most concern to the anesthesiologist is the infant's inability to cough or ventilate effectively, with resultant preoperative pulmonary infection and marked danger of aspiration during anesthesia. Although there is little need for relaxation, absence of abdominal tone makes inflation of the stomach almost unavoidable prior to intubation. Sedation would not be indicated, and choice of anesthesia should be made with the assumption that there is some degree of renal failure. Light levels of halothane with 50% N_2O have been satisfactory in our experience. Intubation of the trachea is easily accomplished without anesthesia. The bladder should be emptied prior to operation and not allowed to become distended during the procedure. Respiratory care after operation will be of maximal importance, and ventilatory assistance may be required. To assist spontaneous respiration after recovery, Hannington-Kiff suggests that small children sit forward with arms extended over a bed table to help pectoral muscles expand the chest.

In *neurogenic bladder,* neurologic deficits, caused primarily by myelomeningocele, result in atonic bladder, infection, reflux, and kidney destruction, as in the case of AMD syndrome, though with fewer associated anomalies. Bladder neck resection, conduit formation, and ureteral reimplantation frequently are necessary. Anesthetic problems are different here, because there is no diaphragmatic deficiency or involvement of thoracic muscles, but danger of increased intracranial pressure will threaten. Patient evaluation should include determination of the level at which sensation is lost, for some children will need hardly any anesthesia if the level is high enough to block sensory supply to the abdomen.

ANESTHESIA FOR PATIENTS IN END-STAGE RENAL FAILURE

The development of dialysis and renal transplantation has brought a new group of patients into the sphere of the anesthesiologist. Patients with renal failure, regardless of their age, have emotional and pathologic problems that demand the combined efforts of psychiatrists, nephrologists, and cardiologists as well as surgeons and anesthesiologists.

The anesthesiologist rarely is concerned with patients who have acute renal failure. Whether caused by hypoxia, trauma, dehydration, or some toxic agent, acute renal failure usually is characterized by severe oliguria or anuria, hyperkalemia, metabolic acidosis, and hypertension, the treatment of which consists chiefly of removing the cause and attempting correction of chemical imbalances. On occasion, if sedation is needed for cystoscopy or peritoneal dialysis, one must observe care in the choice and dosage of agents and provide supportive measures, though few would be required for simple procedures of this nature.

It is the child with chronic renal failure whose many problems harass the anesthesiologist. Chronic renal failure is difficult to describe in exact terms. Dunn (1975) states that

"chronic renal failure (CRF) may be defined as a complex of clinical and laboratory disturbances due to a permanent reduction in renal function, of which the essential feature is a decreased glomerular filtration rate." In preadolescent children, clinical signs seldom appear before the glomerular filtration rate falls below 20 ml/min/m^2, at which time the blood urea nitrogen level will be above 40 mg/dl and the serum creatinine level over 1.6 mg/dl.

These figures represent severe renal pathology, or end-stage renal disease (ESRD). The predisposing diseases leading to CRF listed by Estafanous and associates (1973) in their report of 4164 patients with renal failure showed chronic glomerulonephritis far in the lead, followed by chronic pyelonephritis, sclerosing glomerulonephritis, polycystic disease, systemic lupus erythematosus, malignancy, and other causes.

Surgical procedures

Children with renal failure undergo operations similar to those necessary for adults. Kidney biopsy, nephrectomy, renal transplant, creation of shunts and fistulae, and parathyroidectomy are those most closely related to kidney failure, while hip replacement, due to postnephrectomy osteomalacia, is an unhappy addition to the group.

The surgical requirements for most of these operations are not excessive. The patients have few anomalies that complicate the mechanics of anesthesia. With the exception of cystoscopy and nephrectomy, most of the operations are performed with the children in supine position. Transplantation requires an extensive abdominal wound with full relaxation, but blood loss seldom is enough to require transfusion. Here, and in creation of shunts, the critical need to maintain effective blood flow introduces special difficulties in patients with hypovolemia, as described below.

Evaluation and preparation of patients

It is the condition of the patient, rather than the operation, that creates the worst problems for the anesthesiologist. Children with CRF often are years behind in body development, are under great emotional strain, and carry a variety of serious organic defects, including anemia, acidosis, hyperkalemia, hypocalcemia, hypertension, and distortion of body fluids (Potter and others, 1970, 1970a).

The anesthesiologist may not be aware of the nonsurgical aspect of renal failure therapy that most of these children endure. Dialysis, lasting at least 3 hours two or three times each week, with necessary trips to and from the hospital, consumes a large part of their lives for indefinite periods of months or years. The anxiety level increases with the duration of dialysis therapy, the number of transplants and rejections, and the general home and family situation (Dunn, 1975). The overwhelming combination of the variety of operations they face, the uncertainty of when the next will be needed, and especially the fear of transplant rejection makes the psychologic aspect one of the most difficult and continuing problems related to renal failure. Young school-age children are said to tolerate the situation better than older patients, but it is not surprising that there is an appreciable incidence of suicide that extends down even to the younger patients (Lilly and Starzl, 1971; Grushkin and others, 1972; Sorenson, 1972).

It is a practice in many clinics to have at least one full-time psychiatrist whose entire effort is in this direction. For the same reason, it is advisable for one or more anesthesiologists to be assigned to this group of patients, so that there can be optimal familiarity with both the medical and the emotional situations. It is a great help to the child if he knows in advance that someone he knows and likes is going to take care of him each time he returns to the operating room.

The retarded growth of the child with renal failure is not of itself a major problem for the anesthesiologist, but it must be an added source of discomfort for a 12-year-old to be mistaken repeatedly for a 5- or 6-year-old.

Anemia, of severe degree, is a usual finding in these children (Erslev, 1970). Because of the danger of antibody stimulation that may be caused by repeated transfusion, surgeons prefer to operate in the presence of markedly reduced red blood cells rather than risk transfusion. This comes as a shock to anesthesiologists who have been taught that 10 g/dl is the lower limit of red cell depletion allowable in surgical patients.

It has been argued that the anemia of these patients is of less concern because of the compensatory increase in 2,3-DPG, which should shift the oxygen dissociation curve to the right and increase the delivery of oxygen to the tissues (Torrance and others, 1970). Upon investigation of this assumption, however, it was found that there was little or no increase in 2,3-DPG (Smith and Strieder, 1976; Lichtman and others, 1974). Although such a response would be expected in the presence of any severe anemia, patients with renal failure currently are treated with aluminum hydroxide in order to reduce acidity. The acidity is controlled in this manner, but a side effect is to abolish the desired 2,3-DPG response, and the patient whose hemoglobin is 6 or 7 g/dl is without this assumed protection. Fortunately, experience from many areas has shown very little increased morbidity due to operating on patients with hemoglobin levels of 6 to 9 g/dl. It is now our general practice to regard 8 g/dl as an acceptable lower limit for patients facing transplant and 5.5 to 6 g/dl for those facing lesser procedures. When transfusion is needed, red cells are prewashed five times before use.

Metabolic acidosis is a natural result of decreased renal function, on which elimination of acid metabolites depends. As noted above, aluminum hydroxide is presently the agent used for control of this aspect and the associated osteomalacia.

Hyperpotassemia is the chemical change of most concern to the anesthesiologist, and we regard a blood concentration of 5.5 mEq/L as the definite maximum for any patient who is to receive anesthesia. As previously noted, increases in blood urea nitrogen and creatinine, are important indications for dialysis, as are severe hypertension, acidosis, and reduced levels of sodium, calcium, and magnesium.

It is a general practice to dialyze patients on the day before operation and draw samples for chemistries at the termination of dialysis and again on the morning of operation. Should the serum potassium still be more than 5.5 mEq/L, operation is postponed until further reduction is accomplished. This usually is possible by administration of an enema of the sodium-potassium exchange resin polystyrene sodium sulfonate (Kayexalate). With a dosage of 1 g/kg (1 g dissolved in 3 ml of water, 10% glucose, or 10% sorbitol), a reduction of potassium of 1 mEq/L is expected within 2 to 4 hours (Orloff and others, 1977). Two more factors in evaluation of patients coming to transplantation are the frequency with which they have been requiring dialysis and the weight loss (or gain) usually resulting from dialysis.

Hypertension is one of the most common findings in children with CRF. Although this may have some beneficial effect in maintaining glomerular filtration, excessive pressure elevation, and particularly hypertensive crises, must be avoided. Many children who come to transplantation will be receiving hydralazine (Apresoline) in dosages of 75 to 200 mg/m²/day and propranolol in dosages of 30 mg/m²/day. Others may receive methyldopa (Aldomet), diazoxide (Hyperstat), or similar antihypertensive agents. These drugs are continued through the surgical period (Levin, 1973).

In case of a hypertensive crisis with sudden pressure elevation to 200 or 300 mm Hg, diazoxide, 5 to 10 mg/kg, is given by rapid intravenous injection (Drummond, 1975). Other agents used for this purpose are methyldopa, 10 to 20 mg/kg, and the combination of hydralazine, 0.1 mg/kg, and reserpine, 0.07 mg/kg (maximum dose 2 mg), given together intramuscularly.

In case of cardiac failure, digoxin may be given with care, but the drug is excreted slowly by diseased kidneys. Furthermore, the hypervolemia and apparent edema often mistaken for signs of cardiac failure are more apt to be due to hypernatremia of renal origin.

Other drugs often used in preparation for transplantation are corticosteroids to reduce immune response and antibiotics to control infection. Antibiotics are also excreted more slowly and must be administered as indicated by blood level titration.

An additional factor to consider in evaluation of patients with CRF is the high incidence of infectious hepatitis. Until proved otherwise, it is advisable to take precautions on the assumption that patients with CRF do have the infection. Should hepatitis be known to be present, one might hesitate to use halothane for anesthesia, but the mere possibility would not appear to be a contraindication.

In the anesthetic management of children in acute or chronic renal failure, sedatives and general anesthetic agents are chosen that have minimal effect on the existing renal pathology and that are not appreciably affected by reduced renal function (Aldrete and others, 1971; Cohen and others, 1975; Bastron and Deutsch, 1976). Methoxyflurane is definitely contraindicated on the basis of findings of Crandell and associates (1966), Holaday and associates (1970), Mazze and associates (1972), and others that free fluoride is released in the metabolism of the agent in sufficient amounts to be toxic. Further studies by Bastron and Deutsch (1976) and Mazze and associates (1977) have made the use of enflurane appear inadvisable in the presence of renal pathology. Gallamine has been shown to be excreted entirely by the kidneys (Churchill-Davidson and others, 1967; Feldman and others, 1969) and is ruled out on this count. Ketamine and pancuronium are not toxic, but their hypertensive action makes them undesirable in most situations.

Knowledge that succinylcholine causes marked elevation of serum potassium in the presence of severe tissue injury and other pathologic defects (Tolmie and others, 1967;

Kendig and others, 1972) gives one reason to doubt the safety of succinylcholine in the presence of renal failure. Several studies by Miller and associates (1972), Koide and Waud (1972), and Walton and Farman (1973) have shown that when serum potassium is near the upper level of normality (5 to 6 mEq/L), patients may have an exaggerated response to succinylcholine, but if serum potassium is low or in midrange, administration of succinylcholine is followed by potassium elevation similar to that expected in normal patients.

Based on these concepts, it has been our custom in preparing children for these urologic procedures to reduce the dosage of most agents by 30% to 50% unless experience with individual patients has shown us that a child needs more. In order to reduce the number of injections, an attempt is made to use oral or rectal routes of administration for sedatives whenever possible and to postpone atropine until the child is asleep. Morphine remains one of the better drugs for sedation and serves as the only sedative when an infusion is already established.

The use of regional anesthesia has been recommended by Herrin (1975) for operations other than transplantation and urinary diversions, while Linke and Merin (1976) advocate it for transplantation as well. We believe that regional methods are applicable for creation of shunts and arteriovenous fistulas and have had success with the interscalene block (Winnie, 1970) in a number of cases, but we find that general anesthesia is justifiably safe and is preferred by most younger patients.

Induction of anesthesia may be performed by intravenous or mask technic, and it is often possible to follow the wishes of patients, who frequently develop strong preferences (or aversions). Thiopental, allowable in limited dosage, provides the surest method. When children do not have infusions in place on arrival in the operating room, a suitable vein may be difficult to find. When no others are available, we may use one on the medial aspect of the wrist for induction but feel that this should not be used for a continuing infusion. On occasion one can find a superficial capillary on the surface of the trunk that will receive a 25-gauge hubless needle through which enough thiopental can be injected to put the child to sleep, after which a search for a deeper vein may be undertaken.

For maintenance of general anesthesia, our preference has been use of nitrous oxide and halothane supplemented by d-tubocurarine or metocurine in relatively stable patients, reserving balanced thiopental, nitrous oxide, and morphine for those whose arterial pressure is difficult to maintain. Monitoring of less extensive procedures consists of standard basic apparatus including the ECG, but arterial cannulae and CVP monitors are omitted unless a child is in critical condition. The amount of fluid administered must be suited to the need of the individual patient. In the presence of fluid retention, patients will be limited to approximately 2 ml/kg/hr as a basic allowance.

In order to prevent increasing acid-base imbalance, it is advisable to measure blood gases at the start of critical procedures. If acidosis is present, one should determine its origin and extent and use moderate hyperventilation followed by sodium bicarbonate if the severity of the acidosis warrants it.

As previously noted, surgeons frequently call for more peripheral perfusion during creation of a shunt or fistula. In such a situation, several maneuvers are applicable. Since the circulating blood volume is extremely variable in these patients, one may first check fluid balance. If there are signs of edema or overhydration, more volume is not indicated, but if, as is often the case after dialysis, the child is definitely hypovolemic, the addition of balanced electrolyte, 2 ml/kg, or albumin, 1 ml/kg, may produce a marked improvement in perfusion. One should also attempt to remove any cardiovascular depressant effect of anesthetic agents by reducing or eliminating halothane and d-tubocurarine and substituting nitrous oxide and morphine or possibly Innovar.

Kidney transplantation

A renal transplantation program was initiated at The Children's Hospital Medical Center in 1971 under the direction of Dr. Raphael Levey, surgeon, and Dr. Warren Grupe, nephrologist. A total of 95 patients underwent at least one transplantation between 1971 and 1978. Data are reviewed below. Levey feels that children should be able to tolerate transplantation at least as well as adults because they have fewer associated diseases to complicate their progress. This seems to be borne out in overall results.

DATA ON RENAL TRANSPLANTATIONS, THE CHILDREN'S HOSPITAL MEDICAL CENTER, 1971-1978

Total number of allographs	93
Total number of children	89
Youngest patient	2.4 yr
Oldest patient	24 yr
Mean age	12.6 yr
Total deaths	10
Anesthetic death	1
Total surviving kidneys	70
Lowest preoperative hematocrit	7.5%
Mean preoperative hematocrit	24.9%

PRIMARY DISEASES IN PATIENTS HAVING RENAL TRANSPLANTATION*

Membranoproliferative glomerulonephritis	12
Obstructive uropathy	14
Dysplasia	18
Glomerulonephritis	14
Nephrosclerosis	5
Alport's syndrome	3
Goodpasture's syndrome	2
Lupus erythematosus and immune complex	2
Hypertensive nephropathy	2
Radiation nephritis	2
Hemolytic-uremic syndrome	1
Henoch-Schönlein purpura	1
Cystinosis	1
Polycystic kidneys	1
Other	5

Our plan of management for children coming to transplantation has been similar in general to that described by Katz and associ-

*By permission from Levey, R. H., Ingelfinger, J., Grupe, W. E., and others: Unique surgical and immunologic features of renal transplantation in children, J. Pediatr. Surg. 13:576-580, 1978.

ates (1967), Potter and associates (1970, 1970a), Samuel and Powell (1970), Fine and associates (1973), Firlit (1974), and Salvatierra and associates (1977). The initiating lesions in our series are shown above and include dysplasia, nephrosclerosis, and chronic glomerulonephritis.

Most patients are carried on hemodialysis for several weeks or months before transplantation and often have had a variety of shunts and fistulas for this purpose. Nephrectomy is performed only when required to control excessive hypertension.

The hypertension, anemia, acidosis, and hyperkalemia associated with CRF in adults are also seen in children, who come to operation under controlling medication with steroids, antibiotics, and antihypertensive and antacid drugs and often digitalis as well. The interplay of such combinations is impossible to predict with accuracy. Dialysis is performed the day before operation to stabilize chemical constituents of the blood, and the hemoglobin level is brought up to a minimum of 8 g/dl by administration of frozen washed red blood cells.

Following suitably reduced medication, children are brought to the operating room. Anesthesia is induced with inhalation or intravenous agents as previously described, the trachea is intubated, and anesthesia is maintained under halothane, nitrous oxide, and oxygen supplemented by relaxants. Children are positioned with the side receiving the kidney slightly elevated. Monitors include the stethoscope (precordial instead of esophageal to reduce the risk of irritation, bleeding, and infection), blood pressure cuff (avoiding the arm that carries a shunt or fistula), thermistor probe, ECG and CVP monitors with continuous display, nasogastric tube, urethral catheter, and an infusion. CVP measurement has particular importance here, since the effort made to maintain renal perfusion invites added risk of overloading the heart. Arterial cannulation would be useful, but we try to do without it in order to save the vessel for other use.

During the course of the operation, specific drugs are given for immunosuppressive and supportive effect as follows:

1. Azathioprine (Imuran), 2 mg/kg, is given via drip infusion at the start of the operation for immunosuppression.
2. Mannitol, 1 g/kg, is started by infusion 15 to 20 minutes before expected opening of the circulation through the transplant kidney.
3. Furosemide (Lasix), 3 mg/kg, and methylprednisolone sodium succinate (Solu-Medrol), 10 mg/kg, are given by intravenous push approximately 5 minutes before the circulation is opened.

The new kidney is usually implanted by anastomosis to right or left iliac vessels. Some difficulty may occur when an adult kidney is used for a small child or infant. Fullest relaxation is essential but still may not suffice to make room for a kidney three times the desired size, in which case a temporary skin closure or mesh net repair may be needed for a brief period. A further difficulty is that such a large kidney will demand a much larger share of the cardiac output and may induce cardiac failure, for which rapid digitalization will be required.

Under usual conditions, the new kidney will become pink and will start to put out good quantities of urine within a few minutes after anastomosis has been opened. However, perfusion and urine flow may be delayed minutes, hours, or 2 to 3 days and then gradually begin to appear. Longer anuric spells would call for dialysis while therapy with methylprednisolone sodium succinate (Solu-Medrol) is used to stimulate the return of renal function.

To provide better renal blood flow, the previously mentioned steps are employed. Restoration of blood volume is of first importance. This should be accomplished with albumin rather than blood or electrolyte, and care must be taken not to overinfuse this solution. Measurement of serum protein and osmolality are of some value here.

During the postoperative course and thereafter there will be ongoing danger of infection, hemorrhage, acidosis, and rejection. These patients must be closely watched and usually require therapy for continued immunization and/or hypertension.

ANESTHESIA FOR PLASTIC PROCEDURES
Cleft lip repair (cheiloplasty)

The repair of cleft lip, or harelip, is not one of the most challenging procedures today, but because of the unpleasant facial disfigurement, innumerable attempts at correction have been made since the earliest days of surgery. One finds that many important advances were made by anesthesiologists working in this field, the most outstanding being those of Dr. Philip Ayre of Newcastle-on-Tyne. In looking more closely through the records of past years, one finds that in less skillful hands these operations had a surprisingly high mortality, often reaching 5%, a figure presently acceptable for only the most difficult types of open-heart surgery.

For the high degree of perfection now attainable in facial repair, the surgeon must have clear access to the infant's face, which should be without distortion and immobile. Some surgeons have preferred to face the infant as they work, for better visualization, but the usual approach is for the surgeon to work from the head of the operating table. The duration of the operation and the problems arising vary with the type of defect and the surgeon's experience and technic. A healthy infant with a small single cleft should offer a minimum of problems, and repair should involve less than an hour in any hands. A full double cleft, on the other hand, associated with a cleft palate and possibly additional deformities, may require as much as 4 hours for the fastidious type of repair now performed.

The problems that anesthesiologists have had to meet have consisted chiefly of getting out of the surgeon's way while continuing to control an airway that the surgeon was blocking with hands, instruments, and blood. Among the multitude of methods and devices improvised for these operations, Ayre's T-piece system stands out as the one with the greatest value for all pediatric use (Ayre, 1937, 1937a). Among other descriptions of anesthetic management of these problems are those of Slocum and Allen (1945), Leigh and Kester (1948), Kilduff and associates (1956), Whalen and Conn (1967), Salanitre and Rackow (1962), and others. The historical review of Gordon-Jones (1971) is particularly interesting.

Correction of cleft lip is performed in the neonatal period by some surgeons, whereas others prefer to wait until the infant is 4 to 6 weeks old. Our experience has been primarily with operations performed at 1 month of age. These infants should be in good general condition at the time of operation but often have reduced hematocrit level. Because of their age, some reduction is expected, but an additional factor of decreased nutritional level may be related to abnormal feeding patterns encountered. Hypovolemia also may be a factor in the response of these infants to anesthesia. While it is difficult to evaluate these factors exactly, one does well to bear them in mind during management of anesthesia.

If the surgeon is experienced and skilled, one may expect to get through most procedures within 90 minutes without needing blood replacement. Under other conditions, one must prepare to have blood ready and be sure that a reliable infusion is started at the outset.

Cheiloplasty has been performed with local anesthesia and with many variations of general anesthesia, with and without endotracheal intubation. Having had initial experience with over 1500 cheiloplasties performed under insufflation ether without fatality enables our group to state that this method can be used effectively, but the introduction of halothane and the use of intubation have made the task much easier.

In preparation for operation, the room is warmed and a heating lamp is brought into position. The infant's arms and legs are wrapped, and blood pressure cuff and stethoscope are applied. Using a standard nonrebreathing apparatus, anesthesia is induced with nitrous oxide, oxygen, and halothane, and 0.2 mg of atropine is injected intramuscularly as soon as the infant is asleep. Be-

cause of the malformation of the lip and maxilla, often exaggerated by the presence of a cleft palate, there will be increased obstruction by the tongue and soft tissues, and inhalation induction may be retarded until an airway can be inserted. A pad under the shoulders is definitely helpful at the start of induction but should be removed at the time of intubation. Endotracheal intubation is more difficult in the presence of a single cleft of the maxilla, and the difficulty much greater with a double cleft, especially where there is a freely mobile premaxillary tab in place of the normal rigid upper alveolar ridge (Fig. 17-5). Unless one has had experience with these infants, it may be preferable to avoid induction of apnea for intubation. For teaching and general use, we prefer adequate depth under halothane, often aided by subapneic doses of intramuscular succinylcholine (1.5 mg/kg). On intubation, the blade of the laryngoscope slips into the cleft, rendering it difficult to manipulate. To prevent this, it may help to roll up a sponge or use a piece of dental roll to fill the gap and restore the normal contour of the upper jaw. Following intubation, the tube is taped to the middle of the lower lip, and the anesthesiologist moves to the infant's left side. The infant is positioned for operation with a roll under the shoulders and the head in a soft head-ring. The surgeon's use of a sponge in the back of the mouth helps to keep the endotracheal tube in place. Injection of a limited amount of 1:200,000 epinephrine (2 ml/kg) has been well tolerated when used to control bleeding from the lip.

Anesthesia needs to be only deep enough to keep the child from moving, so we prefer light halothane and nitrous oxide combinations with spontaneous respiration, assisted as necessary to maintain adequate exchange. Here again, the presence of slight biceps tone is an excellent indication of the proper level of anesthesia, while the stethoscope is the most reliable monitor of a patent airway, adequate exchange, and an effective heart. Blood pressure and temperature are also monitored. The ECG serves little practical use during these procedures.

409

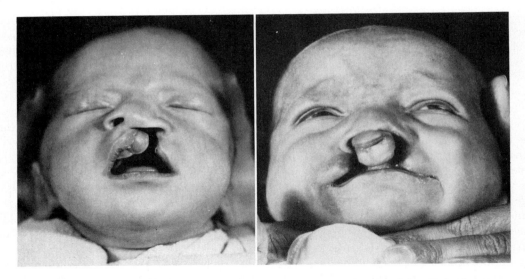

Fig. 17-5. Infants with single and double cleft lip. Presence of the clefts, especially with the free premaxilla and double cleft, makes intubation difficult.

Possible complications during cheiloplasty include displacement of the endotracheal tube, hypothermia, alteration in anesthetic depth, and blood loss, none of which should be allowed to get out of control. Hydration is maintained by infusion of 5% glucose in ¼N saline solution and blood is added in the rare event of its need.

The recovery phase of cheiloplasty may entail the greatest actual danger for these children and requires the best possible care. Three major problems are hypothermia, depression, and airway obstruction, and there are effective methods of preventing all of them. The child is kept warm during operation by warming the room, using a heat lamp, and wrapping, as previously described. A heating blanket has considerably less effect. If the child is warm at the end of the procedure, he will awaken promptly if anesthesia has been correctly administered.

One of the greatest improvements in caring for infants following cleft lip repair, or for any procedure about the mouth, has been for the surgeon to place a traction suture in the infant's tongue just before extubation (see Fig. 10-6). The two ends of the suture are left about 8 inches long and tied in a loop that is easily grasped, providing a most effective means of clearing the child's airway and at the same time affording an equally effective stimulus to breathe and move. The presence of this suture also allows one to extubate the infant somewhat earlier than usual. Before extubation, however, the anesthesiologist moves back to the head of the table and, with combined use of tongue suture and laryngoscope, examines the hypopharynx to confirm removal of the sponge placed there at the beginning of the procedure and to clear away any blood or secretions in the area.

Upon the patient's return to the recovery area, continued expert attendance is necessary, but with the infant placed on his stomach or side and the tongue suture immediately available, complications should be rare. The tongue suture is removed when the infant is ready to leave the recovery area and return to the nursing division.

Cleft palate repair

Repair of cleft palate is usually performed at approximately 1 year of age. By this time these children should have regained normal eating habits and have near-normal red cell counts and blood volume. Because of their facial and upper airway defects, however, one frequently finds that children with cleft

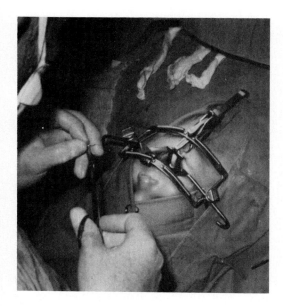

Fig. 17-6. Management of child for repair of cleft palate. Tongue blade of Dingman gag holds endotracheal tube in place. Anesthesiologist is at patient's left side.

palate have almost continuous colds and postnasal discharge, and it may be practically impossible to clear this up prior to operation. In such cases it has seemed reasonable to give these children effective doses of antibiotics for several days and then go ahead with the operation. This has been successful so far.

For performance of cleft palate repair, the surgeon again needs unrestricted access to the child's mouth and face. At our hospital, surgeons work from above the child's head, and the anesthesiologist is positioned at the child's left side.

At this age, a child is given appropriate sedative premedication and a general anesthetic. Halothane and nitrous oxide again are our choice. Induction may be complicated by the presence of draining secretions and abnormal airway, and intubation may be seriously impeded by associated anomalies such as Pierre Robin or Treacher Collins syndromes or other facial deformities. The Pierre Robin syndrome (Robin, 1923; Bougas and Smith, 1958) consists of micrognathia, underdeveloped mandible, and retrocessed tongue. These infants are among the most

difficult to intubate, and it sometimes is impossible to visualize the vocal cords. It has been helpful in several of these cases to use the long, tapered Wis-Foregger laryngoscope blade and look for the glottis at a lower level in the airway. In the Treacher Collins syndrome a variety of facial clefts may interfere with the opening of the child's mouth and visualization of the glottis. On two different occasions we have encountered a child whom we could not intubate.

Under normal circumstances the endotracheal tube is fastened to the lower jaw at the middle of the mouth, as in cheiloplasty. For palate repair, the surgeon uses a mouth gag (Dingman) to hold the mouth open (Fig. 17-6). This also serves to keep the endotracheal tube in place, thereby helping the anesthesiologist, as does the pack that the surgeon places in the hypopharynx.

Palate repair is different from cheiloplasty in that the operation is inside the oral cavity, while cheiloplasty is primarily concerned with structures in front of the teeth. Not only is there much more bleeding during and after palate repair, but it occurs inside the mouth, is harder to control, and naturally gravitates toward the hypopharynx and trachea.

These children usually have relatively accessible veins, and although the use of blood has been a distinct rarity, routine use of intravenous infusions is advisable.

At the conclusion of the operation, which should take from 45 to 90 minutes, it is essential for the anesthesiologist to auscultate both sides of the chest for presence of aspirated blood and then to examine the hypopharynx under direct vision with the aid of a laryngoscope. This must be done with care so as not to disturb the operative site. A tongue suture serves an even more valuable means of airway control here than following cheiloplasty. It is also more important to have these children stay in the prone position during recovery in order to avoid aspiration of blood. The use of jackets with sleeves splinted to prevent elbow flexion (Wellcome sleeves) has been helpful in keeping the children's hands away from their faces (MacCollum and Richardson, 1958).

In view of the problems that have long beset repair of cleft lips and palates, we regard our 35-year series of 4500 operations without fatality as one of our greater achievements.

Other plastic procedures

In addition to correction of harelip and cleft palate, a variety of plastic procedures may be performed in children, including correction of lop ears and webbed fingers and skin grafting. Most of these cause relatively few problems for the anesthesiologist. Otoplasty is performed in smaller children under endotracheal halothane with nonrebreathing technic, whereas intravenous agents may be used in older children if desired. Correction of webbed fingers is usually performed on young children and is a simple but time-consuming operation. Light general anesthesia is well tolerated, but because of the duration one should pay increased attention to maintenance of body temperature, blood pressure, and oxygenation. Endotracheal intubation rarely is necessary. Although easier for the anesthesiologist, it should be remembered that duration of anesthesia is not of itself an indication for intubation and that children between 1 and 3 years of age are most susceptible to postintubation tracheitis (Koka and others, 1977).

Correction of craniofacial deformities

Radical procedures for repair of defects of cranial, orbital, and facial areas developed by Dr. Philip Tessier of Paris (1967, 1971, 1974) now are being performed by American surgeons (Murray and others, 1975; Converse and others, 1975; Munro, 1975). These operations are designed to overcome the disfiguring lesions of children born with Apert's, Crouzon's, and Treacher Collins syndromes, hypertelorism, and other anomalies, as well as defects caused by trauma or by surgical and radiologic treatment of large tumors.

For pediatric anesthesiologists these procedures represent a unique combination of serious difficulties. The requirements of the surgeon in even the simpler procedures, such as mandibular osteotomy, may include wiring the jaws, while the most extensive, the midface advancement, involving as many as 100 surgical steps and consuming 12 to 15 hours, obviously compounds the hazards of airway management, fluid replacement, craniotomy, and cardiorespiratory control during operation and continuing airway and supportive care for several days afterward. It is important for all to bear in mind that such procedures are being undertaken entirely for cosmetic purposes.

Before undertaking the management of any operation of this type, the anesthesiologist should obtain a clear understanding of the intended operation, the possible complications, and the psychologic as well as the medical aspects of the individual situation. The length of the operation, the severe blood loss, and the simultaneous handling of mouth, orbits, and brain in themselves increase the risk greatly, and other problems add further chance of complication.

The variety of defects reported from The Children's Hospital Medical Center and the Peter Bent Brigham Hospital by Murray and associates (1975) is shown below. Among the surgical steps necessary to correct such defects are osteotomy of mandible, maxilla, and zygoma, multiple dental extractions, craniotomy and wide exposure of frontal lobes, medial replacement of orbits, reconstruction of nose and zygomatic arch, and complete mobilization and forward displacement of the maxilla with supporting onlay rib grafts. The last procedure, the midface advancement, or Le Fort III, includes almost all of the steps mentioned and, like several others, requires the additional participation of neurosurgeons and orthodontic surgeons (Murray and Swanson, 1968).

CATEGORIES OF CRANIOFACIAL DEFECTS IN 178 PATIENTS*

Congenital		143
Midface stenosis secondary to:		
Crouzon's, Apert's	28	
Cleft palate	22	

*From Murray, J. E., Swanson, L. T., Strand, R. D., and Hricko, G. M.: Evaluation of craniofacial surgery in the treatment of facial deformities, Ann. Surg. **182:**240, 1975.

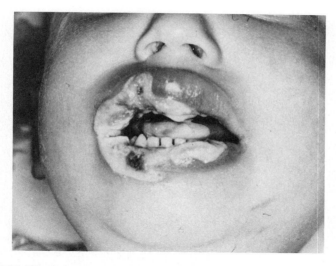

Fig. 17-8. Electric burn of mouth. (Courtesy Dr. Arnold Colodny, Boston, Mass.)

as his health. This is best accomplished by assigning one interested anesthesiologist to be friend, confidante, and guardian of the child and to be responsible for each anesthetic. Sedation and anesthesia are chosen to provide prompt awakening and rapid recovery of appetite in order to maintain nutrition. Sedative requirements decrease as morale climbs, and milder agents may suffice to replace morphine. Sedatives should be chosen that may be given by mouth or by infusion. When atropine is given, it is withheld until the child is asleep. Ketamine is generally preferred for most burn dressings and grafts and often allows children to lie prone without endotracheal intubation (Wilson, 1975). When burns involve the airway, halothane is less apt to cause irritation.

The danger of using succinylcholine in the presence of severe burns is well recognized and is discussed in Chapters 13 and 26.

The concentration of serum potassium is now watched carefully in all patients with burns or other major wounds involving tissue destruction or muscle denervation. Succinylcholine is avoided until wound healing is well established. Relaxants are rarely used with anesthesia, and d-tubocurarine is favored if one is needed.

There have been two major problems in our experience with burn patients: blood loss and heat loss. Blood loss during dressing or grafting of a granulating burn area can be massive and may require repeated transfusions. Heat loss through burned surfaces may cause shivering and hypoxia but has been reduced by warming the operating room, by using heating lamps and warmed intravenous fluids, and in addition by warming any ointments or moist dressings to be applied to the burned areas.

Of the many problems posed by burn contractures, some of the worst are seen in scars around the neck, causing severe retraction of the chin and sometimes making intubation extremely difficult (Fig. 17-9). Awake intubation is most distressing and to be avoided, and relaxants are not indicated in such situations. General anesthesia with spontaneous respiration is acceptable but not always successful. The use of small increments of morphine (0.05 mg/kg), given intramuscularly at intervals of 3 to 4 minutes, and topical spray of 4% lidocaine to the glottis has been successful in patients of all ages, because it dulls anxiety before depressing respiration. If additional help is needed, Epstein and associates (1966) suggest having the surgeon incise the lateral cords of the scar overlying the sternocleidomastoid muscles. This sim-

417

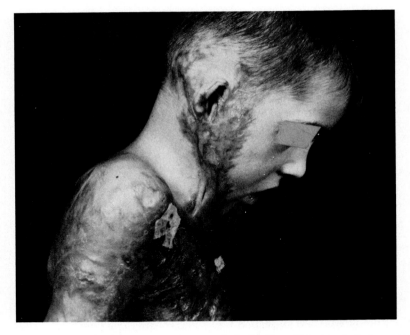

Fig. 17-9. Burn contracture of the neck. (From Epstein, B. S., Rudman, H. L., Hardy, D. L., and Downes, H.: Anesth. Analg. [Cleve.] **45**:352, 1966.)

ple maneuver reportedly facilitates intubation greatly.

BIBLIOGRAPHY

Aisenberg, A. C.: Current concepts in cancer; the staging and treatment of Hodgkin's disease, N. Engl. J. Med. 299:1228, 1978.

Aldrete, J. A., Daniel, W., Higgins, J. W., and others: Analysis of anesthetic-related morbidity in human recipients of renal homografts, Anesth. Analg. (Cleve.) 50:321, 1971.

Aldrete, J. A., Levine, D. S., and Gingrich, T. F.: Experience in anesthesia for liver transplantation, Anesth. Analg. (Cleve.) 48:802, 1969

Allan, C. M., Culley, W. G., and Gillies, D. N. M.: Ventricular fibrillation in a burned boy, Can. Med. Assoc. J. 85:432, 1961.

Antoon, A. Y., Volpe, J. J., and Crawford, J. D.: Burn encephalopathy in children, Pediatrics 50:609, 1972.

Ayre, P.: Anaesthesia for hare-lip and cleft palate operations on babies, Br. J. Surg. 25:131, 1937.

Ayre, P.: Endotracheal anaesthesia for babies; with special reference to harelip and cleft palate operations, Anesth. Analg. (Cleve.) 16:330, 1937.

Baskett, P. J. F., Hyland, J., Deane, M., and Wray, G.: Analgesia for burns dressing in children, Br. J. Anaesth. 41:684, 1969.

Bastron, R. D., and Deutsch, S.: Anesthesia and the kidney, ed. 1, New York, 1976, Grune & Stratton, Inc.

Bennett, W. M., Keeffe, E., Melnyk, C., and others: Response to dopamine hydrochloride in the hepatorenal syndrome, Arch. Intern. Med. 135:964, 1975.

Berger, P. E., Culham, J. A. G., Fitz, C. R., and Harwood-Nash, D. C.: Slowing of hepatic flow by halothane, Radiology 118:303, 1976.

Bernhard, W. F.: The feasibility of partial liver resection under hypothermia, N. Engl. J. Med. 253:159, 1955.

Black, G. W., Coppel, M. B., Hughes, N. C., and Love, S. H. S.: Anaesthesia for cleft palate surgery, Br. J. Plast. Surg. 22:343, 1969.

Bougas, T. P., and Smith, R. M.: Pathologic airway obstruction in children, Anesth. Analg. (Cleve.) 37:137, 1958.

Bush, G. H.: The use of muscle relaxants in burnt children, Anaesthesia 19:231, 1964.

Cannon, W. B., and Rosenblueth, A.: The sensitization of a sympathetic ganglion by preganglionic denervation, Am. J. Physiol. 116:408, 1936.

Churchill-Davidson, H. C., Way, W. L., and deJong, R. H.: The muscle relaxants and renal excretion, Anesthesiology 28:540, 1967.

Churchill-Davidson, H. C., Wylie, W. D., Miles, B. E., and de Wardener, H. E.: The effects of adrenaline, nor-adrenaline and Methadrine on the renal circulation during anesthesia, Lancet 2:803, 1951.

Cohen, E. N., Trudell, J. R., Edmunds, H. N., and Watson, E.: Urinary metabolites of halothane in man, Anesthesiology 43:392, 1975.

Converse, J. M., Wood-Smith, D., and McCarthy, J. G.: Report on a series of 50 craniofacial operations, Plast. Reconstr. Surg. 55:3, 1975.

Crandell, W. B., Pappas, S. G., and MacDonald, A.: Nephrotoxicity associated with methoxyflurane anesthesia, Anesthesiology 27:591, 1966.

Drummond, K. N.: Chronic renal failure. In Vaughan, V. C. III, and McKay, R. J., Jr., editors: Nelson textbook of pediatrics, ed. 10, Philadelphia, 1975, W. B. Saunders Co.

Dunn, J. A.: Role of the physician in prevention of psychologic disorders in the sick child. In Vaughan, V. C. III, and McKay, R. J., Jr., editors: Nelson textbook of pediatrics, ed. 10, Philadelphia, 1975, W. B. Saunders Co.

Ein, S. H.: Abdominal injuries. In Surgical Staff of Hospital for Sick Children, Toronto: Care of the injured child, Baltimore, 1975, The Williams & Wilkins Co.

Ein, S. H., and Stephens, C. A.: Benign liver tumors and cysts in children, J. Pediatr. Surg. 9:847, 1974.

Ein, S. H., and Stephens, C. A.: Malignant liver tumors in children, J. Pediatr. Surg. 91:491, 1974a.

Epstein, B. S., Rudman, H. L., and Downes, H.: Comparison of orotracheal intubation with tracheostomy for anesthesia in patients with face and neck burns, Anesth. Analg. (Cleve.) 45:352, 1966.

Eraklis, A. J., and Filler, R. M.: Splenectomy in childhood; a review of 1,413 cases, J. Pediatr. Surg. 7:382, 1972.

Eraklis, A. J., Kevy, S. V., Diamond, L. K., and Gross, R. E.: Hazard of overwhelming infection after splenectomy in childhood, N. Engl. J. Med. 276:1225, 1967.

Erslev, A. J.: The anemia of chronic renal disease, Arch. Int. Med. 126:774, 1970.

Estafanous, F. G., Porter, J. K., El Tawil, M. Y., and Popowniak, K. L.: Anaesthetic management of anephric patients and patients in renal failure, Can. Anaesth. Soc. J. 20:769, 1973.

Evrard, M.: Anesthesia problems in the infant with acute intestinal intussusception, Anesth. Analg. (Paris) 30:1085, 1973.

Farber, S.: Chemotherapy in the treatment of leukemia and Wilms' tumor. J.A.M.A. 198:826, 1966.

Feldman, S. A., Cohen, E. N., and Colling, R. C.: The excretion of gallamine in the dog, Anesthesiology 30:593, 1969.

Fine, R. N., Korsch, B. M., Riddell, H. G., and others: Second renal transplants in children, Surgery 73:1, 1973.

Firlit, C. F.: Current status of renal transplantation in small children, Urol. Clin. North Am. 1:549, 1974.

Flint, L. M., Mays, E. T., Aaron, W. S., and others: Selectivity in management of hepatic trauma, Ann. Surg. 185:613, 1977.

Furman, E. B.: Anesthesia for right hepatic lobectomy in a child; an exercise in blood volume management (clinical workshop), Anesthesiology 35:436, 1971.

Gordon-Jones, R. C.: A short history of anaesthesia for hare-lip and cleft palate repair, Br. J. Anaesth. 43:796, 1971.

Gross, R. E., Farber, S., and Martin, L. W.: Neuroblastoma sympatheticum; a study and report of 217 cases, Pediatrics 23:1179, 1959.

Grushkin, C. M., Korsch, B., and Fine, R. N.: Hemodialysis in small children, J.A.M.A. 221:869, 1972.

Hannington-Kiff, J. G.: Prune-belly syndrome and general anesthesia; case report, Br. J. Anaesth. 42:649, 1970.

Head, J. M., and Smyth, B. T.: Non-penetrating intra-abdominal injuries in children, J. Pediatr. Surg. 9:69, 1974.

Hendren, W. H.: Megaureter. In Ravitch, M. M., Welch, K. J., Benson, C. D., and others, editors: Pediatric surgery, ed. 3, Chicago, 1979, Year Book Medical Publishers, Inc.

Herrin, J. T.: Preparation of the renal patient for surgery, Int. Anesthesiol. Clin. 13:183, 1975.

Herrin, J. T., and Crawford, J. D.: The seriously burned child. In Smith, C. A., editor: The critically ill child, ed. 2, Philadelphia, 1977, W. B. Saunders Co.

Holaday, D. A., Rudofsky, S., and Treuhaft, D. S.: The metabolic degradation of methoxyflurane in man, Anesthesiology 33:579, 1970.

Holder, T. M., and Ashcraft, K. W., editors: Surgery of infants and children, Philadelphia, W. B. Saunders Co., in press.

Hume, D. M.: Pheochromocytoma in the adult and in the child, Am. J. Surg. 99:458, 1960.

Katz, J., Kountz, S. L., and Cohn, R.: Anesthetic considerations for renal transplant, Anesth. Analg. (Cleve.) 46:609, 1967.

Katz, R. L., and Wolf, C. R.: Pheochromocytoma. In Mark, L. C., and Ngai, S. H., editors: Highlights of clinical anesthesiology, New York, 1971, Harper & Row, Publishers, Inc.

Kaufman, J. M., and Burrington, J. D.: Liver trauma in children, J. Pediatr. Surg. 6:586, 1971.

Kelalis, P. P., and King, L. R.: Clinical pediatric urology, Philadelphia, 1976, W. B. Saunders Co.

Kendig, J. J., Bunker, J. P., and Endow, S.: Succinylcholine-induced hyperkalemia; effects of succinylcholine on resting potentials and electrolyte distribution in normal and denervated muscle, Anesthesiology 36:132, 1972.

Kilduff, C. J., Wyant, G. M., and Dale, R. H.: Anesthesia for repair of cleft lip and palate in infants, using moderate hypothermia, Can. Anaesth. Soc. J. 3:102, 1956.

King, H., and Shumacker, H. B., Jr.: Splenic studies. I. Susceptibility to infections after splenectomy performed in infancy, Ann. Surg. 136:239, 1952.

Koide, M., and Waud, B. E.: Serum potassium concentrations after succinylcholine in patients with renal failure, Anesthesiology 36:142, 1972.

Koka, B. V., Jeon, I. S., Andre, J. M., and others: Postintubation croup in children, Anesth. Analg. (Cleve.) 56:501, 1977.

Kumar, S. M., and Zsigmond, E. K.: Anesthetic management of pheochromocytoma, Anesth. Rev. 5:14, 1978.

Leigh, M. D., and Kester, H. A.: Endotracheal anesthesia for operations on cleft lip and cleft palate, Anesthesiology 9:32, 1948.

Levin, R. M.: Pediatric anesthesia handbook, Flushing, N.Y., 1973, Medical Examination Publishing Co., Inc.

Lichtman, M. A., Murphy, M. S., Byer, B. J., and Freeman, R. B.: Hemoglobin affinity for oxygen in chronic renal disease; the effect of hemodialysis, Blood 43:417, 1974.

Lilly, J. R., Giles, G., Kurwitz, R., and others: Renal homotransplantation in pediatric patients, Pediatrics 47:548, 1971.

Linke, C. L., and Merin, R. G.: A regional anesthetic approach for renal transplantation, Anesth. Analg. (Cleve.) 55:69, 1976.

Lowenstein, E.: Succinylcholine administration in the burned patient, Anesthesiology 28:467, 1967.

MacDonald, D. J. F.: Cystic hygroma; an anaesthetic and surgical problem, Anaesthesia 21:66, 1967.

Martin, L. W., and Woodman, K.: Hepatic lobectomy for hepatoblastoma in infants and children, Arch. Surg. 89:1, 1969.

Masters, F., Hansen, J., and Robinson, D.: Anesthetic complications in plastic surgery, J. Plast. Reconstr. Surg. 24:472, 1959.

Mazze, R. I., Calverley, R. K., and Smith, N. T.: Inorganic fluoride nephrotoxicity; prolonged enflurane and halothane anesthesia in volunteers, Anesthesiology 46:265, 1977.

Mazze, R. I., and Cousins, M. J.: Renal diseases in relation to anesthesia. In Katz, J., and Kadis, L. B., editors: Anesthesia and uncommon diseases; pathophysiologic and clinical correlations, Philadelphia, 1973, W. B. Saunders Co.

Mazze, R. I., Cousins, M. J., and Kosek, J.: Dose-related methoxyflurane nephrotoxocity in rats; biochemical and pathologic correlation, Anesthesiology 36:571, 1972.

McCaughey, T. J.: Hazards of anaesthesia for the burned child, Can. Anaesth. Soc. J. 9:220, 1962.

MacCollum, D. W., and Richardson, S. O.: Care of the child with cleft lip and cleft palate, Am. J. Nurs. 58:211, 1958.

Middleton, H. G., and Wolfson, L. J.: Anaesthesia in burns, Br. Med. Bull. 14:42, 1958.

Miller, R. D., Way, W. L., Hamilton, W. K., and Layzer, R. B.: Succinylcholine-induced hyperkalemia in patients with renal failure? Anesthesiology 36:138, 1972.

Munro, I. R.: Orbito-cranio-facial surgery; the team approach, Plast. Reconstr. Surg. 55:2, 1975.

Murray, J. E., and Swanson, L. T.: Mid-face osteotomy and advancement for craniosynostosis, Plast. Surg. 41:299, 1968.

Murray, J. E., Swanson, L. T., Strand, R. D., and Hricko, G. M.: Evaluation of craniofacial surgery in the treatment of facial deformities, Ann. Surg. 182:240, 1975.

Musgrove, R. H., and Bremmer, J. C.: Complications of cleft palate surgery, J. Plast. Reconstr. Surg. 26:180, 1960.

Orloff, S., Potter, D. E., and Holliday, M. A.: Acute renal failure. In Smith, C. A., editor: The critically ill child, ed. 2, Philadelphia, 1977, W. B. Saunders Co.

Osler, W.: Congenital absence of abdominal muscles associated with distended and hypertrophied urinary bladder, Bull. Johns Hopkins Hospital 12:331, 1901.

Potter, D., Belzer, F. O., Ranes, L., and others: Treatment of chronic uremia in childhood. I. Transplantation, Pediatrics 45:432, 1970.

Potter, D., Larson, D., Leumann, E., and others: Treatment of chronic uremia in childhood. II. Hemodialysis, Pediatrics 46:178, 1970a.

Pratilas, V., and Pratila, M. G.: Anaesthetic management of phaeochromocytoma, Can. Anaesth. Soc. J. 26:253, 1979.

Ravitch, M. M., Welch, K. J., Benson, C. D., and others, editors: Pediatric surgery, ed. 3, Chicago, 1979, Year Book Medical Publishers, Inc.

Rinehart, J. J., Lewis, R. P., and Balcerzak, D. P.: Adriamycin cardiotoxicity in man, Ann. Int. Med. 81:475, 1974.

Robin, P.: La chute de la base de la langue consideré comme une nouvelle cause du gêne dans la respiration naso-pharyngienne, Bull. Acad. Natl. Med. (Paris) 89:37, 1923.

Rosenberg, S. A.: Updated Hodgkin's disease; place of splenectomy in evaluation and management, J.A.M.A. 222:1296, 1972.

Rubin, P.: Updated Hodgkin's disease. A. Introduction, J.A.M.A. 222:1292, 1972.

Salanitre, E., and Rackow, H.: Changing trends in the anesthetic management of the child with cleft lip and palate malformation, Anesthesiology 23:610, 1962.

Salvatierra, O., Feduska, N. J., Cocrum, K. C., and others: The impact of 1,000 renal transplants at one center, Ann. Surg. 186:424, 1977.

Samuel, J. R., and Powell, D.: Renal transplantation; anaesthetic experience of 100 cases, Anaesthesia 25:165, 1970.

Slawson, K. B.: Anaesthesia for the patient in renal failure, Br. J. Anaesth. 44:277, 1972.

Slocum, H. C., and Allen, C. R.: Orotracheal anesthesia for cheiloplasty, Anesthesiology 6:355, 1945.

Smith, R. M., and Strieder, D. J.: Variable oxygen affinity of hemoglobin in children with uremic anemia; paper presented at annual meeting of the American Society of Anesthesiologists, San Francisco, October 1976.

Sorenson, E. T.: Group therapy in a community hospital dialysis unit, J.A.M.A. 221:899, 1972.

Starzl, T. E., Groth, C. G., Brettschneider, L., and others: Orthoptic homotransplantation of the human liver, Ann. Surg. 168:392, 1968.

Steward, D. J., and Creighton, R. E.: Anesthetic management of the injured child. In Surgical Staff of the Hospital for Sick Children, Toronto: Care for the injured child, Baltimore, 1975, The Williams & Wilkins Co.

Stiles, C. M., Stiles, Z. R., and Denson, J. R.: A flexible fiberoptic laryngoscope, J.A.M.A. **221**:1246, 1972.

Taylor, P. H., Filler, R., Nebesar, R., and Tefft, M.: Experience with hepatic resection in childhood, Am. J. Surg. **117**:442, 1969.

Tessier, P.: The definitive plastic surgical treatment of the severe facial deformities of craniofacial dysostosis, Crouzon's and Apert's disease, Plast. Reconstr. Surg. **48**:419, 1971.

Tessier, P.: Orbital clefts and Treacher-Collins syndrome; symposium on surgery of the orbit, Dallas, 1974.

Tessier, P., Guiot, G., Delbet, J. P., and Pastoriza, J.: Ostéotomies cranio-naso-orbito-faciales hypertélorisme, Ann. Chir. Plast. **12**:103, 1967.

Tolmie, J. D., Joyce, T. W., and Mitchell, G. D.: Succinylcholine danger in the burned patient, Anesthesiology **28**:467, 1967.

Torrance, J., Jacobs, P., Restrepo, A., and others: Intraerythrocyte adaptation to anemia, N. Engl. J. Med. **283**:165, 1970.

Turmel, Y., Moussa, S., and Blanchard, H.: Management of major hepatic resection in infants and children; report of sixteen cases, Can. Anaesth. Soc. J. **20**:419, 1973.

Walton, J. D., and Farman, J. V.: Suxamethonium hyperkalaemia in uraemic children, Anaesthesia **28**:666, 1973.

Weiss, C.: Does circumcision of the newborn require an anesthetic? Clin. Pediatr. **7**:128, 1968.

Welch, K. J.: Personal communication, 1979.

Welch, K. J.: Abdominal and thoracic injuries. In Ravitch, M. M., Welch, K. J., Benson, C. D., and others, editors: Pediatric surgery, ed. 3, Chicago, 1979, Year Book Medical Publishers, Inc.

Welch, K. J.: Abdominal musculature deficiency syndrome. In Ravitch, M. M., Welch, K. J., Benson, C. D., and others, editors: Pediatric surgery, ed. 3, Chicago, 1979a, Year Book Medical Publishers, Inc.

Welch, K. J.: Diagnosis of urologic conditions. In Ravitch, M. M., Welch, K. J., Benson, C. D., and others, editors: Pediatric surgery, ed. 3, Chicago, 1979b, Year Book Medical Publishers, Inc.

Whalen, J. S., and Conn, A. W.: Improved technics in anesthetic management for repair of cleft lips and palates, Anesth. Analg. (Cleve.) **46**:355, 1967.

Wilson, J. R.: Dopamine in the hepatorenal syndrome, J.A.M.A. **238**:2719, 1977.

Wilson, R. D.: Anesthesia and the burned child, Int. Anesthesiol. Clin. **13**:203, 1975.

Wilson, R. D., Nichols, R. J., and McCoy, N. R.: Dissociative anesthesia with CI-581 in burned children, Anesth. Analg. (Cleve.) **46**:719, 1967.

Winnie, A. P.: Interscalene brachial plexus block, Anesth. Analg. (Cleve.) **49**:455, 1970.

CHAPTER 18

Anesthesia for pediatric neurosurgery

DIAGNOSTIC AND THERAPEUTIC PROCEDURES

Neurosurgery in infants and children requires anesthesia for the treatment of trauma to the head, spine, and peripheral nerves, correction of hydrocephalus and various congenital defects, excision of tumors and vascular malformations, treatment of brain abscess and complications of bacterial meningitis, cortical resection for epilepsy, and elective procedures performed for relief of pain and involuntary movements (see list below).

Among a variety of diagnostic procedures that may precede neurosurgical operations, several require general anesthesia and carry an appreciable morbidity of their own.

OPERATIVE NEUROSURGICAL PROCEDURES

Diagnostic procedures
  Angiography
  Pneumoencephalography
  Ventricular tap and ventriculography
  Myelography
  Computerized axial tomography (CT scan)

Neurosurgery in the neonate
  Reduction of depressed skull fracture
  Repair of spina bifida, myelomeningocele, dysraphism, meningocele, encephalocele

Surgical requirements

Although there is considerable variation in this group of operations, there are several basic needs that must be fulfilled in order to provide the surgeon with suitable operating conditions. These may include:

1. A completely immobile patient
2. Freedom to work about the head without interference from anesthesiologist or equipment
3. Indefinite time in which to operate
4. Use of diathermy
5. Choice of supine, prone, lateral, or sitting positions
6. Reduction of cerebral blood flow, and maintenance of a "relaxed" brain when desired
7. Provision for rapid, extensive blood replacement
8. Use of vasoconstricting drugs to reduce bleeding from scalp

Characteristic problems in patient care

Special considerations in the management of children with neurosurgical disorders involve the following:

1. Many patients are infants under 1 year of age.
2. Preoperative complications may include traumatic brain damage, coma, advanced malignancy, paraplegia, spasticity, and other disorders.
3. Increased intracranial pressure (ICP) may be present before operation and interfere with induction, may occur during operation and cause coning and cardiorespiratory arrest, or may appear in the postoperative period.
4. Airway management and endotracheal intubation may be complicated in infants with myelomeningoceles or large encephaloceles, in children with advanced hydrocephalus, and in those with craniofacial synostosis.
5. Inaccessibility of the patient during prolonged procedures interferes with monitoring of clinical signs. The anesthesiologist must use considerable ingenuity to remain in contact with the patient and has little chance to follow the course of the operation or to assess the loss of blood.
6. Operations on the brainstem may obscure signs of anesthesia. At other times, the insistence of the surgeon to have the patient continue spontaneous respiration can lead to the development of hypercarbia and increased ICP.
7. Complications associated with these operations include air embolism due to the use of the sitting position and vasomotor collapse associated with induced hypotension.

NEUROLOGIC CONCEPTS AFFECTING ANESTHESIOLOGY

The extensive studies of neurophysiology and neuropharmacology that have been conducted in recent years, as reviewed by Michenfelder and associates (1969), Smith and Wollman (1972), and Shapiro (1975), have been concerned primarily with adults but have established basic concepts that may be applied to pediatric age groups. A more accurate idea of intracranial physiology has been formulated, with measurement of several of the interdependent factors that determine circulatory function, oxygen requirement, and carbohydrate metabolism of the brain. The effect of anesthetic agents on the normal and abnormal brain has been investigated, with highly practical results. Information gained concerning regulation of ICP has been of particular importance in anesthesiology.

Cerebral blood flow (CBF) and the cerebral metabolic rate for oxygen (CMR_{O_2}) appear to be the starting points in evaluation of cerebral activity. In adults, the figures presently accepted as normal for these functions are 44 ml/100 g/min and 3.0 ml/100 g/min, respectively. These and additional related figures are shown in Table 18-1.

Precise measurement of these functions has not been made throughout all stages of development, but it is believed that both CBF and CMR_{O_2} are relatively low at birth and then climb to maximal levels in infancy or early childhood. Using the nitrous oxide uptake technic, Kennedy and associates (1967, 1970) reported a mean CBF of 106.4 ml/g/min and a mean CMR_{O_2} of 5.17 ml/g/min in children 3 to 10 years of age as compared with values of 60.1 ml/g/min and 4.18 ml/g/min, respectively, in young adults.

Definitive developmental evaluation of cerebral function has not been subject to measurement, but Garfunkel and associates (1954) noted that there was a close relationship between CMR_{O_2} and mental ability and that CMR_{O_2} was reduced in the presence of mental retardation, hydrocephalus, and other lesions.

It has been shown that the brain has the capacity to regulate blood flow during considerable variation in perfusion pressure. This feature, termed autoregulation, is effective when perfusion pressures are between 60 and 150 torr (Lassen, 1959). Within these limits, cerebral perfusion pressure has little effect on CBF. However, CBF fails if arterial blood pressure falls below the range of 50 torr or if cerebrospinal fluid (CSF) exceeds 380 to 450 mm H_2O (Greenfield and Tindall, 1965).

Table 18-1. Cerebral blood flow and metabolism: normal values, units, and abbreviations

Full name	Abbreviation	Normal values and units
Cerebral blood flow	CBF	44 ml/100 g/min
Regional cerebral blood flow	rCBF	20-80 ml/100 g/min
Cerebral perfusion pressure*	PP	80 torr
Cerebrovascular resistance†	CVR	1.8 torr/ml/100 g/min
Arteriovenous oxygen content difference	$(A\text{-}V)_{O_2}$	6.8 ml/100 ml
Cerebral metabolic rate for oxygen	CMR_{O_2}	3.0 ml/100 g/min
Cerebral metabolic rate for glucose	$CMR_{glucose}$	4.5 mg/100 g/min
Cerebral metabolic rate for lactate	$CMR_{lactate}$	2.3 mM/100 g/min
Cerebral venous oxygen tension	Pv_{O_2}	35-40 torr
Oxygen glucose index	OGI	90-100%
Lactate glucose index	LGI	0-10%
Cerebral blood flow equivalent	CBF/CMR_{O_2}	14-15 ml blood/ml O_2

From Smith, A. L., and Wollman, H.: Review article; cerebral blood flow and metabolism; effects of anesthetic drugs and techniques, Anesthesiology **36**:378, 1972.
*Defined as mean arterial minus mean cerebral venous pressure or mean arterial pressure minus intracranial pressure.
†Defined as PP/CBF.

Control of ICP and brain volume

Oxygenation and cardiac function are of primary concern during all operative procedures. In neurosurgery, ICP and brain volume are additional factors of primary importance, varying dangerously with the type of lesion, the operative trauma, and the anesthetic management.

Normal ICP in adults varies between 100 and 150 mm CSF (also stated as mm H_2O), or 7 to 11 mm Hg, and is usually midway between arterial pressure and pressure in the jugular bulb. Variations caused by physical factors such as coughing, lifting, or straining may produce temporary elevation to as much as 400 or 500 mm CSF without ill effect, and the ICP of a woman in labor may reach as much as 900 mm CSF (Davson, 1969).

ICP in neonates is in the range of 80 mm CSF, subsequently rising parallel to systemic blood pressure throughout childhood. Although straining does not produce the extreme levels seen in adults, elevation to 600 mm CSF or more is seen in small patients under a variety of circumstances in relation to physical, physiologic, pathologic, or pharmacologic stimuli.

Any exertion that causes closure of the glottis or tension of diaphragmatic and abdominal muscles will compress the venous system and elevate ICP. Struggling during induction of anesthesia, breath-holding, choking, vomiting, or bucking on endotracheal tubes may be equally effective.

Among physiologic factors increasing ICP, hypercarbia comes first and hypoxia follows close behind. Thus, the struggling patient who becomes depressed and hypoxic will be fighting against a combination of destructive forces.

Throughout operation it is highly desirable to maintain a moderate degree of hyperventilation. Naturally, there are certain limitations in the application of hyperventilation that must be observed in order to avoid extreme hypocapnia with resultant respiratory alkalosis and compensatory metabolic acidosis. The desired range of Pa_{CO_2} is considered to be 25 to 35 mm Hg.

Problems may arise when surgeons insist that spontaneous respiration must be retained in order to demonstrate preservation of respiratory function. Management of this situation is described on p. 426.

Table 18-2. Effects of anesthetic drugs on cerebral blood flow, metabolism, and intracranial pressure in man

Anesthetic drug	CBF	CMR_{O_2}	ICP
Nitrous oxide, 70%	0	↓20%	—
Halothane, 1%	↑25%	↓25%	↑
Cyclopropane, 20%	↑50%	↓20%	↑
Enflurane, 2%	0	↓30%	?
Methoxyflurane, 25%	↑30%	↓10%	↑
Thiopental, 35 mg/kg	↓40%	↓50%	?
Morphine, 60 mg	0	↓40%	0
Ketamine, 3 mg/kg	↑60%	↓10%	↑
Innovar, 1 ml/20 lb	↓50%*	↓20%	↓

From Larson, C. P., Jr.: Anesthesia in brain surgery; abnormal intracranial pressure and ischemia call for special approach, Clin. Trends Anesthesiol. 4:1, 1974.
*Studies in dogs.

Pathologic factors causing elevation of ICP in both adults and children include intracranial tumors, hemorrhage from trauma or pathologic lesions, cerebral edema, and vascular anomalies. Children have additional problems in relation to growth of the brain and skull and in relation to CSF production. Early closure of the sutures of the skull (as in craniosynostosis), overproduction of CSF, blockage of the normal passage of CSF from ventricles to spine, and reduced rate of CSF absorption all may result in ICP elevation (Welch, 1975).

On the other hand, if the child has a normal skull, the lack of early fusion allows expansion of tumors and other lesions to abnormally large size before ICP increases enough to produce clinical signs.

The effect of pharmacologic agents on ICP, cerebral metabolism, and blood flow has been brought into much clearer focus, as shown in Table 18-2 (Larson, 1974). Most of the sedatives and hypnotics used intravenously act to reduce ICP, with barbiturates and droperidol being outstanding examples. Ketamine is the principal exception, causing a sharp elevation of ICP unless the response is blunted by preadministration of a counteracting drug such as thiopental.

The effect of most inhalation agents, on the other hand, is an elevation of ICP to varying degrees, chiefly due to dilation of cerebral vessels. Halothane, methoxyflurane, and trichloroethylene are notable examples. When these findings were first published, serious objection was raised to the use of halothane for neurosurgery (Galindo and Baldwin, 1963; editorial, 1969). However, this antagonism receded in consideration of the brief duration of the elevation and the development of several methods of decreasing the response. It is now common knowledge that effective hyperventilation prior to the use of halothane diminishes the usual ICP response by 50% or more, and similar results are obtained by preliminary induction with thiopental or Innovar.

In relation to anesthesia, an especially important finding has been that drugs that induce an insignificant ICP elevation in patients not having intracranial pathology may produce dangerous and sudden ICP increase in patients having space-occupying lesions (Jennett and associates, 1969; Shapiro, 1975).

Control of acid-base balance of CSF has been found to play an important part in neurosurgical lesions. Though less thoroughly understood than the acid-base balance of blood, as noted by Rossanda (1969), in severe systemic acid-base disturbance, analysis of CSF can be extremely valuable in evaluating the degree of involvement and the nature of the change in the central nervous system. Rossanda joins Lassen (1968) and others in emphasizing the danger of attempting to correct acidosis by rapid administration of bicarbonate and advises reliance on hyperventilation to prevent the dangerous progression of cerebral acidosis, edema, and ischemia.

Recognition and treatment of increased ICP

The signs of increased ICP are more easily recognized in conscious patients and may include headache, nausea, dizziness, nuchal rigidity, gait disturbance, seizures, sixth nerve palsy, dilated pupils, and papilledema.

In the unconscious or anesthetized patient most of these signs are lost, but one may have the advantage of visualizing the surface of the brain and the state of vascular engorgement, visible pulsation, and degree of swelling. When the brain is not visible, cardiovascular function gives valuable clues. Bradycardia is a classic sign of increased ICP in both adults and children, and young patients also occasionally show tachycardia as an early sign of increased ICP. Dysrhythmias occur in young and old and, if severe, will lead to a fall in blood pressure. Slow and/or irregular respiration also may be present.

More accurate estimation of ICP is needed for both comatose and anesthetized patients, and several methods have been attempted. The ventricular catheter of Lundberg (1960) and the more recent subarachnoid screw of Vries and associates (1973) offer promise in this direction, but the high incidence of infection has been a complicating factor.

It may be necessary to take steps to reduce ICP before, during, or after operation. The most direct method at any phase, is the removal of CSF, which may be accomplished by ventricular, cisternal, or spinal tap. In preoperative patients, a ventricular drain is frequently connected to a closed system for continuous control of pressure. Steroid therapy may be used for patients with cerebral edema; dexamethasone (Decadron) in doses of 1 to 5 mg at 4-hour intervals is the current choice. Osmotic diuretics also are used in patients with brain swelling due to trauma, fluid overload, or intracranial lesions.

For diuresis, urea has been abandoned in favor of mannitol, which produces greater osmotic effect and less "rebound." A dose of 1.5 g/kg is advised. Side effects may include a brief rise in CBF with resultant decrease in bleeding and an elevation of plasma osmolality of approximately 20 milliosmoles. Hence, osmolality should be monitored, and efforts should be made to keep it below 325 mOsm/L in order to avoid hypernatremia (Gilbert and Brindle, 1966). The bladder should be catheterized whenever diuretics are used during anesthesia.

In the management of patients who have suffered head injuries and are comatose it is important to avoid hypoventilation, airway obstruction, and straining, which cause additional ICP elevation. The use of thiopental for sedation and pharmacologic reduction of ICP, followed by endotracheal intubation (using topical anesthesia, if necessary) and mechanical hyperventilation, provides considerable relief if used in addition to steroid and diuretic therapy.

To reduce ICP during operation, the anesthesiologist's first move is to make sure that the patient is not hypercarbic. This is accomplished by providing definite hyperventilation throughout the entire procedure and by checking for inadvertent kinking or malposition of the endotracheal tube, pulmonary edema, secretions, or external pressure on the body of prone infants. Arterial or venous pH and P_{CO_2} should be measured for definite evaluation of respiratory adequacy. Pa_{CO_2} between 25 and 30 mm Hg, Pv_{CO_2} between 40 and 45 mm Hg, and pH between 7.45 and 7.55 are adequate evidence of the absence of hypercarbia.

A 10° head-up tilt is of some help in patients who have been in horizontal position, and all straining due to light anesthetic level naturally must be eliminated. Other steps that may be taken include removal of fluid from ventricles or spine and the use of steroids and diuretics as previously outlined. At The Children's Hospital Medical Center, patients in whom there is expectation of ICP variation are managed by preoperative insertion of a lumbar puncture needle, which is attached to a drainage bottle by rubber tubing. A clamp on the tube adjusts the rate of escape of spinal fluid and the pressure in the spinal and cerebral fluid. A divided mattress is used for this, allowing a standard spinal needle to remain in place throughout the operation.

In spite of the fact that hyperventilation is highly advantageous in prevention of increased ICP and brain swelling, many surgeons feel that it is even more important to maintain spontaneous respiration during operations involving the floor of the fourth ventricle in order to prevent unrecognized damage to respiratory centers. Michenfelder and associates (1969) pointed out that by ECG monitoring one can remain in excellent control of the situation. However, if one elects to comply with the surgeon's wishes, one must use little or no preoperative sedation, apply topical anesthesia prior to endotracheal intubation, have the surgeon use local anesthesia prior to incision of the skin, and carry the child on nitrous oxide and light halothane mixtures, assisting respiration as necessary and monitoring adequacy of ventilation by repeated measurement of blood gases.

PRINCIPLES OF NEUROSURGICAL ANESTHESIA
Preoperative evaluation

In addition to standard features to be reviewed in all preoperative patients, children scheduled for neurosurgical operations require special attention to details of history, physical examination, and laboratory data that pertain to the central nervous system. Some of particular importance are listed in Tables 18-3 and 18-4.

Premedication and induction

The traditional denial of sedatives for patients prior to neurosurgery has been grad-

ually discarded. The majority of children do not have elevated ICP preoperatively, and use of morphine is permissible if it is not allowed to cause hypoventilation. Use of barbiturate, atropine, and morphine follows similar lines as in other types of pediatric surgery, since precaution is taken, of course, to reduce sedatives where children show depression of neurologic function. Barbiturates have a beneficial effect in neurosurgical patients because of their tendency to reduce ICP and metabolic demand. Consequently, the use of pentobarbital for sedation and thiopental for induction has special advantage. In infants whose veins are difficult to find, induction with nitrous oxide and halothane is usually acceptable. The prescribed use of hyperventilation prior to use of halothane is difficult to manage gracefully in small children. While they often accomplish the same degree of hyperventilation by crying, the additional straining is undesirable.

Children with known elevation of ICP prior to induction deserve special care, and any straining is to be strictly avoided. Here the use of thiopental or methohexital by rectum is particularly advantageous in dosages of approximately 20 mg/kg and 10 mg/kg,

Table 18-3. Special features of preoperative evaluation of neurosurgical patients

History	Physical examination
Apgar score	Ability to stand and
Birth trauma or hyp-	walk normally
oxia	Neuromuscular coor-
Seizures or hyperac-	dination
tivity	Head size
Headache, fainting,	Pupil size, motion,
dizziness, nausea	equality
Difficulty in swallow-	Mental acuity, alert-
ing, coughing	ness
Local or general mus-	Tendon reflexes
cle weakness	Character of cry
Laboratory studies	**X-rays of head or spine**
Cerebrospinal fluid	Angiogram
Pressure	Pneumoencephalo-
Cell count	gram
Osmolality	Ventriculogram
Glucose	Myelogram
Protein	CT scan

Adapted from Gilbert, R. G. B., Brindle, G. F., and Galindo, A., editors: Anesthesia for neurosurgery, Int. Anesthesiol. Clin. 4:819, 1966.

Table 18-4. Constituents of CSF as compared with plasma

	Plasma	CSF
Na, mEq/L	135-145	140
Cl, mEq/L	95-105	126
K, mEq/L	3.5-6.3	2.8-3.9
Cell count		0-2 (0-15 under 6 mo)
Glucose, mg/dl	90	50% of blood level
Protein	7000	30
Volume, ml	3000	200
pH	7.42	7.32
Pa_{O_2}, mm Hg	100	40-55
Pa_{CO_2}, mm Hg	40	49
HCO_3, mEq/L	24	23.5
Osmolarity, mOsm/L	270-300	280-310

Adapted from Gilbert, R. G. B., Brindle, G. F., and Galindo, A., editors: Anesthesia for neurosurgery, Int. Anesthesiol. Clin. 4:819, 1966.

respectively (see Chapter 7), with induction continued subsequently by blowing nitrous oxide and halothane over the child's face until sound asleep.

Not only is it much safer to reduce elevated ICP prior to induction, but it may be mandatory. Induction of anesthesia may be so retarded in the presence of high ICP that patients appear entirely unaffected by inhalation agents, and one is forced to either use intravenous drugs or withdraw fluid from the ventricles.

Final arrangement of monitoring devices and infusions is completed shortly after induction. At least one reliable infusion is necessary for any of these procedures, and CVP and intra-arterial lines occasionally are in order. The stethoscope, blood pressure device, and thermistor are used always, and the ECG is used frequently, but we have limited our use of the electroencephalograph to those procedures involving excision of focal seizure areas. During any prolonged operation the child is catheterized and urine collected in a calibrated container.

Endotracheal intubation

With the possible exception of patients who are undergoing peripheral nerve repair, practically all neurosurgical patients will require endotracheal intubation. In the case of head injury, fracture of the cervical spine, and certain anomalies, there may be considerable difficulty in passage of the endotracheal tube. It has been noted by Eckenhoff (1951) and Colgan and Keats (1957) that the lumen of the airway in the child may be narrower at the cricoid ring than at the glottis, and this may complicate intubation, making it necessary to use tubes one or two sizes smaller than might be expected. These warnings were the result of experience with children with craniofacial deformities, and the problem is familiar to all who have dealt with children with Apert's or Crouzon's syndrome (Fig. 18-1).

Intubation also may be difficult in neonates because of such lesions as encephaloceles or myelomeningoceles. Further problems in maintaining intubation are encountered in use of the prone or sitting position, where

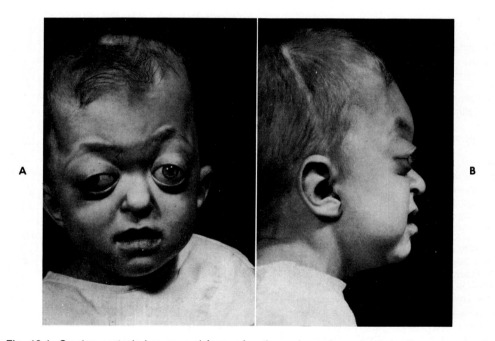

Fig. 18-1. Craniosynostosis has several forms. Apert's syndrome is associated with syndactyly of hands and feet. Crouzon's syndrome, **A** and **B,** shows marked facial deformity and extrusion of eyes due to boney occlusion of orbits. Airway problems are common to all varieties.

there is increased danger of kinking of the endotracheal tube as well as accidental extubation during operation. In fixing of the endotracheal tube, as emphasized by McComish and Bodley (1971), it is especially important that the tape be around the tube itself and not around one of the adapters, which may become detached, allowing the tube to slip into the trachea. Although the mouth is least accessible in the prone position, accidental extubation carries less danger when prone than when sitting or supine. In the prone position, the secretions drain toward the mouth and the tongue falls forward. If spontaneous respiration can be established, it may even be possible to complete an operation without insertion of the endotracheal tube. In supine or sitting position this would be inconceivable.

Protection of the eyes and positioning

Because of the length of neurosurgical procedures, even minor degrees of pressure can cause ulceration and tissue damage. When face down, children can develop particularly unsightly burns and necrotic pressure areas on the forehead, cheeks, and chin as a result of pressure on the headrest and/or strong cleaning fluid used on the scalp that may run down into the face and eyes and remain there throughout the operation. To protect the eyes, some prefer to use oily salves, but these have a tendency to retain irritant fluids, and it seems safer to cover the eyes with gauze shields held in place by waterproof tape.

Surgeon and anesthesiologist share the responsibility of positioning the patient so that the interests of all will be observed. The supine position offers least difficulty, provided that (1) the neck is not too sharply flexed and (2) the endotracheal tube is not allowed to become kinked. Small rolls may be placed under the lumbar area, knees, and ankles to prevent hyperextension.

In the lateral position, a pad is placed under the axilla to prevent pressure on the "down" shoulder, and a thin towel is placed between the knees to prevent chafing.

The prone and sitting positions offer greater problems. In the prone position, ventilation is impeded, and venous return is shunted from abdominal to vertebral channels, thereby often interfering appreciably with operations being performed on the spine (Duflot and Allen, 1956; Slocum and others, 1948; Meridy and others, 1974). When an infant is placed in the prone position, he rests chiefly on his abdomen, with little support from his shoulders. Since respiration in these infants consists to a large extent of diaphragmatic breathing, substantial pads must be fixed under the shoulders and upper thighs in order to decrease the pressure on the abdomen (Fig. 18-2). The head is placed gently in a head ring, which is padded to avoid pressure on or near the eyes, and care is taken to see that the chin does not press against the end of the operating table (Fig. 18-3). When the position is satisfactory, the child is fixed to the table by use of 3-inch adhesive tape passed (1) across the buttocks to either side of the table and (2) from the shoulders, down along the arms, to the sides of the table. The head of the table is then elevated slightly, in position for operation.

Next, the instrument tables are brought up, the patient is prepared, and drapes are applied. This phase is of special concern to the anesthesiologist, for he must not allow the patient to become hidden beneath the drapes. Tables, screens, and covers must be arranged so that the anesthesiologist can visualize the child's body and can reach the airway without difficulty in order to check the apparatus, assist respiration, or use suction when indicated. He must be near enough to monitor the child with a stethoscope, feel his pulse, watch his respiration, and judge the color of his skin. To provide optimal conditions for the patient and team, an instrument table has been constructed that straddles the operating table and the patient, leaving a foot of free clearance over the child. The anesthesiologist sits on a low stool beside the patient.

The sitting position, which is required for most children over 2 years of age undergoing posterior fossa procedures, involves a complicated arrangement of supporting appara-

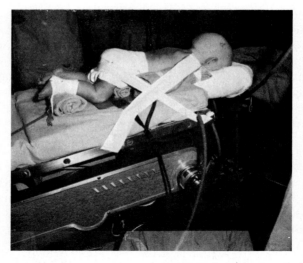

Fig. 18-2. Prone position requires firm support under shoulders and thighs. Adhesive tape prevents infant from slipping during operation. Roll under ankles prevents pressure on feet.

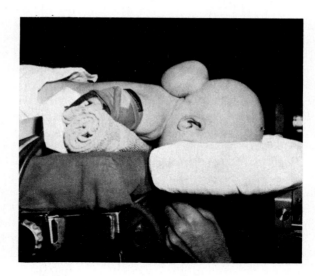

Fig. 18-3. Prone position for removal of encephalocele. Pressure on eyes, face, and chin must be avoided. Suction can easily be applied through the head ring.

tus. The endotracheal tube is brought out in the middle of the mouth to prevent kinking, and care is taken to see that the tube does not descend beyond the carina with flexion of the head. The eyes are carefully covered and doubly protected during application of the head tongs or halo. Pads under the knees prevent hyperextension. Hands and elbows are padded, and the legs are wound with elastic bandages to prevent pooling of blood (Allan and others, 1970) (Fig. 18-4).

Regardless of the position, individual deformities and lesions may lead to further problems, as in the case of extreme hydrocephalus or large encephaloceles (Fig. 18-5).

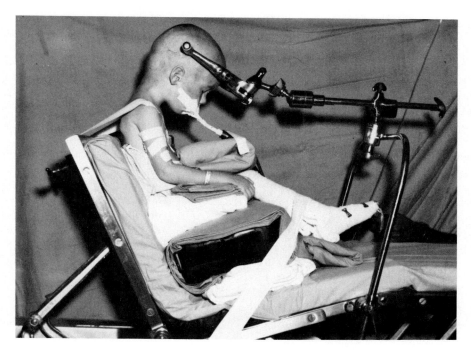

Fig. 18-4. Skull fixation by head tongs ensures stability and prevents pressure on eyes. Elastic bandages prevent venous pooling in legs. Maintenance of airway and of blood pressure becomes more difficult when children are in the sitting position. (Courtesy Dr. D. D. Matson, Boston, Mass.)

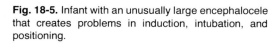

Fig. 18-5. Infant with an unusually large encephalocele that creates problems in induction, intubation, and positioning.

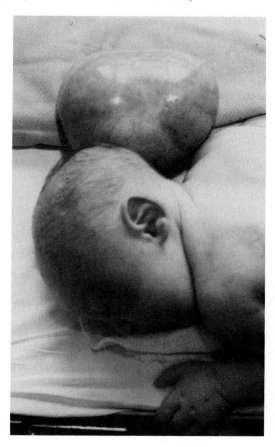

Maintenance of anesthesia

Light, stable anesthesia with minimal cardiovascular depression is highly desirable in infants and small children. The use of hyperventilation, which has had such emphasis in adult neuroanesthesia, is equally valuable for pediatric patients.

In procedures where there is no reason to fear increased ICP there is an even wider choice of anesthetic agents than in general surgery, since there seldom is need to provide relaxation. Thus, halothane and nitrous oxide or various intravenous combinations may be selected at will. Nitrous oxide may be eliminated if one is concerned about its accumulation in enclosed spaces, such as ventricles, and when there is possibility of encountering air embolism.

In the presence or possibility of increased ICP, one avoids ketamine and uses halothane with caution. Intravenous barbiturate-narcotic-relaxant mixtures are preferred, and d-tubocurarine rather than pancuronium is chosen for relaxant.

The neurosurgeon's use of a vasoconstrictor to reduce bleeding from the scalp wound may be upsetting if he expects to inject large quantities of epinephrine. Acceptable alternatives are the substitution of phenylephrine (Neo-Synephrine) for epinephrine or *limitation of the epinephrine to 0.5 ml of 1:200,000 solution per kg.*

The choice of anesthetic technic for pediatric neurosurgery is definitely limited by the surgeon's usurpation of the entire head region of the child. For children over 15 to 20 kg, one may use standard circle absorption apparatus. If the anesthesiologist must be more than 3 feet from the head of the table, double-length breathing tubes (especially those made of lightweight plastic) are helpful, or one may use the Bain (modified Mapleson D) apparatus, as described in Chapter 6. In many procedures a mechanical ventilator may help to maintain a desired degree of hyperventilation.

For small infants, the easy mobility of the various T-tube devices gives them unquestionable superiority over infant circle or adapted circle systems. The addition of warmth and humidification is advisable during long procedures on small children to prevent hypothermia. The use of halothane and/or nitrous oxide over prolonged periods should be an indication for elimination of waste gases by scavenger systems. Another possible consideration is the suspicion that ultraviolet lights, currently used in some operating rooms, might add to the danger of halothane toxicity (Karis and others, 1976). An investigation carried out at our hospital did not confirm this concept.

At the end of intracranial operations, relaxants must be reversed, but since it may be catastrophic if the patient reacts prematurely on the endotracheal tube, reversal and awakening should not be carried out until the dressing has been completed.

One of the more subtle hazards in prolonged operations of this nature is that as patients become colder, more anesthetic is dissolved in their blood, and dangerous overdosage may result although there has been no change in the setting of the vaporizer.

On the other hand, since relaxation is not required, children may be so lightly anesthetized that they react to the presence of the endotracheal tube, suddenly developing bradycardia or dysrhythmias. Once diagnosed, this is easily corrected by increasing the depth of anesthesia and/or administering atropine.

The maintenance of adequate fluid therapy is seldom difficult, the greater danger being that of overhydrating infants and children and inducing cerebral edema. With the exception of children with posterior pituitary lesions, there are scarcely any neurosurgical lesions that call for increased use of fluid. On the other hand, overdosage is extremely dangerous. When the substance of the brain has been disturbed by trauma or surgery, fluid will more easily penetrate the injured tissue, with resultant brain edema. In these situations, the intraoperative and daily fluid allowance should be reduced by 20% to 25%. For the fluid, one can use any one of several mixtures that approximate the electrolyte concentration of normal plasma. Our preference usually is for 5% dextrose to ¼% saline solution.

As previously noted, overhydration can lead to trouble, but attempts to correct it may complicate matters even more by causing hyperosmolality and convulsions. As described previously, it is essential to maintain CSF osmolality between 290 and 325 mOsm/L in order to avoid such problems.

Blood loss

Accurate replacement of blood loss is one of the greatest problems in neurosurgical operations, especially in small infants, since the anesthesiologist cannot see the operative field and the use of continual irrigation makes gravimetric estimation of blood loss practically impossible. Clinical signs of color, temperature, depth of anesthesia, heart rate, blood pressure, heart sounds, distension of neck veins, capillary refill, and urine output plus the judgment of an experienced surgeon must all be taken into consideration.

Other abnormal reactions seen during neurosurgical procedures include sudden cardiorespiratory depression after brainstem irritation (Howland and Papper, 1952) or during repair of myelomeningocele (Bergman, 1957). As noted by Schroeder and Williams (1966), closure of meningocele may lead to elevation of ICP and initiation of cardiorespiratory irregularities.

DIAGNOSTIC PROCEDURES

Before any patient is subjected to an intracranial or intraspinal operation, it is usually advisable to go to some lengths to obtain an accurate idea of the type and location of the lesion. Consequently, patients are frequently put through prolonged studies, some of which introduce appreciable difficulty. Although not all diagnostic procedures are complicated or exhaustive, some, such as pneumoencephalography and arteriography, not only are time-consuming and exacting but also involve significant danger. In children, usual risks are increased by more frequent need of general anesthesia for procedures that adults can tolerate under local anesthesia.

Procedures include ventriculography, angiography, pneumoencephalography, and computerized axial tomography (CT scan) for intracranial lesions and lumbar puncture and myelography for spinal lesions. Although the CT scan has already taken over a large share of this work, all procedures are used to a varying degree.

Angiography

Angiography may be performed by injection of contrast media into the carotid artery or by means of a catheter passed retrograde via the femoral artery. The patient lies supine and requires only enough sedation to overcome anxiety and fatigue. This usually can be accomplished by initial preoperative sedation with morphine and diazepam plus local anesthesia at the site of entry of the catheter. If more analgesic or sedative is needed during the course of the procedure, small doses of either drug may be added via the catheter. Complications that may occur in conjunction with angiography include bradycardia, dysrhythmias, hematoma of cervical vessels with airway obstruction, and cerebral edema or cerebrovascular accident.

Pneumoencephalography

For the diagnosis of tumors in the region of the third ventricle and upper brainstem and for differentiation between those that are intrinsic and those that are extrinsic to the brain, pneumoencephalography still is an essential method of diagnosis. The necessary removal of CSF, injection of contrast gas, and subsequent maneuvering of the patient have resulted in enough morbidity and mortality to create wide respect for the procedure, making it necessary for one to rule out attendant hazards before undertaking the procedure. According to Strand (in press), the principal contraindications to performance of pneumoencephalography are the presence of increased ICP (over 150 torr), the possible presence of posterior fossa tumor, and extreme youth (under 1 year of age).

Prior to pneumoencephalography, children are allowed enough sedation to prevent anxiety (pentobarbital, 2 to 4 mg/kg by mouth or rectum). The immobilization, prolonged duration, extreme positional changes, and headache make general anesthesia an unquestionable choice over local methods for children.

Since the procedure is performed only on children with normal ICP, one has relatively free choice of anesthetic agents. However, many prefer to avoid ketamine for fear of inducing ICP elevation by vasoconstriction and to avoid nitrous oxide because of its tendency to accumulate in gas-filled spaces, with similar increase in ICP. In our experience, both of these agents have been used without known complication. Ketamine has been abandoned in favor of general anesthesia with halothane, but we continue to use nitrous oxide as a supplement to halothane.

Accordingly, anesthesia is induced with nitrous oxide, oxygen, and halothane or with thiopental when there is an available vein. As soon as the child is asleep, a reliable infusion is started on the dorsum of the hand, and a slow drip is started (5% glucose and ¼% saline solution, 2 ml/lb/hr). Atropine is added (0.1 mg + 0.02 mg/kg), then succinylcholine, and the trachea is intubated, with great care being taken to fasten the tube securely. Otherwise, the drag of the breathing tubes and the gyrations of the procedure are apt to pull it out. Precordial stethoscope, blood pressure cuff, and thermometer are used for monitoring.

Next the child is positioned in a specially constructed radiography chair that is movable in all directions. He is strapped securely into the chair, and his head is immobilized by an overhead harness, with the neck slightly flexed to facilitate passage of gas into the cerebral ventricles (Fig. 18-6).

The radiologist inserts the spinal needle near the level of the iliac crests and injects the gas (air, oxygen, helium, or nitrous oxide) in small aliquots (7 ml or less), using a total that seldom exceeds 30 ml. This amount of gas, injected slowly, has rarely caused appreciable response. Following the injection and removal of CSF, however, sudden fall of blood pressure and a shocklike syndrome may occur if the child is moved abruptly.

We maintain anesthesia with equal parts of nitrous oxide and oxygen plus 0.7% to 1.0% halothane during radiologic studies while the child, firmly fixed in a sitting position, is rotated by stages through an entire somersault. As previously mentioned, the endotracheal tube must be very securely fitted in place during this maneuver. Breathing tubes of double length allow the anesthesiologist to stay the necessary distance from the patient. Tubes made of lightweight plastic help to reduce the drag on the endotracheal tube.

It is important to maintain hyperventilation during the entire procedure to prevent increased ICP due to hypercarbia. It is also extremely important to carry out any change

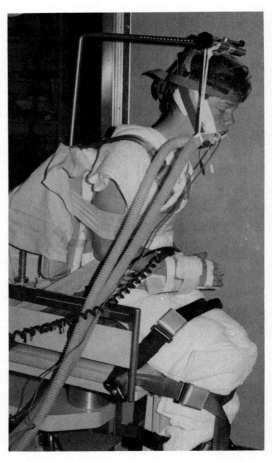

Fig. 18-6. Position of the child for pneumoencephalogram.

in the child's position slowly and smoothly to prevent vascular collapse.

Upon completion of this part of the examination, the child is moved from the chair to a table where more x-ray films are taken in supine and prone positions, again subjecting the endotracheal tube to the danger of kinking and displacement.

After the pneumoencephalogram is finished, the child is returned to his bed where he is kept horizontal for 4 hours and then allowed to move and to resume normal diet as rapidly as he desires. Headache and nausea are the chief postoperative complaints that delay resumption of normal activity.

Complications. Among several known complications of pneumoencephalography, sudden vascular collapse has been of chief concern in our experience, especially in very small infants, and has been most frequently associated with upside-down positioning or other extreme maneuvering. Prevention comes first, but if encountered, this complication should be treated by lowering the infant to horizontal and administering oxygen, followed by intravenous administration of 0.25 ml of 1% solution of either ephedrine or phenylephrine (Neo-Synephrine).

The danger of herniation of the brain, or coning, has been sufficient to establish the presence of increased ICP as a definite contraindication to pneumoencephalography. When ICP exceeds 150 mm CSF, ventriculography or CT scan should be performed in place of pneumoencephalography.

The composition of the gas used for intrathecal injection and the method of injection have been points of particular concern in pneumoencephalography. Air, oxygen, helium, and N_2O have been employed, and all of them may cause gas embolism if injected rapidly. Our intermittent injection of 7-ml aliquots, with delay for x-ray films between each and limit of 30 ml, has been successful to date.

Considerable importance has been placed on the danger of using nitrous oxide for anesthesia when oxygen, nitrogen, or helium is used for intrathecal injection. Diffusion of the more soluble N_2O into the ventricles,

with increased ICP (Saidman and Eger, 1965), or actual bubble formation (Paul and Munson, 1976) presents a real hazard. The use of N_2O for intrathecal injection has been encouraged by Aird (1936) and Newman (1937) as well as the aforesaid, and a series of 475 pediatric patients so managed has been reported by Elwyn and associates (1976). Elwyn's group stressed the greater safety of this method and the advantage of more rapid excretion of N_2O in reducing the postoperative headache and allowing shorter hospitalization.

While the advantages during recovery are clear-cut, the greater safety is less convincing. Use of N_2O for both anesthesia and contrast gas eliminates the danger of N_2O diffusion into the ventricles, but N_2O must be injected in larger quantities and more rapidly than air, thereby increasing the danger of gas embolism. Absorption of the bubbles is delayed by the presence of N_2O in the bloodstream, and the necessary rapid washout of N_2O exposes the patient to cardiovascular collapse and cardiac arrest, as reported by Collan and Ivananien (1969).

The danger of air embolization during pneumoencephalography in patients having ventriculoatrial shunts has been pointed out by Youngberg and associates (1975) and attested to by Paul and Munson (1976). Additional precautionary measures that have been advocated include end-tidal CO_2 monitoring, use of a Swan-Ganz catheter, and ligation of the shunt catheter prior to encephalography.

One is impressed by the apparent inescapability of risk and the complexity of preventive and therapeutic measures. As suggested by Stoelting (1976), avoidance of both contrast media and general anesthesia, frequently possible with the use of tomography, may be the best solution. Unfortunately, CT scan is not ideal nor widely accessible.

In a slightly different approach, Raudzens and Cole (1974) have eliminated the N_2O problem by avoiding its use entirely, employing thiopental and succinylcholine for intubation, followed by maintenance anesthesia with intravenous drip of thiopental and lidocaine. In a relatively small series, the only disadvantage reported was a slight delay in awakening.

The important features in avoiding problems in pneumoencephalography appear to be to avoid rapid injection of contrast gas, to avoid N₂O anesthesia, to avoid N₂O for contrast gas, to avoid pneumoencephalography in the presence of high ICP, and to avoid adding to the risk by use of complex safeguards (Swan-Ganz catheters). One is left with the inference that the only safe method is to avoid pneumoencephalography. However, the record of Elwyn and associates (no deaths in 475 procedures) shows that recognition of the hazards and careful technic overcome many theoretical hazards.

Ventriculography

Ventriculography is considerably safer than pneumoencephalography in patients with increased ICP due to posterior fossa lesions or noncommunicating hydrocephalus. In small children the procedure is usually performed under local anesthesia. The child is held in supine position while the surgeon injects the anesthetic and then inserts an 18-gauge needle through an open coronal suture in small infants or through a small drill hole in older children. After the injection of 25 to 30 ml of gas into the ventricles, films are taken in several positions. Headache during and following the procedure is the principal complication of the operation.

Myelography

While more mature children may tolerate myelography under local anesthesia and moderate sedation, most of the smaller ones will need light general anesthesia in order to obtund the original lumbar puncture and last through the rather prolonged maneuvering, turning, and tilting that often occurs. Standard preoperative sedation, induction with nitrous oxide–halothane, intubation under succinylcholine, and continued halothane–nitrous oxide anesthesia should be suitable for most cases. The chief concerns during these procedures lie in the fact that the room is darkened during much of the time, and in the many positionings and repositionings of the child there is the danger of dislodging the endotracheal tube or the spinal needle.

Computerized axial tomography (CT scan)

For computerized tomography, or the CT scan, the patient lies supine with his head inserted to the eyebrows into a radiographic chamber. As the patient lies thus immobilized, the x-ray unit rotates around the head, taking an impression at each degree of rotation. Rapid improvements are being made in this facility. At this writing the examination requires approximately 5 minutes of immobilization. While this is not long and there is no discomfort, children who are frightened or whose neurologic lesion involves involuntary motion may need sedation or light anesthesia. Since many of the patients who require tomography are critically ill or have been seriously traumatized, no sedative or anesthetic should be administered unless there are full provisions for resuscitation and emergency treatment. Under proper conditions, ketamine, diazepam, thiopental, or inhalation agents may be employed.

NEUROSURGERY IN THE NEONATE
Reduction of depressed skull fracture

Either the application of delivery forceps or the passage through the birth canal may cause an indentation of the skull of the infant, usually about the size of a 50-cent piece and aptly described as a "ping-pong fracture" because of its resemblance to the localized depression of a traumatized ping-pong ball.

The fracture rarely has any immediate effect on the infant, but reduction naturally is desirable and is accomplished within 24 hours after delivery. The operation consists simply of preparing the area, making a ½-inch incision through the skin and skull at the edge of the depression, inserting a blunt instrument, and prying or snapping the inverted area back into normal contour. Closure consists of three or four sutures and a simple dressing.

Absolute immobilization is not mandatory, and local anesthesia should suffice in most instances. The infant must be restrained securely and may be diverted with a nipple, which some like to sweeten with sugar and water or spiritus frumenti.

If the fracture has gone untreated for several days or if there are other complications, it may be preferable to use general anesthesia, which would be accomplished with intramuscular succinylcholine for intubation and light N_2O-halothane for maintenance. At completion, extubation is delayed until the infant is fully reactive and ready to cry.

One should not be tempted to use ketamine in such cases. Although ketamine would provide a satisfactory operating condition, when used in small infants it may cause postoperative respiratory depression at any time during the following 6 or 8 hours.

Spina bifida, myelomeningocele, dysraphism, meningocele, and encephalocele

A variety of lesions of the central nervous system have basic similarity in that they involve abnormal development of spine, vertebrae, or skull, with protrusion or exposure of nervous elements and often with serious functional defects (McQueen and Udvarhelyi, 1979).

In the neonate, the chief consideration is to find out if the lesion has a durable covering of intact skin, if it is covered only by a thin membranous sac, or if it lies open and exposed. The danger of infection is so great that any lesion of this type that is not safely covered must be closed within 24 hours after birth (Sharrard, 1963). It is even considered unsafe to give the infant any oral feeding, since this might initiate the growth of dangerous bacterial flora in the digestive tract (Matson, 1969).

Each of these lesions may be small enough to be barely visible, or may be gigantic. Large size is a bad omen, but the critical factor is the amount of nervous tissue that is involved. Whether a large spinal mass is a true myelomeningocele with inclusion of nerve elements or a simple meningocele may be difficult to determine. In a severe myelomeningocele, however, there may be extensive distortion of the spine and complete loss

of function of the lower half of the body.

In evaluating these infants, one should estimate the degree of function, since some have lost so much sensation that the need for anesthesia will be greatly reduced. One should also share the responsibility of honestly evaluating the child's chance for future development, since there may be overwhelming deformities of skeletal, gastrointestinal, neuromuscular, and genitourinary systems. Reasoning parents may prefer to forego operation.

Operation on infants with some promise of future improvement entails drawing skin over the midline defect. This may require the raising of rotation flaps in several stages, with the definite possibility of the development of hydrocephalus (Schroeder and Williams, 1966). The first operation will be in the first 24 hours after birth and will require general endotracheal anesthesia and between 1 and 4 hours of surgery, during which blood replacement should be anticipated. Management will include intubation under intramuscular succinylcholine and maintenance with N_2O-halothane, as with other neonates.

During any operation on or near the spinal cord there will be danger of major cardiorespiratory disturbances due to compression or irritation of the fourth ventricle or nerve tracts. This is especially true in large myeloceles, where the nerves leaving the spine often are grossly misplaced and distorted and the spine is exposed to easy injury. In addition to cardiovascular depression, sudden rise of blood pressure may occur, as noted by Bergman (1957) and Ciliberti and associates (1954).

If more than one operation is needed in these patients, there may be signs of increasing ICP because of the removal of the expansile area that had allowed for accumulation of fluid. These infants often face a lifetime of pressure-reducing maneuvers, starting with establishment of some form of shunt and followed by repeated shunt revision and replacement. As with other neurosurgical procedures, particular care must be taken to reduce ICP before operation if possible, to avoid drugs that increase ICP, to maintain hyperventilation, and to monitor carefully, ready to meet signs of increasing pressure with diuretics, steroids, and other devices.

Excision of meningocele. Operation for excision of meningocele may be extensive but usually is less complicated than that for myelomeningocele, with reduced risk of infection and less nerve involvement. Anesthetic management is similar in both lesions, and complications and blood loss offer sufficient cause for concern.

Excision of encephalocele. Occipital encephaloceles that are as large as an infant's head may be encountered. Although unsightly, repair is less urgent than in myelomeningocele, since encephaloceles are usually covered by normal scalp.

The prognosis of the infant depends on the content of the encephalocele. Some contain only fluid, and the loss of the entire mass will cause no harm. Others contain a varying amount of brain tissue, loss of which may cause blindness as well as motor and sensory impairment. If the encephalocele contains an appreciable amount of brain tissue, the infant will not survive.

There may be some difference in the response of these infants to anesthesia, depending on the degree of loss of brain substance, but the greatest anesthetic problem may be in intubation, since the head cannot be held in the usual manner. Prior to anesthesia the infant's body can lie supine, prone, or on either side. At the time of intubation, one will find it very important to have the infant lying with the right side of the face uppermost (*right side up*), for in this position the base of the laryngoscope will displace the tongue downward rather than make it necessary to lift the tongue out of the way to pass the tube. This makes a significant difference, especially among infants because of their large tongues.

A light plane of anesthesia, with hyperventilation, should suffice. The anesthesiologist should be alert to changes that might be due to removal of brain tissue, e.g., changes of cardiac rate or rhythm, blood pressure, respiratory function, or motor activity. As with the related lesions, many of these infants will develop hydrocephalus.

NEUROSURGERY IN INFANTS AND CHILDREN

For the many neurosurgical procedures that are seen during infancy and childhood, anesthetic management follows rather well-established principles that are planned to serve two fundamentally different groups: those who have normal ICP and those who have increased ICP.

Anesthesia for children with normal ICP

The management of most young patients during neurosurgical operations is similar to that for other types of surgery, differing chiefly in positioning and provision for adequate field of operation.

Repair of craniosynostosis. Premature closure of cranial sutures demands early operation in order to prevent increasing pressure on brain substance. The operation involves removing a strip of skull on either side of the fused suture and lining it with polyethylene film in order to prevent early reclosure. In 1968 Shillito and Matson reported 519 operations for repair of craniosynostosis performed at The Children's Hospital Medical Center, and the repair of sagittal synostosis outnumbered other types by 5:1. By 1972 a total of 682 operations had been performed here. In the entire series only two deaths occurred. The fact that both deaths were related to bleeding correctly suggests that blood loss is the major hazard. Active hemorrhage from the longitudinal sinus always involves the threat of rapid exsanguination, but the main source of blood loss in our experience has been continued bleeding from bone edges. Although the dura is not opened, these small infants lose an average of 200 ml of blood during the operative and postoperative periods. Previously encountered danger of pressure injury to the face in prone position has been eliminated by placing the head in the lateral position.

In most cases that are diagnosed early, the anesthetic requirement consists merely of light, steady anesthetic level, with attention concentrated on blood replacement. If the condition has progressed to the state where there is severe restriction of the expansion of the brain, however, there may be brain damage, blindness, and markedly increased ICP, and one will have to use an entirely different approach, as outlined in treatment of patients with increased ICP.

Craniofacial synostosis: Crouzon's and Apert's syndromes. In simple cranial synostosis, the facial bones are not affected, but craniofacial synostosis involves distortion of the entire skull, usually including hypertelorism, retrocession of the maxilla with resul-

tant choanal atresia, and malocclusion of the jaws. Craniofacial synostosis without other defects is known as Crouzon's syndrome, while that involving additional syndactyly of hands and feet and joint contractures is known as Apert's syndrome (Fig. 18-7). Operation for these patients now consists of the more extensive Tessier midface advancement, described in Chapter 17.

Topectomy and hemispherectomy. Patients with uncontrollable seizure disorders may require cortical exploration and resection of part or all of one half of the brain. This is a long, but not necessarily overwhelming, operation. It calls for well-controlled light

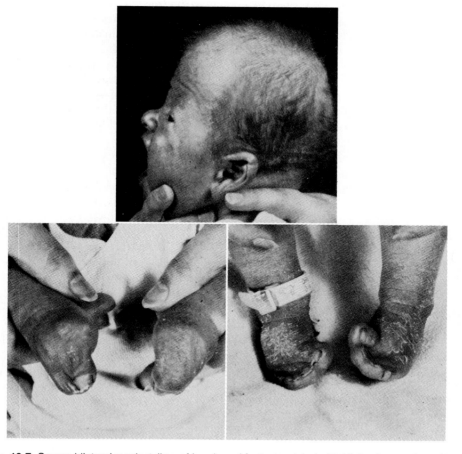

Fig. 18-7. Severe bilateral syndactylism of hands and feet associated with bilateral premature closure of the coronal suture in a newborn (Apert's syndrome). (From Matson, D. D.: Neurosurgery of infancy and childhood, ed. 2, Springfield, Ill., 1969, Charles C Thomas, Publisher.)

anesthesia during which 15 to 20 electro-encephalographic sensors are placed in contact with the exposed cortex to localize the seizure focus. The patient must be practically awake during this part of the procedure. To accomplish this effect, the anesthesiologist may order morphine and diazepam for sedation, induce anesthesia with nitrous oxide and halothane, anesthetize the larynx with lidocaine, intubate, and then maintain the patient on nitrous oxide supplemented by relaxant and morphine. The halothane is excreted rapidly, and thereafter the patient can be awakened merely by reducing the nitrous oxide. For procedures such as this that may last 8 or 10 hours, more extensive monitoring will be necessary, including arterial cannulation for blood gas determination, ECG, nerve stimulator, urinary catheter, and electroencephalograph.

Operation for arteriovenous aneurysm. The operation for arteriovenous aneurysm is considered to be the prime indication for induction of hypotension in order to facilitate exposure and prevent exsanguinating hemorrhage. In the past, trimethaphan (Arfonad) has been used successfully for this procedure, but this agent is relatively difficult to control, and children develop tachyphylaxis rather quickly. Our present preference is for sodium nitroprusside, given in a 0.01% solution, as described in Chapter 14.

With this particular technic of induced hypotension, one must take additional measures of monitoring, including arterial cannulation and urethral catheterization.

Since the danger of sudden, profuse hemorrhage is especially prominent here, it is of primary importance to prepare for this by establishment of an infusion with at least two large-bore plastic cannulae, CVP monitor, and an ample supply of fresh blood.

Anesthesia for children with increased ICP

Among the many lesions that may entail added problems of increased ICP are hydrocephalus, advanced craniosynostosis, tumors, traumatic conditions, hemorrhage from intracranial aneurysms, and encephalitis.

The anesthetic management of adults having elevated ICP before or during operation, as described in detail by Gilbert and associates (1966), Michenfelder and associates (1969), Shapiro and associates (1972), Shapiro (1975), and others, applies in general to pediatric situations.

Operative treatment of hydrocephalus. During the past 20 years, operations for the treatment of hydrocephalus have occupied a large share of the pediatric neurosurgeon's time. Hydrocephalus, as defined by Matson (1969), is an increase in the amount of CSF that is, or has been, under increased pressure. Matson listed 17 causes of hydrocephalus, which he grouped under the headings congenital, neoplastic, infectious, traumatic, and operative, thereby emphasizing his point that hydrocephalus is not a disease in itself.

In the actual accumulation of CSF, three potential factors include increased formation of fluid, obstruction to its natural circulation, and reduced rate of absorption. The only known cause of excess production of CSF is choroid plexus adenoma, a relatively rare tumor, but one that occurs predominantly in the first year of life (Eisenberg and others, 1974).

There are a great many causes of obstruction to the circulation of CSF (noncommunicating hydrocephalus), including tumors, cysts, hematomas, vascular anomalies, and abnormal brain development. For extensive studies of CSF and hydrocephalus, the works of Davson (1969) and Welch (1975) are recommended. Communicating hydrocephalus, due to reduced rate of resorption of CSF, makes up some 20% to 25% of cases and is caused by defective arachnoidal granulations (Shillito and Ojemann, 1973).

Deliberative examination must be made to determine whether resection of a tumor or other lesion can correct the cause of the hydrocephalus. Failing this, operation is planned to relieve the accumulation of CSF by one of several possible shunting procedures. Following early use of the Torkildsen shunt and Matson's ventriculoureteral shunt, several valved devices were introduced allowing release of CSF into the bloodstream or body cavities. The ventriculoatrial shunt was used extensively (Fischer and others, 1972), but requirement for accurate placement was not compatible with the rapid growth of small children, and frequent revision was necessary. Current local preference is for the use of a drain that leads from the ventricle to a Rickham reservoir at the surface of the brain and then is connected to a long plastic catheter that extends well into the peritoneal cavity, with reversal of flow being controlled by a Hakim valve. The catheter leading into the peritoneum can be long enough to allow for many years' growth, and replacement seldom is necessary.

In the anesthetic management of these children, one's first consideration is of the possibility of increased ICP. This frequently, but not always, is present and calls for appropriate adaptation of technic. So great is the concern about infection, however, that relief of increased pressure by any form of direct drainage is avoided until the operation. Even under strict precautions, a high incidence of infection has been the chief complication of this procedure. Instillation of gentamycin currently promises excellent results.

In the presence of significant elevation of ICP, rectal or intravenous thiopental facilitates quiet induction, after which one may use *d*-tubocurarine for intubation and continue with a relaxant-thiopental combination for maximal avoidance of ICP elevation or introduce halothane and nitrous oxide if conditions permit.

Because of separation of shunts, malposition, or malfunction, repeated operations have frequently been necessary. These procedures seldom take more than an hour and do not present serious problems unless signs have gone unnoticed as pressure developed.

Excision of intracranial tumors. Matson's explicit descriptions of the management of neurosurgical conditions in infants and children are especially valuable in regard to tumors. In 750 operations for excision of brain tumors performed at this hospital between 1940 and 1969, the incidence of 418 posterior fossa tumors was in line with the usual preponderance of infratentorial tumors in the

younger age groups. The types of tumor, as seen in Table 18-5, were primarily astrocytoma, medulloblastoma, brainstem glioma, and ependymoma.

The relatively late appearance of obvious symptoms results in the development of high ICP prior to operation. This contraindicates use of pneumoencephalography for diagnosis. Ventriculography is performed under local or light general anesthesia, with provision for immediate operation if necessary.

Operation in children under 2 years of age is performed in the prone position with a support under the upper chest and the neck slightly flexed to give maximum exposure to the cervical region and the occiput.

As previously noted, preparation of patients with high ICP may require preoperative treatment with osmotic diuretics and corticosteroids over a period of several days and steroid therapy throughout the course of operation.

Preoperative sedation in infants over 6 months of age consists of pentobarbital suppositories, with the use of atropine delayed until the infant is asleep. The speed and potency of halothane and the resultant reduction of struggling override the disadvantage

Table 18-5. 750 intracranial tumors in children—tumor type*

Astrocytoma (grade I-II)	202
Medulloblastoma	139
Brainstem glioma (many unverified)	79
Craniopharyngioma	68
Ependymoma	66
Astrocytoma (grade III-IV) (and mixed gliomas)	64
Optic pathway glioma	27
Choroid plexus papilloma	23
Dermoid cyst	12
Teratoma	11
Miscellaneous	60

Data from Matson, D. D.: Neurosurgery of infancy and childhood, ed. 2, Springfield, Ill., 1969, Charles C Thomas, Publisher.

*Distribution of 750 consecutive intracranial tumors in the Pediatric Neurosurgical Department of The Children's Hospital Medical Center, Boston.

of its pharmacologic effect in increasing ICP, and infants tolerate it well.

Operations for posterior fossa tumors in children over 2 years of age are done in the sitting position, adding the problems of airway control, vasomotor control, and air embolism to those of ICP and interference with respiratory and vasomotor control centers in the floor of the fourth ventricle.

Venous air embolism. The danger of venous air embolism has been emphasized and perhaps exaggerated. Allan and associates (1970) named it as "the most common cause of complications and death following exploration of the posterior fossa in the upright position." Although striking in its suddenness and unique in character and reported in 15 of Marshall's series of 34 cases (1965), the considerable experience of anesthesiologists at the Mayo Clinic, as reported by Michenfelder and associates (1966, 1969, 1972), shows an incidence of 3.8% in over 600 posterior fossa explorations, with no resultant mortality. In our experience in over 450 posterior fossa explorations in children, there have been no known deaths attributable to air embolism, and our calculated incidence of the occurrence of air embolism would limit it to a maximum of ten recognized incidents, none of which were of significant consequence.

It is possible that subclinical amounts of air entered the venous system that were not diagnosed. It also seems possible that the threat is reduced in smaller patients. One reason for this could be that the veins of younger patients might have less tendency to remain open, and another possibility is that there would be less negative pressure in the smaller patient's wound, since the distance above the heart, or potential column of air, would be appreciably less in small children than in adults. Regardless of the frequency of its appearance, one should take reasonable precautionary steps for its prevention, prompt diagnosis, and immediate treatment should it occur.

For the prevention of air embolism, one relies on the surgeon to avoid opening large diploic veins and venous sinuses, to close all vessels, and to secure all venous bleeding immediately. Anesthesiologists place considerable importance on maintaining controlled ventilation in order to eliminate negative pressure. Although this seems reasonable, most of the cases in our institution have been accomplished with assisted spontaneous ventilation. Since we cannot be sure whether our success was due to good technic or good luck, others should not rely on our experience in face of known dangers.

Methods of diagnosis of air embolism have greatly improved. The classic sign of air embolism has been the sudden appearance of a rough mill wheel murmur, audible by precordial or esophageal stethoscope. Since the adaptation of Doppler-designed ultrasound apparatus, it has been possible to recognize air embolism much earlier in its formation and to initiate treatment more promptly (Maroon and others, 1968; Michenfelder and others, 1972). This apparatus is now used routinely for patients in the sitting position.

Other signs of possible significance in detecting air embolism are the abrupt appearance of cardiac arrhythmias, drop in blood pressure, and change in respiratory pattern. Withdrawal of air from a central venous catheter affords the positive evidence to clinch the diagnosis as well as the definitive means of treatment.

Treatment of air embolism must be prompt to be effective and should include as many of the following steps as possible: notify the surgeon, who will attempt immediate closure of open venous channels; apply positive ventilatory pressure; shut off N_2O, if being used; compress jugular vessels and ventilate with oxygen; monitor cardiac action and blood pressure and add isoproterenol (Isuprel) if arterial pressure remains at shock level; lower patient and turn onto his left side. The last move is not well suited to neurosurgical procedures and need not be performed at once, but it may be helpful in some circumstances.

Tumors of cerebral hemispheres. Contrary to findings in adults, the incidence of supratentorial tumors in children is considerably less than that of infratentorial, or posterior fossa, tumors. Unfortunately, those that do occur in children are apt to be tremendous, involve high ICP, and present great difficulty to the surgeon. Operation is usually performed either with the child supine, the head turned to one side, and the shoulder partly elevated or through a frontal approach with the body supine and the head in a neutral position. In the presence of increased ICP, preoperative control with diuretics and steroids may be indicated. ICP also can be controlled by use of an inlying lumbar intrathecal needle attached to a drainage bottle, with the amount of drainage regulated by a screw-clamp. Use of a split mattress allows the needle to stay in place with the patient supine.

Craniopharyngioma. In 1932 Cushing said that craniopharyngiomas "offered the most baffling problem which confronts the neurosurgeon." Although the scene had changed considerably by 1976, Shillito still felt much the same, stating that "one of the most challenging, frustrating and humbling benign intracranial tumors of childhood is the craniopharyngioma. . . . Lurking beneath the optic chiasm, it leads the neurosurgeon on only to defeat his dissection, outmaneuver his microscope, and defy his ambition."

The tumor that has so harassed the neurosurgeon has been equally interesting to the anesthesiologist. Craniopharyngiomas occur primarily in children and make up about 13% of intracranial tumors in that age group. Until 1950, all attempts at surgical removal had resulted in fatality. Although they are not neoplastic, the cellular composition is ectodermal in origin, and they grow by proliferation of epithelial tissue that desquamates, accumulates, and solidifies. By reason of its position in the suprasellar region, the tumor presses on ocular, hypophyseal, and hypothalamic pathways, inducing visual disturbances, intracranial hypertension, hypophyseal disorders, and hypothalamic dysfunction. Visual disturbance may progress from hemianopsia to complete blindness, increased ICP may caused marked hydrocephalus, and hypophyseal and hypothalamic disorders often include dwarfism, pituitary

cachexia, diabetes insipidus, and other disturbance of adrenal, thyroid, and gonadotropic hormones.

With the advent of steroid therapy, pituitary function could be sufficiently regulated to support children through surgery, and operative success became possible (Matson and Crigler, 1960), but preoperative damage, operative difficulty, and postoperative complications still pose major problems. As noted in the review of Katz (1975), of 51 patients operated on at The Children's Hospital Medical Center between 1950 and 1968, 22 of 34 in whom total removal was performed at the initial procedure now survive, while of 24 who were admitted for reoperation only 7 survive.

The diagnosis of craniopharyngioma seldom is difficult. Headache, visual disturbances, diabetes insipidus, and radiographic evidence of suprasellar calcification make further study unnecessary.

Surgical approach is subfrontal, with the patient supine and the head level or slightly elevated. Although prolonged and delicate dissection is necessary, hemorrhage has not been a problem, and induced hypotension is not mandatory. Because of the poor survival rate associated with repeated operation, the surgeon will make an all-out attempt to perform complete removal at the initial operation and may injure optic nerves or further disrupt pituitary function.

Anesthetic management demands some understanding of the physiologic derangements involved and careful preoperative evaluation of the child, who may be markedly debilitated, with increased ICP and a variety of hormonal problems. A thorough study of the patient is made by the endocrinologist, who plays a major part in the entire management of the child. Tests related to neuroendocrine function, as suggested by Matson and Crigler (1969), are shown on p. 444. For the anesthesiologist, those pertaining to sodium and fluid control are especially important, because abnormal antidiuretic hormone secretion is prominent at all stages of the operative treatment. Patients are regulated in relation to cortisone treatment before operation, and dosage is increased substantially on the day of operation. In addition to the usual care of neurosurgical patients, all of these children must have urethral catheters and frequent calculation of fluid gain and loss as well as serum and urine sodium and osmolality. Vasopressin (Pitressin) is added to therapy several days after operation; it is apt to lead to confusion if added before that time. Hyperosmolality has been the greatest early problem in the aftercare of these children since prevention of adrenal collapse has been possible, while visual disturbances and panhypopituitarism, particularly disturbances of growth, have remained the chief long-term problems.

NEUROENDOCRINE DYSFUNCTION IN CHILDREN—CLINICAL AND LABORATORY EVALUATION*

Signs and symptoms

Altered growth rates (heights, weights)
Altered maturation (skeletal, sexual)
Polydypsia and polyuria
Fever, labile temperature responses
Behavioral changes

Laboratory evaluation of hormonal regulation

ADH: fluid balance, serum electrolytes or osmolalities, urine specific gravities
Thyrotropin: PBI, resin T_3, cholesterol, thyroidal ^{131}I uptake, BMR, bone age
ACTH: urinary 17-OH and 17-KS (adolescents) response to metyrapone; response to water load (20 ml/kg)
Gonadotropins (FSH, LH): urinary or serum (immunologic) assays, vaginal smears, testicular biopsies
Growth hormone: serum immunologic assay (IRGH) response to induced hypoglycemia or arginine-HCl infusion with simultaneous measurements of blood sugar, plasma free fatty acids and immunoreactive insulin (IRI), BUN, alkaline phosphatase

ANESTHESIA FOR TRAUMA

The rapidly increasing proportion of traumatized children makes it essential for the anesthesiologist to be prepared to deal with the severely injured, regardless of the type of hospital in which he practices.

While the emergency treatment of head

*From Matson, D. D., and Crigler, J. F., Jr.: Management of craniopharyngiomas in childhood, J. Neurosurg. **30:**377, 1969.

injuries is basically the same for patients of all ages, the type of injury and the child's response to it differ in many respects from those of the adult. Several types of trauma in children are not recognized for some time because of the infant's inability to verbalize and the gradual onset of recognizable signs. The softer skull can expand in response to increased ICP before acute signs are evident. As mentioned earlier, a segment of the skull of the neonate may simply invert instead of crack in response to force. Other head injuries characteristic of the infant and child include extradural and subdural hematomas and compound fractures, while injuries of the spine include compression fracture with damage to the cord at any level.

Hematomas

Extradural, or epidural, hematomas are those classically described in which the child strikes his head, is momentarily unconscious, but then awakens, to fall back into a deepening coma that is only relieved by prompt surgical relief of the pressure and control of the bleeding vessel. In a small infant this may be a vein as well as an artery. Matson (1969) stated that the trauma causing extradural hemorrhages is usually so forceful that the child rarely has the brief lucid period following the first unconsciousness.

Subdural hematoma follows a distinctly different course. Often the original trauma is believed to occur during the infant's delivery, caused by a tear of the bridging veins, which continue to bleed over the course of many days, forming a hematoma under the dura. This grows to occupy a large area within the infant's skull, giving rise to characteristic symptoms of irritability, poor eating, vomiting, and enlargement of the head. Diagnosis is confirmed by tapping the fluid, and continual daily withdrawal of fluid is carried out rather than an attempt being made to remove fluid and hematoma all at once, a method that proved unrewarding. A bone flap is raised, and the membrane is removed. For these children, operation is not an emergency, and there should be sufficient opportunity to build the child up into suitable condition for operation. One of the most common defects found in infants prior to operation is anemia, which often should be treated before the operation is begun.

Compound skull fracture

The relatively weak calvarium of growing children is easily either penetrated or stove in. It is essential to debride and close the wound promptly and replace the depressed fragments in their normal positions as much as possible.

Common factors causing head injury are falls from household chairs, stairs, and beds, traffic accidents, and the unhappy situation of the battered child.

Not all compound fractures are matters of great concern. If the wound is not large and the fragments are not driven deeply into brain substance, there may be a minimum of brain damage and little fluid to replace. On the occasion of a full kick of a horse, however, there may be a massive wound, crushing the entire side of a child's head.

Following a severe head injury, there usually will be an indefinite period of unconsciousness. The immediate treatment of a comatose child should be to clear the airway of blood, vomitus, or other debris, intubate the trachea, establish effective ventilation, and then treat the child for shock and blood loss. Operation is undertaken as soon as cardiovascular stability has been achieved. Operation will include cleaning and debriding the scalp wound, removing broken bone fragments, and trimming and irrigating jagged edges of the remaining skull. The wound is closed, but if there has been extensive loss of skull, only a simple skin closure is attempted at first, with a metal plate to be implanted at a later date (Humphreys and others, 1975).

If the child with severe head injury is conscious, anesthesia is induced cautiously with small amounts of thiopental, followed by muscle relaxant and light halothane after establishment of the endotracheal tube. If the child is comatose, the endotracheal tube is inserted as a primary step in emergency treatment, and anesthetic induction obvious-

ly will be unnecessary. In either case, however, relatively heavy barbiturate sedation and hypothermia may be elected as a means of protecting the brain from hypoxic damage (Shapiro and others, 1974; Michenfelder and others, 1976).

During repair of severe head injuries, it will be essential to control arterial and CSF pressures. Consequently, monitoring will be of increased importance. Blood gases should be obtained at intervals to maintain adequate oxygenation and to hold Pa_{CO_2} between 25 and 35 mm CSF (Miller and Sullivan, 1979).

Should CSF pressure rise, one proceeds to use of osmotic diuretics, use of steroids, removal of CSF, or occasionally use of induced hypotension or hypothermia, in the same manner as described for adults. In all cases, mild hyperventilation and control of blood and fluid volume and acid-base balance are required, with constant urinary drainage.

As noted by Steward and Creighton (1975), the ECG aids in detection of arrhythmias caused by change in ICP, excessive hyperventilation may induce increased intracranial bleeding, and postoperative hyperthermia should be anticipated by use of careful thermometry and circulating water mattresses.

Injuries to the spinal cord

Because of the child's heavy head and the ease with which his small body may be thrown about on contact, injury to the spine is not uncommon. Two main features of treatment concern the danger of adding further injury by moving the child injudiciously and the danger of sudden potassium release in paraplegic or quadriplegic patients. The small size and the pitiful plight of the injured child make it difficult for the observer to resist the impulse to pick him up to comfort him and thereby perhaps transect the cord. Obviously, extreme caution must be used in the management of any spinal cord injury, regardless of the age of the patient.

The danger of sudden increase of serum potassium and cardiac arrest is well known (Tolmie and others, 1967). For this reason, one should avoid use of succinylcholine for intubation of patients who have many types of severe nerve damage, myoneural dysfunction, or tissue destruction. While patients who have long-standing nerve lesions have on occasion tolerated succinylcholine, one should use it only with full realization of the possible consequences and would do well to avoid it if preoperative serum potassium is in excess of 5.0 mEq/L.

BIBLIOGRAPHY

Aird, R. B.: Experimental encephalography with anesthetic gases, Arch. Surg. **32:**193, 1936.

Alexander, S. C., Wolman, H., Cohen, P. J., and others: Cerebrovascular response to Pa_{CO_2} during halothane anesthesia in man, J. Appl. Physiol. **19:**61, 1964.

Allan, D., Kim, H. S., and Cox, J. M.: The anaesthetic management of posterior fossa explorations in infants, Can. Anaesth. Soc. J. **17:**227, 1970.

Bergman, N. A.: Problems in anesthetic management in patients with spina bifida, Anesth. Analg. (Cleve.) **36:**60, 1957.

Bethune, R. W. M., and Brechner, V. L.: Detection of venous air embolism by carbon dioxide monitoring (abstract), Anesthesiology **29:**178, 1968.

Ciliberti, B. J., Goldfein, J., and Rovenstine, E. A.: Hypertension during anesthesia in patients with spinal cord injuries, Anesthesiology **15:**273, 1954.

Colgan, F. J., and Keats, A. S.: Subglottic stenosis; a cause of difficult intubation, Anesthesiology **18:**265, 1957.

Collan, R., and Ivananien, M.: Cardiac arrest caused by rapid elimination of N_2O from cerebral ventricle after encephalography, Can. Anesth. Soc. J. **16:**519, 1969.

Cushing, H.: Intracranial tumors; notes upon a series of two thousand verified cases with surgical-mortality percentages pertaining thereto, Springfield, Ill., 1932, Charles C Thomas, Publisher.

Davson, H.: The cerebrospinal fluid. In Lajtha, A., editor: Handbook of neurochemistry, New York, 1969, Plenum Publishing Corp.

Devivo, D. C., and Dodge, P. R.: Diagnosis and management of head injury. In Smith, C. A., editor: The critically ill child, ed. 2, Philadelphia, 1977, W. B. Saunders Co.

Duflot, L. S. M., and Allen, C. R.: Anesthesia for pediatric neurosurgery, South. Med. J. **49:**1502, 1956.

Eckenhoff, J.: Some anatomic considerations of the infant larynx influencing endotracheal anesthesia, Anesthesiology **12:**401, 1951.

Editorial; halothane and neurosurgery, Br. J. Anaesth. **41:**277, 1969.

Einspach, B. C., and Clark, K.: Further studies on the effectiveness of agents used to lower intracranial pressure, J. Neurosurg. **23:**45, 1965.

Eisenberg, H. M., McComb, J. G., and Lorenzo, A. V.: Cerebrospinal fluid overproduction and hydrocepha-

lus associated with choroid plexus papilloma, J. Neurosurg. **40:**381, 1974.

Elwyn, R. A., Ring, W. H., Loeser, E., and Myers, G. G.: Nitrous oxide encephalography; 5-year experience with 475 pediatric patients, Anesth. Analg. (Cleve.) **55:**402, 1976.

Fischer, E. G., Shillito, J., Jr., and Schuster, S.: Ventriculo-direct atrial shunts; a clinical evaluation, J. Neurosurg. **36:**438, 1972.

Fitch, W., and McDowall, D. G.: Effect of halothane on intracranial pressure gradients in the presence of intracranial space-occupying lesions, Br. J. Anaesth. **43:**904, 1971.

Galindo, A.: Basic concepts in neurosurgical anesthesia. Int. Anesthesiol. Clin. **4:**713, 1966.

Galindo, A., and Baldwin, M.: Intracranial pressure and internal carotid blood flow during halothane anesthesia in the dog, Anesthesiology **24:**318, 1963.

Garfunkel, J. M., Baird, H. W., and Ziegler, J.: The relationship of oxygen consumption to cerebral functional activity, J. Pediatr. **44:**64, 1954.

Gilbert, R. G. B., and Brindle, G. F.: Control of brain volume and intracranial pressure. In Gilbert, R. G. B., Brindle, G. F., and Galindo, A., editors: Anesthesia for neurosurgery, Int. Anesthesiol. Clin. **4:**819, 1966.

Gordon, E., editor: A basis and practice of neuro-anesthesia. Monograph in anaesthesiology, vol. 2, New York, 1975, Elsevier North-Holland, Inc.

Greenfield, J. C., and Tindall, G. T.: Effect of acute increase in intracranial pressure on blood flows in the internal carotid artery of man, J. Clin. Invest. **44:**1343, 1965.

Henriksen, H. T., and Jörgensen, P. B.: The effect of nitrous oxide on intracranial pressure in patients with intracranial disorders, Br. J. Anaesth. **45:**486, 1973.

Howland, W. S., and Papper, E. M.: Circulatory changes during anesthesia for neurosurgical operations, Anesthesiology **13:**343, 1952.

Humphreys, R. P., Hendrick, E. B., and Hoffman, H. J.: Head injuries. In Surgical Staff of the Hospital for Sick Children, Toronto, editors: Care of the injured child, Baltimore, 1975, The Williams & Wilkins Co.

Jennett, W. B., Barker, J., Fitch, W., and McDowall, D. G.: Effects of anaesthesia on intracranial pressure in patients with space-occupying lesions, Lancet **1:**61, 1969.

Jorgensen, P. B., and Henriksen, H. T.: The effect of fluroxene on intracranial pressure in patients with intracranial space-occupying lesions, Br. J. Anaesth. **45:**599, 1973.

Karis, J. H., Menzel, D. B., Donia, A., and Bennett, P. B.: Increase of halothane toxicity by ultraviolet irradiation, paper presented to American Society of Anesthesiologists, San Francisco, October 11, 1976.

Katz, E. L.: Late results of radical excision of craniopharyngioma in children, J. Neurosurg. **42:**86, 1975.

Kennedy, C., Grave, G. D., Jehle, J. W., and Sokoloff,

L.: Blood flow to white matter during maturation of the brain, Neurology **20**:613, 1970.

Kennedy, C., and Sokoloff, L.: An adaptation of the nitrous oxide method to the study of the circulation in children; normal values for cerebral blood flow and metabolic rate in childhood, J. Clin. Invest. **36**:1130, 1967.

Koos, W. T., and Miller, M. H. L.: Intracranial tumors of infants and children, St. Louis, 1971, The C. V. Mosby Co.

Larson, A. G.: Deliberate hypotension, Anesthesiology **25**:682, 1964.

Larson, C. P., Jr.: Anesthesia in brain surgery; abnormal intracranial pressure and ischemia call for special approach, Clin. Trends Anesthesiol. **4**:1, 1974.

Lassen, N. A.: Cerebral blood flow and oxygen consumption in man, Physiol. Rev. **39**:183, 1959.

Lassen, N. A.: Brain extracellular pH; the main factor controlling cerebral blood flow, editorial, Scand. J. Clin. Lab. Invest. **22**:247, 1968.

Lundberg, N.: Continuous recording and control of ventricular fluid pressure in neurosurgical practice, Acta Psychiatr. Neurol. Scand. (Suppl.) **36**(Suppl. 149):1, 1960.

Maroon, J. C., Goodman, J. M., Horner, T. L., and Campbell, R. L.: Detection of minute venous air emboli with ultrasound, Surg. Gynecol. Obstet. **127**: 1236, 1968.

Marshall, B. M.: Air embolus in neurosurgical anesthesia, its diagnosis and treatment, Can. Anaesth. Soc. J. **12**:255, 1965.

Matson, D. D.: Neurosurgery of infancy and childhood, ed. 2, Springfield, Ill., 1969, Charles C Thomas, Publisher.

Matson, D. D., and Crigler, J. F., Jr.: Radical treatment of craniopharyngioma, Ann. Surg. **152**:699, 1960.

Matson, D. D., and Crigler, J. F., Jr.: Management of craniopharyngiomas in childhood, J. Neurosurg. **30**: 377, 1969.

McComish, P. B., and Bodley, P. O.: Anaesthesia for neurological surgery, Chicago, 1971, Year Book Medical Publishers, Inc.

McDowall, D. G., Barker, J., and Jennett, W. B.: Cerebrospinal fluid pressure measurements during anaesthesia, Anaesthesia **21**:189, 1966.

McQueen, D., and Udvarhelyi, G.: Congenital anomalies of the neuraxis and related maldevelopmental disorders. In Ravitch, M. M., Welch, K. J., Benson, C. D., and others, editors: Pediatric surgery, ed. 3, Chicago, 1979, Year Book Medical Publishers, Inc.

Meridy, H. W., Creighton, R. E., and Humphreys, R. P.: Complications during neurosurgery in the prone position in children, Can. Soc. J. **21**:445, 1974.

Michenfelder, J. D., Gronert, G. A., and Rehder, K.: Review article; neuroanesthesia, Anesthesiology **30**: 65, 1969.

Michenfelder, J. D., Milde, J., and Sundt, T.: Cerebral protection by barbiturate anesthesia, Arch. Neurol. **33**:345, 1976.

Michenfelder, J. D., Miller, R. H., and Gronert, G. A.: Evaluation of ultrasonic device (Doppler) for the diagnosis of venous air embolism, Anesthesiology **36**: 164, 1972.

Michenfelder, J. D., and Terry, H. R., Jr.: Current practices and trends in neuroanesthesia, Clin. Neurosurg. **13**:252, 1965.

Miller, J. D., and Sullivan, H. G.: Severe intracranial hypertension, Int. Anesthesiol. Clin. **17**:19, 1979.

Murray, J., and Swanson, L.: Mid-face osteotomy and advancement for craniosynostosis, J. Plast. Reconstr. Surg. **41**:299, 1968.

Newman, H.: Encephalography with ethylene, J.A.M.A. **108**:461, 1937.

Paul, W., and Munson, E. S.: Gas embolism during encephalography, Anesth. Analg. (Cleve.) **55**:141, 1976.

Raudzens, P., and Cole, A. F. D.: Thiopentone/lidocaine anaesthesia for pneumoencephalography, Can. Anaesth. Soc. J. **21**:1, 1974.

Rosomoff, H. L.: Protective effects of hypothermia against pathological processes of the nervous system, Ann. N.Y. Acad. Sci. **80**:475, 1959.

Rosomoff, H. L.: Effect of hypothermia and hypotonic urea on distribution of intracranial contents, J. Neurosurg. **18**:753, 1961.

Rossanda, M.: Clinical value of cerebrospinal fluid acid-base management, Int. Anesthesiol. Clin. **7**:701, 1969.

Saidman, L. J., and Eger, E. I. II: Change in cerebrospinal fluid pressure during pneumoencephalography under nitrous oxide anesthesia, Anesthesiology **26**: 67, 1965.

Schroeder, H. G., and Williams, N. E.: Anesthesia for meningocele surgery; some problems associated with immediate surgical closure in the neonate, Anaesthesia **21**:57, 1966.

Shapiro, H. M.: Intracranial hypertension; therapeutic and anesthetic considerations, Anesthesiology **43**:445, 1975.

Shapiro, H. M., Wyte, S. R., Harris, A. B., and Galindo, A.: Acute intraoperative intracranial hypertension in neurosurgical patients; mechanical and pharmacologic factors, Anesthesiology **37**:399, 1972.

Shapiro, H. M., Wyte, S. R., and Loeser, J.: Barbiturate augmented hypothermia for reduction of persistent intracranial pressure, J. Neurosurg. **40**:90, 1974.

Sharrard, W. J. W.: Meningomyelocele; prognosis of immediate operative closure of the sac, Proc. R. Soc. Med. **56**:510, 1963.

Shillito, J., Jr.: The treatment of craniopharyngiomas of childhood. In Morley, T. P., editor: Current controversies in neurosurgery, Philadelphia, 1976, W. B. Saunders Co.

Shillito, J., Jr., and Matson, D. D.: Craniosynostosis; a review of 519 surgical cases, Pediatrics **41**:829, 1968.

Shillito, J., Jr., and Ojemann, R. G.: Hydrocephalus. In Youmans, J., editor: Neurological surgery, Philadelphia, 1973, W. B. Saunders Co.

447

Slocum, H. C., O'Neal, K. C., and Allen, C. R.: Neurovascular complications from malposition on the operating table, Surg. Gynecol. Obstet. **86:**729, 1948.

Smith, A. L., and Wollman, H.: Cerebral blood flow and metabolism; effects of anesthetic drugs and techniques, Anesthesiology **36:**378, 1972.

Steward, D. J., and Creighton, R. E.: Anesthetic management of the injured child. In Surgical Staff of the Hospital for Sick Children, Toronto, editors: Care of the injured child, Baltimore, 1975, The Williams & Wilkins Co.

Stoelting, R. K.: Comment, Anesth. Analg. (Cleve.) **55:** 143, 1976.

Strand, R. D.: Gas ventriculography and pneumoencephalography with comments on anesthesia in pneumoencephalography by R. M. Smith. In Amador, L. V., editor: Brain tumors in the young, Baltimore, The Williams & Wilkins Co., in press.

Tessier, P.: The definitive plastic surgical treatment of the severe facial deformities of craniofacial dysostosis; Crouzon's and Apert's diseases, J. Plast. Reconstr. Surg. **48:**419, 1971.

Tolmie, J. D., Joyce, T. W., and Mitchell, G. D.: Succinylcholine danger in the burned patients, Anesthesiology **28:**467, 1967.

Vries, J. K., Becker, D. P., and Young, H. F.: A subarachnoid screw for monitoring intracranial pressure, J. Neurosurg. **39:**416, 1973.

Welch, K.: The principles of physiology of the cerebrospinal fluid in relation to hydrocephalus including normal pressure hydrocephalus. In Friedlander, W. J., editor: Advances in neurology, New York, 1975, Raven Press.

Wollman, H., Alexander, S. C., Cohen, P. J., and others: Cerebral circulation during general anesthesia and hyperventilation in man, Anesthesiology **26:** 329, 1965.

Youngberg, J. A., Kaplan, J. A., and Miller, E. D.: Air embolism through a ventriculoatrial shunt during pneumoencephalography, Anesthesiology **42:**487, 1975.

CHAPTER 19

Anesthesia for orthopedic surgery

Operations and underlying conditions
Features of orthopedic surgery that concern
  anesthesia
Fundamental anesthetic management
Anesthetic maintenance
Anesthetic management of specific problems

OPERATIONS AND UNDERLYING CONDITIONS

Among the several fields of surgery that have developed special interest in the pediatric group, orthopedic surgery led most others by some 50 years. Because of the urgency of broken bones and osteomyelitis and the compelling need of children with severe deformities, many surgeons were drawn into this field, and numerous corrective procedures were developed and standardized before 1920. Until 1940 the greater part of the operating schedules in pediatric hospitals consisted of orthopedic procedures, with the usual addition of tonsillectomies, mastoidectomies, and incision of abscesses. An important factor in the early development of orthopedic surgery was the fact that open-drop ether met most of the current surgical requirements and, except for an occasional overdose, aspiration, or convulsion, left little to be desired.

Following World War II, the introduction of antibiotics and better understanding of physiology and anesthesiology enabled surgeons to take great new strides, first in infant surgery and then in cardiac surgery, thereby ending the dominance of orthopedic surgeons. Antibiotics eliminated osteomyelitis, leaving poliomyelitis as the greatest concern of the orthopedic field. At least half of the time and effort of many surgeons was occu-

pied in the care of children during the acute or chronic forms of this disease.

The introduction of poliomyelitis vaccine reduced the work of the orthopedic surgeon but did not change the picture as drastically as might have been expected. The last major epidemic in 1955, and many that preceded it, left enough crippled children to occupy orthopedic surgeons for many years. In addition, new concepts were originated that opened the way for more ambitious procedures, especially in the treatment of scoliosis and bone tumors.

In a children's hospital that has an active orthopedic service, numerous operations are performed on bones, joints, muscles, and tendons. These procedures include open and closed reduction of fractures and dislocations, tendon release and transplant, osteotomy or fusion of long bones and spine, bone graft, amputation, and many others. A representative list of operative orthopedic lesions is given below. These and others are described in standard texts of pediatrics and orthopedic surgery (Ferguson, 1957; Tachdjian, 1972; Vaughan and McKay, 1975; Moe and others, 1978). In addition, Katz and Kadis (1973) have compiled an excellent reference that describes the pathophysiology and anesthetic management of a variety of the less common disorders, many of which affect muscle, bone, or connective tissue. The index of syndromes by Jones and Pelton (1976) is also extremely helpful.

CONDITIONS ENCOUNTERED IN PEDIATRIC ORTHOPEDIC SURGERY

Traumatic conditions

Fractures, dislocations (simple, compound, single or multiple)

449

Congenital anomalies
Congenital clubfoot
Congenital dislocated hip
Torticollis
Sprengel's deformity
Klippel-Feil syndrome
Congenital scoliosis

Infections
Acute hematogenous osteomyelitis
Rheumatoid arthritis
Septic arthritis

Disturbances of growth or metabolism
Arachnodactyly (Marfan's disease)
Arthrogryposis multiplex
Achondroplasia
Legg-Perthes disease
Leg length discrepancy
Morquio-Ullrich syndrome
Osteogenesis imperfecta
Streeter's dysplasia
Idiopathic scoliosis

Neuromuscular disorders
Poliomyelitis
Werdnig-Hoffmann disease
"Amyotonia congenita"
Myotonia congenita
Myotonic dystrophy
Progressive muscular dystrophy
Charcot-Marie-Tooth syndrome

Neurologic disorders
Cerebral palsy
Neurofibromatosis

Bone cysts and tumors
Bone cysts
Tumors of bone
Benign
Malignant

As suggested in the above list, the pediatric hospital attracts children with unusual and bizarre syndromes that seldom are encountered elsewhere. The anesthesiologist must be alert to the nature of these rarities and be able to distinguish between those in which the total lesion is obvious and unrelated to other organ systems and those in which underlying conditions may be of considerably greater significance than the orthopedic condition for which the operation is performed.

During the past decade, the greatest interest has been in the treatment of all forms of scoliosis, especially the more severely affected children, many of whom had previous-ly been considered too crippled to be corrected or too frail to survive operation. The accomplishments brought about by the introduction of internal fixation of the spine have been enough to regain for the orthopedic surgeon his prior place of eminence and to present to the anesthesiologist sufficient challenge to make this one of our most interesting areas of endeavor.

The management of trauma becomes an ever-increasing problem, whether due to city traffic or farm machinery. Among the most demanding situations are those involving replacement of severed limbs, often requiring all-out effort of orthopedic, vascular, and plastic surgeons.

Other fields of increased intensity in orthopedic surgery include the study and treatment of an extensive variety of metabolic and pathologic lesions, chief among which are bone tumors. An aggressive approach combining surgery, radiation, and medical therapy is now offering children greater hope of survival and recovery, presently at the cost of repeated mutilating operations but with promise of significant and continuing advances. Anesthetic management of the emotional and physical problems encountered in these patients calls for psychologic insight, intraoperative support, and extremely critical postoperative management.

FEATURES OF ORTHOPEDIC SURGERY THAT CONCERN ANESTHESIA

Each type of surgery has a pattern of its own. In general, orthopedic operations performed on children have the following characteristics:

1. The children often are chronically ill or have had prolonged immobilization and, in addition to their operative lesion, may have defects of the cardiorespiratory system and endocrine, metabolic, or enzyme disorders.
2. Many have deep-rooted psychiatric problems due to crippling disease; others are faced with the overwhelming emotional shock of unexpected major amputation.
3. Operations are often of relatively long duration (4 hours or more).

4. Many patients must return for a series of operations.
5. Deep relaxation is seldom necessary.
6. Use of cautery and x-ray may be expected.
7. A tourniquet is frequently used on arm or leg to control bleeding.
8. Casts and apparatus may limit postoperative positioning.

FUNDAMENTAL ANESTHETIC MANAGEMENT

The management of anesthesia is determined by adapting pediatric methods to fit the special considerations mentioned above.

Preoperative considerations

The anesthesiologist's preoperative visit is especially important in orthopedic surgery. The underlying disease may be an unusual disorder, the significance of which will not be recognized. The anesthesiologist should learn the nature and the extent of the disease before accepting the child as his responsibility. In a lesion such as Streeter's dysplasia (Fig. 19-1), the deformities of the limb usually represent the only pathology, but in Marfan's syndrome, major cardiac defects often complicate the problem (Cooke, 1968; Murdoch and others, 1972).

In addition to standard preoperative examination and musculoskeletal evaluation, specific tests of heart, lungs, and electrolytes often are needed. Black patients must have sickle cell tests, especially if a tourniquet is to be applied. Special enzyme tests used to determine muscular disorders include aldolase, creatine phosphokinase (CPK), serum glutamic pyruvic transaminase (SGPT), serum glutamic oxaloacetic transaminase (SGOT), and lactic dehydrogenase (LDH). Electromyograms also may be of value in diagnosis of muscular disorders. Details of preoperative studies of scoliotic patients are described later.

The fact that children often must return for several operations makes it necessary to spend extra time with them in order to bolster their morale and help them overcome apprehension. It is especially helpful if the same anesthesiologist can care for the child during successive operations and also if he can find out whether any experiences were particularly upsetting during the first anesthetic so that they may not be repeated. Pre-

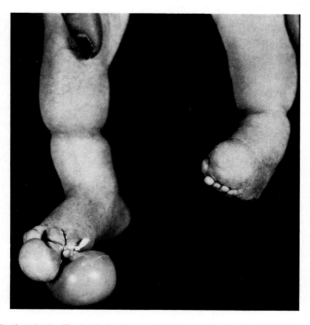

Fig. 19-1. Streeter's dysplasia. Typical circular constriction in legs, with distal deformities.

operative sedation may be a problem in a child who is apprehensive or has poor respiratory exchange because of muscular weakness. In such cases it is advisable to use a light sedative at bedtime and repeat it preoperatively. Pentobarbital (2 mg/kg) would be suitable.

A child who is unexpectedly confronted by the loss of an arm or leg may present an even more difficult emotional problem than the child with congenital heart disease who enters for potentially lethal cardiac surgery.

ANESTHETIC MAINTENANCE

During orthopedic operations, the dangers associated with long procedures are especially feared. A slight degree of hypoventilation gradually leads to serious hypoxia and hypercapnia. Similarly, insidious blood loss during an "uneventful" 4-hour operation may go unnoticed until severe hypovolemia suddenly becomes evident. Since there is a tendency for anesthesiologists to overestimate blood loss and for surgeons to underestimate it, measurements are definitely advisable in these procedures.

Whether the high incidence of repeat operations increases the danger of halothane toxicity is still an unanswered question (Davidson and others, 1966). At The Children's Hospital Medical Center, we have had three patients who were believed to have had halothane hepatitis. A 9-year-old girl who recovered and an 11-year-old girl who died were both reported in the study of Carney and Van Dyke (1972). An 18-year-old boy who recovered was not considered a pediatric patient.

Since all three of these were orthopedic patients and because there is greater latitude in choice of anesthetic agent for such procedures, we refrained from using halothane in any orthopedic procedure for 4 years. However, since the 9-year-old is the only child under 10 known by us, either through the literature or by hearsay, to have had a convincing story of halothane hepatitis, we have discontinued this restriction in prepubertal patients (p. 454).

Some surgeons prefer to keep children in plastic jackets or body casts during anesthesia and surgery (Denton and O'Donoghue, 1955). The danger of respiratory embarrassment, the greater difficulty in endotracheal intubation, and the inaccessibility of the chest in case of cardiac arrest make this practice one to be avoided whenever possible.

The danger of pressure areas and nerve injury makes it imperative to position patients carefully and to check them frequently. Masks should be removed, and the face should be massaged gently every 10 to 15 minutes to prevent pressure injury. In addition, special care must be taken to protect the eyes. When a patient is face down, the head should be repositioned every 15 minutes.

One of the greatest hazards of modern anesthesia lies in the increasing duration of operations; surgeons apparently are taking less and less notice of the passing hours. Not only does this entail direct danger of physiologic disturbance in the patient, but it introduces a very real danger of anesthesiologist fatigue. In relatively uncomplicated operations, monotony and inattention become increasingly dangerous unless special measures are taken. Such measures, as outlined in Chapter 9, include the following of a strict routine of checkpoints, frequent visits by instructors or colleagues, and the use of minor changes in anesthetic technic to provide additional interest in the case. Monitors with alarms would be especially desirable in such operations. If monitors could warn the entire surgical team when the heart rate, blood pressure, or temperature pass outside of normal range, there would be fewer serious complications.

Tourniquets, sickle cell anemia, and tourniquet pain

Many elective and emergency orthopedic operations are performed on the extremities, and the use of tourniquets usually is helpful and often deemed mandatory by the surgeons.

The danger of sequestration and stagnation of blood in patients with sickle cell anemia is well known. As previously stated, all black patients should be tested for the presence of sickling before tourniquets are applied for surgical use (Gilchrist, 1973; Gillies, 1974) (this does not deny their use for blood pressure determination). There has been considerable indecision concerning the danger involved. However, there now is ample evidence that *the presence of sickle cell disease is a definite contraindication to the use of a surgical tourniquet, but there has not been sufficient evidence to deny the use of tourniquets on patients who have the sickle cell trait only* (Searle, 1973). A finer definition now followed is to limit the use of tourniquets to patients having less than 40% hemoglobin S by electrophoresis.

A minor reaction is seen in normal patients operated on with the use of tourniquets. After the tourniquet has been inflated for 30 to 60 minutes, patients often show gradually increasing heart rate and blood pressure (Fig. 19-2). This response appears to be due to stimulation of sympathetic nerves that occupy the arterial sheaths, causing so-called tourniquet pain, which has been known to penetrate light levels of anesthesia. The stimulation may require an increasing concentra-

tion of anesthesia, which, upon release of the tourniquet and cessation of stimulation, may be followed by sudden hypotension and anesthetic depression. Three factors that may contribute to this complication are the excessive pressure often used to inflate surgical tourniquets, hypovolemia, and continuing administration of a high concentration of anesthetic. Instead of the use of 250 and 500 mm Hg pressure on arm and leg tourniquets, respectively, as seems customary, it would appear rational to measure a child's blood pressure and set the tourniquets at pressures not more than 50 mm Hg above those figures. The importance of maintenance of blood volume and prompt reduction of anesthetic concentration immediately after release of the tourniquet is self-evident. (For references on pneumatic tourniquets, see Flewellen and Jarem [1978].)

Recovery

The immediate postoperative period can carry special risks for orthopedic patients. Many children are immobilized in casts or traction apparatus that prevent them from turning, exposing them to extreme danger

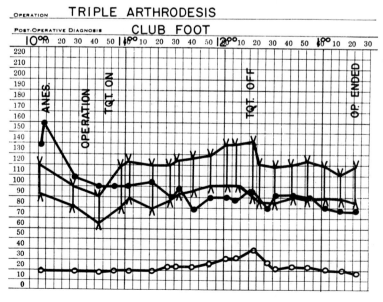

Fig. 19-2. Anesthesia chart of 6-year-old girl showing gradual rise in blood pressure during operation with tourniquet inflated to 500 psi and distinct fall upon release of tourniquet.

of vomiting and strangulation. Other children have variable degrees of neuromuscular coordination or weakness that carry similar risk.

Most of these children should be kept in the operating room with endotracheal tube in place until their gag reflex has returned and they are actually awake. In some it may be preferable to leave the endotracheal tube in place for a longer period and support respiration by use of a ventilator. Extubation should be carried out under maximum precautions. To facilitate prompt recovery in the operating room, quickly excreted or reversible agents should be used. It also is advisable to empty the stomach of such patients shortly before they awaken.

Since the recovery pattern of patients with different types of amyotonia is less predictable, the period of special recovery care should be considerably prolonged.

Agents and technics

Children under ten years of age. The choice of agent and technic is not strictly limited in anesthesia for pediatric orthopedic procedures. Use of adaptations of the Ayre system for children under 10 kg and circle absorption for larger patients has been our practice, though there are many different preferences.

If a small child has an intravenous infusion already established on arrival in the operating room, this is used for induction. Otherwise, an inhalation method is usually more acceptable, especially if the child has poor veins. For short procedures, inhalation anesthesia often is more practical, allowing one to avoid intubation and providing more prompt awakening if one has not depressed the child. As previously mentioned, there seems to be little reason to restrict the use of halothane in children under 10 to 12 years of age. Two situations that are considered to be contraindications to halothane in all patients are (1) when there is increased possibility of malignant hyperthermia and (2) when use of halothane would increase the risk of litigation.

Intravenous anesthetic agents have increased advantage in 6- to 10-year-olds, especially when intubation is needed. Ketamine is employed sparingly, mostly for induction of poor-risk or uncontrollable smaller children.

Endotracheal intubation is certainly not required for all orthopedic procedures and should be avoided when reasonable. The belief that intubation is indicated simply because an operation is expected to last more than 1 or 2 hours is often based more on the welfare of the anesthesiologist than on that of the patient. A child's ventilation is usually quite easily maintained by mask when he is lying supine with an oral airway in place.

Children over ten years of age. Many orthopedic procedures are performed on teenage patients and call for slightly different management. Circle absorption systems have been almost universally indicated for general anesthesia, but local and regional blocks have definite value.

Sensitivity to halothane, or posthalothane hepatitis, if such does exist, seems to increase with the onset of secondary sexual characteristics, and whatever precautions one believes are indicated for adults should be applied from puberty onward.

Our tendency has been to use intravenous agents for adolescents. Veins are more frequently available and relaxant-narcotic combinations are well suited. Innovar, consisting of the combination of fentanyl and droperidol, was popular briefly, but as noted by Foldes and associates (1966), the mixture of two such divergent drugs does not seem logical. Our usual approach is to start with thiopental or nitrous oxide and to continue with d-tubocurarine and morphine, using a 50-50 mixture of nitrous oxide and oxygen. With the present concern over waste gases, we try to maintain total gas flows at 3 to 4 L/min or less. In addition to general anesthesia, one finds increased indications for local and regional blocks in this age range; axillary and intravenous regional blocks far outnumber all others (see Chapter 11).

ANESTHETIC MANAGEMENT OF SPECIFIC PROBLEMS
Traumatic lesions and other emergencies

Severe injuries involving a crushed chest or fractures of the skull, vertebrae, pelvis, or long bones may be associated with shock, hemorrhage, or brain injury, all of which demand specific treatment similar to that used for adults. Following blood replacement and adequate stabilization, emergency measures may be accomplished under local or regional block, ketamine (in smaller patients), morphine–nitrous oxide, or halogenated agents (Steward and Creighton, 1975).

Although accidents claim a tremendous number of children's lives, the child's ability to survive major trauma is a continual source of wonder, as exemplified by the 2-year-old girl who was run over by her father in a 2-ton truck, her only injury being tire marks and a broken pelvis, and the 1- and 3-year-old brothers who fell out of a window to the pavement four stories below, the total damage being two broken legs and one slight concussion.

More frequently, children require treatment for such minor accidents as simple Colles' fractures. Since one can never be sure that children have not eaten recently, it may be safer to forego general anesthesia and employ a brachial block, preferably by the axillary route. If general anesthesia is chosen, one should apply the concepts described under management of full stomach in Chapter 22.

A relatively common orthopedic emergency is the child with an *infected hip*. The surgeons often insist that there is pus that must be removed promptly in order to prevent necrosis of the head of the femur and that they need only 15 minutes of anesthesia while they aspirate it. The child is dehydrated, febrile, and in a toxic condition and usually is a chubby 1-year-old with no visible veins. The prone position may be necessary to allow access to the hip joint. Very frequently the surgeons find that aspiration is not adequate and that incision and drainage

are necessary, thereby prolonging the operation by at least an hour and often involving need of transfusion.

With this probable sequence in mind, one should insist on full preparation of such children, with initiation of antibiotics, establishment of a reliable infusion, appreciable rehydration, control of fever, and preparation of blood for infusion before starting the anesthesia.

Elective surgery of the hip

The hip is the site of several operations that may worry the anesthesiologist. In congenital dislocation of the hip, the initial operation may be nothing more than a closed manipulation under mask anesthesia. If it is an open reduction, the operation often requires blood replacement, in preparation for which one should always have blood previously typed and crossmatched and an infusion running.

It may not be the operation itself that provides the difficulty as much as the application of spica casts at repeated intervals after operation. For these procedures the infant is suspended by one small support under the coccyx and another at the scapular level. While the surgeons apply the plaster, the anesthesiologist is expected to provide anesthesia and relaxation and, at the same time, to push on the infant's shoulders to keep his perineum against the vertical strut between his legs. This is almost impossible unless there is a full-time assistant to push the infant caudalward throughout the entire procedure. It is also a particular duty of the anesthesiologist to see that adequate space is provided within the spica for the infant to breathe. This the surgeon should do by making a "belly pad" of several folds of stockinette, which is placed next to the stomach and kept there until the cast is completed. If of sufficient size, its removal should then allow "breathing room" for the diaphragm.

Operations involving pinning, nailing, and application of plates to the hip, as well as osteotomies of femur and ilium, are encountered in children for treatment of Legg-Perthes disease, slipped femoral epiphyses, old congenital hip dislocations, and other problems. It is almost always an extremely overweight youth who needs pinning of one or both hips for slipped femoral head. Time, relaxation, and blood are the prime requisites for these procedures.

Hip replacement

In adult orthopedics there is much activity now in relation to total hip replacement. This procedure is infrequently performed in children but is necessary occasionally, particularly following renal transplantation. The anesthesiologist certainly should be aware of the danger of blood loss as well as the problem of sudden fall in arterial pressure caused by acrylic bone cement (Berman and others, 1974). Investigation by Cohen and Smith (1971) suggests that the best prevention of this complication is to maintain circulating blood volume at or above normal level, because the greatest incidence of mortality has been related to loss of peripheral resistance in the presence of reduced blood volume. Although we have not used induced hypotension for hip replacement, the technic has been advocated to reduce operating time and blood loss. In addition, Fahmy and Laver (1976) believe that it reduces the hypotensive response to methyl methacrylate.

Scoliosis

Spinal fusion. As previously mentioned, the greatest progress in pediatric orthopedics in recent years has been in the correction of scoliosis. The introduction of internal metallic fixation of the spine by means of Harrington rod instrumentation (Harrington, 1962) or the Dwyer anterior approach and cable fixation (Dwyer and others, 1969), with additional skeletal traction procedures, has enabled surgeons to produce greatly improved results and to help many children previously believed to be inoperable.

The problems faced by participating anesthesiologists involve maximum-risk patients who must be carried through one and often several operations of greater magnitude than previously known in pediatric orthopedic

surgery. For any degree of success, the anesthesiologist must have a clear idea of the underlying pathology, know how to evaluate the patient's chance of survival, be cognizant of the previous operations, and be expert in anesthetic management. In addition, he must be able to carry borderline patients through days or weeks of postoperative ventilatory support and be able to make diagnoses and decisions concerning complications arising during the critical period of recovery (Nickel and others, 1957; Hardy, 1974).

Etiologic factors. Keim (1972) defined scoliosis as one or more lateral-rotary curvatures of the spine and went on to classify different curves according to nonstructural and structural characteristics. The variety of causative lesions is shown in the listing of 72 possible causes by Riseborough (1973). The most common type is that termed "idiopathic," which accounts for 65% of all scoliosis and occurs primarily in otherwise healthy teenage girls. The remaining 35% Riseborough divided into the following groups: congenital skeletal abnormalities (15%), neuromuscular abnormalities (10%), and neurofibromatosis (5%), plus a scattering of such rarities as spinal tumors, spondylolisthesis, Sjögren's syndrome, and Refsum's disease (Fogan and Munsat, 1974).

Patients differ widely in respect to anatomic, physiologic, and etiologic factors of the scoliosis and the associated lesions. The first consideration, from the anatomic standpoint, is the curvature that the fusion is intended to correct, reduce, or simply arrest. The scoliosis may occur at cervical, thoracic, or lumbar levels, and although there usually are two curves, there may be as many as four, with varying degrees of angulation, rotation, and kyphosis or lordosis.

The level of the curve has important bearing on the risk of the situation. Curvature of the cervical spine suggests destructive disease, trauma, or congenital deformity, each of which entails special underlying problems, and the technical management is particularly demanding for both surgeon and anesthesiologist.

Thoracic and thoracolumbar curves produce maximal physiologic effect on cardiac and respiratory function. Extreme curves so limit ventilation and cardiac output that death may occur in childhood. The age of onset, etiology, rate of progression, and angle of curve are among the most important factors. One of the best criteria of patient viability remains the patient's exercise tolerance. It is essential to know whether a child can walk, run, and jump or if he has never been able to sit up in bed.

Curvature of the lower lumbar spine causes the least physiologic handicaps, but correction often requires the more difficult Dwyer anterior fusion.

The degree of thoracolumbar curvature is used as an indication of the degree of ventilatory limitation and also as a guide to the need for operation (Zorab, 1966; Makley and others, 1968; Shannon and others, 1971). Surgery is seldom indicated in patients with curvature of less than 35°. While operation may be indicated for a slightly greater degree of curvature, children with curves under 65° who have only idiopathic scoliosis rarely show clinical evidence of respiratory impairment. However, patients with congenital scoliosis may have marked respiratory limitation and even less skeletal angulation.

Curvature of between 65° and 90° usually causes some reduction, and curvature of over 90° causes marked limitation of ventilation, especially in relation to increasing ratio of residual lung volume to total lung capacity (Riseborough and Davis, 1974).

A fixed vertebral curve, whether due to congenital block or long-standing disease, adds considerably to operative difficulty and functional restriction and may necessitate one or more additional operations for removal of a wedge of bone and application of halofemoral apparatus for several weeks of traction.

In a detailed description of the evaluation of ventilatory involvement, Nickel and associates (1957) stressed the importance of an effective cough and the increased handicap of children who are subject to repeated pulmonary infections, have spastic or rigid thorax, or are unable to cooperate adequately.

It is essential to recognize the major problems before operation (Hardy, 1974). Among the most difficult cases are those whose deformities are associated with muscle weakness or paralysis. Whether due to amyotonia, neurifibromatosis, tumor, or transection, these patients have reduced tolerance to positional change, operative trauma, and postoperative stresses. The presence of spasticity is no less restrictive than lesions involving weakness. Thus, cerebral palsy is one of the principal complicating factors in patients undergoing spinal fusion (MacEwen, 1974).

Spinal fusion for congenital scoliosis or myelomeningocele may be necessary in infants under 2 years old. Many of these involve cervical lesions; others are complicated by paraplegia. Most of them present marked difficulty in positioning, monitoring, and support during operation and in postoperative management.

Specific tests of pulmonary function, if based on arm spread rather than height, have proved to be of practical value (Hardy, 1974). Relton and Conn (1963) recommended measurement of tidal volume, minute volume, vital capacity, and maximum breathing capacity, but some rely chiefly on vital capacity. Patients usually tolerate 50% reduction of vital capacity, sometimes tolerate 50% to 70% reduction, but rarely tolerate over 70% reduction without tracheostomy or prolonged tracheal intubation and ventilatory support (Stiles, 1975).

Blood gases may be of more significance than ventilation studies. Tidal volume and total lung capacity have been found to be only slightly reduced in some patients who show significant reduction of arterial oxygen, and this hypoxia is exaggerated by exercise. Shannon and associates (1971), Dollery and associates (1965), and Zorab (1966) have shown that scoliotic curvature has more effect on ventilation-perfusion ratios, resulting in lowered arterial oxygenation, decreased respiratory reserve, and areas of increased dead space.

Riseborough and Davis (1974) state that patients having curves of over 65° may show

Pa_{O_2} reduction to 80 mm Hg and even lower with exercise. In advanced scoliosis, Pa_{CO_2} may exceed Pa_{O_2} (55 and 50 mm Hg, respectively), while patients with severe ventilatory restriction have been found with Pa_{O_2} as low as 28 mm Hg when breathing room air. Since blood loss is a major consideration, special attention is paid to platelet count, template bleeding time, aggregometry, prothrombin time (PT), partial thromboplastin time (PTT), and history of aspirin medication (Kevy, 1979).

Relationship of age and respiratory pathology. Scoliosis that does not appear until late in the growth period has minimal effect on cardiorespiratory function but is of greater concern in relation to body mechanics. In contrast to this are the forms such as congenital scoliosis, where curvature is severe prior to completion of lung development.

At birth, a normal infant's lung contains 50,000 to 100,000 alveoli, which increase to the maximum of 300,000 by 2 years of age, after which time alveoli continue to increase in size until 15 years of age. When curvature appears early in life, the compressed lung may reach only one-third normal size, being defective in both number and size of alveoli (Reid, 1966). As the child grows, there is decreasing lung volume, dead space, respiratory reserve, and compliance and increasing pulmonary vascular resistance. Decreasing alveolar ventilation produces increasing hypoxia, hypercapnia, and respiratory acidosis. Pulmonary hypertension follows as a result of reduced vascular bed and vasoconstriction secondary to hypoxia, with final development, in fatal cases, of cor pulmonale and right ventricular failure, usually ending with terminal pneumonia (Bergofsky and others, 1959).

Preoperative evaluation: recapitulation. Anesthesiologists should be familiar with all of the preceding considerations. In the preoperative evaluation, the essential features that should be specifically determined prior to spinal fusion include the following:

1. The level and angulation of the spinal curve or curves and the approximate number of vertebrae involved in each.

2. The primary etiology of the curve, in particular whether there is any generalized neuromuscular weakness.

3. Exercise tolerance, specifically what type of activity the patient has been able to maintain.

4. The restriction of ventilation, estimated by spinal angulation, ventilation studies, and/or blood gas determinations.

5. The type of and indication for intended operation or operations.

6. The history of previous operations, especially those for scoliosis, with particular reference to blood loss, postoperative ventilatory adequacy, and emotional experiences.

7. The presence of underlying complications or intercurrent infections.

Surgical considerations in correction of scoliosis. The correction of different types of scoliosis may call for the use of either posterior fusion or anterior fusion alone or performance of anterior fusion with subsequent posterior fusion. Furthermore, performance of wedge resection followed by halo-femoral or halo-pelvic traction may be required prior to either type of fusion, whether one or both types of fusion are planned. The essential aspects of posterior and anterior fusion are outlined below.

BASIC PROCEDURES IN POSTERIOR AND ANTERIOR SPINAL FUSION

Posterior spinal fusion: Harrington rod instrumentation

Indications:
  Curve 85°, normal patient
  Curve 65°, weak patient
Operative position: prone, on frame
Incision:
  Midline, along vertebral spines
  Posterior iliac graft
Procedure:
  Inject epinephrine solution
  Incise, clear vertebrae
  Rongeur spinous processes, decorticate vertebrae, raise iliac graft, control bleeding
  Place rod, apply distracting force
  Awaken patient to test for function of spinal cord
  Lay on graft
  Close wound
Expected duration: 3 to 5 hours (teaching hospital)
Blood loss: 0.4 to 0.6 TBV or more
Postoperative ventilation: seldom

Anterior spinal fusion: Dwyer cable fixation

Indications:

 Fixation of spine by kyphos or boney block (congenital or old lesion) unapproachable by posterior route

 Inability to use rods because of absence of laminae (myelomeningocele, tumor, etc.)

 Low lumbar curve in healthy patient

Position: on side, convex curve up

Incision: thoracoabdominal

Procedure:

 Expose and strip 4 to 8 vertebrae involved, remove intervertebral disks, fix cleats and screw eyes to vertebrae, insert cable, cut and fix cable

 Repair diaphragm, close chest and abdomen

Expected duration: 5 to 8 hours

Blood loss: 0.2 to 0.3 TBV

Postoperative ventilation: usual

Posterior spinal fusion. Since 1911, operative treatment of scoliosis has consisted of decortication of vertebral laminae and laying on of bone grafts taken from tibia or ilium. The additional use of internal metallic fixation produces greater correction and immediate stability.

For Harrington rod instrumentation the patient is anesthetized and then positioned prone on a supporting frame (Figs. 19-3 and 19-4). A long midline incision is made, followed by exposure of the affected vertebrae. The spinous processes are rongeured away, and the laminae are decorticated. Bone grafts are taken from ilium or tibia, and bleeding is controlled. The large metal Harrington rod is fixed in place on the concave side of the curve, with the aid of metallic hooks that are inserted under the laminae of the designated vertebrae, and then jacked apart, straightening the curve. In some patients a compression rod is placed on the convex side of the curve in addition to the distraction rod on the concave side (Fig. 19-5).

When the full force of the apparatus has been applied, it is now our custom to arouse the patient enough to demonstrate ability to move both feet, thus showing that the tension exerted has not been enough to injure the spinal cord (Sudhir and others, 1976). Anesthesia is restored, bone chips are laid along the site of fusion, bleeding is con-

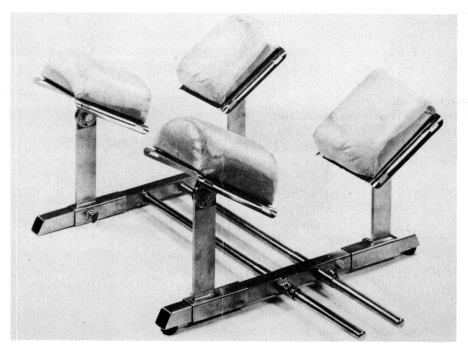

Fig. 19-3. Relton-Hall frame for posterior spinal fusion.

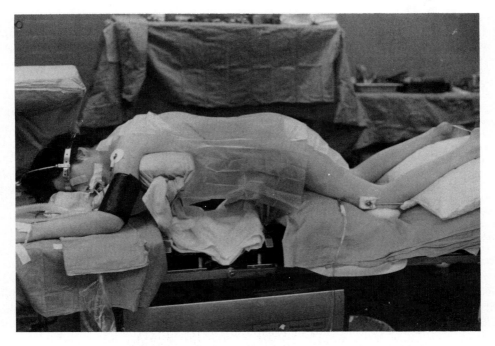

Fig. 19-4. Patient positioned on frame for Harrington rod posterior spinal fusion.

trolled, and the wound is closed. These patients do not ordinarily require postoperative ventilatory support. Consequently, at the end of the operation they are awakened and extubated in the operating room and then moved to a Stryker frame for transport to the recovery room.

The greatest problem during these operations is blood loss, which often is in the range of 0.4 to 0.6 times the total blood volume and sometimes considerably more (Jones and Gonski, 1967).

Anterior fusion with Dwyer cable fixation. The essential features of the Dwyer anterior fusion technic include lateral positioning of the patient on the operating table with the convexity of the spine uppermost (Fig. 19-6), thoracoabdominal incision, exposure and stripping of the involved vertebrae, and removal of the intervertebral disks and adjoining surfaces of the vertebral bodies. Large staples are then screwed to the vertebrae to be corrected by means of heavy screw eyes, through which a braided steel cable is

passed and then tightened, thereby bringing the vertebrae into line (Fig. 19-7).

Candidates for anterior fusion generally are more debilitated, often having serious underlying handicaps. Exceptions to this are healthy adolescents with low lumbar curves that are not adaptable to correction by Harrington rod. The operations require 5 to 8 hours, most of that time with an open chest, and are followed by several days of mechanical ventilation. The principal dangers are related to hypoxemia, ventilation, and trauma and are greatest when the lesions involve upper thoracic vertebrae.

Anesthetic management: posterior approach. Preparation of these patients requires careful examination, as outlined. Special care should be directed toward control of apprehension and preparation for blood replacement.

Severe deformity, multiple operations, and restricted ventilation often combine increased need of sedation with increased danger of depression. Chief reliance should be

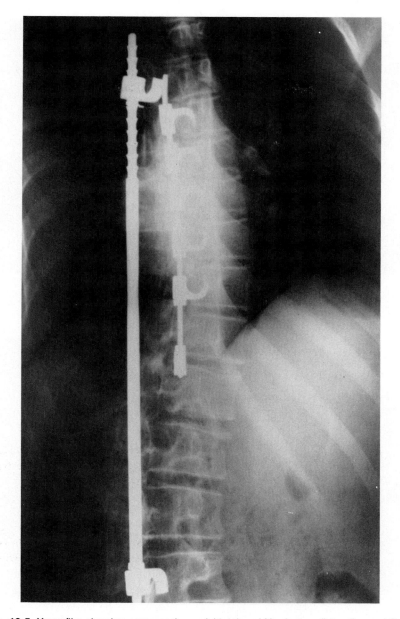

Fig. 19-5. X-ray film showing compression rod *(right)* and Harrington distraction rod *(left).*

placed on psychotherapy, where possible. Sedation may be used sparingly. Nondepressing agents such as hydroxyzine, in doses of 2 to 3 mg/kg, may be tried at 6- to 8-hour intervals, starting 24 hours before operation, to eliminate anxiety. Morphine and atropine may be used for premedication. Substitution of fentanyl for morphine during operation has been associated with reduced bleeding.

Blood is ordered to suit predicted needs. Normally, fresh whole blood (not more than 2 days old) is prepared the night before operation. For normal adolescents, we order 250 ml of whole blood per vertebra to be fused.

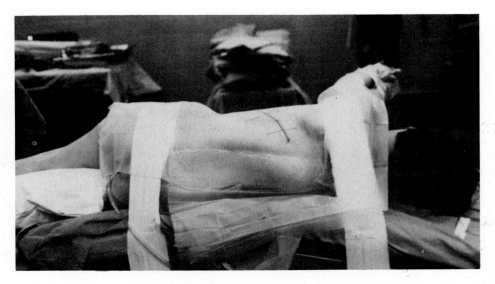

Fig. 19-6. Lateral position of patient for anterior (Dwyer) spinal fusion. Patient lies with convex curve uppermost. Site of incision is marked on skin.

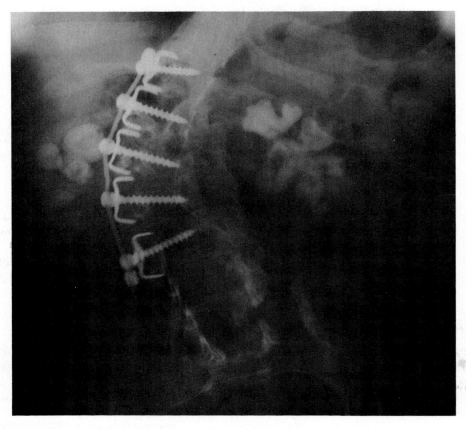

Fig. 19-7. X-ray film showing Dwyer screws and cable. Screws pierce the entire body of the vertebrae from side to side.

Three to six extra units may be ordered for patients expected to require more replacement. Among these would be patients known to have bleeding or coagulation defects, those who have had previous spinal fusion procedures, and especially those who have bled profusely during previous spinal fusions. Fresh-frozen plasma should always be available within 15 to 20 minutes, but platelets must be specially procured and should be ordered ahead of time, allowing several hours for preparation.

Placement of infusions. Two intravenous lines are established in all patients undergoing spinal fusion. A central venous line is essential for poor-risk patients but is not considered mandatory for healthy teenagers with idiopathic scoliosis. One or more of the intravenous lines may be started before the patient is brought into the operating room, and additional tranquilizer may be added as indicated. If the patient is not disturbed by the procedure, the central line may be inserted at this time. Otherwise, it is preferable to wait until the patient is asleep.

Veins on the dorsum of the hand or wrist are preferable for placement of simple infusions, using 16- or 18-gauge plastic cannulae. We prefer to avoid cannulation of the internal jugular veins for CVP monitoring. Antecubital veins often are satisfactory, but we have found cannulation of the external jugular vein in the neck to be safe, reliable, and practical when cannulation is accomplished with the aid of a J catheter guide, as described by Blitt and associates (1974).

Anesthetic induction is carried out with the patient on the transport stretcher rather than on the operating table. Thiopental is used for stronger patients, and repeated small doses of morphine or ketamine are used for more debilitated patients, followed by a muscle relaxant.

For endotracheal intubation, succinylcholine is chosen if not contraindicated by the presence of denervated musculature. When relaxation has been gained, the anesthesiologist sprays the airway with 4% lidocaine and then intubates using cuffed endotracheal tubes for children taking sizes larger than 5.0 mm ID. Orotracheal intubation is used unless the patient is expected to need mechanical ventilation following operation.

Should more relaxant be needed before a very weak patient is turned, a second dose of succinylcholine is given. *d*-Tubocurarine is avoided for fear of inducing further hypotension during change of position. Pancuronium maintains blood pressure but has been avoided because of resultant increase in blood loss.*

Any patient lying face down with tubes inserted in his nostrils runs a real risk of pressure ulceration of nasal cartilage, a remarkably disfiguring mark to bear. When possible, the oral route is chosen for all tubes. The endotracheal tube is fixed toward the middle of the mouth to prevent angulation and kinking, then the gastric suction tube and the esophageal stethoscope are placed, and finally the esophageal thermistor probe is placed, its stiffer body being more easily pushed through the other apparatus. To prevent overcrowding and pressure in the hypopharynx, an oral airway is not used. Instead a bite block made of 2 or 3 sponges rolled, taped, and moistened with saline solution is fixed between the teeth in one corner of the mouth. The endotracheal tube is secured with extra care, since the prone position often allows saliva to run down the tube and loosen the tape.

In poor-risk patients an arterial cannula may be inserted, and the ECG is attached prior to turning. In good-risk patients an arterial cannula is not inserted unless hypotensive methods are to be used, and the ECG is attached after turning. The bladder is catheterized in all patients undergoing spinal fusion.

After the eyes are taped shut and the blood pressure is rechecked, the patient is ready to be lifted from the stretcher, turned, and positioned on the operating table.

To prevent dislodgement of the endotracheal tube, we prefer to hyperoxygenate the child and then disconnect the endotracheal tube during actual turning.

---

*Metocurine is well suited to this use.

Turning these patients may induce cardiovascular stress and must be accomplished with care. The child is encumbered by wires and tubes and often has marginal vasomotor reserve. Four persons usually are required for atraumatic turning and positioning of the average scoliotic patient.

Criteria for optimal position of these patients have changed greatly. Anesthesiologists once insisted on supporting the chest and pelvis to favor ventilation at the expense of maximum exposure for the surgeon. Under controlled respiration, less bolstering is now required, and positioning is designed to combine maximal exposure with reduction of blood loss.

It has been demonstrated that blood normally returning via the inferior vena cava is diverted by abdominal pressure to an alternative route through a network of valveless venous plexuses surrounding the spine (Batson, 1940). Supporting the patient so as to minimize abdominal pressure now appears to be of high priority. Though some favor traditional pads and sandbags, special supporting frames have been developed. The frame designed by Relton and Hall (1967) (Fig. 19-3), which raises the body on 10-inch supports under the anterior chest and pelvis, allows the abdomen complete freedom without limiting ventilation. It also provides adequate support to allow the exposure and heavy operative manipulation required in such procedures.

Since the legs are not elevated by this device, the reduced circulating blood volume may either facilitate surgery or promote shock. In patients with limited reserve, elastic bandages may be indicated.

The head is supported on a soft foam-rubber cushion, and the face is turned and kept in view of the anesthesiologist to prevent injury or pressure. The arms are brought forward and supported with elbows flexed (Fig. 19-4). A second intravenous infusion is started in the dorsum of the hand or wrist of the arm not previously cannulated.

Maintenance. After the patient is stabilized, anesthesia is continued using *d*-tubocurarine or metocurine for relaxant, with fentanyl supplementation. Most anesthetic agents are permissible, except for droperidol, since its alpha-adrenergic blocking effect counteracts the epinephrine used for hemostasis (8 ml of 1:500,000 epinephrine in saline solution per kg injected along the area of incision).

Important considerations during maintenance include provision of adequate ventilation, cardiovascular stability, blood replacement, temperature control, and testing for spinal cord damage.

Ventilation. Ventilation is usually controlled by mechanical ventilator, which is set to provide 10 to 15 ml/kg/min. Since mechanical ventilation is subject to errors of malfunction, continuous monitoring of exchange is maintained by *esophageal stethoscope*, and arterial blood gases are measured at regular intervals to maintain ventilation and acid-base control. Arterial cannulation is employed in patients with impaired oxygenation of any type but often is avoided in healthy individuals undergoing uncomplicated procedures. In good-risk patients, venous sampling for pH gives satisfactory assessment of ventilation.

As an attempt to avoid increased venous pressure, a slight negative pressure (-2 cm H_2O) is used with expiration, chiefly to prevent the end-expiratory pressure of 2 to 5 cm H_2O that is often present in ventilators. Measurement of CVP by means of a catheter inserted in the antecubital or external jugular vein and extending to the superior vena cava is of assistance in evaluating the venous pressure above the diaphragm but is of little value in evaluating any congestion developing in the paravertebral sinuses.

Cardiac stability. Cardiac stability is maintained by monitoring heart rate and blood pressure, by avoiding light anesthesia, straining, depressing drugs, and sudden turning, and by preventing hypovolemic shock. ECG monitoring is routine but actually is of less value than stethoscope and blood pressure apparatus. For best guidance in poor-risk patients, the continuous tracing of arterial and venous pressures is recommended.

Blood replacement. Bleeding has been a

major problem during posterior spinal fusion, obstructing the surgeon's progress and requiring large amounts of replacement. As shown in Table 19-1, estimates of blood loss vary widely. It is essential to be aware of the many factors that contribute to blood loss (see list below) so that one will not make the mistake of relying on any single, potentially dangerous device to correct the entire problem.

MAJOR FACTORS IN THE ETIOLOGY OF BLOOD LOSS DURING POSTERIOR SPINAL FUSION

Surgical wound

Length of wound (determined by the number of vertebrae requiring fusion)

Lateral extent and degree of soft-tissue and bone dissection

Bone graft: site, size, and phase of operation during which graft is taken

Hemostatic technic

Duration of operation

Patient response

Local vasoconstrictive response and coagulation mechanisms

General response: arterial blood pressure, venous blood pressure

Anesthetic management

Bleeding increased by elevation of arterial pressure in presence of hypoxia, hypercarbia, inotropic or adrenergic drugs, morphine, and pancuronium

Bleeding increased by elevation of venous pressure in presence of straining, light anesthesia, anxiety, abdominal pressure, intrathoracic pressure, head-down position

Bleeding decreased by elimination of above and additional maneuvers to reduce arterial and venous pressure by induced hypotension, hypothermia

Table 19-1. Estimated blood losses during posterior spinal fusion

Author	Amount
Gartsman (Boston Children's)*	300-4500 ml, av. 2057 ml
Relton and Conn (Toronto)	200-3200 ml, av. 2230 ml
McNeill and associates (Chicago)	Normotensive, 2270 ml
	Hypotensive, 1380 ml
Harrington (Houston)	70-2300 ml, av. 900 ml

*These figures relate to 1963. Present losses are reduced by 50% by methods described in the text and elimination of intraoperative morphine and pancuronium.

Aspects to be considered in the management of bleeding include (1) factors that may contribute to operative blood loss during spinal fusion, (2) methods of estimating blood loss, (3) methods of replacing blood, and (4) concepts of reduction of blood loss.

The principal factors contributing to blood loss during spinal fusion are related to the extent of the operative wound, the surgeon's technic of hemostasis, the patient's local vasoconstrictive response and coagulation mechanism, and additional effects of anesthetic and ventilatory management. Avoidance of the causes of increased blood loss is the first goal, after which one can consider methods of reducing normal bleeding.

The surgical wound must be made. Since the length of the wound will depend on the number of vertebrae to be fused, this is predetermined by the degree of scoliosis in each case. The width to which the wound is extended varies with the surgical technic, however, as does the amount of decortication of vertebral bodies, the site from which the graft is taken, and the manner of its performance.

The handling of the wound is of some significance. Cautery serves as the most economical technic wherever possible. Attempts to control local bleeding by injection of large amounts of vasoconstrictive agents may be of use in developing the initial incision, and firm pressure-packing at sites of decortication of bone is definitely essential.

Easily the most important surgical factor in relation to blood loss is the duration of operation, as will be discussed later.

Patient features contributing to excess bleeding include abnormal vasoconstrictive responses, deficiency in clotting factors, neurofibromatosis, and recent ingestion of aspirin. Patients with history of previous spinal fusions often bleed profusely, though the cause is not clear. Indicated steps should be taken to correct coagulation defects well in advance of the operation. Elimination of aspirin 4 days before operation is believed to be adequate (Kevy, 1979).

Anesthetic management can increase or decrease bleeding by alteration of physiologic and pharmacologic responses. Before operation, anxiety will increase stress and arterial pressure but can be reduced by proper reassurance and sedation. A difficult induction with excitement, resistance, coughing, or straining, followed by light, uneven anesthetic level, can elevate both arterial and venous pressure. During maintenance, further elevation of arterial pressure may be caused by hypoxia or hypercarbia, while elevation of venous pressure may be caused by airway resistance or pressure on the abdomen, unless care is taken to avoid such problems.

Anesthetic drugs that may increase bleeding by stimulation of heart rate, cardiac output, and arterial pressure include ketamine, pancuronium, and atropine, and even morphine may contribute to the hypertensive effect. Ketamine and pancuronium are easily omitted. The preoperative use of atropine will be retained by many, but its action is brief, and neither it nor preoperative morphine is believed to have enough inotropic effect to cause trouble. Morphine is no longer used during spinal fusions at our hospital.

One more important cause of increased bleeding may be hypervolemia due to excessive administration of fluid or blood.

In our work, we respect these considerations and, in cooperation with the surgeons, carry out the following specially directed maneuvers: (1) the patient is positioned on the Relton-Hall frame to prevent venous stasis and increased paravertebral bleeding, (2) the surgeon injects 1:500,000 epinephrine solution, 8 ml/kg, into and around the site of the intended incision, (3) a negative pressure (-2 cm H_2O) is used at the end of expiration, and (4) a loss of at least 10% of the patient's blood volume is allowed before replacement is started, if the patient's condition justifies it (see below for special technics).

We consider these maneuvers rather conservative, but with the help of an excellent blood bank, this method has been effective in the accomplishment of 92 anterior spinal fusions and 400 posterior fusions in the past 5 years.

ESTIMATION OF BLOOD LOSS. In extensive procedures, especially when one is dealing with increased-risk patients, the danger of overreplacement is as great as that of underreplacement, and real effort should be made to evaluate both the total amount of blood that is lost and the rate at which the loss is occurring.

For the estimation of blood losses, one can use clinical signs, measure the actual blood by direct technics, or calculate the loss by laboratory determination of altered blood constituents. Clinical signs should always be observed and respected but are more difficult to follow when patients are prone and mostly covered.

Measurement of blood loss seldom approaches accuracy but is definitely worthwhile during spinal fusion. Use of dry sponges gives greater credibility to gravimetric measurement, and this, added to blood in the suction bottle, should produce a total within 20% to 25% of the actual loss. Since losses may range from 10% to 150% of total volume, an estimate within 25% can be of much assistance.

In the management of patients with near-normal blood pressure, we have been able to rely on clinical signs and the direct measurement of blood loss, adding an additional 25% to the total measured loss in our final replacement. When signs and measurement do not agree, we rely on signs and take additional measurements.

When one is dealing with patients under induced hypotension, hemodilution, or other specialized methods, the serial determination of hematocrit, red cell mass, and blood volume is advised. Although hematocrit determinations on peripheral blood are unreliable, those taken by arterial or central venous sampling provide more accurate guidance.

METHOD OF BLOOD REPLACEMENT. Procedures in replacement of blood are based on common goals of patient safety, economy of blood, and facilitation of surgery but vary in respect to materials used and the amount and timing of replacement. Methods that may be used include the following:

1. Immediate administration of whole blood to replace or stay ahead of blood losses.

2. Allowance of 10% loss of estimated blood volume (EBV), with replacement of subsequent loss with whole blood.
3. Similar methods of replacement using large quantities of crystalloid, gradually producing hemodilution.
4. Withdrawal of 20% to 30% of blood volume at the start, and replacement with a 3:1 ratio of Ringer's lactate solution for initial establishment of hemodilution, blood to be replaced toward the end of the procedure with simultaneous diuresis of fluid excess.

We prefer the second method. A tally of the blood loss is recorded by the circulating nurse on a wall board. Good-risk patients are maintained with a deficit of approximately 500 ml of blood. An infusion of 5% dextrose in 0.25% saline solution is run at 4 to 6 ml/kg/hr throughout the procedure.

Blood loss is appreciable as the muscles are stripped from the vertebrae but becomes maximal during decortication of the vertebrae and raising of the iliac bone graft. Blood is administered to keep the systolic pressure above 80 mm Hg. Speed in performance of this part of the operation is especially helpful in reducing blood loss.

As shown in Table 19-2, a study of 26 procedures performed in our hospital showed that the average patient lost 42% of total blood volume during posterior spinal fusion. "Massive blood loss" usually denotes any amount in excess of 30% of EBV and, if not replaced, may be lethal, especially if it occurs rapidly. The more gradual loss and simultaneous replacement that occur with spinal fusion require concerned attention, but patients tolerate considerably greater loss without showing signs of shock or significant stress.

Our practice is to use whole blood as replacement and to have much of it freshly drawn (within 4 hours) when dealing with patients expected to have increased bleeding. All blood is warmed by electric heating devices, and blood that is more than 3 days old is passed through a micropore filter. Other fluids are taken from warmed storage cabinets.

With increasing amounts of blood loss,

Table 19-2. Comparable data on blood loss during posterior and anterior spinal fusion (normotensive)

	Posterior fusion	Anterior fusion
Number	20	6
Average blood loss (%TBV)	42.4	37
Average duration (hr)	4.36	6.5
Loss/hour (%TBV)	9.5	5.8

Data compiled by Gartsman, G., The Children's Hospital Medical Center, Boston, 1963.

several procedures are followed. Extra blood that is used is drawn fresh, if possible, and usually is not more than 48 hours old when infused. Fresh-frozen plasma is added after each fourth unit of fresh blood or after each third unit of older blood. Calcium is used as indicated by measurement of ionized calcium, or if measurements are not made, 500 mg of $CaCl_2$ is administered with every two units of blood.

If blood loss exceeds 50% of EBV, a coagulogram is performed to determine template bleeding time, PT, and PTT. If platelets number less than $125,000/mm^3$, an infusion of 250 ml is ordered. Similarly, if oozing appears to be excessive, blood is tested for fibrinolysins. Positive findings here are also considered an indication for platelet infusion. Transfusion usually should be continued following operation to replace postoperative bleeding and should total 10% to 25% more than measured loss, occasionally much more.

Concepts of reduction of blood loss. Conservative methods of reducing blood loss obviously include all practical means of avoiding the causes of blood loss, such as:

1. Reduction of the size of the wound
2. Reduction of the amount of tissue and bone dissection
3. Improved hemostasis
4. Avoidance of light or unstable anesthesia
5. Avoidance of iatrogenic elevation of arterial or venous blood pressure
6. Preoperative correction of bleeding and coagulation defects

7. Use of whole blood, platelets, and calcium as needed
8. Delayed replacement of lost blood
9. Reduction of operating time

In our experience, the factor that most closely relates to blood loss has been duration of operation. It has been shown that after 4 hours, the rate of blood loss accelerates significantly (Gartsman, 1963). While the exact reason for this is not clear, it is evident that the most effective way to reduce blood loss is to reduce the duration of operation. Actually, several elements contribute to this, especially the extent of the operation. A two-vertebrae lumbar fusion cannot be compared with a 12-vertebrae thoracolumbar fusion. However, it has been evident that the same type of fusion that requires 6 hours for an inexperienced surgeon can be done by some highly skilled surgeons in half the time, with one-quarter the blood loss.

HEMODILUTION, HYPOTENSION, AND HYPOTHERMIA. More aggressive methods of blood loss reduction have included hemodilution, hypotension, and hypothermia, all of which may be applied in different combinations and to variable degrees. The extent to which these must be carried to produce appreciable effect is not predictable, nor is the level at which the hazards become significant.

Induced hypotension using sodium nitroprusside or trimethaphan, with supplementary halothane, has been described in Chapter 14. Early enthusiasm for this technic was dulled by unexpected deaths that alerted users to the importance of dose-related toxicity and the individual differences in tolerance to sodium nitroprusside. This technic now is employed for spinal fusion in many areas. Reduction of mean arterial pressure to 40 mm Hg with hemodilution to a hematocrit of 10% to 12% has been used successfully in a limited number of cases (Furman, 1977). More often the induced changes approximate 25%, 30%, or 40% reduction of mean arterial pressure to 60 to 80 mm Hg.

We have used light halothane anesthesia to control intraoperative hypertension, preferably maintaining systolic pressure at or below 100 mm Hg. We regard the optimal systolic pressure for combined patient safety and economy of blood to be between 80 and 100 mm Hg.

The use of hemodilution, accomplished without the use of potentially hazardous drugs, appears less formidable than hypotension. With patients at normal body temperature, it is believed reasonable to dilute the blood to a hematocrit of 25%, and this may be carried considerably further with induction of hypothermia. Some consider it reasonable to lower the hematocrit 1% with each 1° C reduction of body temperature, aiming at a temperature of 25° to 27° C and a hematocrit of 20% to 25%. While one avoids the danger of nitroprusside toxicity and reduced cardiac output inherent in induced hypotension, the use of invasive monitors represents a hazard not often present in fusions performed at normal body temperatures. As emphasized by Laver and Bland (1975), removal of blood at the beginning of the hemodilution process probably is less disturbing than removal of excess fluid at the end of operation, with attendant danger of upsetting fluid balance and electrolyte concentrations.

In summary, it appears that there is reason for the considerable differences in the amount of blood lost during spinal fusion and in the technics employed to facilitate surgery and conserve blood. The rapid, skilled surgeon, cutting a few corners, needs no alteration of physiology. Those with less experience and those using more extensive exposure of tissue and bone, especially when dealing with complicated cases, will encounter increased bleeding. If adequate stores of blood are available and problems of replacement are minimal, it probably will be safer to refrain from use of hypotension or hemodilution. If bleeding is excessive and the quantity and/or quality of replacement blood is not adequate, and if there are experts in the field of induced hypotension or hemodilution available, these technics would appear to have some justification.

Before using these technics, however, one should make sure that all suitable precautions are observed and that indications are clearly evident. Alteration of any body function involving oxygen transport in order to facilitate surgery or reduce blood replacement represents a direct insult to the patient to produce an indirect benefit. While tolerated by robust young patients, such methods would reduce the margin of safety in a paralytic child or in any patient who encounters the severe stress of hypoxia, hemorrhage, or additional hypotension.

It certainly must be borne in mind that the success of spinal fusion is not measured by either the amount of blood replacement or the speed of the surgeon but by the survival of the patient and the success of the operation. In posterior spinal fusion, the principal measure of success lies in the minimal incidence of pseudarthrosis. Our opinions are based on experience, during which there have been no deaths related to blood loss and the incidence of pseudarthrosis has been among the lowest in the country.

Problems in anesthetic management. Air conditioning and the infusion of quantities of cold blood may reduce the patient's temperature to 34° or 35° C. This can be prevented by inserting a warming blanket into the space between the patient's abdomen and the supporting frame and by warming blood, supplemental fluids, and the operating room. Body temperature is monitored by esophageal, rectal, or axillary probe.

Marked hyperthermia has also been observed during and immediately after spinal fusion. In two instances, the children were known to have been operated on in body casts. Those occurring at termination were unexplained, and although the temperature of one reached 42° C, all receded within a few hours in response to conservative treatment.

The real danger of fat embolism has been attested to by Weisz and Barzilai (1973), who reported on five children, of whom two had Harrington rod instrumentation and a third had the Dwyer procedure. The best diagnostic clue was found to be reduction of Pa_{O_2} below 75 mm Hg.

Intraoperative testing for spinal cord function. The increased amount of force that can be applied by Harrington instrumentation introduces the danger of damaging the spinal cord. Several approaches have been attempted in order to determine whether excessive force has been applied so that it may be adjusted at once, thereby saving considerable time and preventing what might be serious injury to the spinal cord.

The method used in our institution has been reported by Sudhir and associates (1976) and consists of keeping the patient lightly anesthetized with nitrous oxide, fentanyl, and relaxant until the surgeon has fixed the rod in place. The anesthesiologist then turns off the nitrous oxide and within 3 minutes the patient usually awakens sufficiently to obey commands to move hands and feet. If the hands are moved but not the feet, the force on the rod is reduced until hands and feet are equally mobile. The patient is put back to sleep with diazepam and thiopental, with relaxant added as needed. To date this has been carried out in over 250 cases. On follow-up, only one patient reported any distressing effect, and most did not remember being awakened. Temporary paralysis was corrected in four patients who otherwise might have had permanent cord injury.

Some who have used this method have been bothered by the sudden awakening of the patients, with inadvertent tracheal extubation or displacement of the Harrington rods. By measuring transmission of nervous impulses from head to foot or spine to foot, one can test function without awakening the patient. This computerized measurement of somatosensory evoked potential, as described by Engler and associates (1978), involves a more sophisticated noninvasive technic and has been used successfully in several hundred patients.

At the end of the operation, most patients can tolerate reversal of muscle relaxants and tracheal extubation. They are moved to Stryker frames and transported to the recovery room, where blood and electrolyte solutions are continued, as previously noted.

Suitable analgesic medication is ordered in small, frequent intravenous dosage, oxygen is administered by plastic mask, and blood gases are checked. In addition, patients are encouraged to breathe deeply and cough. After 5 or 6 hours, they are transferred to the orthopedic special care room.

During recovery from spinal fusion, two complications that one should watch for are excessive bleeding and pneumothorax. A third complication that has occurred several times is early postoperative hyperpyrexia (to 103° and 105° F), which has responded to symptomatic treatment but has not been explained by blood culture, chest film, fat stain, urine culture and analysis, or other tests and has receded over 48 or 72 hours without further incident.

Anesthetic management: anterior (Dwyer) approach. There are two distinctly different types of patients requiring anterior fusion, and it is important for one to make this distinction before starting anesthesia. The majority of patients are significantly handicapped by severe angulation and ventilatory restriction. However, there are some, as previously mentioned, who are perfectly healthy and in whom the indication for anterior fusion is a low lumbar curve that is not amenable to correction by Harrington rods. Several of the special precautionary measures essential for the weaker patients will be unnecessary with this group.

Prior to anterior fusion, patients are lightly medicated and brought to the waiting area, where an infusion is started. In the operating room, they are placed directly on the operating table, and blood pressure apparatus, stethoscope, and ECG are fixed in place. Anesthesia is induced with thiopental (or successive doses of morphine in maximum-risk patients).

With the exception of the healthy type of patients previously mentioned, most of those having anterior fusion will require postoperative ventilatory assistance; consequently, these patients are intubated by nasal route.

A second infusion is established for CVP measurement, an arterial cannula is placed, and a urethral catheter is inserted. The patient is then positioned on his side, with the convex curvature uppermost.

Maintenance anesthesia for prolonged procedures is accomplished by intravenous combinations using nitrous oxide, thiopental, morphine, and relaxants. A mechanical ventilator (without negative phase) is used intraoperatively. Since no epinephrine solution is injected prior to incision, the restrictions on use of droperidol and halothane for posterior fusion do not apply here.

Operation begins with a wide thoracoabdominal incision and development of entry by taking down half of the diaphragm. With each major physiologic change, one should look for disturbance of oxygenation and blood pressure and correct them promptly by manipulation of ventilatory or fluid input.

Among several hazards of this operation, those of hypoxemia and traumatic shock are most evident. The exposed lung is partially collapsed for 5 or 6 hours and must be reinflated at frequent intervals. Reduced arterial oxygenation often suggests more frequent expansion than would have been expected. The problems of blood replacement are much less than during posterior fusion, since there is neither decortication nor bone graft. However, following the preparation of vertebral bodies and placement of staples, screws, and cable, the forceful compression, often aided by heavy manual pressure on the protruding vertebrae, can be distinctly upsetting and must be undertaken only when the child is well stabilized.

Closure of the chest and abdomen, though requiring considerable time, should not present critical problems. The chest is drained as in any thoracotomy.

Following anterior fusion, respiration is usually supported by mechanical ventilator. Consequently, the endotracheal tube is left in place and the relaxants are not reversed.

Immediately following operation, x-ray films are obtained to confirm the position of the endotracheal tube and adequate expansion of both lungs. The duration of mechanical assistance varies considerably and may be required for a week or more. The patient's survival often is in question and dependent on the combined efforts of expert nurses, respiratory therapists, and physicians, working together in an area provided with all the essentials of an intensive therapy unit. Arterial blood gas determinations are often necessary at 15- to 30-minute intervals during the early stages of recovery, and cardiorespiratory function must be controlled with as much finesse as that of any patient who has undergone open-heart surgery.

During this phase, the dangers of pneumonia and atelectasis are paramount, especially in those with previously damaged lungs, and premature extubation or discontinuation of ventilatory support must be avoided. The hazard of taking these steps at times when a full complement of skilled personnel is not on hand is one too frequently disregarded.

Additional lesions of concern to pediatric anesthesiologists

Congenital clubfoot. This is one of the more common orthopedic problems of young children. It may involve a child who is otherwise normal, but it also is frequently found in children with cerebral palsy, myelomeningocele, or other deformities. Repeated anesthetic experience for cast change and manipulation of foot is upsetting, and the postoperative pain caused by manipulation and cast often is troublesome.

Torticollis. Commonly termed "wry neck," torticollis is caused by contracture of the sternocleidomastoid muscle, which tilts the head forward and to one side, and may present some difficulty in induction and tracheal intubation.

Klippel-Feil syndrome. Here congenital fusion of two or more cervical vertebrae results in shortening and widening of the neck and limitation of its mobility. Surgical treatment may include Z-plasty to reduce the wide skin folds, with muscular and fascial release to improve mobility. It may be associated with Sprengel's deformity. Whether it occurs by itself or is complicated by other problems, the lesion makes airway management a real challenge (Tachdjian, 1972).

Sprengel's deformity. This is characterized by upward displacement of one or both scapulae, with fixation to cervical vertebrae. Sprengel's deformity results in elevation of the affected shoulder, with limitation of arm-raising above the horizontal. The airway is unaffected, but prone positioning for release of scapulae may be difficult (Greville and Coventry, 1956).

Osteomyelitis. Now only occasionally seen, osteomyelitis most often occurs as a complication of compound fracture, decubitus ulcer, or similar problem involving poor wound healing or chronic illness. Anemia, chronic illness, and sepsis increase the risk factor.

Septic arthritis. Any joint may become involved, but the septic hip of the infant, previously described, is of most concern to the anesthesiologist.

Rheumatoid arthritis. Here chronic illness, limitation of joint mobility, and prolonged therapy with steroids and aspirin combine to endanger the patient. Additional steroid should be given during the operative period, and aspirin should be discontinued a minimum of 4 to 7 days prior to surgery if the patient can do without it (Davies and Steward, 1977; Kevy, 1979).

Arachnodactyly (Marfan's disease). This is an inherited dominant trait consisting of abnormally long extremities and digits, with recurrent joint dislocations, combined with kyphosis, pectus excavatus, subluxation of the optic lenses, and severe congenital cardiac defects (Woolley and others, 1967). Aortic insufficiency and danger of aortic dissection make maintenance of stable blood pressure mandatory.

Arthrogryposis multiplex. This consists of fixed joints of limbs and vertebrae with reduced musculature, causing severe distortion and crippling. The neuropathic form shows decreased anterior horn cells and reduced size of spinal cord and nerve roots. The myopathic form shows fibrous and fatty degeneration of muscles, with normal nervous components. Surgery may be aimed at improving mobility of any part of the head, body, or limbs. Anesthesia is complicated by fixation of jaw, neck, or limbs plus moderate incidence of congenital cardiac defects (Friedlander and others, 1968; Tachdjian, 1972).

Achondroplasia (chondrodystrophia fetalis). Characterized by lack of cartilage production, this is the most common type of dwarfism. While body structures show obvious disproportion and create anatomic problems for the anesthesiologist, organic function and intelligence usually are unaffected.

Legg-Perthes disease. This is softening of the head of the femur. It occurs in children in the active growing period and is caused by inadequate blood supply. Treatment is by nailing or immobilization for 6 to 8 weeks.

Leg length discrepancy. In this, unequal growth leaves one leg longer than the other. Operation surprises the uninitiated, because the *good* leg is the one that is corrected. Operation consists of epiphyseal arrest.

Morquio-Ullrich syndrome. Severe dwarfing is caused by atlanto-occipital subluxation and acute kyphoscoliosis, leading to increasing cardiac and pulmonary dysfunction early in life (mucopolysaccharidosis IV) (Gilbertson and Boulton, 1967; Birkinshaw, 1975).

Osteogenesis imperfecta. Due to impaired osteoblastic activity, the bones of children with this disease break easily and frequently, with such marked deformity of head and limbs that they are often mistaken for patients with Morquio's syndrome. Great care must be observed in positioning them, for an innocent attempt to extend a misshapen arm or leg could easily cause additional fractures. Stehling (1978) has warned of platelet dysfunction affecting the operative course of these patients and the frequent occurrence of moderate degrees of hyperthermia, presumably related to the generalized condition of hypermetabolism.

Streeter's dysplasia. This growth disturbance is caused by formation of a tight fibrous band encircling a limb or digit, with circulatory disturbance and marked deformity beyond the band (Fig. 19-1). There are no associated defects or anesthetic problems (McKusick, 1972).

Amyotonia congenita. This is a nonspecific term now including several "floppy baby" syndromes that may be caused by neurologic or myopathic diseases, including cerebral palsy, glycogen storage disease, transverse myelitis, and peripheral neuropathies (Walton, 1964; Byers and Banker, 1961; Tachdjian, 1972). Surgery usually is confined to muscle biopsy for diagnosis.

Werdnig-Hoffmann disease. This is a specific cause of the flaccid infant that is due to lesions of the anterior horn cells. Infants have difficulty swallowing; hence, aspiration is common, and the airway must be carefully protected during and after anesthesia. Response to relaxants is unpredictable. Light, controlled anesthesia is indicated (Cobham and Davis, 1964; Jones and Pelton, 1976).

Poliomyelitis. Until 1955, poliomyelitis was the most common orthopedic surgical lesion, but it has since become a rarity in this country, occasionally found as residual weakness from long-standing paralysis. It is caused by an anterior horn cell defect.

Myotonia congenita (Thomsen's disease). This congenital, nonprogressive, intermittent type of myotonia (cause unknown) improves with activity. Muscle hypertrophy occurs with growth of the child. Response to stimulation and to depolarizing drugs is prolonged tonicity. Succinylcholine should be avoided* (Ellis, 1974).

Myotonic dystrophy. This is a progressive form of myotonia involving muscles of the face, tongue, and upper limbs particularly. Myotonic spasm initiated by activity and succinylcholine is not relieved by nondepolarizing agents. Muscles gradually atrophy (Ravin and others, 1975).

Progressive muscular dystrophy. Several forms of this syndrome have the same basic pattern of progressive atrophy and weakness of muscles, varying in the distribution of the muscles and rate of progression, but none involve myotonia (Wislicki, 1962; Cobham and Davis, 1964; Walton, 1964). Avoid relaxants and watch for poor respiratory function and aspiration.

Charcot-Marie-Tooth syndrome. This is atrophy of the peroneal muscle due to de-

---

*NOTE: Although the relationship is uncertain, there is probably some increased risk of malignant hyperthermia in any patient with a neuromuscular disease.

generation of the peroneal nerve. Operation is performed for transfer of muscles to do the work of the peroneal muscle. There are no related organic defects or anesthetic problems (Tachdjian, 1972).

Cerebral palsy. Children with spastic deformities frequently require repeated procedures to increase their mobility. Many of these children have been so incapacitated that they have been unable to move about, and their tolerance for anesthesia will be considerably reduced. The fact that their spasticity will call for deeper planes of anesthesia to accomplish relaxation accentuates this hazard.

It is particularly important to remember that cerebral palsy does not always affect the mind, and some of the most unfortunate patients are those who have very little ability to communicate but are completely perceptive. In attending any patient with cerebral palsy, at the outset one should make sure of both the level of the child's intelligence and the degree of his anxiety.

Neurofibromatosis (Von Recklinghausen's disease). This is a relatively common (1/3000) familial disease in which fibromatous nodules arise from nerve sheaths in all parts of the skeleton, soft tissues, and skin, causing pressure and physiologic changes. They often invade the head, airway, lungs, brain, and spine and cause scoliosis in nearly 20% of cases. Those coming to operation present increased risk due to additional presence of tumors in other parts of the body as well as pressure and destruction of the spinal cord. All should have myelogram prior to fusion. Neurofibromatosis occasionally occurs in association with pheochromocytoma (Chaglassian and others, 1976). Due to unknown cause, blood loss has been excessive in patients with neurofibromatosis.

Cysts and tumors of the bone. Bone cysts usually are benign, but when they occupy a large area of bone there may be extensive blood loss involved in curetting the cyst and filling it with bone graft.

More radical surgery is now being attempted in children with malignant bone tumors and may involve shoulder or hind-quarter amputation or replacement of the femur or the knee joint and associated malignant tumor with metallic prostheses (Watts, 1979).

The danger of operating on patients who have received doxorubicin (Adriamycin) was brought to our attention by an associated fatality. Doxorubicin is a popular antineoplastic agent known to have cardiotoxic effect (Rinehart and others, 1974). An accumulated dose of more than 300 mg/m² puts the patient at increased risk. The drug is generally stopped at or before a total dose of 450 mg/m² for fear of development of cardiac enlargement and congestive failure. The toxic effects are present for at least 6 months after discontinuation of the drug. It is a set rule in our institution that any patient coming to surgery after having more than 300 mg of doxorubicin per m² should have cardiac evaluation and echocardiogram within 2 weeks of anesthesia. Halogenated drugs are usually avoided in such patients.

Amputation is definitely one of the most shattering tragedies faced by a child and his parents. In addition to guidance by a skilled psychiatrist, treatment should include particular care by the anesthesiologist. Additional sedation the day before, during, and after operation, as well as much personal attention, frequently is needed.

Reflex sympathetic dystrophy, or causalgia. The syndrome of reflex sympathetic dystrophy, or causalgia, has been seen very infrequently in children in the past, but the increasing emphasis on organized sports for younger children appears to be associated with a marked increase in this problem. As described by Fermaglich (1977), the symptoms in children are similar to those in adults and consist of continuous pain, extreme sensitivity to light touch, edema, and discoloration in either upper or lower extremity, usually starting with mild or moderate trauma.

Eight cases in our recent experience have aroused our appreciation of this syndrome. Ranging in age from 9 to 18 years of age, seven were girls. The one boy was 17 years old. All patients associated their problem with a relatively mild injury—one to overuse of her fifth finger in playing the saxophone, several to turning an ankle. None involved fractures or immobilization in casts, as might be expected.

Symptomatology was similar in nature but different in degree. All had hyperalgesia; in several cases it was extreme and probably related to their personal pain threshold or parental indulgence, but definitely marked. The degree of edema and discoloration varied considerably, some showing no visible evidence of either but several having obvious, stocking-type swelling and erythema. The thin, bluish shiny skin was much less noticeable than in older patients.

Casten and Betcher (1955), Bonica (1973), Carron and McCue (1972), and others stress the importance of early, continuous treatment for these patients, but unfortunately an injury of this type seldom appears serious at the outset, and patients rarely are seen until several weeks after the original injury.

There often seems to be definite emotional or psychologic involvement in these cases, and one should start with a very thorough history of the trauma, the surrounding events, and the pressures and family background of the situation. The 17-year-old basketball player appeared to have been the object of maternal pressure to achieve. One young girl, a brilliant 9-year-old with excruciating pain following a sprained ankle, was believed to have become "sensitized" in part by the fact that her mother was partially crippled. It is important to look for such possibilities but to refrain from blaming them for the entire problem and attempt to treat them along with the anatomic injuries.

Early treatment for sprains and strains includes immediate application of cold, subsequent heat therapy, and immobilization, with recourse to steroids, if indicated. These have usually been tried by the time the anesthesiologist is consulted. At this point, sympathetic block is requested. In our experience, three patients with hand and forearm dystrophies responded quickly and completely to stellate blocks—two patients requiring two blocks and one requiring three—given preferably 48 hours apart in order to

allow time for soreness to wear off before repeating.

All five of the patients with lower limb dystrophies presented far greater difficulties. To minimize the duration and discomfort involved in the procedure of lumbar sympathetic block, low spinal anesthesia was performed on three as initial treatment and was adequate in one. In the remaining four patients, we had to perform repeated epidural blocks, using 12 to 24-hour continuous epidural blocks in three and finally resorting to acupuncture and hypnotism in two before definite improvement was obvious. Although these patients are brought to the anesthesiologist with a general attitude of waiting and watching, our experience has been similar to that of others in finding that prompt therapy is important and that in the use of blocks, one should establish an effective block and maintain it until symptoms begin to show definite response. Complete cure may require weeks or months, but the patients may be discharged as soon as they begin to show definite improvement. Their return to normal surroundings and activities is believed to be an important stimulus to recovery.

BIBLIOGRAPHY

Batson, O. V.: The function of the vertebral veins and their role in the spread of metastases, Ann. Surg. 112: 129, 1940.

Bergofsky, E. H., Turino, G. M., and Fishman, A. P.: Cardiac failure in kyphoscoliosis, Medicine 38:263, 1959.

Berman, A. T., Prince, H. L., and Han, J. F.: The cardiovascular effects of methylmethacrylate in dogs, Clin. Orthop. 11:265, 1974.

Birkinshaw, K. J.: Anaesthesia in a patient with an unstable neck; Morquio's syndrome, Anaesthesia 30:46, 1975.

Blitt, C. D., Wright, W. A., Petty, W. C., and others: Central venous catheterization via the external jugular vein; a technique employing the J-wire, J.A.M.A. 229:817, 1974.

Bonica, J. J.: Causalgia and other reflex sympathetic dystrophies, Postgrad. Med. 53:143, 1973.

Byers, R. K., and Banker, B. Q.: Infantile muscular atrophy, Arch. Neurol. 5:140, 1961.

Carney, F. M. T., and Van Dyke, R.: Halothane hepatitis; a critical review, Anesth. Analg. (Cleve.) 51:135, 1972.

Carron, H., and McCue, F.: Reflex sympathetic dystrophy in a ten year old, South. Med. J. **65:**631, 1972.

Casten, D. F., and Betcher, A. M.: Reflex sympathetic dystrophies; criteria for diagnosis and management, Anesthesiology **16:**994, 1955.

Chaglassian, J. H., Riseborough, E. J., and Hall, J. E.: Neurofibromatosis; natural history and results of treatment of thirty-seven cases, J. Bone Joint Surg. (Am.) **58:**695, 1976.

Cobham, I. G., and Davis, H. S.: Anesthesia for muscular dystrophy patients, Anesth. Analg. (Cleve.) **43:** 22, 1964.

Cohen, C. A., and Smith, N. T.: The intraoperative hazard of acrylic bone cement; report of a case, Anesthesiology **35:**547, 1971.

Cooke, R. E., editor: The biologic basis of pediatric practice, New York, 1968, McGraw-Hill Book Co.

Davidson, C. S., Babior, B., and Popper, H.: Concerning hepatotoxicity of halothane, N. Engl. J. Med. **275:**1497, 1966.

Davies, D. W., and Steward, D. J.: Unexpected excessive bleeding during operation; role of acetylsalicylic acid, Can. Anaesth. Soc. J. **24:**452, 1977.

Denton, M. V. H., and O'Donoghue, D. M. A.: Anaesthesia and the scoliotic patient, Anaesthesia **10:**366, 1955.

Dollery, C. T., Billiam, P. M. S., Hugh-Jones, P., and Zorab, P. A.: Regional lung function in kyphoscoliosis, Thorax **20:**175, 1965.

Dwyer, A. F., Newton, N. C., and Sherwood, A. A.: An anterior approach to scoliosis, Clin. Orthop. **62:**192, 1969.

Ellis, F. R.: Neuromuscular disease and anaesthesia, Br. J. Anaesth. **46:**603, 1974.

Engler, G. L., Spielholz, N. I., Bernhard, W. N., and others: Somatosensory evoked potentials during Harrington instrumentation for scoliosis, J. Bone Joint Surg. (Am.) **60:**528, 1978.

Fahmy, N. R., and Laver, M. B.: Pulmonary vascular effects of bone cement during total hip replacement in man, paper presented at annual meeting of American Society of Anesthesiologists, San Francisco, October, 1976.

Ferguson, A. B.: Orthopedic surgery in infancy and childhood, ed. 1, Baltimore, 1957, The Williams & Wilkins Co.

Fermaglich, D. R.: Reflex sympathetic dystrophy in children, Pediatrics **60:**881, 1977.

Flewellen, E. H., and Jarem, B.: Pneumatic tourniquets, Anesthesiol. Rev. **5:**31, 1978.

Fogan, L., and Munsat, T. L.: Spinocerebellar degenerative diseases. In Hardy, J. H., editor: Spinal deformity in neurological and muscular disorders, St. Louis, 1974, The C. V. Mosby Co.

Foldes, F. F., Kepes, E. T., Kronfeld, P. P., and Shiffman, H. P.: A rational approach to neuroleptanesthesia, Anesth. Analg. (Cleve.) **45:**642, 1966.

Frankel, L. S., Damme, C. J., and Van Eys, J.: Childhood cancer and the Jehovah's Witness faith, Pediatrics, **60:**916, 1977.

Friedlander, H. L., Westin, G. W., and Wood, W. L.: Arthrogryposis multiplex congenita, J. Bone Joint Surg. (Am.) **50:**89, 1968.

Furman, E. B.: Proceedings of World Congress of Anesthesiology, Japan, September 1973.

Furman, E. B.: Anesthetic management and blood conservation during scoliosis surgery, paper presented before American Academy of Pediatrics, New Orleans, April 17, 1977.

Gartsman, G.: Unpublished data, 1963.

Gilbertson, A. A., and Boulton, I. B.: Anaesthesia in difficult situations; influence of disease on pre-op preparation and choice of anaesthetic, Anaesthesia **22:**607, 1967.

Gilchrist, G. S.: Preoperative hematologic evaluation and management. In Gans, S. J., editor: Surgical pediatrics, New York, 1973, Grune & Stratton, Inc.

Gillies, I. D. S.: Anaemia and anaesthesia; a review, Br. J. Anaesth. **46:**549, 1974.

Greville, N. R., and Coventry, M. G.: Congenital high scapula (Sprengel's) deformity, Mayo Clin. Proc. **31:** 465, 1956.

Hall, J. E.: The anterior approach to spinal deformities, Orthop. Clin. North Am. **3:**81, 1972.

Hardy, J. H., editor: Spinal deformity in neurological and muscular disorders, St. Louis, 1974, The C. V. Mosby Co.

Harrington, P. R.: Treatment of scoliosis; correction and internal fixation by spinal instrumentation, J. Bone Joint Surg. (Am.) **44:**591, 1962.

Jones, A. E. P., and Pelton, D. A.: An index of syndromes and their anaesthetic implications, Can. Anaesth. Soc. J. **23:**207, 1976.

Jones, C. S., and Gonski, A.: Reduction of blood loss during spinal surgery, Med. J. Aust. **2:**382, 1967.

Katz, J., and Kadis, L. B.: Anesthesia and uncommon diseases; pathophysiologic and clinical correlations, Philadelphia, 1973, W. B. Saunders Co.

Keim, H. A.: Scoliosis, Ciba Found. Symp. **24:**1, 1972.

Kevy, S. V.: Surgical implications of hematologic disorders. In Ravitch, M. M., Welch, K. J., Benson, C. D., and others, editors: Pediatric surgery, ed. 3, Chicago, 1979, Year Book Medical Publishers, Inc.

Laver, M. B., and Bland, J. H. L.: Anesthetic management of the pediatric patient during open-heart surgery, Int. Anesthesiol. Clin. **13:**149, 1975.

Lin, H. Y., Nash, C. L., Herndon, C. H., and others: The effect of corrective surgery on pulmonary function in scoliosis, J. Bone Joint Surg. (Am.) **56:**1173, 1974.

MacEwen, G. D.: Cerebral palsy and scoliosis. In Hardy, J. H., editor: Spinal deformity in neurological and muscular disorders, St. Louis, 1974, The C. V. Mosby Co.

Makley, J. R., Herndon, C. H., Inkley, S., and others: Pulmonary function in paralytic and non-paralytic scoliosis before and after treatment, J. Bone Joint Surg. (Am.) **50:**1379, 1968.

McKusick, V. A.: Heritable disorders of connective tissue, St. Louis, 1972, The C. V. Mosby Co.

McNeill, T. W., DeWald, R. L., Kuo, K. N., and

others: Controlled hypotensive anesthesia in scoliosis surgery, J. Bone Joint Surg. (Am.) **56**:1167, 1974.

Messmer, K.: Hemodilution, Surg. Clin. North Am. **55**:659, 1975.

Moe, J. H., Bradford, D. S., Winter, R. B., and Lonstein, J. E.: Scoliosis and other spinal deformities, Philadelphia, 1978, W. B. Saunders Co.

Murdoch, J. L., Walker, B. A., Halpern, B. L., and others: Life expectancy and causes of death in the Marfan syndrome, N. Engl. J. Med. **288**:804, 1972.

Nickel, V. L., Perry, J., Affeild, J. E., and Dail, C. W.: Elective surgery on patients with respiratory paralysis, J. Bone Joint Surg. (Am.) **37**:189, 1957.

Nickel, V. L., Perry, J., Garrett, A., and Heppenstall, M.: The halo, a spinal skeletal traction device, J. Bone Joint Surg. (Am.) **50**:1400, 1968.

Oliverio, J. R.: Anesthetic management of intramedullary nailing in osteogenesis imperfecta; report of a case, Anesth. Analg. (Cleve.) **52**:232, 1973.

Orzalesi, M. M., Reynolds, E. O. R., and Cook, C. D.: Lung function in scoliosis and pectus excavatum, Cesk. Pediatr. **20**:404, 1965.

Ravin, M., Newmark, Z., and Saviello, G.: Myotonia dystrophica; an anaesthetic hazard; two case reports, Anesth. Analg. (Cleve.) **54**:216, 1975.

Reid, L.: Autopsy studies of the lung in kyphoscoliosis. In Zorab, P. A., editor: Proceedings of a symposium on scoliosis, London, 1966, Vincent House.

Relton, J. E., and Conn, A. W.: Anaesthesia for the surgical correction of scoliosis by the Harrington method in children, Can. Anaesth. Soc. J. **10**:603, 1963.

Relton, J. E., and Hall, J. E.: An operation frame for spinal fusion, J. Bone Joint Surg. (Br.) **498**:327, 1967.

Rinehart, J. J., Lewis, R. P., and Balcerzak, D. P.: Adriamycin cardiotoxicity in man, Ann. Int. Med. **81**:475, 1974.

Riseborough, E. J.: The anterior approach to the spine for the correction of deformities of the axial skeleton, Clin. Orthop. **93**:298, 1973.

Riseborough, E. J., and Davis, N.: Anesthesia. In Hardy, J. H., editor: Spinal deformity in neurological and muscular disorders, St. Louis, 1974, The C. V. Mosby Co.

Riseborough, E. J., and Herndon, T. H.: Scoliosis and other deformities of the axial skeleton, Boston, 1975, Little, Brown & Co.

Salem, M. R., Wong, A. Y., Bennett, E. J., and others: Deliberate hypotension in infants and children, Anesth. Analg. (Cleve.) **53**:975, 1974.

Scott, J. C.: Scoliosis and neurofibromatosis, J. Bone Joint Surg. (Br.) **47**:240, 1965.

Searle, J. F.: Anaesthesia in sickle cell states; a review, Anaesthesia **28**:48, 1973.

Shannon, D. C., Riseborough, E. J., and Kasemi, H.: Ventilation-perfusion relationship following correction of kyphoscoliosis, J.A.M.A. **217**:579, 1971.

Siegel, I. M.: Charcot-Marie-Tooth disease; a diagnostic problem, J.A.M.A. **228**:873, 1974.

Stehling, L.: Anesthesia for children requiring orthopedic surgery, Anesthesiol. Rev. **5**:19, 1978.

Steward, D. J., and Creighton, R. E.: Anesthetic management of the injured child. In Surgical Staff of the Hospital for Sick Children, Toronto, editors: Care of the injured child, Baltimore, 1975, The Williams & Wilkins Co.

Stiles, C. M.: Personal communication, 1975.

Sudhir, K. G., Smith, R. M., Hall, J. E., and Hansen, D. D.: Intraoperative awakening for early recognition of possible neurologic sequelae during Harrington rod spinal fusion, Anesth. Analg. (Cleve.) **55**:526, 1976.

Tachdjian, M. O.: Pediatric orthopedics, Philadelphia, 1972, W. B. Saunders Co.

Vaughan, V. C. II, and McKay, R. J., Jr., editors: Nelson textbook of pediatrics, ed. 10, Philadelphia, 1975, W. B. Saunders Co.

Walton, J. N.: Disorders of voluntary muscle, Boston, 1964, Little, Brown & Co.

Walts, L. F., Finerman, G., and Wyatt, G. M.: Anaesthesia for dwarfs and other patients of pathological small stature, Can. Anaesth. Soc. J. **22**:703, 1975.

Watts, H. G.: Bone tumors. In Ravitch, M. M., Welch, K. J., Benson, C. D., and others, editors: Pediatric Surgery, ed. 3, Chicago, 1979, Year Book Medical Publishers, Inc.

Weisz, G. M., and Barzilai, A.: Nonfulminant fat embolism; review of concepts on its genesis and physiopathology, Anesth. Analg. (Cleve.) **52**:303, 1973.

Westgate, H. D., and Moe, J. H.: Pulmonary function in kyphoscoliosis before and after correction by the Harrington instrumentation method, J. Bone Joint Surg. (Br.) **51**:935, 1969.

Wislicki, L.: Anaesthesia and postoperative complications in progressive muscular dystrophy; tachycardia and acute gastric dilatation, Anaesthesia **17**:482, 1962.

Woolley, M. W., Morgan, S., and Hays, D. M.: Heritable disorders of connective tissue; surgical and anesthetic problems, J. Pediatr. Surg. **2**:325, 1967.

Zorab, P. A.: The lungs in kyphoscoliosis, Dev. Med. Child Neurol. **4**:339, 1962.

Zorab, P. A.: Assessment of cardiorespiratory function in kyphoscoliosis. In Zorab, P. A., editor: Proceedings of a symposium on scoliosis, London, 1966, Vincent House, pp. 54-56.

CHAPTER 20

Anesthesia for ophthalmic surgery

KATHRYN E. McGOLDRICK

GENERAL ASPECTS AND OBJECTIVES

The successful management of anesthesia for ophthalmic surgery demands comprehensive knowledge of ocular pharmacology and physiology as well as competence in technical details of anesthetic administration. Thorough familiarity with the patient's medical history is of paramount importance, because drugs frequently used in ophthalmology may drastically alter reactions to anesthesia. Of course, anesthesiologist-ophthalmologist communication is mandatory, for anesthetic drugs and methods may dramatically change intraocular dynamics.

Such factors as the pathology of the eye, depth of anesthesia, Pa_{CO_2}, size of the pupil, change in tone of the extraocular muscles, hydrational state of the patient, and use of adjuvant drugs including muscle relaxants interact to determine the effect of anesthesia on the eye (Rosen, 1962; Goldman, 1966; Smith, 1973). Therefore, a detailed understanding of the normal maintenance of intraocular pressure, as well as the effect of adjuvant drugs and technics on intraocular pressure, is essential to competent manage-

ment. The text by Harley (1975) is recommended for general information on surgical aspects of pediatric ophthalmology.

INTRAOCULAR PRESSURE
Importance of normal values

Normal intraocular pressure is stated to vary between 10 and 22 torr and is considered pathologic above 25 torr. Intraocular pressure far exceeds not only tissue pressure (2 to 3 torr) but also intracranial pressure (7 to 8 torr). Apparently the maintenance of such a relatively high pressure in the eye is demanded by the optical properties of refracting surfaces; the corneal surface should be kept at a constant curvature, and the stroma must be under constant high pressure to maintain a uniform refractive index (Aboul-Eish, 1973). However, an abnormally high pressure may lead to opacities by interfering with normal corneal metabolism.

During anesthesia or postoperatively, a rise in intraocular pressure can result in permanent loss of vision. If the intraocular pressure is already elevated, a further rise can precipitate an acute attack of glaucoma. If the eyeball is opened suddenly when the intraocular pressure has been too high, rupture of a blood vessel with subsequent hemorrhage may occur. Once the globe has been opened, the intraocular pressure becomes atmospheric, and any sudden increase in pressure can lead to loss of vitreous and prolapse of the lens or iris (Ivankovic and Lowe, 1971). Thus, the appropriate control

477

of intraocular pressure is of vital importance in ophthalmic anesthesia.

Central nervous system control mechanism

The mechanism for maintenance of intraocular pressure is under the control of the central nervous system. Therefore, ocular hemodynamics can be altered via nerve impulses or hormonal effects, or both, to meet the needs of a given situation. It is felt that general anesthesia lowers the intraocular pressure by depressing certain diencephalic areas that are associated with changing intraocular pressure (Adler, 1970).

Pathologic factors influencing intraocular pressure

Three pathologic factors influence intraocular pressure: (1) pressure on the eye from outside by various entities, such as orbital tumor, venous congestion of orbital veins (as may be associated with vomiting and coughing), and contraction of the orbicularis oculi muscle, (2) scleral rigidity, and (3) changes in the intraocular contents that are semisolid (lens, vitreous, any intraocular tumor) or fluid (blood and aqueous humor) (Aboul-Eish, 1973).

This last category is of considerable interest to the anesthesiologist. For example, changes in semisolid contents may significantly affect intraocular pressure. The lens size gradually and progressively increases with age, an increase that is well tolerated. However, if a sudden increase in lens size occurs, as in traumatic cataract, an acute rise in intraocular pressure may occur that is secondary to rapid increase in lens size as well as to pressure on the iris, leading to obstruction of the angle of the eye and interference with aqueous drainage.

The vitreous is basically an unstable gel with a fine, fibrous supporting structure. Hydration of the normal vitreous can be increased by excessive fluid intake; thus, the vitreous may increase its water content when a patient is overhydrated. It is customary, therefore, to keep glaucoma patients slight-ly dehydrated before and during surgery.

Important as the semisolid contents are in influencing intraocular pressure, the major control of intraocular tension is via the fluid contents (blood and aqueous humor), in particular the aqueous humor. Since other ocular constituents are rather incompressible and scleral distensibility is limited, a variation in the volume of one of these two fluids should be accompanied by an equal and opposite change in the volume of the other to maintain constant intraocular pressure.

The volume of blood—determined mainly by the state of vessel dilation or contraction in the spongy layers of the choroid plexus—contributes significantly to the intraocular pressure. While changes in both arterial and venous pressure may secondarily affect intraocular pressure, variations in arterial pressure are rather insignificant compared with venous fluctuations. It is said that essential hypertension is not a cause of glaucoma, for in sustained arterial hypertension the ocular tension returns to its normal level after a period of adaptation because of (1) increased flow of aqueous humor from the eye as a result of elevated intraocular pressure and (2) compression of the blood vessels in the choroid plexus as a result of elevated intraocular pressure. Thus, an important feedback mechanism exists to diminish the total volume of blood and protect the eye by keeping the intraocular pressure constant in a patient with systemic hypertension (Adler, 1970; Aboul-Eish, 1973).

However, if the venous return from the eye is disturbed at any point between Schlemm's canal and the right atrium, the intraocular pressure rises markedly. This is secondary to increased intraocular blood volume and distension of orbital vessels as well as to interference with aqueous drainage. Straining or coughing greatly increases intraocular pressure by raising the venous pressure. For example, a mild cough can elevate the intraocular pressure by 34 to 40 torr (Kornblueth and others, 1959), and the intraocular pressure of a crying child easily reaches 50 torr. Thus, the deleterious implications of breath-holding and straining during anesthesia seem apparent.

Aqueous humor and intraocular pressure

The anterior and posterior chambers of the eye are filled with a clear fluid called aqueous humor, the volume of which depends on the balance between the rate of formation and the rate of drainage (2 μl/min at equilibrium). While the amount of protein is as low as 0.02 g/ml and the urea, glucose, and bicarbonate concentrations are lower than in the blood, the concentrations of chloride, sodium lactate, and ascorbate are higher. The pH is 7.1 to 7.2, and the specific gravity is 1.003 (Adler, 1970; Aboul-Eish, 1973).

Aqueous humor, formed mainly in the posterior chamber by the epithelial cells of the ciliary process, is the only source of nutrition for the lens and the posterior part of the cornea, since these elements are devoid of blood vessels. From the posterior chamber, the aqueous humor circulates to the anterior chamber through the pupil, to be drained at the angle of the eye, traversing numerous small channels called Fontana's spaces and then draining into Schlemm's canal. From Schlemm's canal, the aqueous is carried by small ducts, called ophthalmic veins, to the episcleral veins, which end in the ophthalmic veins draining into the cavernous sinus inside the skull. The ophthalmic veins have additional communications with veins outside the skull; the superior ophthalmic vein anastomoses with the facial vein, and the inferior ophthalmic vein anastomoses with the pterygoid plexus through the inferior orbital fissure. Thus, aqueous humor as well as intraocular blood is ultimately drained by the external and internal jugular veins to the innominate veins to the superior vena cava and thence to the right side of the heart (Grant, 1962; Aboul-Eish, 1973). Therefore, obstruction of blood flow in any part from the eye to the right side of the heart will impede aqueous drainage and concomitantly elevate intraocular pressure.

Two-thirds of the aqueous humor is formed in the posterior chamber by the ciliary body in an active secretory process, and one-third is formed in the anterior chamber by simple filtration through the anterior surface of the iris. In the posterior chamber, sodium is actively transferred from the blood to the aqueous humor via the sodium pump. This sodium pump is helped by carbonic anhydrase and cytochrome oxidase enzymes. Since pumped sodium must be replaced by another positively charged ion, an immediate source for this is the hydrogen ion liberated from the reaction that is accelerated by carbonic anhydrase:

$$CO_2 + H_2O \rightarrow H_2CO_3 \rightarrow HCO_3^- + H^+$$

The total solutes in the aqueous humor are higher than those in the plasma by an amount equal to 5 mmole/L of sodium chloride, and therefore the osmotic pressure difference between the aqueous humor and the plasma is equal to 10 mOsm/L (Aboul-Eish, 1973). Since 1 osmole exerts a pressure of 22.4 atmospheres of 17,000 torr (760 $\times$ 22.4), 10 mOsm exert a pressure of 170 torr. The intraocular pressure can be calculated from the following formula (Aboul-Eish, 1973):

$$IOP = K \left[(OP_{aq} - OP_{pl}) + CP \right]$$

where

$$
\begin{aligned}
K &= \text{coefficient of outflow} \\
OP_{aq} &= \text{osmotic pressure of aqueous humor} \\
OP_{pl} &= \text{osmotic pressure of plasma} \\
CP &= \text{capillary pressure}
\end{aligned}
$$

Normally:

$$
\begin{aligned}
IOP &= 0.1 \left[(5170 - 5000) + 30 \right] \\
&= 0.1 \times 200 \\
&= 20 \text{ torr}
\end{aligned}
$$

This equation underscores the fact that the most important factor for the formation of aqueous humor is the difference between the osmotic pressure of the aqueous and the plasma (Aboul-Eish, 1973). That a slight change in the solute concentration of the plasma can markedly affect the formation of aqueous humor and subsequently the intraocular pressure is the basis for using intravenous hypertonic solutions such as mannitol

479

tion anesthetic agents, intravenous hydroxy-dione sodium succinate (Viadril) depresses intraocular pressure in proportion to the depth of anesthesia (Magora and Collins, 1962; Duncalf and Foldes, 1973). During deep anesthesia with any inhalation anesthetic agent, the intraocular pressure approaches a common value of 8 to 10 torr under conditions of normocarbia. This decreased pressure has been attributed primarily to an increased facility of aqueous outflow.

In contradistinction to curare, succinylcholine increases intraocular pressure (Schwartz and deRoeth, 1958; Craythorne and others, 1960; Gesztes, 1966; Katz and Eakins, 1969). It has been reported that 0.3 mg of succinylcholine per kg administered during light thiopental anesthesia was associated with an average rise in intraocular pressure of 7.9 torr. The intraocular pressure returns to initial values within 5 minutes, even in wide-angle glaucoma (Lincoff and others, 1955).

A specific histologic structure called *Felderstruktur* has been found in extraocular muscles. In contrast to other skeletal muscles, these muscles contain large numbers of fibers that, when immersed in depolarizing solutions or exposed to stimuli of acetylcholine, respond with slow tonic contraction (Duncalf and Foldes, 1973).

Drugs that abolish the fasciculations produced by succinylcholine might also be expected to prevent the rise in intraocular pressure. Surprisingly, in the past it was reported that an increase in intraocular pressure still occurs when the intravenous administration of succinylcholine is preceded by either the intravenous injection of *d*-tubocurarine (Whalin, 1960) or hexafluorenium dibromide (Sobel, 1962). However, more recent studies suggest that some nondepolarizing muscle relaxants under certain circumstances are able to inhibit succinylcholine-induced increases in intraocular pressure. That is, increases in intraocular pressure after succinylcholine in both healthy and glaucomatous eyes were prevented by the intravenous administration of 20 mg of gallamine or 3 mg of curare (Miller

and others, 1968). The prior administration of acetazolamide (Carballo, 1965) and of the beta-adrenergic blocking agent propranolol also abolished succinylcholine-induced intraocular hypertension (Kaufman, 1967).

In recent years it has become increasingly apparent that, under normal conditions, the rise in intraocular pressure following succinylcholine is *dissipated before surgery commences*. The peak action in anesthetized patients with normal eyes was noted between the second and fourth minutes and had subsided by the sixth minute (Pandey and others, 1972).

It no longer seems tenable that succinylcholine be used only with great reluctance in ocular surgery. However, succinylcholine is definitely contraindicated in patients with penetrating ocular wounds. The initial response of intraocular pressure to succinylcholine is maximum with the first dose of the drug; supplementary doses cause a much reduced response. Consequently, in elective operations in which the eyeball is to be opened, succinylcholine may be given before the eyeball is opened and repeated after it is opened. Initial use of the drug after the eyeball is opened, however, should be avoided. Of interest is Jampolsky's (1965) recommendation that succinycholine not be used in strabismus patients undergoing reoperation, because the forced duction test does not return to normal for 30 minutes following succinylcholine.

DRUG INTERACTIONS
Antihypertensive drugs

Although encountered rather infrequently, hypertension is by no means a stranger to the pediatric age group, and it is incumbent upon the anesthesiologist to be aware of certain pharmacologic points. For example, thiazide diuretics could cause sufficient renal tubular loss of potassium such that an increased sensitivity to nondepolarizing muscle relaxants might occur (Dundee and McDowell, 1971), and also signs of digitalis toxicity might be manifest.

Long-term reserpine therapy with its effect of catecholamine depeletion at the neurovascular end-plate results in diminished responsiveness to indirect-acting vasopressors such as ephedrine and metaraminol. Therefore, should a vasopressor be required intraoperatively, a direct-acting drug such as phenylephrine or methoxamine should be selected. In contrast, patients on guanethidine therapy may be hyperreactive to direct-acting vasopressors.

Monoamine oxidase (MAO) inhibitors lead to increased brain and tissue levels of catecholamines. When vasopressor drugs are administered to patients on MAO inhibitors, hypertensive crises may develop. In addition to the potentiation of pressor drugs, an interaction with various narcotics may be associated with severe hypotension (Dundee and McDowell, 1971). Since the actions of general and local anesthetics, barbiturates, belladonna drugs, ganglionic blockers, and insulin may all be potentiated in patients treated with MAO inhibitors, it is recommended that MAO-inhibitor therapy be discontinued 10 days prior to elective surgery (Collins, 1970).

Anticholinesterase agents

Long-acting anticholinesterase agents such as echothiophate iodide (Phospholine Iodide) may prolong the action of succinylcholine (Humphreys and Holmes, 1963). These long-acting drugs used in the treatment of glaucoma are absorbed into the systemic circulation following instillation in the conjunctival sac. It is reported that after 5 to 7 weeks of therapy, serum cholinesterase levels are drastically reduced and may take as long as 6 weeks to return to normal following discontinuance of the drug (Ellis and Esterdahl, 1967). Therefore, these patients, if given succinylcholine, are likely to have prolonged apnea. The anesthesiologist must also expect these patients to display a delay in the metabolism of local anesthetic agents of the ester variety such as procaine.

Anticholinergic agents: atropine

As mentioned previously, glaucoma is not a contraindication to the use of anticholinergic agents, provided that the usual clinical doses are not exceeded. In such cases, topical miotics are recommended on the morning of surgery. The effect of atropine on the eyes of patients with Down's syndrome is described in Chapter 24.

Epinephrine

Many feel that it is inadvisable to use topical epinephrine in the eye in patients being anesthetized with a halogenated hydrocarbon. However, Smith and associates (1972) reported on the administration of epinephrine into the anterior chamber of patients undergoing cataract surgery by phacoemulsification and aspiration. The authors concluded that it is apparently safe to administer epinephrine into the anterior chamber in doses up to 68 μg/kg in adults undergoing cataract aspiration with halothane anesthesia. It was postulated that the iris with its rich supply of adrenergic receptors may be able to capture with extreme rapidity the epinephrine injected into the eye.

However, serious drug interactions may occur when exogenous epinephrine or other catecholamines are administered under certain circumstances. Patients taking the following drugs may display increased sensitivity: cocaine, guanethidine, tricyclic antidepressants (imipramine [Tofranil]), reserpine, MAO inhibitors, and methyldopa (Aldomet) (Linn and Smith, 1973). This list, while representative, is still incomplete.

OPHTHALMIC REQUIREMENTS OF GENERAL ANESTHESIA

The majority of patients who undergo eye surgery are either under 10 years of age or over 55 years of age. Operations on the ocular adnexa, including lid surgery, repair of lacrimal apparatus, and repair of extraocular muscles, are especially frequent in the pediatric age group. However, surgery on the anterior segment, such as cataract removal, glaucoma procedures, and trauma repair, are certainly not confined to the adult population.

Most ocular procedures require profound analgesia but minimal muscle relaxation. The child's airway must be protected from obstruction, and the anesthesiologist must concomitantly remove himself and his apparatus from the surgical field. Although local anesthesia is successfully employed for many ophthalmic operations, reliable general anesthesia with endotracheal intubation is probably the method of choice in most pediatric eye procedures. However, if the operation is of especially brief duration, such as probing of lacrimal ducts, insufflation rather than intubation may be elected safely.

Two special challenges confront the anesthesiologist: the avoidance of high intraocular tension and the specter of the oculocardiac reflex.

Avoidance of high intraocular tension

Intraocular hypertension may result in complications that could seriously compromise the success of surgery. These complications include extrusion of ocular contents and intraocular hemorrhage. Loss of vitreous is the most common complication and may eventually result in retinal detachment and blindness, poor wound healing with a higher incidence of postoperative iris prolapse, and increased incidence of intraocular hemorrhage.

A large rise in venous pressure, and hence in intraocular pressure, is associated with coughing, vomiting, and straining, as in the screaming of a frightened child. In such situations, if the eyeball is lacerated, loss of vitreous is almost certain to occur. Thus, the importance of a quiet induction cannot be overemphasized. As described on p. 111, rectal thiopental is excellent for this purpose.

Oculocardiac reflex

The oculocardiac reflex, first described in 1908, is elicited by pressure on the globe, and many have used this maneuver in attempts to control persistent hiccoughs. During surgical procedures, three types of stimulus are particularly apt to initiate the reflex: grasping of the conjunctiva, traction on the extraocular muscles, especially the medial rectus, and enucleation. The afferent limb of the oculocardiac reflex is trigeminal,

and the efferent limb is vagal (Bosomworth and others, 1958). Numerous methods suggested to abolish or obtund this reflex include retrobulbar block and the use of gallamine, but none has been as effective as intravenous atropine administered within 30 minutes before surgery (Taylor and others, 1963). Lidocaine, 1 mg/kg, may be given by intravenous route if the arrhythmia persists. Because several cardiac arrests have been associated with the oculocardiac reflex, preoperative atropine is given routinely by most pediatric anesthesiologists (Nagel and others, 1973; Danis, 1975).

An interesting study of 191 pediatric patients scheduled for surgical correction of strabismus at Columbia Presbyterian Medical Center was reported by Katz and Bigger (1970). The incidence of oculocardiac reflex was 72%; a retrobulbar block decreased this to 35%, while intramuscular or intravenous atropine decreased it to 30% (Katz and Bigger, 1970). However, following atropine the arrhythmias were more severe and prolonged than those in the untreated patients. Thus, both atropine and retrobulbar block were abandoned, and the current practice at Columbia is to monitor ECG and if a persistent arrhythmia develops, the surgeon temporarily stops manipulation. This method has been safely employed with over 2,000 patients during the past 6 years. Of interest is the observation of Moonie and associates (1964) that with repeated handling of the extraocular muscles, bradycardia is less likely to occur, probably because of fatigue of the oculocardiac reflex at the level of the cardioinhibitory center.

CLINICAL MANAGEMENT OF ANESTHESIA

The management of anesthesia for children undergoing ophthalmic procedures in our institution follows the general principles just described. The variety of surgical operations performed is suggested in Table 20-1. Correction of strabismus occupies 80% of the operating time of the Department of Ophthalmology.

Preparation of the children must include

Anesthesia for ophthalmic surgery

Table 20-1. Surgical lesions and procedures in pediatric ophthalmology

Lesions	Procedures
Strabismus	Correction by recession and/or resection
Esotropia (ET)	
Exotropia (XT)	
Ptosis	Levator repair
	Fascial sling
Cataract	
Congenital	Iridectomy
Down's syndrome	Discission of pupillary membrane
Galactosemia	Cataract aspiration
Steroid-treated asthma	
Glaucoma	Trabeculectomy
Iritis	Steroid injection
Anomalies of tear duct	Tear duct probing
	Dacryocystorhinostomy
	Dacryocystogram
	Myectomy
Cysts and tumors	
Congenital cysts	Excision
Cysts of eyelids	Excision
Retinoblastoma	Enucleation
	Exenteration
Chalazion	Excision
Trauma	
Foreign body	Removal
Laceration of eyeball	Repair
Scleral perforation	
Blow-out fracture	
Anesthesia examination	Measurement of intraocular pressure
	Examination of lens, cornea, anterior and posterior chambers
	Gonioscopy

identification of underlying diseases, such as diabetes, renal disease, or long-standing asthma, and particular effort to prepare the child emotionally for the recovery period, when he will wake up with one or both eyes closed by bandages. This is important not only to save him from reasonable fear and anxiety but also to prevent much of the activity and thrashing about that fright might cause, to the disadvantage of the eye.

For elective procedures, preoperative sedation is chosen carefully. Atropine, if ordered, should not be given more than 30 minutes before operation. Induction is usually started with nitrous oxide, followed by halothane, which is believed to be preferable for most operations of this type. Atropine is usually repeated, by intravenous injection, as soon as the child is asleep. For major procedures, orotracheal intubation is preferred, aided by succinylcholine unless the child has been receiving echothiophate or similar drugs. The endotracheal tube is liberally coated with lidocaine jelly to reduce the sensitivity of the child's pharynx, and the ECG is added to the standard monitoring devices. As previously stated, arrhythmias occur more frequently during eye surgery and may be severe. Rather than an attempt being made to correct them at once, it has appeared much safer to have the surgeon desist long enough to stop the arrhythmia and to add atropine, if none had been given within the previous 30 minutes. One should avoid the administration of atropine while the vagal reflex is still active, or one should expect to encounter some very bizarre cardiac tracings.

485

Maintenance of anesthesia should be deep enough to avoid reflexes. Some help in this may be obtained by liberal application of anesthetic jelly to the endotracheal tube and/or spraying of the hypopharynx and upper airway with topical anesthetic.

Similarly, responses should be avoided, if possible, when the child awakens, and extubation should occur well before there is a tendency to cough. If both eyes are covered with bandages on awakening, one person should be constantly at the child's bedside to comfort him and to restrain arms and legs, if necessary. Vomiting is to be avoided at all costs.

For most pediatric procedures in this category, halothane has been widely favored because it is rapidly effective and only slightly irritating to the trachea and stomach. It also reduces intraocular pressure. The management of the child for repair of lacerated eyeball is described on p. 111.

Ophthalmic procedures in ambulatory surgery

As noted by Nagel and associates (1973), several procedures about the eye may be performed on an outpatient basis. These include such simple procedures as tear duct probing, removal of sutures, excision of small cysts, and some of the simpler eye examinations. Measurement of intraocular pressure can be performed under light sedation aided by application of proparacaine ointment, a rapidly acting nonirritant ointment that is an excellent adjunct for home or professional use. For more complete examination of the cornea or the anterior or posterior chambers of the eye, general endotracheal anesthesia is usually necessary.

Anesthesia for extended daily x-ray treatments of ocular tumors

Retinoblastoma may call for daily x-ray therapy over a course of 2 to 3 weeks. This is one situation in which ketamine has unrivaled preference (Cronin and others, 1972; ApIvor, 1973). Using an intramuscular dose of 3 to 5 mg/kg or an intravenous dose of 1 to 2 mg/kg, one may treat small children daily for an apparently unlimited time without encountering dangerous side effects. The required dosage will vary in some and may show a tendency to increase over prolonged use, but it often shows little change. Children must be given atropine prior to ketamine administration, particularly if they are to remain supine during treatment, lest secretions accumulate in the pharynx. With modern equipment, the duration of treatment is usually not more than a few minutes, but the child must be monitored with absolute certainty that the airway is clear and ventilation unobstructed. It is not adequate to watch the child's chest move, for the chest may move in the absence of exchange if the airway is occluded. The safest method is to use a simple precordial stethoscope and lengthen the tubing as necessary, even to 20 feet, through which breath as well as heart sounds may be heard distinctly. After treatment, the child must be attended in a suitable recovery area until he is fully able to control all his motor coordination and has mental clarity.

BIBLIOGRAPHY

Aboul-Eish, E.: Physiology of the eye pertinent to anesthesia. In Smith, R. B., editor: Anesthesia in ophthalmology, Boston, 1973, Little, Brown & Co.

Adler, F. H.: Physiology of the eye; clinical applications, ed. 5, St. Louis, 1970, The C. V. Mosby Co.

Adriani, J.: The chemistry and physics of anaesthesia, ed. 2, Springfield, Ill., 1967, Charles C Thomas, Publisher.

Agarwal, L. P., and Mathur, S. P.: Curare in ocular surgery, Br. J. Ophthalmol. 36:603, 1952.

ApIvor, D.: Ketamine in paediatric ophthalmological surgery, Anaesthesia 28:501, 1973.

Ausinsch, B., Rayburn, R. L., Munson, E. S., and Levy, N. S.: Ketamine and intraocular pressure in children, Anesth. Analg. (Cleve.) 55:773, 1976.

Bosomworth, P. D., Ziegler, C. H., and Jacoby, J.: Oculo-cardiac reflex in eye muscle surgery, Anesthesiology 19:7, 1958.

Carballo, A. S.: Succinylcholine and acetazolamide in anaesthesia for ocular surgery, Can. Anaesth. Soc. J. 12:486, 1965.

Collins, V. J.: Principles of anesthesiology, Philadelphia, 1970, Lea & Febiger.

Corssen, G., and Hoy, J. E.: A new parenteral anesthetic—CI-581; its effect on intraocular pressure, J. Pediatr. Ophthalmol. 4:20, 1967.

Craythorne, N. W. B., Rottenstein, H. S., and Dripps, R. D.: Effect of succinylcholine on intraocular pressure in adults, infants and children during general anesthesia, Anesthesiology 21:59, 1960.

Cronin, M. M., Bousfield, J. D., Hewett, E. B., and others: Ketamine anaesthesia for radiotherapy in small children, Anaesthesia 27:135, 1972.

Danis, M. H.: Anesthesia in the pediatric patient for surgery of the eye. In Harley, R. D., editor: Pediatric ophthalmology, Philadelphia, 1975, W. B. Saunders Co.

deRoeth, A., and Schwartz, H.: Aqueous humor dynamics in glaucoma; effect of ganglionic blocking agents and thiopental sodium on aqueous humor dynamics, A.M.A. Arch. Ophthalmol. 55:755, 1956.

Drucker, A. P., Sadove, M. S., and Unna, K. R.: Ocular manifestations of intravenous tetraethylammonium chloride in man, Am. J. Ophthalmol. 33:1564, 1950.

Duncalf, D., and Foldes, F. F.: Effect of anesthetic drugs and muscle relaxants on intraocular pressure. In Smith, R. B., editor: Anesthesia in ophthalmology, Boston, 1973, Little, Brown & Co.

Duncalf, D., and Weitzner, S. W.: Ventilation and hypercapnia on intraocular pressure during anesthesia, Anesth. Analg. (Cleve.) 43:232, 1963.

Dundee, J. W., and McDowell, S. A.: Influence of drug therapy on anaesthesia. In Gray, T. C., and Nunn, J. F., editors: General anaesthesia; clinical practice, vol. 2, New York, 1971, Appleton-Century-Crofts.

Ellis, E. P., and Esterdahl, M.: Echothiophate iodide therapy in children; effect upon blood cholinesterase levels, Arch. Ophthalmol. 77:598, 1967.

Galin, M. A., Aizawa, F., and McLean, J. M.: Intravenous urea in the treatment of acute angle glaucoma, Am. J. Ophthalmol. 50:379, 1960.

Gesztes, T.: Prolonged apnea after suxamethonium associated with eye drops containing an anticholinesterase agent, Br. J. Anaesth. 38:408, 1966.

Goldman, E. J.: Anesthesia for ophthalmology. In Benson, D. W., editor: Surgical specialties, Philadelphia, 1966, F. A. Davis Co.

Grant, B.: Grant's atlas of anatomy, ed. 5, Baltimore, 1962, The Williams & Wilkins Co.

Grant, W. M., and Trotter, R. R.: Diamox (acetazolamide) in the treatment of glaucoma, A.M.A. Arch. Ophthalmol. 51:335, 1954.

Harley, R. D.: Pediatric ophthalmology, Philadelphia, 1975, W. B. Saunders Co.

Hill, D. W.: Physics applied to anaesthesia, New York, 1968, Appleton-Century-Crofts.

Humphreys, J. A., and Holmes, J. H.: Systemic effects produced by echothiophate iodide in treatment of glaucoma, Arch. Ophthalmol. 69:737, 1963.

Ivankovic, A. D., and Lowe, H. J.: Eye procedures with methoxyflurane, Chicago, 1971, Abbott Laboratories.

Jampolsky, A.: Strabismus; surgical overcorrections, Highlights Ophthalmol. 8:78, 1965.

Katz, R. L., and Bigger, J. T.: Cardiac arrhythmias during anesthesia and operation, Anesthesiology 33:193, 1970.

Kaufman, L.: General anaesthesia in ophthalmology, Proc. R. Soc. Med. 60:1280, 1967.

Kornblueth, W., Aladjemoff, L., Magora, F., and Gabbay, A.: Influence of general anesthesia on intraocular pressure in man; the effect of diethyl ether, cyclopropane, vinyl ether, and thiopental sodium, A.M.A. Arch. Ophthalmol. 61:84, 1959.

Lincoff, H. A., Ellis, C. H., DeVoe, A. G., and others: Effect of succinylcholine on intraocular pressure, Am. J. Ophthalmol. 40:501, 1955.

Linn, J. G., and Smith, R. B.: Intraoperative complications and their management. In Smith, R. B., editor: Anesthesia in ophthalmology, Boston, 1973, Little, Brown & Co.

Magora, F., and Collins, V. J.: The influence of general anesthetic agents on intraocular pressure in man; the effect of non-explosive agents, Arch. Ophthalmol. 66:806, 1962.

Miller, R. D., Way, W. L., and Hickey, R. F.: Inhibition of succinylcholine-induced increased intraocular pressure by non-depolarizing muscle relaxants, Anesthesiology 29:123, 1968.

Moonie, G. T., Rees, D. I., and Elton, D.: The oculocardiac reflex during strabismus surgery, Can. Anaesth. Soc. J. 11:621, 1964.

Nagel, E. L., Forster, R. K., Jones, D. B., and MacMahon, S.: Outpatient anesthesia for pediatric ophthalmology, Anesth. Analg. (Cleve.) 52:558, 1973.

Ophthalmologic Staff of the Hospital for Sick Children, Toronto: The eye in childhood, Chicago, 1967, Year Book Medical Publishers, Inc.

Pandey, K., Badola, R. P., and Kumar, S.: Time course of intraocular hypertension produced by suxamethonium, Br. J. Anaesth. 44:191, 1972.

Rosen, D. A.: Anaesthesia in ophthalmology, Can. Anaesth. Soc. J. 9:545, 1962.

Schwartz, H., and deRoeth, A.: Effect of succinylcholine on intraocular pressure in human beings, Anesthesiology 19:112, 1958.

Smith, R. B., editor: Anesthesia in ophthalmology, Boston, 1973, Little, Brown & Co.

Smith, R. B.: Anesthesia for surgery of strabismus, Bull. N.Y. Acad. Med. 51:382, 1975.

Smith, R. B., Douglas, H. N., Petruscak, J., and Breslin, P.: Safety of intraocular adrenaline with halothane anaesthesia, Br. J. Anaesth. 44:1314, 1972.

Snow, J. C., Kripke, B. J., Norton, M. L., and others: Corneal injuries during general anesthesia, Anesth. Analg. (Cleve.) 54:465, 1975.

Sobel, A. M.: Hexafluorenium, succinylcholine, and intraocular tension, Anesth. Analg. (Cleve.) 41:399, 1962.

Taylor, C., Wilson, F. M., Roesch, R., and Stoelting, V. K.: Prevention of oculocardiac reflex in children, Anesthesiology 24:646, 1963.

Whalin, A.: Clinical and experimental studies on effects of succinylcholine, Acta Anaesthesiol. Scand. (Suppl.) 5:1, 1960.

CHAPTER 21

Anesthesia for ear, nose, and throat surgery

General aspects and objectives
Operations about the ear
Operations about the nose
Tonsillectomy and other operations on the
  pharynx, larynx, and esophagus
Diagnostic procedures

GENERAL ASPECTS AND OBJECTIVES

The vast number of tonsillectomies performed during recent decades under the most varied anesthetic talents suggests that this phase of anesthesia is not especially demanding. The record of deaths resulting from this approach should correct this impression.

In more complicated situations involving airway emergencies, aspirated foreign bodies, or posttonsillectomy "bleeders," both the danger and the need for anesthetic skill are second to none (McKenzie, 1963; Merifield, 1972).

For suitable operating conditions in this type of surgery, anesthesia usually should provide the following:

1. Complete analgesia and immobility but relatively little relaxation
2. Protection of the patient's airway from blood, loose tissue, and operative manipulation
3. Minimal obstruction of operative field by the anesthesiologist and his equipment
4. Increased protection against hyperactive vagal reflexes
5. Avoidance of straining or vomiting during recovery from specified operations

Since many of these patients are admitted

on a short-term basis, there may be increased danger of hurried, inadequate work-up. The anesthesiologist must insist that no details be neglected and that history, physical examination, and essential laboratory work supply the necessary information. Previous concern over the measurement of bleeding and clotting times prior to tonsillectomy has been redirected toward tests for PT and PTT.

Preoperative medications, including sedative and belladonna agents, are usually administered. Innumerable variations have been recommended, but for tonsillectomy one of the least upsetting technics is to use a barbiturate suppository (pentobarbital, 5 mg/kg) and add atropine (0.2 to 0.4 mg) immediately after the child is put to sleep, thus avoiding the usual needling that is so abhorrent to all. To prevent excitement during recovery, it is usually advisable to add a narcotic during anesthesia (morphine, 0.1 mg/kg).

For better antiemetic effect, chlorpromazine (0.1 mg/kg) may be preferable before operations where postoperative vomiting involves increased danger (Smith, 1972). Droperidol and perphenazine also are effective for prevention of emesis, and acetaminophen (Tylenol) is effective for correction of emesis.

Local anesthesia, once popular for surgery about the face and head, is rarely used as the primary anesthetic for small children. However, cocaine in 4% strength may be used for children prior to nasal procedures and usually becomes the principal agent in adolescents undergoing septoplasty. Although Chung and associates (1978) state that co-

488

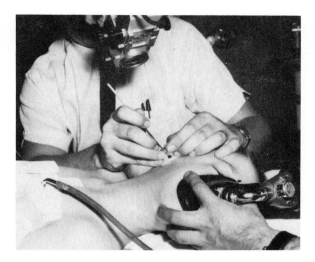

Fig. 21-1. Myringotomy is usually performed as an elective procedure, and patients should be well prepared for general anesthesia. Mask administration should serve well for this purpose.

caine does not sensitize the heart to halothane, at The Children's Hospital Medical Center we have encountered several episodes of tachycardia and bizarre arrhythmias under such circumstances and believe that cocaine should be used with reasonable economy. General anesthesia, usually with endotracheal intubation, is chosen for most operative procedures of this class. Preference for purely inhalation or intravenous technics depends on the individual situation.

OPERATIONS ABOUT THE EAR
Myringotomy

Myringotomy, paracentesis tympani, or incision of the tympanic membrane requires only a momentary period of analgesia and immobilization without relaxation. Another 30 seconds may be needed if myringotomy tubes are to be inserted.

Formerly, myringotomy was most often performed on an emergency basis, with the membrane bulging and the child feverish and unprepared. If the child had eaten, the procedure was best performed with morphine plus 50% nitrous oxide and oxygen, so that the gag reflex would remain intact. At present, myringotomy is more frequently scheduled electively, and the child is more adequately prepared (Fig. 21-1). Though pre-

operative sedation is hardly necessary, having the child afebrile and with an empty stomach is a great improvement. Mask administration of oxygen, nitrous oxide, and halothane gives effective, controllable anesthesia, and prompt ambulation can be expected.

Mastoidectomy and tympanoplasty

One finds several variations in operations about the inner ear (Jackson and Jackson, 1945; Ferguson and Kendig, 1972). In general, they require 1 to 3 or more hours of surgery and permit a fairly uniform anesthetic approach. For simple mastoidectomy there are no particular restrictions to the choice of anesthesia or technic. In the performance of tympanoplasty the use of nitrous oxide should be avoided during and after placement of the tympanic graft, because the accumulation of nitrous oxide in any free space increases the ambient pressure and in this case tends to lift the graft away from its new site.

There seems to be no objection to halothane-oxygen mixtures in young children. In teenagers, if one prefers to avoid halogens, one may use nitrous oxide–relaxant methods and, if a tympanic graft is to be used, substitute fentanyl (0.01 mg/kg) in repeated doses

489

or add halothane for this limited period. Thiopental, though not an analgesic, can be used here to provide the desired effect of keeping the child asleep and reducing postoperative excitement. Other inhalation combinations, as well as intravenous methods, may be employed. As in any long procedure, special precautions should be maintained to monitor temperature and provide adequate fluids. The danger of heat retention is increased in patients such as these who are enveloped in drapes and who often are scheduled for operation in late afternoon.

OPERATIONS ABOUT THE NOSE
Reduction of nasal fracture

This operation requires only light analgesia and scarcely more time than was required for the injury. The chief danger in such cases lies in the possibility that the child's stomach may contain undigested food plus an unknown quantity of blood from the injured nose. Premedication plus light nitrous oxide anesthesia will afford adequate analgesia for reduction in most cases. If a more prolonged procedure is necessary, endotracheal intubation under one of the general anesthetics may be indicated. The pharynx should be packed to prevent passage of more blood into the hypopharynx, and the endotracheal tube should be left in place until the child has awakened in order to prevent postoperative regurgitation and aspiration.

Since both thiopental and ketamine often precipitate serious laryngotracheal reflexes, they should definitely be avoided here. Because of its minimal airway irritation, halothane would be the current agent of choice.

Correction of deviated septum, polypectomy, and other intranasal operations

These operations usually are best performed under oral endotracheal anesthesia, again using nonrebreathing methods in younger children. Nitrous oxide induction followed by halothane probably would be best for such procedures. Thiopental may cause objectionable sneezing or coughing if used for operations on the nose and consequently seems a poor choice. Packing of the pharynx is indicated in most intranasal operations. As previously mentioned, 4% cocaine may be used as a topical application for supplementary anesthesia in younger patients or as primary anesthesia in teenagers if supplemented by sedation.

Special consideration should be given to the management of children with *cystic fibrosis* in whom nasal polyps often occur as a relatively late complication. The polyps are multiple, recur following removal, and frequently are superimposed on considerable local infection. Obviously these children have severe underlying disease, and all anesthetics carry disadvantages (Smith, 1965).

Our experience with use of ketamine for children with cystic fibrosis, consisting of two attempts that led to uncontrollable, near-fatal coughing, convinced us that ketamine was contraindicated in this disease. To date, our most satisfactory technic has been the use of nitrous oxide and *d*-tubocurarine with endotracheal intubation. This combination allows the surgeon to use epinephrine and electrocautery and precludes the need for atropine, which may make it increasingly difficult for patients to raise the heavy secretions that block their airways.

Children having cystic fibrosis may be expected to be in critical condition because of pulmonary pathology, cor pulmonale, and anemia (p. 531). Those operated on for nasal polyps often bleed profusely during and occasionally after operation, and blood should always be prepared for transfusion.

Nasal packs, usually required during early recovery, lead to further problems in oxygenation. This situation is partially relieved if the surgeon first introduces a nasopharyngeal catheter and then packs around it. In any condition, early, full postoperative recovery of ventilatory function is mandatory to enable patients to overcome their several handicaps.

NOTE: Nasal polyps in otherwise normal children should be approached with caution, since a nasal encephalocele is identical in appearance (Matson, 1969; Schmidt and Leyendiijk, 1974).

Choanal atresia

Occasionally infants are born with boney occlusion of one or both posterior nares, or choanae (Fig. 21-2) (Fearon and Dickson, 1968; Ferguson, 1972). This may be unrelated to other lesions but frequently is associated with craniofacial synostosis (Apert's and Crouzon's syndromes). Since infants depend chiefly on nasal breathing, neonates may suffocate unless an airway is strapped into the mouth. Operation on these infants must be performed in the first few days of life. Other infants may have only unilateral obstruction, which will not be diagnosed for months or years and may only be noticed by the presence of unilateral nasal discharge.

Surgical approach is possible through the nostrils, but the lesion is difficult to expose.

By entering through the mouth and turning down a flap of palate, the boney obstruction can be visualized more easily and can be chiseled away. These patients tolerate halothane fairly well and may be maintained on oral endotracheal Ayre technic.

TONSILLECTOMY AND OTHER OPERATIONS ON THE PHARYNX, LARYNX, AND ESOPHAGUS

For several decades, tonsillectomy greatly outnumbered all other pediatric operations (Davies, 1964). Not only was the operation performed with little or no indication (often on siblings as a prophylactic measure), but it was assumed that any physician could operate and that any human could anesthetize (Compton and others, 1955). It is not sur-

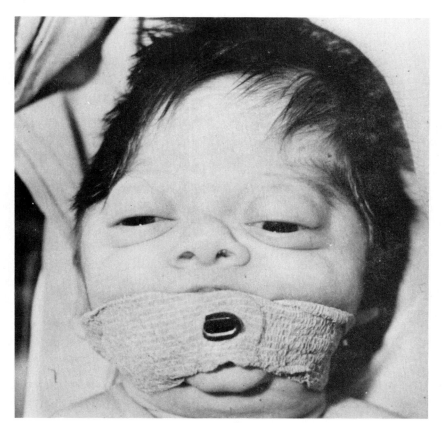

Fig. 21-2. Newborn with Apert's syndrome and choanal atresia. Normally a nose-breather at birth, an infant with choanal atresia may die unless the mouth is kept open with an oral airway.

prising that such conditions led to many preventable deaths. Mortality figures have been difficult to obtain, and those available probably reflect the more successful records (Cummings, 1954). Alpert and associates (1968) estimated one death per 1800 operations, while Tate (1963) estimated one in 15,000. The fact that tonsillectomy can be safe has been attested to by a series of 35,000 tonsillectomies performed without mortality at the Pittsburgh Eye and Ear Infirmary (Smith and Petruscak, 1974).

The situation today is considerably improved but not entirely corrected. Since the operation is questioned by some and openly condemned by others, it is being performed more carefully and much less frequently. However, in some areas it was being performed in the sitting position without intubation as recently as 1978.

Formerly, surgeons who admitted children to the hospital on the day of operation were open to criticism. The more concerned admitted their patients the day before, though all were hospitalized for 24 hours after surgery. The latest development is to perform tonsillectomy as an outpatient procedure (Ahlgren and others, 1971). Under the careful precautions observed this appears to be justified, though few have adopted the practice.

The indication for tonsillectomy today is seldom mere hypertrophy. Some degree of hearing loss or recurrent infection is more often listed as justification (Haggerty, 1968).

In the preoperative examination one naturally examines the tonsils for degree of enlargement or inflammation. One should also have the child breathe with the mouth closed to estimate adenoidal hypertrophy. Not only does marked airway obstruction promise greater technical difficulty during anesthesia, but Noonan (1965) recognized that longstanding obstruction by hypertrophied tonsils and adenoids could cause cor pulmonale and cardiac failure. Talbot and Robertson (1973) collected a total of 40 such cases with 10% mortality. Suspicion of such a situation should be aroused in any child with extremely large tonsils. Liver enlargement, disten-

sion of cervical veins, and other signs call for definitive cardiac and ventilation studies and appropriate corrective measures prior to operation (Edison and Kerth, 1973).

It is also particularly important to inspect the teeth, since tonsillectomy often is performed on children who are losing their primary dentition. Any teeth missing before operation should be carefully noted. A tooth that is loose should be pointed out to parent and child, with explanation that it may be necessary to remove it. Sometimes the anesthesiologist is asked to remove it while the child is asleep (be sure to save it). It is also quite possible for the surgeon to dislodge or chip teeth in the application of a mouth gag or during other intraoperative manipulation.

Classic studies by Eckenhoff (1953), Jackson and associates (1953), and others have demonstrated that children may have severe emotional disturbances following tonsillectomy and require the same careful management as children facing more serious procedures.

As previously described, the anesthetic management usually includes mild sedation and use of atropine for drying of secretions and for vagal depression, followed by induction with nitrous oxide–oxygen and halothane or with thiopental in larger children (Burnap, 1962). Thousands of tonsillectomies were reasonably performed under ether on supine patients without intubation, but with replacement of ether by such depressant agents as halothane, intubation became mandatory and now is the accepted standard practice.

Intubation is easily performed under nitrous oxide and halothane, but succinylcholine may be used either intravenously (1.5 mg/kg) or intramuscularly (1.5 to 2 mg/kg) to facilitate the procedure. The endotracheal tube should be as small as is feasible in order to increase the surgeon's mobility, and it is positioned in the middle of the mouth (Fig. 21-3). It is usually held in place by the groove-bladed tongue depressor that is part of the Ring adaptation of the Brown-Davis gag (Fig. 21-4). The endotracheal tube should be long enough to be kept out of the

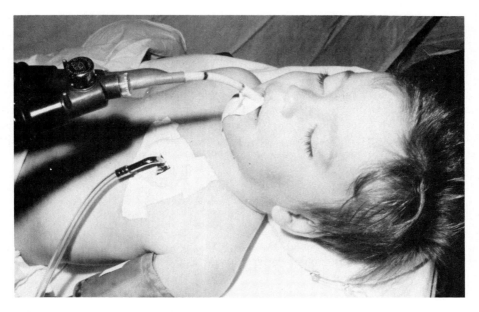

Fig. 21-3. For tonsillectomy, the endotracheal tube is fixed to the middle of the lower lip.

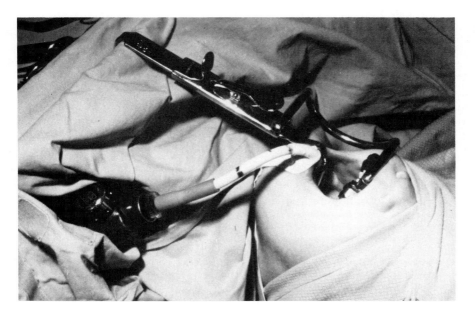

Fig. 21-4. Patient in position for tonsillectomy. Brown-Davis mouth gag, supported by instrument table, holds mouth open, and groove in the tongue blade holds endotracheal tube in place.

surgical field. We prefer endotracheal tubes in sizes less than 5.5 mm ID to be uncuffed.

Whatever technic is used, the endotracheal tube can become compressed, angulated, or dislodged. Thus, observation of ventilatory exchange, which may be either assisted or controlled, is of particular importance throughout the entire operation, and continuous precordial stethoscopic monitoring is mandatory.

493

Cardiac arrhythmias have been observed frequently during tonsillectomy. In a group of 29 children, Soule and Mazuzan (1969) reported 8 with nodal rhythm or wandering pacemaker, 13 with premature ventricular contractions, 8 with pulsus bigeminus, and 4 with multifocal tachycardia. None of these arrhythmias produced hypotension, however, and 10,000 tonsillectomy procedures were reported without mortality. This experience, and that of others, confirms the high incidence of disturbing arrhythmias during tonsillectomy and their lack of major significance. Careful stethoscopic monitoring and observation of blood pressure have been successful in our own work over the past 30 years, and ECG has not been considered essential in healthy children.

If the operation requires only 15 to 20 minutes, thermometric temperature monitoring does not seem necessary, provided that the anesthesiologist observes skin temperature with intelligence. Children who are operated on early in the morning may start taking fluids in time to prevent dehydration, but infusions usually are started for administration of atropine and postoperative sedatives.

Use of epinephrine by surgeons during tonsillectomy must be carefully restricted but is not absolutely prohibited. Three or four drops of 1:200,000 epinephrine solution used in the adenoidal bed speeds hemostasis and has not caused significant cardiac irritability in our experience. The adult limit (10 ml of 1:100,000 epinephrine in 10 minutes) recommended by Katz and associates (1962) seems a reasonable guide. However, by substituting 1:100,000 phenylephrine, surgeons can use twice as much with equally good results and without the hazards encountered when epinephrine is used (Katz, 1965).

Bleeding during operation seldom is excessive, but exsanguinating hemorrhage has occurred with tearing of carotid vessels, and careful measurement in routine cases can show surprising data (McNeill, 1967). Nowill and Ridall (1969) found that out of 2055 children undergoing tonsillectomy during a 5-year study, 43% lost more than 10% of their total blood volume!

Before a child regains active reflexes toward completion of operation, the anesthesiologist should auscultate both sides of the chest to rule out the presence of aspirated blood or secretions and, under direct laryngoscopic visualization, should check mouth and pharynx for blood or other debris that could cause irritation following extubation.

Laryngeal spasm following extubation can be quite troublesome after tonsillectomy. Methods for avoiding this include extubation while the child is either quite deeply or very slightly anesthetized and use of either a narcotic or a topical anesthetic to reduce the child's sensitivity to stimulation. Baraka (1978) recommends intravenous administration of lidocaine, 2 mg/kg, prior to extubation. Steward (1978) reports use of ephrane for tonsillectomy, in place of halothane, with complete elimination of extubation spasm. Subapneic doses of succinylcholine have also been recommended.

One method that reduces the incidence of spasm is to spray 4% lidocaine around the endotracheal tube on completion of the operation and then delay extubation until the child is nearly awake. The child is turned face down for transportation and postoperative nursing ("T & A" position, p. 220).

Postoperative tonsillectomy: the "tonsil bleeder"

Occasionally bleeding will continue after tonsillectomy, and it will be necessary to reanesthetize the child in order to remove clots and to pack or suture the bleeding area. This situation involves several hazards, and as noted by Alexander and associates (1965), failure to initiate prompt action in this situation has been one of the chief sources of tonsillectomy death. Atropine certainly should be repeated, and more sedation often may be needed. By this time, the child may have been without fluids for several hours and should receive an infusion before the second anesthetic is started. The anesthesiologist must look for evidence of excess bleeding and shock. There may be blood in the bed, but often the child has swallowed most of the blood, and the loss can only be guessed by pulse, blood pressure, and the color of the skin and mucous membranes. Transfusion may be necessary prior to reoperation (Holden and Maher, 1965).

The presence of blood in the patient's stomach introduces the hazard of regurgitation and aspiration, just as if the patient had eaten recently. In this situation my preference would be to induce the child rapidly with an inhalation agent, preferably halothane, intubate the trachea, and leave the tube in place until the child is truly awake, so that there can be no danger of aspirating vomited blood clots. One should attempt to suction the stomach while the patient is still anesthetized. A large tube must be used if clots are to be removed. Davies (1964a) also emphasized the importance of this complication but reported only one death in 546 cases. He, too, stresses the danger of using relaxants for this procedure and favors halothane, but the appropriately termed "crash" induction is widely accepted.

Pharyngeal abscess

Rarely seen but always a major threat to life is a large pharyngeal abscess that can release great quantities of pus to flood the pharynx and occlude the larynx and trachea.

If the abscess does not obstruct the airway and is not on the point of breaking, general anesthesia with endotracheal intubation is a reasonable choice. With a large, "ripe," obstructing abscess, however, induction and intubation invite obvious hazards that are better avoided. In this situation, essential points include the following:

1. Establish effective atropinization.
2. Position the child on his side.
3. Keep an approach to the pharynx available with a bite block.
4. Prepare strong "suction" with a rigid "tonsil" suction tip.
5. Retain gag reflex

With these essentials, several approaches may be used. Bennett (1943) advocated nitrous oxide analgesia with retention of the gag reflex, now somewhat of a lost art. The proposal of Leigh and Belton (1948) to apply topical anesthesia and then aspirate the abscess still makes a great deal of sense, especially if one uses enough sedation to make the child manageable (without reducing the cough reflex). Here the better understanding of morphine comes into excellent use, for it can be well controlled, involves few side effects, and preserves patient cooperation, and moderate analgesia usually precedes significant respiratory depression. Divided doses of morphine, 0.10 mg/kg, (or meperidine, 0.25 mg/kg) by intravenous infusion can be used to establish the desired effect over a 10- or 15-minute period and can be promptly reversed when desired with naloxone (Narcan), which has been shown by Fischer and Cooke (1973) to be safe and reliable for infants and children in doses of 0.005 mg/kg to 0.01 mg/kg.

Ludwig's angina

Involving quite a different problem of equal danger is Ludwig's angina, a diffuse cellulitis often originating from dental infection and spreading to involve the floor of the mouth in such a firm and massive swelling that a child cannot open his mouth (Gross and Nieburg, 1977). For the anesthesiologist, visualization of the hypopharynx or glottis may be impossible, even with the child under general anesthesia. Furthermore, the inflammatory nature of the process is believed to make the carotid sinus more sensitive to stimulation and increase the risk of sudden cardiac asystole.

The usual operative procedure for this condition has been deep incision under the ramus of the jaw, requiring a moderate degree of analgesia. The degree of involvement naturally varies, and preoperative evaluation of swelling and restriction of jaw mobility is essential. If the swelling is minimal, inhalation induction may be permissible for intubation. If the condition is full-blown, however, most anesthetic agents invite considerable risk. Intravenous barbiturates, relaxants, and ketamine would seem to be definitely contraindicated, and general anesthesia is extremely hazardous. In 1941, when this problem was seen more frequently, Williams and Marcus advised preliminary incision of pretracheal tissues under local anesthesia, with exposure of the trachea, so that instant tracheotomy could be performed. With this precaution, just enough thiopental was administered to allow the necessary incision for drainage of the infected area.

Operations on the larynx

Some years ago, only relatively short procedures were attempted on the larynx of infants and children, but the field has expanded to include not only excision of polyps and other momentary operations but also repair of laryngeal defects of larger proportions and use of the laser. All three types of surgery require special methods of anesthesia to provide satisfactory working conditions and at the same time furnish adequate ventilation.

The removal of laryngeal polyps and papillomas (Fig. 21-5) has been accomplished in the past by means of snares or cauterization. The presence of any kind of tumor in the upper airways involves the danger of respiratory obstruction from the outset, with sudden complete occlusion if the tumor should unexpectedly become inverted and trapped between the vocal cords.

For the simple use of snares or excision and cauterization of such lesions, the usual procedure has been to begin with full atropinization and minimal sedation and to induce anesthesia with halothane and oxygen. In order to provide maximal oxygenation, the customary nitrous oxide is reduced or eliminated, depending on the degree of obstruction present. Airway obstruction also complicates the picture by slowing anesthetic induction quite noticeably. It is decidedly helpful in all types of airway obstruction to maintain 10 to 20 cm H_2O of positive pressure on the breathing bag throughout the respiratory cycle in order to distend the upper airway and promote exchange. An oral airway, liberally anointed with lidocaine jelly, and subsequent spraying of pharynx and glottis with 4% lidocaine also are helpful.

When the pupils have become centrally fixed and slightly constricted, the trachea is intubated with a tube of minimal allowable size in order to give the surgeon optimal working space. If the lesion is small, the surgeon may be able to introduce instruments beside the endotracheal tube and complete his task. If the surgeon needs more room or wishes to dilate the larynx, it may be neces-

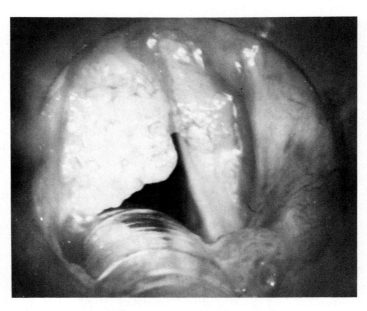

Fig. 21-5. Laryngeal papillomas. Endotracheal tube wound with aluminum foil is seen entering the glottis.

sary to remove the endotracheal tube. Then it usually is advisable to establish a relatively deep plane of anesthesia with halothane and supplement this with topical anesthetic. Adequate relaxation and analgesia will be provided for a short procedure, and the time may be prolonged simply by creating ventilation by external compression of the chest.

Tracheal resection and other major procedures

Use of the suspension laryngoscope for microlaryngeal surgery, resection of subglottic stenosis, and other major procedures has stimulated the development of several new approaches to anesthetic management as well as the adaptation of more familiar ones. As described by the Finnish team of Savolainen and Grahne (1973), lesions of the upper trachea may be handled by using a low tracheostomy for anesthesia and ventilation. Lesions of the lower trachea are more difficult to manage. These authors described unsuccessful trials of several agents due to failure to control coughing or other reflexes, but

they finally decided on the use of methoxyflurane (Penthrane) supplemented with clobutinol chloride (Silomat), which was most effective as an antitussive.

Several methods for insufflating gases into the trachea have been devised in this country. The Sanders ventilating bronchoscope (1967) was one of the first instruments introduced for continued ventilation during instrumentation of the larynx. Carden and Ferguson (1973) and Carden and Vest (1974) used short cuffed endotracheal tubes placed below the vocal cords combined with ventilation by a high-pressure jet that is attached to the cuff. Carden and associates (1976) also suggested percutaneous transtracheal insertion of a high-pressure jet device for use in microlaryngeal surgery.

Laser surgery of the larynx

The introduction of the laser for removal of laryngeal papillomas has required the introduction of several modifications in anesthesia (Fig. 21-6).

The laser beam burns through any soft ma-

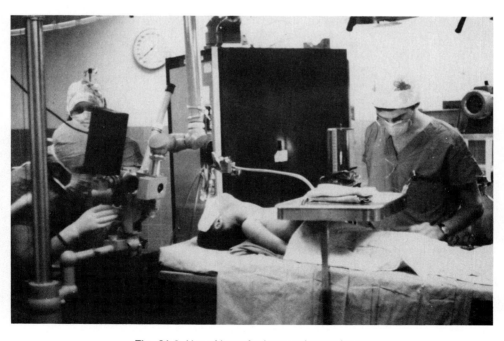

Fig. 21-6. Use of laser for laryngeal procedures.

terial, such as body tissues, rubber airways, and plastic endotracheal tubes, and ignites flammable plastic. When the beam strikes metal objects, however, including aluminum foil, the beam is deflected and dispersed. The technic devised by Snow and associates (1974) and Norton and associates (1976) consists of using nonflammable rubber endotracheal tubes that are wound with protective aluminum foil (Fig. 21-7), obtainable at radio equipment shops as sensing tape, or using the flexible metal endotracheal tube introduced by Norton in 1978 (Fig. 21-8).

For the initial removal of papillomas in the anterior glottis, the child is intubated with the nonflammable endotracheal tube (of smaller than usual dimensions) and carried on nonrebreathing technic while the suspension laryngoscope is positioned. The eyes must be covered by thick pads strapped securely in place. Glottis and trachea are sprayed with lidocaine, and dexamethasone (0.1 mg/kg) is administered intravenously to prevent glottic swelling. Succinylcholine is given either by intermittent injection or by 0.2% drip, and a nasogastric tube is inserted. With the endotracheal tube lying in the posterior angle of the glottic chink, most of the obstructing papillomas can be removed without difficulty. If the endotracheal tube impedes access to masses in the posterior part of the glottis, Norton's technic has been to arrange a Venturi system by mounting a jet needle on a clamp that is then positioned inside the lumen of the laryngoscope. With an H-tank of oxygen, a two-stage reducing valve, 6 feet of plastic tubing, and a modified Speedaire Blo-gun* (Fig. 21-9), the child's chest is expanded rhythmically by manual operation of the Blo-gun. At pressures of 4 to 6 kg, sufficient force is developed by Venturi to expand the chest, even though the tip of the jet is 3 or 4 inches above the vocal cords and inside the lumen of the laryngoscope. With this management, the surgeon has unlimited time to operate. At the end of the procedure, all surgical and anesthetic apparatus is disassembled, an orotracheal airway is inserted, and ventilation is supported by bag and mask until adequate return of spontaneous respiration. Any gas remaining in the stomach is removed, and the nasogastric tube is withdrawn. In the recovery room the child is placed in an oxygen tent with heavy mist until ready for discharge to the nursing division.

In an occasional situation there is enough glottic swelling to require reinsertion of the endotracheal tube for 2 or 3 hours, after which time the swelling is reduced enough to allow extubation without further difficulty.

*No. 2X492, Dayton Electric Mfg. Co., Chicago, Ill.

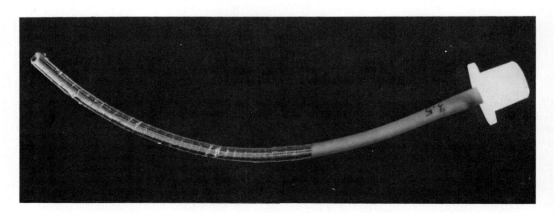

Fig. 21-7. Red rubber tube with aluminum tape to disperse the incident light beam. (From Norton, M. L., and de Vos, P.: Ann. Otol. Rhinol. Laryngol. **87**:554, 1978.)

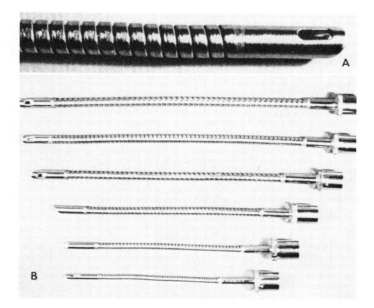

Fig. 21-8. A, Enlargement of the tip of a metal endotracheal tube. **B,** Endotracheal tubes of various sizes (2.4 mm ID through 6.4 mm ID). (From Norton, M. L., and de Vos, P.: Ann. Otol. Rhinol. Laryngol. **87**:554, 1978.)

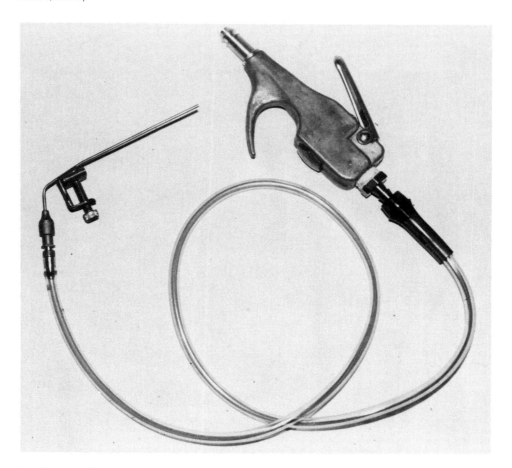

Fig. 21-9. Modified Speedaire Blo-gun *(right)* and jet needle. (From Norton, M. L., Strong, M. S., Snow, J. C., and others: Ann. Otol. Rhinol. Laryngol. **85**:656, 1976.)

Technics of laser surgery were described by Strong and associates (1976).

Anesthesia for performance of tracheostomy

In acute severe upper airway obstruction, when the patient is cyanotic and near death, no anesthesia is needed, but an airway must be established at once. Passage of an endotracheal tube with immediate ventilation will usually be the most rapid method available (Smith, 1972). If a bronchoscope is available, this may be forced through an obstruction that will not yield to an endotracheal tube, but the risk of severe trauma will be greater. Once in place, the bronchoscope offers a better guide to the surgeon as he cuts into the neck toward the trachea, which can be difficult to locate.

After ventilation has been reestablished by endotracheal tube or bronchoscope, a tracheostomy can be performed without haste (Fig. 21-10). There is a good chance that the patient might awaken as soon as oxygenation is restored and that anesthesia would be needed. This can be provided by local infiltration of the wound with 1% lidocaine or procaine or by administration of nitrous oxide and halothane by endotracheal route.

When the surgeon is ready to insert the tracheostomy tube, the endotracheal tube (or bronchoscope) is retracted but not removed, since several trials may be necessary before a satisfactory fitting is made. After the tracheostomy tube is in place, the anesthesia inflow tubing is transferred from the endotracheal tube to the tracheostomy tube for further ventilation or anesthesia.

Situations may arise in which glottic swelling makes intubation impossible, or an emergency may arise when there is no bronchoscope or endotracheal tube at hand (Reed

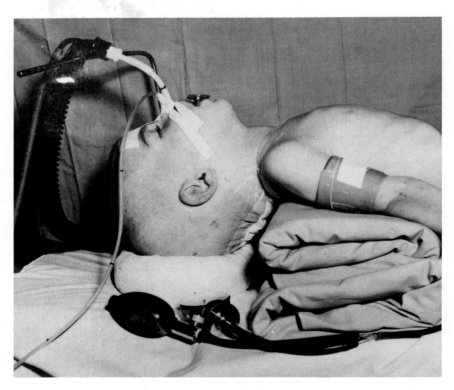

Fig. 21-10. Child prepared for elective tracheostomy.

and others, 1954). Sheldon and Pudenz (1957) advocated a spear-pointed tracheostomy set for emergency use, but as reported by Smith (1957) and Ivankovic and associates (1969), this can cause disastrous accidents by perforation of the trachea, esophagus, or great vessels. Insertion of a 15- or 16-gauge needle (Reed and others, 1954) into the trachea allows one to blow enough oxygen through it to sustain life while tracheostomy is performed, but this has also led to perforation of the esophagus and other complications. If the need should arise for instant relief of obstruction, probably the surest method is to make an incision at the cricothyroid interspace, where the trachea lies immediately under the skin, and establish an orifice. Then a short hollow tube, such as the barrel of a ball-point pen, can be inserted into the trachea to ventilate the child.

When children are not in severe respiratory distress prior to tracheostomy, induction of general anesthesia is advisable. Care must be taken not to increase the respiratory obstruction by either excitement or irritation. Mild sedation is indicated, and induction with oxygen and halothane is chosen, since this offers minimal stimulation. Once adequate depth of surgical anesthesia is reached, an endotracheal tube or bronchoscope can be introduced and oxygen and halothane continued during tracheostomy.

Tracheostomy may be indicated in patients suffering from meningitis, cervical cord injury, or terminal illness. For those who are already receiving respiratory support, it will usually be necessary to detach the ventilator and use the anesthesia machine to induce anesthesia. For those who are conscious, intravenous thiopental may facilitate induction, followed by maintenance with halothane and oxygen.

When children requiring continuous nasotracheal ventilatory support are to have tracheostomy, one can substitute a manual ventilating bag for the power-driven ventilator, take the child to the operating room, connect him to an anesthesia machine, and induce light anesthesia with halothane and oxygen.

In the most severely weakened patients it may be safest to perform the tracheostomy under local infiltration, although this usually is an uncomfortable procedure.

Anesthesia after tracheostomy

When tracheostomy has already been performed on a child, anesthesia is considerably facilitated. If the tracheostomy is well established, one may take out the tube and insert a shortened endotracheal tube into the stoma. If the stoma is not well healed, it may be necessary to start induction with the tracheostomy tube in place. The inner tube may be removed and a small endotracheal tube inserted in its place (Fig. 21-11). Usually it is possible to remove the entire tube after the child is asleep and insert a larger endotracheal tube. In either case, gas flows should be reduced to about half those used by mask in order to reduce tracheal irritation. Since odors are less noticeable, children seldom object to this form of induction.

Foreign bodies in trachea or esophagus

Inhalation or ingestion of foreign bodies is common in younger children, especially those in the exploratory years between 2 and 4 (Tucker, 1964). Removal of articles from the esophagus is not usually a complicated procedure. One first tries to determine what object has lodged in the esophagus and where it is, and then one inquires as to what food might be in the stomach. Allowance is made for digestion of gastric contents, sedation is provided, and either inhalation or intravenous anesthesia with endotracheal intubation should offer little difficulty. The use of a relatively small endotracheal tube and intermittent doses of succinylcholine facilitate the endoscopy.

Unless the anesthesiologist is reasonably sure that there is no food in the child's stomach, the endotracheal tube is left in place after operation until the child is awake.

As an emergency measure when foreign bodies obstruct the upper airway, the Heimlich maneuver (1975) is recommended for patients of all ages before resorting to inversion

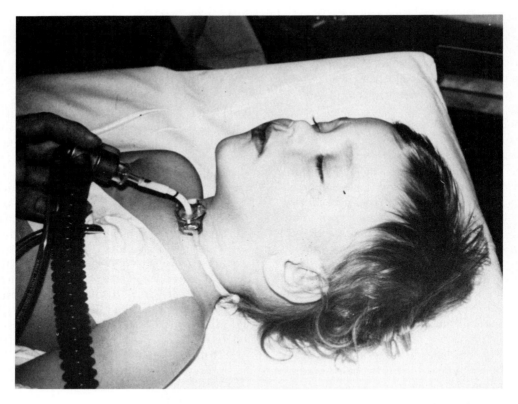

Fig. 21-11. Induction of anesthesia in child with established tracheostomy. (From Smith, R. M.: Anesthesia for pediatric otolaryngology. In Ferguson, C. F., and Kendig, E. L., Jr., editors: Pediatric otolaryngology, Philadelphia, 1972, W. B. Saunders Co.)

or back-slapping. General anesthesia is used for removal of foreign bodies that do not cause acute hypoxia.

When foreign bodies lodge in the larynx, trachea, or bronchi (Fig. 21-12), the situation is much more complicated and dangerous, first because respiration may be seriously obstructed by the presence of the foreign body and second because the use of an endotracheal tube will not be possible. Without question, the removal of foreign bodies from the respiratory tract is one of the most exciting and exacting procedures known, and success depends greatly on excellent anesthesia. Numerous approaches to this interesting problem have been suggested by Robinson and Mushin (1956), Burrington and Cotton (1972), Smith (1972), Baraka (1974), Law and Kosloske (1976), and others.

When possible, it is particularly important to wait for digestion of gastric contents before removal of foreign bodies from the airway is attempted.

Since the abandonment of ether and methoxyflurane, it is no longer possible to depend on spontaneous respiration during bronchoscopic procedures in children. Instead, one starts with effective atropinization and induces anesthesia with halothane and oxygen (using nitrous oxide if the child is not hypoxic) until anesthesia is deep enough to allow endotracheal instrumentation. At this time the glottis, trachea, and carina are sprayed with 4% lidocaine (up to 5 mg/kg).

Halothane is administered for approximately 5 minutes at 2.0% to 3.0% to establish sufficient tissue level, an infusion is

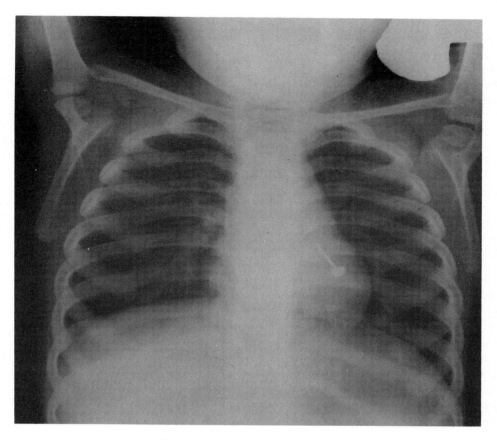

Fig. 21-12. Foreign body in bronchus.

started, and the surgeon is allowed to proceed using either a ventilating bronchoscope or a bronchoscope with a side arm through which oxygen and anesthetic gases can be introduced. An even plane of anesthesia with satisfactory oxygenation should be possible. However, if the bronchoscope is advanced far down one bronchus, distribution may be severely reduced, and partial withdrawal of the instrument may be required. Should ventilation via bronchoscope become inadequate, an anesthesia assistant should be present to add external thoracic compression. Monitoring by stethoscope is definitely mandatory, since the airway is in constant danger and the room may be darkened for fluoroscopic guidance. An audible pulse monitor is also valuable, and any reduction in heart rate calls for immediate procedures to improve oxygena-

tion plus administration of more atropine if indicated.

To find and grasp the foreign body may require many minutes during which adequate ventilation and immobility usually can be provided by continued halothane-oxygen anesthesia with supplementary morphine, though Baraka (1974) and others have advocated muscle relaxant technics throughout.

Whatever the anesthetic technic, the crucial moment comes when the surgeon finally believes he has grasped the object and attempts to remove it. If the vocal cords are not in complete relaxation, a large insecurely grasped object is easily lost at this point. It may fall back down into a bronchus or worse yet may remain in the trachea and completely obstruct exchange. This can be fatal unless the surgeon has the presence of mind to push the object back down into a bronchus, allowing ventilation in the other lung.

To prevent such a problem and provide the best possible conditions for removal of a large foreign body, we prefer to let the surgeon grasp the object and then have him wait while a full-relaxant intravenous dose of succinylcholine (2 mg/kg) provides maximal glottic opening and optimal opportunity to deliver the foreign body. If, after successful removal of the object, the surgeon desires further bronchoscopic manipulation, the child should be reoxygenated briefly with bag and mask before the bronchoscope is reinserted. If the child is still apneic after completion of bronchoscopy, it may be advisable to intubate the trachea and control respiration until adequate spontaneous ventilation returns (Robinson and Mushin, 1956).

Following instrumentation of trachea or larynx, a child should be placed in humidified oxygen and receive intravenous fluids and steroids (dexamethasone, 0.1 mg/kg) plus racemic epinephrine if signs of tracheal edema develop.

Anesthetic management of children with epiglottitis

A more complete discussion of the problems of epiglottitis is found in Chapter 27, but it seems appropriate to mention them briefly in relation to other otolaryngologic topics.

The rapid development of epiglottitis demands a well-planned approach and the co-operation of representatives of several different specialties—usually pediatrics, otolaryngology, and anesthesiology and occasionally surgery. In our institution, the Anesthesiology Department sends a member of the staff to meet the patient as he is brought into the emergency room. It is the anesthesiologist's responsibility to oxygenate the child initially, to supervise his transportation to the operating room (without visualizing the larynx or stopping for x-ray films), and to have the determining voice in deciding if and when the child should undergo anesthesia and intubation.

When intubation is undertaken, the child is brought into the operating room, usually sitting on a stretcher, and anesthesia is induced with the child still in the sitting position using oxygen and halothane. After the child has become drowsy, an infusion is started, and atropine is administered. No injection or blood sampling is performed before the child is asleep for fear of upsetting him further. The chief problem is maintaining sufficient exchange to oxygenate the child and coax enough halothane through the obstructed airway to produce anesthesia. One must assist ventilation with considerable pressure but avoid inflating the stomach. A higher concentration of halothane is required, and it often takes three or four times as long to reach the state where relaxation and *centrally fixed pupils* indicate that the child is ready for intubation. Neither nitrous oxide nor any relaxant is used prior to intubation.

As now practiced in many institutions, we insert an oral endotracheal tube when a child has been acutely hypoxic and change to a nasal tube after the child has become oxygenated and stabilized. Thus far, we have not had great difficulty in passing an oral endotracheal tube. Standard plastic tubes are used without a stylet, the use of which we feel is apt to be more traumatic. In several cases where the lumen of the glottis was entirely occluded, it was possible to find the proper point of entry by having an assistant compress the chest forcibly and noticing where the expiratory passage opened. By aiming the tip of the endotracheal tube at that spot and advancing the tube with a gentle twisting motion, we were able to insert the tube in the glottis. At other times we have simply aimed the tip of the tube so that it passed between and just above the arytenoids, which almost always are discernable even when the epiglottis is greatly swollen.

The treatment of epiglottitis by intubation has been so successful that we now are more concerned by the occasional need to intubate a child with laryngotracheitis. As seen in Fig. 21-13, subglottic inflammation characteristic of laryngotracheitis carries a real threat of leading to tracheal stenosis if the patient is

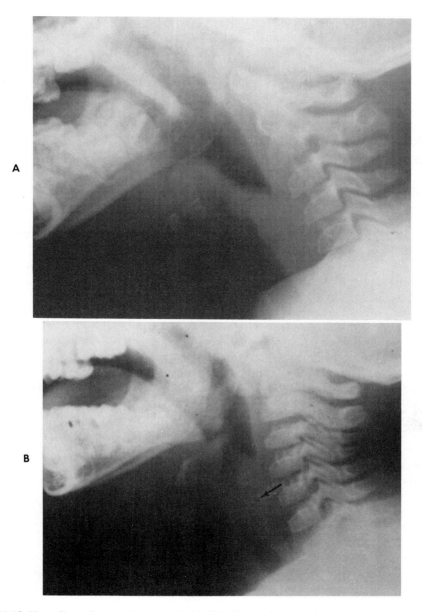

Fig. 21-13. X-ray films of upper airway. **A,** Epiglottitis. Upper airway is obstructed by marked swelling of epiglottis. Note also the loss of normal curvature of cervical spine. **B,** Laryngotracheitis. Arrow points to airway constriction below the vocal cords. (Courtesy Department of Radiology, The Children's Hospital Medical Center, Boston.)

subjected to the trauma of prolonged intubation, while epiglottitis bears little or no danger of this complication, with extubation in 24 to 48 hours almost invariably followed by complete recovery.

DIAGNOSTIC PROCEDURES

Laryngoscopy and tracheoscopy are frequently indicated for diagnosis of the etiology of stridor and other problems. Laryngoscopy can be performed without anesthesia or with topical anesthesia, but if relaxation is desired, general (halothane) anesthesia is preferable.

Tracheography may be desired for further diagnostic details. In small infants this is most safely done without anesthesia. With the aid of a laryngoscope or an anterior commissure laryngoscope, a small (19-gauge) plastic catheter is passed through the larynx, 2 or 3 ml of radiopaque material are injected, the catheter is withdrawn, and x-ray films are taken (Flake and Ferguson, 1955; Wittenborg and others, 1967).

For older children it is preferable to induce general anesthesia with a nondepressant agent that does not incite laryngeal irritation.

After induction, anesthesia is discontinued, allowing several minutes for instillation of oil and the x-ray exposures. Thorough clearing of the airway is necessary before the child is returned to his bed (Austin, 1963).

For diagnostic bronchoscopy, children are handled as described for removal of foreign bodies. Here, however, the risk is related more to the child's underlying disease than to the problem of instrumentation. Halothane and topical anesthesia are effective together and may be supplemented further by intermittent doses of succinylcholine. Ventilation is assisted or controlled by occlusion of the bronchoscope with a finger or coverglass and rapid gas flow, by use of a ventilating bronchoscope (Sanders, 1967), or by manual compression of the thorax. If x-ray films are taken, a standard metal precordial stethoscope will interfere with the picture. We have found that this problem is nicely overcome by substituting a stethoscope head fashioned out of radiolucent plastic material (see Fig. 9-7).

If an entirely quiet chest is required, repeated doses of succinylcholine may be used. Active coughing is often preferred for diagnosis and therapy, however, and can be induced by limiting initial topical anesthesia and succinylcholine. Prior to extubation, coughing should be encouraged to allow generous oxygenation and clearing of secretions.

When bronchography is combined with bronchoscopy, the obstruction of airways by radiopaque material and the turning of the child back and forth in a darkened room add up to a sizable risk. Here, we believe, the anesthesiologist needs a competent assistant to help with monitoring, positioning, and administration of agents.

Bronchography usually follows bronchoscopy. Thus, as soon as the bronchoscope is withdrawn, the anesthesiologist passes an endotracheal tube and attaches the desired circle apparatus or T-system, to which we add a curved adapter with an open-end extension for suction (Rovenstine elbow adapter). The open end is fitted with a perforated rubber nipple. For introduction of opaque material into the bronchial tree, a plastic catheter is introduced through the perforated nipple and advanced inside the endotracheal tube to the desired location in the trachea (Fig. 21-14). Thus, an airtight system is maintained throughout the entire study, and complete ventilatory control is always possible by intermittent succinylcholine supplementation of halothane and oxygen. This is especially helpful during injection of the dye, since the catheter can be located under fluoroscopy without haste or hypoxia, and respiration can be halted at any stage of inspiration or expiration for individual films. With this method, the ability to work slowly allows more precision and also enables the endoscopist to add the dye gradually, often markedly reducing the total amount.

Again, monitoring is of maximum importance. The plastic precordial stethoscope is of tremendous assistance. Next best is an esophageal stethoscope, but this may interfere somewhat with intubation and bronchoscopy. Blood pressure measurement is essential, but other monitors may be impractical.

It often helps to have an assistant keep a finger on the child's femoral pulse, and while the room is darkened, a video screen makes the activity of lungs, diaphragm, and heart visible to all.

After films are completed, an attempt is made to remove the dye and other secre-

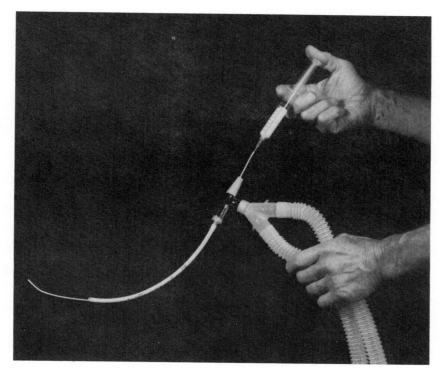

Fig. 21-14. Technic for performance of bronchogram. Dye is injected through catheter that enters system through perforated rubber stopper, maintaining an airtight system that allows use of controlled ventilation.

tions, but one should not expect much in return and should refrain from traumatizing the airways. After full return of spontaneous respiration and cough reflex as well as ample oxygenation, the endotracheal tube is removed, and the child is returned to the recovery room and given oxygen, mist, and dexamethasone (0.1 mg/kg). Any appearance of postoperative respiratory irritation or obstruction should be regarded with alarm. Inhalation treatment with racemic epinephrine (1 ml of 2.5% racemic epinephrine in 8 ml of water) is advised to suit individual requirements (Adair and others, 1971).

BIBLIOGRAPHY

Adair, J. C., King, W. H., and Jordan, W. S.: Ten-year experience with IPPB in the treatment of acute laryngotracheobronchitis, Anesth. Analg. (Cleve.) **50:**649, 1971.

Ahlgren, E. W., Bennett, E. J., and Stephen, C. R.: Outpatient pediatric anesthesiology; a case series, Anesth. Analg. (Cleve.) **50:**402, 1971.

Alexander, D. W., Graff, T. W., and Kelley, E.: Factors in tonsillectomy mortality, Arch. Otolaryngol. **82:**409, 1965.

Alpert, J. J., Peterson, O. L., and Colton, T.: Tonsillectomy and adenoidectomy, Lancet **1:**1319, 1968.

Austin, S.: Anesthesia for bronchoscopy and bronchography in children, Anesth. Analg. (Cleve.) **42:**632, 1963.

Baraka, A.: Bronchoscopic removal of inhaled foreign bodies in children, Br. J. Anaesth. **46:**124, 1974.

Baraka, A.: Intravenous lidocaine controls extubation laryngospasm in children, Anesth. Analg. (Cleve.) **57:**506, 1978.

Battaglia, J. D., and Lockhart, C. H.: Management of acute epiglottitis by nasotracheal intubation, Am. J. Dis. Child. **129:**334, 1975.

Bell, T. H.: Bronchography in children, Arch. Dis. Child. **42:**55, 1967.

Benjamin, B., and O'Reilly, B.: Acute epiglottitis in infants and children, Ann. Otol. Rhinol. Laryngol. **85:**565, 1976.

Bennett, J. M.: Anesthetic management for drainage of submandibular space (Ludwig's angina), Anesthesiology **4:**25, 1943.

Bethmann, W., and Hochstein, H. J.: Anesthesiological experience in 4000 operations on infants and children for cleft lip and palate, Plast. Reconstr. Surg. **41:** 129, 1968.

Bougas, T. P., and Smith, R. M.: Pathologic airway obstruction in children, Anesth. Analg. (Cleve.) **37:**137, 1958.

Burnap, T. K.: Anesthesia for operations in ophthalmology and otolaryngology, Int. Anesthesiol. Clin. **1:**195, 1962.

Burrington, J. D., and Cotton, E. K.: Removal of foreign bodies from the tracheobronchial tree, J. Pediatr. Surg. **7:**119, 1972.

Carden, E., Becker, G., and Hamood, H.: Percutaneous jet ventilation, Ann. Otol. Rhinol. Laryngol. **85:** 652, 1976.

Carden, E., and Ferguson, G. B.: A new technique for micro-laryngeal surgery in infants, Laryngoscope **83:** 691, 1973.

Carden, E., and Ferguson, G. B.: Large tracheal papillomas; a difficult anesthetic problem and an apparent cure; a case report, Ann. Otol. Rhinol. Laryngol. **84:** 233, 1975.

Carden, E., and Vest, H. R.: Further advances in anesthetic technics for microlaryngeal surgery, Anesth. Analg. (Cleve.) **53:**584, 1974.

Catlin, F. I., and Bordley, J. E.: Otolaryngologic disorders. In Ravitch, M. M., Welch, K. J., Benson, C. D., and others, editors: Pediatric surgery, ed. 3, Chicago, 1979, Year Book Medical Publishers, Inc.

Chung, B., Naraghi, M., and Adriani, J.: Sympathomimetic effects of cocaine and their influence on halothane and enflurane anesthesia, Anesth. Rev **5:**16, 1978.

Cohen, S. R., and Chai, J.: Epiglottis; twenty-year study with tracheotomy, Ann. Otol. Rhinol. Laryngol. **87:** 461, 1978.

Collins, V. J., and Granatelli, A.: Anesthesia for tonsillectomy in children; endotracheal technic with cardiovascular observations, J.A.M.A. **161:**5, 1956.

Compton, J., Bader, M. N., Haas, M. V., and Lange, M.: Who is administering anesthesia today? Hosp. Management **80:**48, 1955.

Cummings, G. O.: Mortalities and morbidities following 20,000 tonsil and adenoidectomies, Laryngoscope **64:** 647, 1954.

Davies, D. D.: Anaesthetic mortality in tonsillectomy and adenoidectomy, Br. J. Anaesth. **36:**110, 1964.

Davies, D. D.: Reanesthetizing cases of tonsillectomy and adenoidectomy because of persistent postoperative hemorrhage, Br. J. Anaesth. **36:**244, 1964a.

Eckenhoff, J. E.: Preanesthetic sedation of children; analysis of the side effects of tonsillectomy and adenoidectomy, Arch. Otolaryngol. **57:**411, 1953.

Eden, A. N., and Larkin, V. D.: Corticosteroid treatment of croup, Pediatrics **33:**768, 1964.

Edison, B. D., and Kerth, J. D.: Tonsilloadenoid hypertrophy resulting in cor pulmonale, Arch. Otolaryngol. **98:**205, 1973.

Fearon, B., and Cotton, R.: Surgical correction of subglottic stenosis of the larynx, Ann. Otol. Rhinol. Laryngol. **81:**1, 1972.

Fearon, B., and Dickson, J.: Bilateral choanal atresia in the newborn; a plan of action, Laryngoscope **78:** 1487, 1968.

Ferguson, C. F.: Congenital choanal atresia. In Kendig, E. L., editor: Disorders of the respiratory tract in children, ed. 2, Philadelphia, 1972. W. B. Saunders Co.

Ferguson, C. F., and Kendig, E. L.: Pediatric otolaryngology. In Kendig, E. L., editor: Disorders of the respiratory tract in children, ed. 2, Philadelphia, 1972, W. B. Saunders Co.

Fink, B. R.: The etiology and treatment of laryngeal spasm, Anesthesiology **17:**569, 1956.

Fink, B. R.: The human larynx; a functional study, New York, 1975, Raven Press.

Fischer, C. G., and Cooke, D. R.: The respiratory and narcotic antagonistic effects of naloxone in anesthetized infants, paper presented at annual convention of American Society of Anesthesiologists, San Francisco, 1973.

Flake, C., and Ferguson, C. F.: Tracheography and bronchography in infants and children, Pediatr. Clin. North Am. **2:**279, 1955.

Frazer, J. E.: The development of the larynx. J. Anat. **44:**156, 1910.

Graff, T.: Acid base balance during halothane anesthesia for tonsillectomy, Anesth. Analg. (Cleve.) **43:**620, 1964.

Gross, S. J., and Nieburg, P. I.: Ludwig angina in childhood, Am. J. Dis. Child. **131:**291, 1977.

Haggerty, R. J.: Diagnosis and treatment; tonsils and adenoids; a problem revisited, Pediatrics **41:**818, 1968.

Hast, M. G.: Applied embryology of the larynx, Can. J. Otolaryngol. **3:**4, 1974.

Heimlich, H. J.: A life-saving maneuver to prevent foodchoking, J.A.M.A. **234:**398, 1975.

Holden, H. G., and Maher, J. J.: Some aspects of blood loss and fluid balance in pediatric tonsillectomy, Br. Med. J. **2:**1349, 1965.

Holinger, P. H., and Brown, W. T.: Congenital webs, cysts, laryngoceles and other anomalies of the larynx, Ann. Otol. Rhinol. Laryngol. **76:**744, 1967.

Holinger, P. H., Schild, J. A., Kutnick, S. L., and Holinger, L. D.: Subglottic stenosis in infants and children, Ann. Otol. Rhinol. Laryngol. **85:**591, 1976.

Ivankovic, A. D., Thomsen, S., and Rattenborg, C. C.: Fatal haemorrhage from the innominate artery after tracheostomy; a case report, Br. J. Anaesth. **41:**450, 1969.

Jackson, C., and Jackson, C. L.: Diseases of nose, throat and ear, Philadelphia, 1945, W. B. Saunders Co.

Jackson, K., Winkley, R., Faust, O. A., and others: Behavior changes indicating emotional trauma in tonsillectomized children, Pediatrics **12:**23, 1953.

Jordan, W. S., Graves, C. L., and Elwyn, R. A.: New therapy for postintubation laryngeal edema and tracheitis in children, J.A.M.A. **212:**585, 1970.

Katz, R. L.: Effects of alpha and beta adrenergic blocking agents on cyclopropane-catecholamine cardiac arrhythmias, Anesthesiology **26:**289, 1965.

Katz, R. L., Matteo, R. S., and Papper, E. M.: The injection of epinephrine during general anesthesia, Anesthesiology **23:**597, 1962.

Law, D., and Kosloske, A. M.: Management of tracheobronchial foreign bodies in children, Pediatrics **58:**362, 1976.

Lee, J. A., and Atkinson, R. S.: A synopsis of anaesthesia, ed. 7, Bristol, 1973, John Wright & Sons Ltd.

Leigh, M. D., and Belton, M. K.: Anesthesia for ear, nose and throat operations in infants and children, Anesth. Analg. (Cleve.) **27:**41, 1948.

Love, S. H. S., and Morrow, W. F. K.: Anaesthesia for bronchography in children, Anaesthesia **9:**74, 1954.

Matson, D. D.: Neurosurgery of infancy and childhood, Springfield, Ill., 1969, Charles C Thomas, Publisher.

McKenzie, W.: Risks of tonsillectomy, Lancet **2:**958, 1963.

McNeill, C. G.: A method of control for postoperative adenoidal bleeding, Can. Anaesth. Soc. J. **14:**483, 1967.

Merifield, D. O.: Anesthesiology 1970, Arch. Otolaryngol. **96:**282, 1972.

Mushin, W. W., and Lake, R.: Anaesthesia for bronchography in children, Anaesthesia **6:**88, 1951.

Noonan, J. A.: Reversible cor pulmonale due to hypertrophied tonsils and adenoids; studies in two cases, Circulation **32**(Suppl. 2):164, 1965.

Norton, M. L., and de Vos, P.: New endotracheal tube for laser surgery of the larynx, Ann. Otol. Rhinol. Laryngol. **87:**554, 1978.

Norton, M. L., Strong, M. S., Snow, J. C., and others: Endotracheal intubation and Venturi (jet) ventilation for laser microsurgery of the larynx, Ann. Otol. Rhinol. Laryngol. **85:**656, 1976.

Nowill, W. K., and Ridall, E. G.: Blood loss during adenotonsillectomy, Surgery **66:**856, 1969.

Pallister, W. K.: Anesthesia for bronchography. In Gray, T. C., and Nunn, J. F., editors: General anaesthesia, Borough Green, Kent, 1971, Butterworth & Co., Ltd.

Parkin, J. L., Stevens, M. H., and Jung, A. L.: Acquired and congenital subglottic stenosis in the infant, Ann. Otol. Rhinol. Laryngol. **85:**573, 1976.

Reed, J. P., Kemph, J. P., Hamelberg, W., and others: Studies with transtracheal artificial respiration, Anesthesiology **15:**28, 1954.

Robinson, C. L., and Mushin, W. W.: Inhaled foreign bodies, Br. Med. J. **2:**324, 1956.

Sanders, R. D.: Two ventilating attachments for bronchoscopes, Del. Med. J. **39:**170, 1967.

Savolainen, V. P., and Grahne, B.: Anaesthesia in operations for laryngeal and tracheal stenosis, Acta Otolaryngol. (Stockh.) **75:**385, 1973.

Schmidt, P. H., and Leyendijk, W.: Intranasal meningoencephalocele, Arch. Otolaryngol. **99:**402, 1974.

Sheldon, C. H., and Pudenz, R. H.: Percutaneous tracheostomy, J.A.M.A. **165:**2068, 1957.

Singer, O. R., and Wilson, W. J.: Laryngotracheobronchitis; 2 years experience with racemic epinephrine, Can. Med. Assoc. J. **115:**132, 1976.

Smith, R. B., and Petruscak, J.: Tonsillectomy mortality, J.A.M.A. **227:**557, 1974.

Smith, R. M.: Anesthetic management of patients with cystic fibrosis, Anesth. Analg. (Cleve.) **44:**143, 1965.

Smith, R. M.: The management of airway emergencies. In Green, M., and Haggerty, R. J., editors: Ambulatory pediatrics, Philadelphia, 1968, W. B. Saunders Co.

Smith, R. M.: Anesthesia for pediatric otolaryngology. In Ferguson, C. F., and Kendig, E. L., Jr., editors: Pediatric otolaryngology, Philadelphia, 1972, W. B. Saunders Co.

Smith, V. M.: Perforation of trachea during tracheostomy performed with Sheldon tracheotome, J.A.M.A. **165:**2074, 1957.

Snow, J. C., Kripke, B. J., Strong, M. S., and others: Anesthesia for carbon dioxide laser microsurgery on the larynx and trachea, Anesth. Analg. (Cleve.) **53:**507, 1974.

Soule, A. B., and Mazuzan, J. E., Jr.: Cardiac arrhythmias in the pediatric surgical patient, paper presented at Annual Convention of the American Medical Association, New York, June 1969.

Spoerel, W. E., and Greenway, R. E.: Techniques of ventilation during endolaryngeal surgery under general anaesthetic, Can. Anaesth. Soc. J. **20:**369, 1973.

Steward, D. J.: Personal communication, 1978.

Strong, M. S., Vaughan, C. W., Cooperland, S. R., and Clemente, M. A.: Recurrent respiratory papillomatosis; management with the CO_2 laser, Ann. Otol. Rhinol. Laryngol. **85:**508, 1976.

Talbot, A. R., and Robertson, L. W.: Cardiac failure with tonsil and adenoid hypertrophy, Arch. Otolaryngol. **98:**277, 1973.

Tate, N.: Death from tonsillectomy, Lancet **2:**1090, 1963.

Tucker, G. F.: The age of incidence of lodgement of single coins in the esophagus, Ann. Otol. Rhinol. Laryngol. **73:**1116, 1964.

Westley, C. R., Cotton, E. K., and Brooks, J. G.: Nebulized racemic epinephrine by IPPB for the treatment of croup; a double-blind study, Am. J. Dis. Child. **132:**484, 1978.

Williams, A. C., and Marcus, P. S.: Choice of anesthesia in Ludwig's angina, Anesth. Analg. (Cleve.) **20:**160, 1941.

Wittenborg, M. H., Gyepes, M. T., and Crocker, D.: Tracheal dynamics in infants with respiratory distress, stridor and collapsing trachea, Radiology **88:**653, 1967.

CHAPTER 22

Anesthesia for outpatient and emergency surgery

Anesthesia for elective outpatient procedures
Anesthesia for emergency and unscheduled
  operations

ANESTHESIA FOR ELECTIVE OUTPATIENT PROCEDURES

Outpatient surgery, whether elective or emergency, has frequently held special disadvantages for the anesthesiologist. Operations performed in outpatient areas have usually entailed relatively little surgical risk, while the use of general anesthesia, wherever administered, must involve major hazards that are significantly increased in such situations.

The anesthesiologist working in outpatient areas frequently has been handicapped by poor working facilities, reduced equipment, inadequately prepared patients, insufficient personnel, and poor recovery facilities. Yet he has been expected to provide a smooth induction, an even anesthetic, and a rapid, uncomplicated recovery and to then ensure a safe trip home with no unpleasant aftereffects. He often failed. Against such odds, anesthesia could only be undertaken for a limited variety of procedures without unjustified risks.

Changing role of outpatient care

Through a fortunately timed combination of external pressures and increasing anesthetic capability, a fundamental change is underway in outpatient surgery (Davenport and others, 1971; Ahlgren, 1973).

Though no longer a factor, an acute shortage of bed space was the first important stimulus to increased outpatient services. This was followed by greater and more lasting financial pressure as well as growing concern over cross-infection of hospitalized patients (Izant, 1958; Rita and Seleny, 1974) and the emotional stress involved in separating young children from their parents (Bowlby, 1953; Smith, 1964; Nagel and others, 1973).

Increasing anesthetic capability has consisted to a large extent of greater precision in anesthetic technics, augmented by greater control over total patient management and increased participation in overall organization of the outpatient effort. It is now evident that development of an outpatient system as one of the major hospital functions requires drastic revision of expenditure for space, equipment, and personnel.

Facilities: space, equipment, and personnel. If 10 to 30 outpatients are to be operated on daily, there should be rooms to examine patients (prior to the day of surgery, if possible) with laboratory services, a reception area, a preoperative area for patients, and waiting rooms for parents. Operating room facilities must be equal to those for major procedures, with few, if any, exceptions. Complete equipment for anesthesia, monitoring, support, and resuscitation should be fundamental. Major changes essential to reduction of anesthetic risks may be necessary in establishing modern standards of recovery care for outpatients. A specially designated area should be suitably equipped and staffed by professional personnel trained for this type of care. Particular attention must be paid to these patients, since their recovery must be carried to the point where they can leave the hospital without further professional assistance.

Improved staffing of outpatient departments has been an essential factor in raising accomplishment. This includes more professional personnel at advanced levels as well as a full cadre of secretaries, aides, and technicians (Epstein, 1973).

The increased potential of adult outpatient surgery was impressively demonstrated by the SurgiCenter of Phoenix, Ariz. (Ford and Reed, 1969), where many procedures were performed for which hospitalization previously had been thought necessary. Similar methods have been applied to pediatric work in Dallas (Ahlgren and others, 1971), Toronto (Steward, 1973, 1975), and other areas. The volume and scope of the work accomplished will vary with the facilities available, as illustrated by Steward's 1973 figures showing that 20% of all the operations at Toronto's Hospital for Sick Children were performed on an outpatient basis. It must be recognized, of course, that these figures do not reflect the much shorter duration of most outpatient procedures.

Selection of cases. Patients are selected first on the basis of the required operation, but additional requisites must be fulfilled. The child should be in good general health and of reasonable emotional and behavioral makeup. The parents must be moderately intelligent and entirely reliable and preferably should live within 20 to 30 miles of the hospital in case of complications after discharge.

In many pediatric hospitals, the same basic outpatient procedures are performed, such as repair of minor lacerations, extraction of deciduous teeth, cystoscopy, myringotomy, fundus examinations, opening of abscesses, and difficult dressing changes. This general type of procedure can be extended considerably without increasing the risk of operative or postoperative complications.

Natural limitations to outpatient proce-
dures have been related to magnitude of operation (no entry of major body cavities), condition of patient (only ASA physical status I or II), duration (not over 45 minutes), and avoidance of special hazards of bleeding or airway involvement (exclusion of tonsillectomy). Endotracheal intubation has been used by Slater and Stephen (1949) and others for outpatient pediatric dentistry for some time, but fear of postoperative tracheitis influenced us to limit intubation to relatively few procedures.

The boundaries for outpatient procedures are being pushed aside. After some debate, herniorrhaphy is practiced even in such conservative areas as Boston, and use of endotracheal anesthesia is definitely increasing. Although some of us recall the family doctor removing tonsils in the kitchen, today tonsillectomy is regarded as a justifiable outpatient procedure by a few, but only the more heroic.

At The Children's Hospital Medical Center, the volume of outpatient procedures has increased rapidly. Of approximately 9000 operations performed yearly, 18% to 22% were accomplished on an outpatient basis in the years 1972 to 1975 and increased to 29% in 1976. Herniorrhaphy is performed frequently, endotracheal intubation occasionally, and tonsillectomy not yet. (The average duration of outpatient operations was 21 minutes, the range 3 to 65 minutes; that of procedures in the main operating room was 74 minutes, the range 15 minutes to 15 hours.)

Anesthetic management for elective surgery

Successful anesthesia demands establishment of standards and their maintenance. Standards in preoperative preparation of children treated as outpatients are especially critical because of (1) the general tendency to take shortcuts in their workup, and (2) the uncertainty as to whether parents have been able to deny the child all oral intake before operation.

A child should appear for operation with completed history and physical examination and essential laboratory work performed within the preceding 10 days either by the pediatrician or at the hospital. Parents are given explicit printed instructions not to feed the child after midnight unless the operation is to start after 11:00 AM, in which case he may have half a cup of cola or apple juice.

After checking in at the desk, child and parent are taken to a small waiting room where the child is undressed and allowed to lie down prior to operation.

Preoperative sedation is individualized. A quiet, unafraid child receives no medication, apprehensive children may be given morphine, 0.1 mg/kg, and an actively resistant 3-year-old may require the quieting influence of thiopental or methohexital by rectal instillation. Dental patients have done well on elixir of chloral hydrate, 10 mg/kg, plus excellent coaching by the dental staff. Fentanyl, 0.001 mg/kg, of shorter duration and a most effective sedative-analgesic, is well suited to outpatient use and is gaining general approval. Atropine is not assumed to be mandato.y but is used with halothane for operations on small infants, prior to endotracheal intubation, and for procedures in the region of the head and neck. With intravenous barbiturates or ketamine, atropine is needed for vagolytic and drying action.

Parental presence. I have no doubt that parents can be extremely helpful during both the induction and recovery phases of outpatient anesthesia. An intelligent, reassuring parent is often invited to stay with an apprehensive child as he is put to sleep, thereby reducing the child's fear and the amount of sedative that would be necessary. The same holds true during recovery (Shulman and others, 1967).

Anesthetic agents and technics. Of the methods and materials described in previous chapters, the nitrous oxide–oxygen and halothane combination is a heavy favorite for outpatient pediatric procedures. It is less irritating than enflurane (Rita and Seleny, 1973) and isoflurane, easily controllable, and rapidly expelled, and there is little in pediatric anesthesia for which it is not well suited. Occasionally, however, a frightened child

can be put to sleep with less emotional upheaval by intravenous thiopental.

The precautions necessary in anesthesia for outpatient procedures are the same as those observed for hospitalized children. In addition, one should double-check on the child's abstinence from eating and have a final inspection of his mouth for concealed food and chewing gum. Precordial stethoscope and blood pressure apparatus are standard monitoring items, but temperature monitoring seems less imperative for shorter cases. A regulation anesthesia chart is required for all patients regardless of the brevity of the procedure.

Alternatives to general anesthesia do exist and include local infiltration for suturing of minor lacerations and occasional nerve blocks for work on extremities if a child has eaten recently. Intravenous thiopental and methohexital definitely are valuable for older children who have an easily accessible vein. Ketamine, initially expected to be ideal for outpatient work, has caused delay in complete recovery; we have relegated its use to occasional procedures about the face or when the child is prone, ketamine serving as a substitute for endotracheal intubation.

Although intubation is not definitely contraindicated for outpatient use, we observe the following precautions:

1. Patients living within a radius of 20 miles from the hospital are observed for at least 2 hours after operation before discharge.
2. Patients who live at a distance of more than 20 miles from the hospital are observed for 4 hours or are kept overnight.
3. Parents are told to watch for signs of respiratory obstruction and are instructed about the necessary steps should they appear.

Although acupuncture does not appear to be of appreciable value for minor pediatric surgery, hypnosis can be invaluable. Children frequently make fine subjects, and as described below, many of the hazards of general anesthesia can be eliminated by application of this technic.

During recovery all patients are attended continuously by trained personnel until return of reflexes and consciousness. Parents are allowed to sit with children as they regain general control. This helps to avoid sedatives, which we prefer to omit, and speeds attainment of discharge status.

Discharge. Suitability for discharge varies with the age and condition of the child. Older children, who will walk, climb onto buses, and such, must regain total mental and neuromuscular control. Children who will be carried require less complete recovery but must definitely have regained all protective reflexes, consciousness, and full respiratory exchange, though complete muscular coordination is not essential.

Airway obstruction from any cause and vomiting are the most frequent reasons for delayed discharge. Horne and Ahlgren (1973) reported the incidence of recovery vomiting to be 5%, 3%, and 4% following halothane, enflurane, and isoflurane, respectively.

Should recovery involve such complications as bleeding, protracted vomiting, or airway obstruction, overnight hospital admission must always be seriously considered. To date, only one of the children anesthetized as an outpatient at our hospital has required overnight observation, this because of a brief period of intraoperative hypotension. The child had been receiving doxorubicin (Adriamycin), an antileukemic agent later recognized as having marked cardiotoxic properties (Vaisrub, 1977).

ANESTHESIA FOR EMERGENCY AND UNSCHEDULED OPERATIONS

For many years, children were rushed to the hospital for "emergency surgery" that included treatment of lacerations, burns, fractures, appendicitis, peritonitis, intestinal obstruction, abscesses, and a number of other conditions. In the belief that immediate treatment was all-important and because of the surgeon's desire to get the unwelcome interruption out of the way as soon as possible, history and physical examination were omitted, preparation was neglected, and various other shortcuts compounded the errors, often changing a minor accident into a major catastrophe.

Actually, there are very few conditions that demand "emergency surgery." Respiratory obstruction, uncontrolled hemorrhage, and acute head injury may deserve immediate treatment. In most types of acute pathology, however, time must be taken to examine the child thoroughly for other illness or injury, to treat shock or fluid imbalance, to administer sedatives and antibiotics, and to take any other indicated measures to get the child into suitable condition for anesthesia and operation. Thus, haste must not lead us into stupid, preventable errors. The former attitude of "emergency surgery—hurry" has been replaced by that of "emergency surgery—watch out."

Problems in minor operations

In the management of children with lacerations, simple fractures, and other minor injuries, the anesthesiologist meets two major problems: *control of fear* and *management of the full stomach.*

Fear. A bloody, grimy little boy with a gashed head who has been rushed to the hospital by frantic parents is much different from a well-prepared child who is brought into the same department for elective circumcision.

Every effort must be taken to control the child's emotions before any treatment is undertaken. Simply putting the child on a bed in a quiet room and allowing his parents to sit down by him will help considerably. Further reassurance of the parents and sedation of the child will be repaid by their feeling of relief and grateful confidence. Although morphine is of some benefit to these children, it will be ineffective in controlling truly excited patients unless excessive doses are given. Other approaches must be considered.

For the screaming, unmanageable child who is more frightened than hurt, rectal administration of thiopental (25 mg/kg) or methohexital (10 mg/kg) combines gentleness with effectiveness. The child stops crying, becomes drowsy, and falls off to sleep in 8 to 10 minutes without struggling, resistance, or physiologic disturbance, and his watching parents are equally pacified. Following this mild initiation, supplementation with inhalation agents is extremely simple, and it will be found that recovery is not greatly delayed if additional sedatives and narcotics are avoided.

Depending on the circumstances, ketamine probably has more place in quieting an uncooperative, resistant child for whom the added insult will change relatively little than one who had become calm and could be badly upset by this renewed assault.

Again, hypnosis in the hands of an expert may be spectacular, and the development of this talent should be encouraged.

The "full stomach" problem. One of the most dangerous situations in anesthesia is the patient who faces operation with the stomach overloaded with food or distended by unrelieved intestinal obstruction. While most anesthesiologists have had firsthand experience with this problem, there are numerous references in the literature to the technics, morbidity, and mortality involved (Morton and Wylie, 1951; Smith, 1956; Collins, 1960). Two articles by Salem (1970) and Salem and associates (1972) are especially pertinent.

In pediatric anesthesia the situation differs somewhat from that in adults. Children are less adaptable to such alternative methods as local and regional anesthesia and awake endotracheal intubation. Children also have more irregular eating habits than most adults and give less reliable information about what and how much they have ingested.

To children's advantage is their less forceful fasciculation following succinylcholine and apparently decreased reaction to aspirated gastric content (see below).

Ongoing debate as to the preference for intravenous or inhalation induction in patients with a full stomach suggests uncertainty in their management. While it is true that there is disagreement about details, the following essential safety factors are generally accepted:

1. Awareness of the danger involved, i.e., *fatal aspiration of gastric content*
2. Avoidance or delay of general anesthesia, if possible
3. Extensive preparation if anesthesia is required

4. Preanesthetic relief of gastric distension, if present
5. Endotracheal intubation by method of choice
6. Evacuation of stomach during operation
7. Delay of tracheal extubation until patient is awake and eyes are open

The fact that we are aware of the danger is a great step toward safety, for it means that we are forewarned and should have a definite plan of action in mind.

General anesthesia can often be avoided, especially if a few additional maneuvers are included. Local and regional anesthesia can be rendered more acceptable by preliminary establishment of an infusion by which morphine, diazepam, or other nonirritative sedatives may be administered (not barbiturates or ketamine).

Delaying anesthesia is an important consideration, but it is difficult to judge how long to wait for a child to digest his gastric contents (Inkster, 1963). Twelve hours may be insufficient following a large meal, but a child who has merely borrowed half a glass of cola from his neighbor should not require surgical postponement for more than an hour. It is well known that when an accident occurs shortly after a meal, the food may lie unchanged for many hours. Conversely, when a child has been calm and drowsy or has had a night's sleep, emptying of the stomach should progress normally. A wide variation in individual management is necessary here. The use of gastric antacids has been advocated by Taylor (1975), Wheatley and associates (1979), and many others. Lack of evidence of benefit coupled with definite evidence of increased vomiting has justified our disinterest in this maneuver.

The preparations for operation consist primarily of ensuring extensive suction equipment. Setting up suction should be the first thing an anesthesiologist does when he prepares for a case. It is certainly inexcusable to start without a full complement of airways, endotracheal tubes, laryngoscope, and stethoscope, but *suction is the most indispensable item in the anesthesiologist's entire effort.* One, and often two, strong, reliable suction devices should be present and actually in operation prior to induction. Three suction catheters small enough to pass easily through the endotracheal tube, three large catheters to clean mouth and pharynx, and two metal or rigid plastic "tonsil" suction tips should be on hand, plus five or six wooden tongue depressors, which are invaluable for opening clenched jaws. A large-bore suction device, consisting of a short endotracheal tube fitted to a wide-bore adapter (Fig. 22-1), is easily improvised. A bite block is useful to prevent the jaws from clamping together at the time of recovery. Equipment for bronchoscopy and tracheostomy should be easily available (Whalen, 1955).

Premedication should include enough sedative to overcome anxiety and fright and enough atropine to prevent vagal responses.

For induction, intravenous barbiturates carry increased risk for patients with full stomach, while danger of severe protracted laryngospasm is so great with ketamine that we consider this agent to be contraindicated in such circumstances.

It has been suggested that an attempt be made to empty the stomach in *all* children with question of "full stomach" by methods including induction of vomiting by apomorphine and other maneuvers, passage of stomach tubes, and blocking of the esophagus by passage of a balloon-carrying gastric tube (Guiffrida and Bizzari, 1957). These methods are not recommended, for they seldom are reliable and always are too upsetting to be employed as a standard technic.

However, if a child's stomach is actually distended by gas, liquid, or solid, this distension must be relieved prior to use of any general inhalation or intravenous anesthetic. Passage of a large naso- or orogastric tube with several holes and repeated rinsing with saline solution should remove all gas, much liquid, and some solids and reduce the danger sufficiently to justify proceeding with inhalation or intravenous induction if

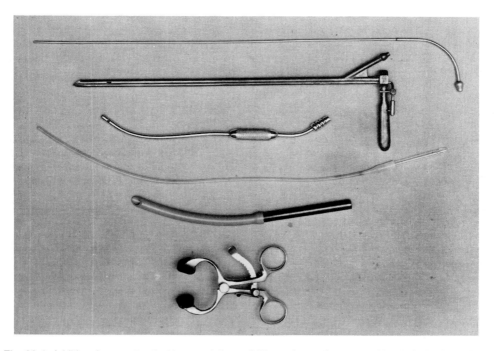

Fig. 22-1. Additional apparatus that is especially useful for patients who are vomiting includes bronchoscope, metal pharyngeal suction tube, stiff plastic suction catheter for the trachea, wide-bore suction catheter, and dental bite block.

one uses consummate skill and meticulous care.

Fortunately, very few patients considered to have "full stomach" have enough gastric content or pressure to present maximum danger, so that the survival rate is relatively good when basic precautions are observed.

The forces that affect vomiting and regurgitation have been discussed at length (Atkinson, 1962; Clark, 1963; Salem, 1970), especially those dealing with intragastric pressure and its response to succinylcholine. Intragastric pressure in resting adults was reported by Roe (1962) as ranging from 4 to 16 cm H_2O (mean 11.9) and by LaCour (1969) as ranging from 1 to 17 cm H_2O (mean 7.0). While fasciculation caused by succinylcholine was found by Roe (1962) to exceed 19 cm H_2O in some patients, straining or coughing was found by Salem (1970) to raise pressures above 80 cm H_2O.

Salem and associates (1972), measuring intragastric pressures in 30 infants and children, found a mean of 13.8 cm H_2O, slightly above those noted for adults. Administration of succinylcholine, however, caused much less fasciculation and an actual drop in mean pressure to 11.3 cm H_2O (range 4.5 to 25) 1 minute after injection. These data were presented as justification for use of succinylcholine for intubation of children with full stomach without prior administration of an antidepolarizing agent. That a rather small dose of succinylcholine (1.0 mg/kg) was used and that children with full or distended stomach might have higher intragastric pressure than those tested was not discussed.

Salem recommends cricoid compression of the esophagus (Sellick maneuver, 1961) to add to the safety of intravenous induction. While this may help to prevent regurgitation, forceful vomiting against such compression might rupture the esophagus.

It would appear that there are two dangerous processes that occur in full-stomach asphyxiation: first, passage of stomach content from stomach to pharynx, and second, passage of content from pharynx into trachea. In respect to both of these, halothane seems safer than succinylcholine. It causes neither the fasciculation nor the flaccidity that allows material to reflux into the pharynx, and the gag reflex remains active throughout most if not all of induction, thereby preventing passage of material from the pharynx into the trachea.

The head-up position has been proposed to reduce the danger of regurgitation (Snow and Nunn, 1959) and the head-down position to reduce the danger of aspiration, but Roe (1962) showed that vomiting could easily overcome a head-up tilt, which would then increase the hazard of aspiration. It was obvious, also, that head-down tilt increases the hazard of regurgitation. Consequently, most anesthesiologists feel that it is best for the patient to be level during induction, with the head turned well to the side to enable secretions to flow into the cheek and escape.

Inhalation induction can be unhurried, since vomiting is extremely rare during halothane induction. When the patient is moderately relaxed (not flaccid) and respiration becomes depressed, respiration can be assisted without danger of inflating the stomach, unless excessive anesthetic concentrations are used. Any passage of gas into the stomach will be heard by a stethoscope placed low over the left anterior thorax and, if heard, will signify sufficient relaxation for endotracheal intubation.

Topical anesthetic spray is contraindicated because of the danger of obtunding the gag reflex. The operating table is flat, and the child's head is in the usual sniffing position. If exposure of the glottis does not show complete glottic relaxation, deeper anesthesia should be achieved, because glottic spasm must be avoided. When an open glottis is seen, the tube is passed. One may use the Sellick maneuver, but under inhalation methods esophageal relaxation is not sufficient to require this step.

The endotracheal tube should be large enough to ensure the airway and to block passage of particulate matter from the pharynx to the trachea, but it should not have to be forced past the vocal cords. Cuffed tubes may be used in children 6 or more years of age. Leakage of a small amount of fluid around the tube into the larynx and trachea is to be feared less than pressure necrosis.

Once the endotracheal tube is fixed in place, relaxants may be given as desired. It is usually advisable to pass either a large nasogastric tube or an even larger orogastric tube in an attempt to evacuate the stomach contents, using saline solution as rinse material. After use, the large tube may be replaced by a regular nasogastric tube, as deemed necessary.

Upon completion of operation, most important of all is to keep the endotracheal tube in place until the patient is truly awake and, if curarized, until completely reversed. As they awaken, children may move their arms, legs, and head, roll, retch, vomit copiously, and grimace, but often they do not open their eyes for 5 or 10 minutes. It is the eyes that must be watched, for there is no reliable sign of returning gag reflex in the gradual recovery until the opening of the eyes and return of consciousness (Fig. 22-2).

During the excitement of lighter stages, it may be difficult to keep the endotracheal tube in place and at the same time prevent the child from biting down on it. An airway that extends into the pharynx increases the irritation considerably and is better withdrawn until it merely serves to keep the teeth apart. One may also use two or three wooden tongue depressors or a bite block, but these must be held firmly in place while strong active children are thrashing about. After the tube is removed, the airway reestablished, and the mouth cleared effectively and the child complies with spoken demands, the bite block may be removed.

To illustrate the variety of patients who may be referred to as having a full stomach, the following cases are presented:

1. A 12-year-old boy fractured his wrist 20 minutes after eating a hamburger. *Treatment:* give fentanyl, 0.02 mg/kg IM, and perform axillary block without further waiting.
2. A 1-year-old infant brought to the outpatient department for circumcision is found to have been given 6 ounces of milk by mistake. *Treatment:* cancel case.
3. A 6-year-old has eaten a hard candy half an hour before operation. *Treatment:* proceed without delay.

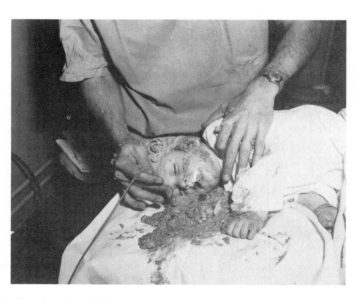

Fig. 22-2. Aspiration of vomitus is the greatest hazard in pediatric anesthesia. It can be avoided by induction with inhalation agents and by endotracheal intubation. The endotracheal tube must be left in place until the child is *actually awake.* (From Smith, R. M.: N.Y. J. Med. **56:**2213, 1956.)

4. An 8-year-old with acute appendicitis has not eaten for 6 hours but has vomited; stomach shows no gas or distension. *Treatment:* give thiopental followed by intravenous or inhalation induction for tracheal intubation; pass a nasogastric tube during anesthesia; delay extubation until the child opens his eyes (there should not be enough material in the stomach to interfere with induction, but added care is needed during recovery).

5. A 6-year-old girl who aspirated a bone during a large fish dinner shows good ventilatory exchange, but the sharp bone threatens to perforate the right main bronchus. *Treatment:* sedate with morphine and atropine by intravenous infusion; induce with nitrous oxide–halothane and intubate the trachea; then introduce a large gastric tube and wash out the stomach exhaustively. The endotracheal tube may then be removed to allow passage of a bronchoscope under continued inhalation anesthesia. At the time of extraction of the bone, succinylcholine is given for complete relaxation of the glottis. Immediately after the bone is extracted, the endotracheal tube is reinserted and not removed until the child awakens.

Major traumatic conditions

Respiratory emergencies. When children are admitted following severe injuries, the anesthesiologist first checks ventilation and cardiac activity. If needed, immediate assistance is effected by clearing the airway and providing mouth-to-mouth resuscitation or cardiac massage by external compression of the chest. Respiratory exchange may be endangered by head injury or by local injury to the upper airway or chest. The airway can be established by passage of an endotracheal tube or a bronchoscope (see Chapter 27). Following initial aeration, a tracheostomy is performed if necessary. Subsequent ventilatory assistance may also be supplied if respiration is depressed.

Shock. The treatment of children in shock follows the same rules used for adults. The patient is placed in a horizontal or slight Trendelenburg position, and blood volume is restored as rapidly as possible. The best substance to use for blood volume replacement undoubtedly is whole blood. Until this can be procured and crossmatched, however, we believe that 5% albumin solution is the most valuable substitute (Kevy, 1979). This material is prepared easily by any standard blood bank and is available commercially. It can be kept prepared in solution, can be stocked for long periods, does not carry hepatitis virus, and does not interfere with crossmatching, as does dextran. Ringer's lactate solution also can be used for rapid replacement of fluid volume.

When active bleeding occurs, it must be controlled; otherwise, operative procedures are delayed until the child's blood pressure and pulse are within normal limits and his condition is sufficiently improved to tolerate anesthesia.

Anesthesia for patients recovering from shock carries definite restrictions. With reduced circulating blood volume, the uptake of inhaled anesthetics will be more rapid, and excessive depth may be attained without warning. Obviously, an intravenous infusion should be running prior to induction of anesthesia. Intravenous barbiturates, spinal anesthesia, and ether are best avoided. Cyclopropane formerly was a popular agent but has given way to ketamine for induction of hypovolemic patients; narcotic analgesia, nitrous oxide, and oxygen may suffice for many. Halothane and relaxants are not contraindicated but must be used with increased caution. Pancuronium and metocurine are favored over *d*-tubocurarine.

Children with severe burns rarely require anesthesia during the acute phase of injury. Sedation is allowed, but these patients appear to be shocked into a state of analgesia and do not suffer as much as would be expected.

If burns involve the face or airway, however, anesthesiologists may immediately be concerned with supportive management. As outlined by Wilson (1970), this requires a comprehensive therapeutic approach for a variety of pathologic lesions, including upper airway obstruction, irritation of tracheobronchial tree, and shock lung.

Acutely ill patients

In children with acute appendicitis and peritonitis, with intestinal obstruction, large abdominal tumors, brain abscess, and other conditions involving high fever, and with loss of weight, protracted vomiting, and other debilitating conditions, the problem is not one of speed but of adequate preparation for operation. To rush these patients to the operating room as soon as the diagnosis is made is the surest way to kill them.

Any patient who has a high fever or rapid pulse and who is dehydrated or anemic must be sent not to the operating room but to the ward and treated there until given fluids, antibiotics, and specific therapy sufficient to bring him into a reasonably safe condition for operation. These measures are described in Chapter 25.

After such sick children have been brought to optimum condition, premedication and anesthetic must be chosen. Acutely ill children often require little sedation. Certainly each patient must be considered individually, and sedative should be given in reduced quantities. If there has been a recent temperature elevation, atropine is withheld until the time of anesthetic induction and then is given intravenously. This precaution is taken to avoid an iatrogenic pulse elevation that could not be distinguished from one caused by sudden exacerbation of the underlying disease.

Anesthesia for small infants who are critically ill may well consist of local infiltration. If relaxation is needed, halothane combines controllability with rapid recovery and is well tolerated. In very sick children it is better to use a very light concentration of general anesthetic and supplement it with a relaxant than to attempt a greater depth with inhalation agent alone.

Sick children 3 or more years of age who come to the operating room following special preparatory treatment usually have an infusion running. Induction is most humanely accomplished by adding thiopental (approximately 1 mg/lb) to the infusion. After the child has fallen asleep, anesthesia may be continued with halothane or nitrous oxide–relaxant combinations. Spinal anesthesia and epidural anesthesia have been recommended for appendectomy and other abdominal operations in sick children. If the patient is adequately hydrated and prepared, these methods may be used, but an ill, poorly prepared child is no better candidate for spinal anesthesia than for general anesthesia.

The problem of high fever in the patient requiring emergency surgery is familiar to all. It is generally recognized that it is extremely dangerous to operate on a child with elevated temperature, yet few have arrived at a reasonable solution. Our approach is to administer fluids, antibiotics, and rectal aspirin until normal hematocrit and urinary flow give evidence of adequate hydration (hematocrit, 30% to 35%; urine specific gravity, 1.005 to 1.035).

If the temperature remains elevated, the child is taken to the operating room. Anesthesia is induced with thiopental, and the trachea is intubated under succinylcholine and halothane so that surface cooling with ice, alcohol, and water mattress can be performed without causing discomfort or shivering. The operation is delayed until the temperature has been brought down below 102° F and is definitely under control. Operation may then proceed, but the temperature is closely monitored throughout the entire operative and recovery period, for hyperthermia may recur after the child has been covered with heavy drapes.

The anesthetic agent for patients who have had a high fever is less important than the supplementary methods of temperature control. Most agents are safe if the temperature remains below 102° F, but few, if any, are safe if the temperature rises above that. Since halothane promotes dissipation of body heat, this is recommended. If there is any suspicion of the possibility of malignant hyperthermia, both succinylcholine and halothane are contraindicated (see Chapter 26).

Unscheduled operations on newborns

The infant who is born with a cystic lung, diaphragmatic hernia, or intestinal obstruction sends no warning in advance; therefore, these situations fall into the class of emergency or unscheduled surgery. Operations for these conditions actually make up a large part of the unscheduled procedures in most pediatric surgical services and present the anesthesiologist with many problems. Although the anesthetic management of the newborn has already been discussed (Chapter 15), it may be repeated that any anesthesiologist who deals with infants and children must be prepared to care for critically ill newborns. When preparation is made for such cases, two factors are of great importance: (1) to have a complete stock of equipment on hand for infant anesthesia and (2) to have a clear understanding of the special pathologic problems involved.

BIBLIOGRAPHY

Ahlgren, E. W.: Pediatric outpatient anesthesia; a 4-year review, Am. J. Dis. Child. **126:**36, 1973.

Ahlgren, E. W., Bennett, E. J., and Stephen, C. R.: Outpatient pediatric anesthesiology; a case series, Anesth. Analg. (Cleve.) **50:**402, 1971.

Atkinson, M.: Mechanisms protecting against gastro-oesophageal reflux, Gut **3:**1, 1962.

Bowlby, J.: Some pathological processes engendered by early mother-child separation. In Senn, M. F. E., editor: Infancy and childhood, transaction of the Seventh Conference of Josiah Macy, Jr., Foundation, New York, March 23-24, 1953.

Clark, M. M.: Aspiration of stomach contents in a conscious patient, Br. J. Anaesth. **35:**133, 1963.

Cohen, D. D., and Dillon, J. B.: Anesthesia for outpatient surgery, Springfield, Ill., 1970, Charles C Thomas, Publisher.

Collins, V. J.: Fatalities in anesthesia and surgery, J.A.M.A. **172:**549, 1960.

Davenport, H. T., Shah, C. P., and Robinson, G. C.: Day surgery for children, Can. Med. Assoc. J. **105:**498, 1971.

Edwards, G., Morton, H. J. V., Pask, E. A., and Wylie, W. D.: Deaths associated with anaesthesia; a report of 1000 cases, Anaesthesia **11:**194, 1956.

Epstein, B. S.: Outpatient anesthesia, lecture presented at Annual Convention of American Society of Anesthesiologists, San Francisco, 1973.

Fahy, A., and Marshall, M.: Post-anaesthetic morbidity in out-patients, Br. J. Anaesth. **41:**439, 1969.

Ford, J. L., and Reed, W. A.: The surgicenter; an innovation in the delivery and cost of medical care, Arizona Med. **26:**801, 1969.

Gilman, S., and Abrams, A. L.: Prevention of aspiration of gastric contents during general anesthesia, N. Engl. J. Med. **255:**508, 1956.

Guiffrida, J. G., and Bizzari, D.: Intubation of the esophagus; its role in the prevention of aspiration pneumonia and asphyxial death, Am. J. Surg. **86:**329, 1957.

Horne, J., and Ahlgren, E. W.: Halothane, enflurane and isoflurane for outpatient surgery, paper presented at Annual Convention of American Society of Anesthesiologists, San Francisco, 1973.

Inkster, J. W.: The induction of anaesthesia in patients likely to vomit, with special reference to intestinal obstruction, Br. J. Anaesth. **35:**160, 1963.

Izant, R.: Nosocomial infections in a children's hospital, paper presented at the twenty-seventh Ross Paediatric Research Conference, Chicago, 1958.

Kay, B.: Out-patient anaesthesia, especially for children, Acta Anaesthesiol. Scand. (Suppl.) **17:**421, 1965.

Kevy, S. W.: Surgical implications of hematological disorders. In Ravitch, M. M., Welch, K. J., Benson, C. D., and others, editors: Pediatric surgery, ed. 3, Chicago, 1979, Year Book Medical Publishers, Inc.

LaCour, D.: Rise in intragastric pressure caused by suxamethonium fasciculations, Acta Anaesthesiol. Scand. **13:**255, 1969.

Merrill, R. B., and Hingson, R. A.: A study of incidence of maternal mortality from aspiration of vomitus during anesthesia occurring in major obstetric hospitals in the United States, Anesth. Analg. (Cleve.) **30:**121, 1951.

Morse, T. S.: Triage, technics and teaching in a children's emergency room, J. Surg. **8:**701, 1973.

Morton, H. J. V., and Wylie, W. D.: Anaesthetic deaths due to regurgitation or vomiting, Anaesthesiology **6:**190, 1951.

Nagel, E. L., Forster, R. K., Jones, D. B., and MacMahon, S.: Outpatient anesthesia for pediatric ophthalmology, Anesth. Analg. **52:**558, 1973.

Newman, M. G., Frieger, N., and Miller, J. C.: Measuring recovery from anesthesia; a simple test, Anesth. Analg. (Cleve.) **48:**1, 1969.

O'Mullane, E. J.: Vomiting and regurgitation during anaesthesia, Lancet **1:**1209, 1954.

Otherson, H. B., Jr., and Clatworthy, H. W.: Out-patient herniorrhaphy for infants, Am. J. Dis. Child. **115:**78, 1968.

Rita, L., and Seleny, F. L.: Pediatric outpatient anesthesia; premedication versus no premedication and the choice of anesthetic agent, Anesthesiol. Rev. **1**(8):9, 1974.

Roe, R. B.: The effect of suxamethonium on intragastric pressure, Anaesthesia **17:**179, 1962.

Salem, M. R.: Anesthetic management of patients with "a full stomach"; a critical review, Anesth. Analg. (Cleve.) **49:**47, 1970.

Salem, M. R., Wong, A. Y., and Lin, Y. H.: The effect of suxamethonium on the intragastric pressure in infants and children, Br. J. Anaesth. **42:**166, 1972.

Sellick, B. A.: Cricoid pressure, Lancet **2:**404, 1961.

Shulman, J. L., Foley, J. M., Vernon, D. T. A., and Allan, D.: A study of the effect of the mother's presence during anesthesia induction, Pediatrics **39:**111, 1967.

Slater, H. M., and Stephen, C. R.: Anesthesia in prolonged dental cases, Anesth. Analg. (Cleve.) **28:**339, 1949.

Smith, R. M.: Some reasons for the high mortality in pediatric anesthesia, N.Y. State J. Med. **56:**2212, 1956.

Smith, R. M.: Anesthesia for emergency surgery in pediatrics, Clin. Anesth. **2:**99, 1963.

Smith, R. M.: Children, hospitals and parents, Anesthesiology **25:**461, 1964.

Snow, R. G., and Nunn, J. F.: Induction of anaesthesia in the foot-down position for patients with a full stomach, Br. J. Anaesth. **31:**493, 1959.

Steward, D. J.: Experiences with an out-patient anesthesia service for children, Anesth. Analg. (Cleve.) **52:**877, 1973.

Steward, D. J.: Outpatient pediatric anesthesia, Anesthesiology **43:**268, 1975.

Taylor, G.: Acid pulmonary aspiration syndrome after antacids, Br. J. Anaesth. **47:**615, 1975.

Vaisrub, S.: Anthracycline antibiotics and the heart, J.A.M.A. **238:**60, 1977.

Vernon, D. T. A., Schulman, J. L., and Foley, J. M.: Changes in children's behavior after hospitalization, Am. J. Dis. Child. **37:**581, 1966.

Whalen, J. S.: Emergency paediatric anaesthesia, Can. Anaesth. Soc. J. **2:**366, 1955.

Wheatley, R. G., Kallus, F. T., Reynolds, R. C., and Giesecke, A. H., Jr.: Milk of magnesia is an effective preinduction antacid in obstetric anesthesia, Anesthesiology **50:**514, 1979.

Wilson, R. D.: Respiratory problems in the acutely burned patient, Anesth. Analg. (Cleve.) **49:**714, 1970.

Wylie, W. D.: The use of muscle relaxants at the induction of anaesthesia of patients with a full stomach, Br. J. Anaesth. **35:**168, 1963.

CHAPTER 23

Anesthesia for dentistry in children

ROBERT J. BERKOWITZ and ROBERT M. SMITH

Problems in dental anesthesia
Evolution of dental management technics
Mortality in dental anesthesia

PROBLEMS IN DENTAL ANESTHESIA

The continuing problems of anesthesia in adult dentistry are also encountered in children. These include whether anesthesia is indicated, what anesthesia should be given, who should give it, and where the procedure should take place.

Although certain dental procedures are well tolerated without analgesia, few adults deny the need for analgesia in more extensive dental procedures. When children undergo office dentistry, their need of possible adjuncts to control pain equals that of adults. In addition, the anxiety of the child, his inability to cope with fear, and his consequent lack of sufficient cooperation to sit through a dental procedure are often so great that continued patient management is required to reduce the child's anxiety.

The great importance of patient cooperation thus comes into full view in pediatric dentistry, and dentists who work in this demanding area must assume the management of the child's behavior along with his dental problems.

It is obvious that dental practitioners interested in children take a more active role than surgeons or physicians in allaying patient anxieties. The deeper interest of pedodontists in gaining the cooperation of their pa-tients is evident in their studies of the child's behavior and fears and the methods of controlling them.

Several workers (Lang, 1965; Carrel, 1968) have focused on familiar technics of sedation, while Croxton (1967), Chambers (1970), and others have probed the psychologic origins of the child's anxieties to develop approaches for controlling them. They question the indiscriminate use of sedatives in the belief that a child gains poise and self-confidence through responding appropriately to conservative office dentistry, while sedation promotes development of evasive technics.

Of special interest to all pediatric anesthesiologists are the views of pedodontists on the effect of parental presence. The beneficial effect with physically and mentally compromised patients is highly valued. However, the problems and hazards of allowing overpermissiveness are equally stressed, and definite limitations are set on the degree of parental participation.

EVOLUTION OF DENTAL MANAGEMENT TECHNICS

During recent years, several different approaches to management of pedodontic patients have developed in response to appreciation of the importance of early dental care, growing concern over the child's sensibility, and greater skill in controlling his psychic and somatic sensitivity. For the most part, these may be separated into office dentistry with local anesthesia, outpatient dentistry with general anesthesia, hospitalization and general anesthesia, and outpatient dentistry with combinations of oral sedation, regional anesthesia, and 30% to 50% nitrous oxide–oxygen. Many pedodontists also utilize intramuscular narcotics for behavior management of uncontrollable children (for review, see Wright, 1975). This type of behavior management technic should be used most judiciously in light of the potential complications associated with this approach (Benusis and others, 1979).

Office dentistry with local anesthesia

This is the basic approach whereby the child enters the dental treatment area and sits in the traditional dental chair. With appropriate behavior management and well-administered local anesthesia, most normal, healthy, cooperative children can usually tolerate the demands of reconstructive dentistry and minor oral surgery.

The amount of work that can be accomplished by this approach in a fully conscious child can be extended quite remarkably by the skill and personal management of the dentist. Further refinements of patience and understanding that build a child's confidence, plus a dash of salesmanship and a hint of hypnosis, can enlarge the scope of this approach tremendously, thereby reducing time, trouble, and expense and eliminating many potential hazards introduced by sedatives and general anesthetics.

Conversely, with mentally retarded children and those with severe behavior problems, the use of this approach is greatly reduced. Although much effort has been expended by Diner (1968) and others in developing special technics of managing such patients, use of sedation and general anesthesia may be required for relatively minor procedures.

The use of mild sedatives or analgesics given by mouth prior to office visits seems a reasonable step to take with less cooperative children. As yet our attempts in this direction have been disappointing but deserve continued investigation.

Outpatient dentistry with general anesthesia

Short procedures that are truly stressful (e.g., the extraction of several permanent teeth) are considered appropriate for the outpatient department, provided that the children are relatively healthy and manageable and that the procedure will not require tracheal intubation.

For such procedures, children are considered to be in the same category as other surgical outpatients and must have an adequate preoperative history, physical examination, and blood and urine analysis including sickle cell tests for black children. The examination may be performed by a reliable physician outside the hospital if within 48 hours of the procedure, but preferably it takes place at a preliminary outpatient visit where the parents are given specific information about the operation. Particular emphasis is always placed on the importance of strict compliance with instructions (written) to avoid oral intake prior to general anesthesia.

The use of preanesthetic sedation for this type of outpatient procedure is questioned by some. In any group of unmedicated children, however, there will always be a highly vocal minority.

For unmedicated or inadequately sedated children, it is often helpful to invite a reasonable parent to stand beside the child and hold his hand, preferably without speaking, until the child is asleep.

If a sedative is used, short-acting agents that can be given by mouth will make the next visit more acceptable to any child. A palatable syrup makes an excellent medium, or a suppository may be used for those who are less cooperative. At The Children's Hospital Medical Center, a suspension of chloral hydrate (Chloralixin) containing 88 mg of chloral hydrate and 0.1 mg of atropine per ml has been practical, the dose being 0.5 mg/kg not to exceed 10 ml. This medication is given when the child arrives at the hospital and is effective in 20 minutes.

Among many other sedatives, narcotics, and tranquilizing agents that have been suggested, hydroxyzine and diazepam have been popular recently, but dose response has been highly variable. The success that we have had using mild sedatives has been due in large degree to the presence of members of the dental staff who have already established an excellent relationship with the patients.

In our management of these children, anesthesia is administered by a member of the regular anesthesia staff.

With complete operating room facilities and resuscitative apparatus at hand, anesthesia is induced under nitrous oxide–halothane anesthesia, with stethoscopic and blood pressure monitoring. Anesthesia is carried to a depth adequate for intubation prior to any operative maneuvering. At this time, the anesthesiologist can change to a small nasal mask or preferably pass a short nasopharyngeal tube into the hypopharynx and continue anesthesia in this manner. The dentist then opens the child's mouth, applies a bite block, places a sponge pack in the mouth to catch blood and debris, and proceeds to the extractions.

This procedure inevitably involves pressure on the jaw, which must be supported actively by the anesthesiologist to prevent airway obstruction. Such procedures take only 2 or 3 minutes, after which bite block and mouth pack are removed and bite pads are inserted at extraction sites as the child awakens on the table. He is then moved to a stretcher (on his side) on which he is taken to the recovery room, where he rests, under trained supervision, for at least 30 minutes.

As far back as 1949, Slater and Stephen advocated intubation (nasal) of children for outpatient dental procedures, and in the present rapid expansion of outpatient services, many are now practicing routine outpatient tracheal intubation, thereby extending the safe limit of operative time and facilitating both anesthesia and operation. For many years we limited the use of endotracheal intubation to exceptional cases, but we have recently extended our outpatient practice to include 2-hour dental rehabilitation procedures under nasotracheal intubation and nitrous oxide–halothane anesthesia in a selected group of patients.

In contrast to our conservative approach is the report of Venn (1971), whose management of 208 children consisted of induction (without premedication) with propanidid, 10 mg/kg, followed by alcuronium, 0.2 mg/kg, and atropine, 0.3 to 0.6 mg, nasotracheal intubation, halothane-propanidid maintenance during operation, reversal of relaxant, careful pharyngeal suction, extubation, and discharge of the patient within 5 to 20 minutes.

Hospitalization and general anesthesia

In 1948, the concept of dental rehabilitation was initiated by Dr. Paul Losch of The Children's Hospital Medical Center. Under this plan, children who required extensive work were admitted to the hospital and six or eight extractions and a dozen or more fillings accomplished under general anesthesia during a single 2- or 3-hour operation; thus, what would have required numerous office visits was completed in one session.

To subject a child to a prolonged general anesthetic "just for dental work" was criticized at the outset, and only children with severe cardiac disease, mental retardation, and similar problems were managed in this way. The method proved to be safe, however, and was gradually expanded to include any child who needed extensive treatment that could not be rendered by other outpatient technics (e.g., nitrous oxide–oxygen with oral premedication). Other clinics reported on the success of this method, especially for children with behavior problems (Scott and Allan, 1970; Troutman and Mayer, 1971; Marcy, 1974), and our own series grew to 3500 without mortality or serious complication.

The specific management has consisted of admission and full anesthetic preparation on the day before operation. Since many of these children have special medical or psychiatric problems, additional evaluation or therapy may be needed, a large proportion requiring cardiac consultation, radiologic reevaluation, and electrocardiography.

Children with neurologic disorders also require special management. With patients receiving anticonvulsant medication, the question arises as to the effect of anesthesia on the incidence of seizures and whether the medication should be discontinued prior to operation. Except for ketamine and enflurane, most anesthetics reduce seizure activity, but it is generally believed preferable to continue anticonvulsant medication and add regular sedation. Additional care may be needed to avoid injury to the gums of these children, since anticonvulsants often produce gingival hypertrophy.

The needs of the pedodontist are not excessive. His preference for tracheal intubation by nasal route is reasonable, but with children under 2 years of age or those who have large adenoids or facial maldevelopment, it may be necessary to use the oral route. Choice of agent and technic is limited only by problems of individual patients. Our usual method consists of premedication with a barbiturate, narcotic, and atropine (p. 99) and either inhalation technic using nitrous oxide–oxygen and halothane or intravenous technic using thiopental-succinylcholine for intubation, followed by relaxant–nitrous oxide–morphine maintenance. In general, the inhalation technic has been more suitable for children under 10 years old, and intravenous methods have been more suitable for older children.

Several factors deserve special consideration. The head and face are usually covered with drapes that may press the endotracheal tube against the nostril with enough force to cause ulceration and scar contracture of the nostril unless care is taken to tape the tube down to the upper lip and leave the entire nostril in view.

Full-length draping of the patient also promotes heat retention, making temperature monitoring and fluid therapy of increased importance.

Patients with cardiovascular disease, especially those with valvular and septal defects, are exposed to the risk of incurring bacteremia and endocarditis. Consequently, procaine penicillin, 300,000 to 600,000 units, is administered and continued four times daily for 3 days.

Several authors have reported increased incidence of cardiac arrhythmias during dental surgery. Miller (1970) has stressed the importance of atropine for prevention, while Plowman and associates (1974) find local anesthetic block an effective prophylactic.

At completion of operation, particular care must be taken prior to extubation to expose the mouth and hypopharynx and clear secretions or debris under direct vision and to make sure that all sponges have been removed. Since some bleeding may be expected during recovery, keeping the child in lateral or prone position will be mandatory.

A higher incidence of sore throat and tracheitis may be expected following prolonged dental procedures. In our experience, three children have required 48 hours of mist and steroid therapy, one has required reintubation for 12 hours, but none has required tracheostomy.

Although a large proportion of these children have had severe underlying diseases, and the average duration of procedure has been 150 minutes, there has been no mortality in 3500 procedures.

In spite of the success of this method, the rapidly rising cost of hospitalization and related services stimulated the development of other methods by which these children might be treated. That of analgesic sedation has shown great promise.

Outpatient dentistry with oral sedation, regional anesthesia, and 30% to 50% nitrous oxide

General anesthesia given in dental offices and clinics has caused reasonable doubts, especially when intravenous anesthetics have been employed. Shane (1966, 1966a), Carrel (1968), and others have reported favorably on their use, but agents so administered act rapidly, promote airway problems, and are difficult to control.

The concept variously termed analgesic sedation, conscious sedation (Bennett, 1978), or relative analgesia (Diner, 1968) avoids the use of potent intravenous anesthetics but combines oral sedation, regional anesthesia, and subhypnotic concentrations of nitrous oxide and produces a calm, cooperative child. This enables the pedodontist to work with children on an outpatient basis, at minimal risk, for an hour or more at a time. This practice, recently instituted at our hospital, was carried out on 120 children within the first 8 months, most of these children being drawn from the group that would have required hospitalization.

The method used has consisted of oral medication on arrival of the child with hydroxyzine, 1 mg/kg, and chloral hydrate, 25 mg/kg. The child is seated in the dental chair 45 minutes later. The dental surgeon, who has had basic training in anesthesia and resuscitation, administers nitrous oxide in 30% to 50% concentration by nasal mask. With this anesthetic, the child is kept light enough to retain consciousness and gag reflex, but enough analgesia and sedation can be provided to allow the dental surgeon to place a block without the pain and anxiety usually associated with local anesthesia.

Procedures accomplished under this management have included multiple restorative fillings and extractions, excision of dentigerous cysts and papillomas, gingivectomy, and other operations, most of which required 15 to 45 minutes for completion. There have been no significant complications to date, and the process appears highly worthwhile.

Many of the children in this group previously would have required hospitalization. Those requiring full hospitalization management have been reduced to the most severely handicapped and the very young.

MORTALITY IN DENTAL ANESTHESIA

Statistics gained from the medical literature usually reflect the records of successful experiences. As with tonsillectomy, we find reports of several thousand dental anesthetics without mishap; those with less shining records show less urge to publish. Actuarial records give unbiased figures. One source lists the following data for the United States in 1973:

Total deaths during general anesthesia for dental procedures	74

Anesthesia deaths	64
Those occurring in dental office	59
Anesthesia by trained individuals	4
Anesthesia by untrained individuals	54
Those occurring in hospitals	5

In one of the most inclusive studies of death in dental anesthesia, Tomlin (1974) surveyed available British figures and estimated one death per 300,000 office anesthetics and one death per 15,000 hospital procedures. The higher incidence of the latter is because of the greater risk usually involved.

His data show 48 dental anesthesia deaths in approximately 8 million patients during 6 years, 17 of which occurred in a hospital and 29 in a dental office. Of 28 patients described in detail, seven were under 10 years of age.

The discrepancy between American and British figures suggests great errors in data and/or anesthetic management.

An enlightening survey in practices and technics of 120 pedodontists (Bowers and Hibbard, 1971) reflects attitudes concerning use of anesthesia in the office, behavior management, and anesthetic training requirements for dental anesthesia.

BIBLIOGRAPHY

Bennett, C. R.: Conscious sedation in dental practice, ed. 2, St. Louis, 1978, The C. V. Mosby Co.

Benusis, K., Kafaun, D., and Furman, L.: Respiratory depression in a child following premedication; report of a case, J. Dent. Child. 46:50, 1979.

Bowers, D. F., and Hibbard, E. D.: Technique for behavior management; a survey, J. Dent. Child. 38:368, 1971.

Carrel, R.: A supplement to an intravenous amnesia technique in pediodontic cases, Anesth. Prog. 15:39, 1968.

Chambers, D. W.: Managing the anxieties of young dental patients, J. Dent. Child. 37:363, 1970.

Croxton, W. L.: Child behavior and the dental experience, J. Dent. Child. 34:212, 1967.

Diner, H.: Relative analgesia in the handicapped child. In Langa, H., editor: Relative analgesia in dental practice, Philadelphia, 1968, W. B. Saunders Co.

Kaufman, L.: Cardiac arrhythmias in dentistry, Lancet 2:287, 1965.

Lang, L. L.: An evaluation of the efficacy of hydroxyzine (Atarax-Vistaril) in controlling the behavior of child patients, J. Dent. Child. 32:253, 1965.

Langa, H.: Relative analgesia in dental practice; inhalation analgesia with nitrous oxide, Philadelphia, 1968, W. B. Saunders Co.

Love, S. H.: The complications of dental anesthesia, Lancet 1:754, 1966.

Marcy, J. H.: Anesthesia for dental procedures in the pediatric patient. In Bennett, C. R.: Monheim's general anesthesia in dental practice, ed. 4, St. Louis, 1974, The C. V. Mosby Co.

Miller, J. R.: Factors in arrhythmia during dental outpatient general anesthesia, Anesth. Analg. (Cleve.) 49:701, 1970.

Plowman, P. E., Thomas, W. J. W., and Thurlow, A. C.: Cardiac dysrhythmias during anaesthesia for oral surgery; the effect of local blockade, Anaesthesia 29:571, 1974.

Scott, J. G., and Allan, D.: Anaesthesia for dentistry in children; a review of 101 surgical procedures, Can. Anesth. Soc. J. 17:391, 1970.

Shafto, C. E.: Continuous intravenous anaesthesia for pediatric dentistry, Br. J. Anaesth. 41:407, 1969.

Shane, S. M.: Intravenous amnesia for total dentistry in one sitting, J. Oral Surg. 24:27, 1966.

Shane, S. M.: Intravenous amnesia to obliterate fear, anxiety and pain in ambulatory dental patients, J. Maryland State Dent. Assoc. 9:94, 1966a.

Slater, H. M., and Stephen, C. R.: Anesthesia in prolonged dental cases, Anesth. Analg. (Cleve.) 28:339, 1949.

Tomlin, P. J.: Death in outpatient dental anaesthetic practice, Anaesthesia 29:551, 1974.

Troutman, K. C., and Mayer, B. W.: Pedodontic oral rehabilitation; dental and anesthetic considerations, J. Am. Dent. Assoc. 82:388, 1971.

Venn, P. H.: General anaesthesia for dental conservation in children, Anaesthesia 26:90, 1971.

Wright, G. Z.: Behavior management in dentistry for children, Philadelphia, 1975, W. B. Saunders Co.

CHAPTER 24

Special problems in pediatric anesthesia

Toxic and critically ill patients
Presence of acute or chronic respiratory
  disease
Metabolic disorders
Endocrine disorders
Dermatologic disorders: epidermolysis bullosa
Separation of conjoined (Siamese) twins

There are several types of patients who present special problems for pediatric anesthesiologists. These may include dangerously sick patients, such as those in late stages of malignant disease; children in respiratory, cardiac, or renal failure; and those with rare diseases whose response to anesthesia is unusual or carries increased risk and who require unusual forms of treatment.

The number of rare diseases that may be encountered in infants and children is so great that only a few will be mentioned here, but several hundred may be found in such standard references as the *Nelson Textbook of Pediatrics* (1975) as well as definitive texts such as those by Stanbury and associates (1966) and Warkany (1971). Articles on the anesthetic management of different bizarre cases have been scattered through the literature over many years. The volume by Katz and Kadis (1973), devoted entirely to this subject, has been most helpful, and the tabulated information of Jones and Pelton (1976) offers a quick source of information and a rich supply of references. Articles by Gilbertson and Boulton (1967), Ellis (1974), and Brown and associates (1975) also are valuable.

Many of the rare varieties have already been described, including Apert's and Crouzon's syndromes, Pierre Robin and Treacher Collins syndromes, and several of the orthopedic anomalies. The patients to be discussed here include a few of those who are seen with some frequency, and whose anesthetic management involves increased risk, and those of unusual interest.

TOXIC AND CRITICALLY ILL PATIENTS

Although a child with acute appendicitis and peritonitis may be nursed into fair condition by preoperative hydration and antibiotics prior to operation, one who has advanced malignancy (Fig. 24-1) may not respond to any form of preoperative therapy and may require operation while in extremely poor condition. One must consider all possible alternatives in such situations. One should first consider the possibility that such a patient should be sent to another institution where more adequate personnel and facilities are available. In many instances this would apply to postoperative care rather than surgical or anesthetic care. One should also weigh the possible gain in such a procedure against the probable prolongation of suffering involved, for all-out attempts to keep patients alive are not uncommon in teaching hospitals.

In the preoperative review of patients who have been receiving prolonged tumor therapy, one should examine the record to find out what drugs have been used, in what dosage, how recently, and for how long. The antineoplastic agent currently of particular

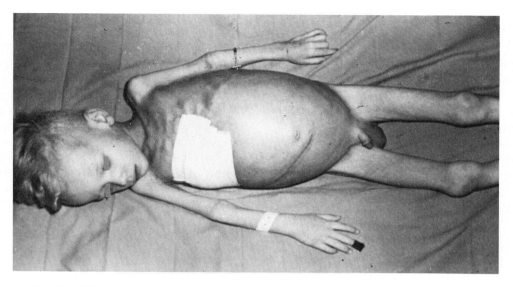

Fig. 24-1. Children with advanced malignancy require minimal amounts of anesthetic agents.

interest to anesthesiologists is doxorubicin (Adriamycin). As described in relation to bone tumors on p. 473, doxorubicin is known to be a cardiotoxic agent with cumulative effect, and the limit of safe dosage is believed to be approximately 250 mg/m². Precautions to be observed with this drug are described in the above reference.

Preoperative sedation may present a problem in management of chronically ill patients (Wilson and others, 1969). They may be expected to be distressed, but their illness may have reduced their tolerance to medication. On the other hand, if they have been receiving analgesics for pain control, they may have built up an appreciable tolerance to both sedatives and narcotics. One must question the patient or his parents and examine the record rather closely or risk making a bad mistake. A trial of the intended sedative on the night before operation helps the anesthesiologist judge the correct preoperative dose and usually is needed by the patient.

In choosing an anesthetic for poor-risk patients one should not forget the advantages of local anesthesia. Seriously ill patients may have reduced sensitivity to pain and require relatively little analgesia. Whether local or

general anesthesia is used, it is advisable to begin with smaller amounts than usual, because the constricted plasma volume distributes agents less widely and a higher concentration than usual reaches the brain. In patients with poor tissue perfusion due to shock or edema, drugs given by intramuscular or subcutaneous injection may take effect very slowly but have a prolonged duration of action.

PRESENCE OF ACUTE OR CHRONIC RESPIRATORY DISEASE

A troublesome and extremely common situation arises when a child who is scheduled for operation appears to have a cough, a runny nose, or a slight fever (100° to 101° F). If the operation is elective, the presence of fever, pharyngeal inflammation, or signs of upper respiratory tract or pulmonary infection should call for postponement of the procedure. If possible, such a child should not be readmitted until he has been clear of all such signs for at least a week. The greatest danger, however, is in the first days of the cold.

If the operation is considered to be urgent, it is often necessary to proceed. One should

529

then reconsider the choice of anesthesia and evaluate the several possible alternatives, including local, inhalation, intravenous, and spinal anesthesia. Inhalation often is the best choice, and nitrous oxide and halothane cause less irritation than most agents. Unless endotracheal anesthesia is mandatory, opinions differ as to its advisability. The tube may cause more irritation, and for that reason be considered inadvisable, but if used would provide better airway control and easy access for clearing secretions involved in the infection. Final decision would depend on individual situations. Either course would appear to carry appreciable risk. Administration of suitable antibiotics should be carefully considered, especially if spinal anesthesia is chosen.

Bronchial asthma is seen relatively frequently in children and will vary in degree from an insignificant finding to an incapacitating affliction. Although all agents have been administered to such patients, it seems advisable to avoid thiopental, which is known to aggravate laryngeal spasm. Ketamine has been recommended for therapeutic effect in patients with severe asthma (Betts and Parkin, 1971), but experience in using this agent with other forms of respiratory pathology has fortified my impression that ketamine is not the best agent to give to asthmatics. Earlier use of tribromoethanol and ether has given way to halothane, which is the agent of choice for most forms of airway irritation or obstruction. If there is exacerbation of airway obstruction during the course of the anesthetic, the intravenous administration of aminophylline (3 to 5 mg/kg) should reduce bronchial spasm. If one prefers to use epinephrine as a bronchodilator, it would be advisable to use balanced intravenous agents. Although both morphine and d-tubocurarine are known to be bronchoconstricting agents, their use for support of patients in status asthmaticus is well known, and they have been found to be more reliable than such alternatives as pancuronium and meperidine. Metocurine is now considered preferable to d-tubocurarine.

Patients known to be chronic asthmatics should be thoroughly questioned about their use of steroids. Those who have been receiving steroids continuously or who have been given a course of steroid therapy within 6 months usually should have hydrocortisone, 2 to 4 mg/kg, immediately prior to anesthesia. For other known asthmatics, preparation with aminophylline is recommended using a loading dose of 6 mg/kg over 15 to 30 minutes to obtain a serum level of 10 μg/kg, followed by infusion of 0.9 mg/kg/hr to maintain a serum level of 5 to 15 μg/kg. Additional information on the anesthetic management of patients with asthma may be found in Converse and Smotrilla (1961), Gold (1966, 1970), and Hirshman and Bergman (1978).

Cystic fibrosis

Cystic fibrosis (mucoviscidosis, pancreatic fibrosis) is a generalized disease involving the mucus-secreting glands of the entire body. It is inherited as an autosomal recessive trait and is lethal, in most cases, during adolescence, although some are now being carried into the third decade (Shwachman, 1960; Taussig and Landau, 1976). Between 1952 and 1977, 2500 patients were treated for cystic fibrosis at The Children's Hospital Medical Center. The mean age of death between 1940 and 1948 was 1½ years, while that in 1976 was 16 years (Shwachman and others, 1977).

Four characteristics of the disease, according to Vaughan and McKay (1975), are increased electrolyte content of sweat, absent pancreatic enzymes, chronic pulmonary involvement, and family history of the problem. Different aspects of cystic fibrosis have already been discussed. The earliest form of the disease is meconium ileus, seen in the neonatal period. An infant who survives this will be easy prey to several other phases of the illness. As the disease progresses, the child appears malnourished and develops an emphysematous chest and a protruding abdomen (Fig. 24-2).

Although lack of intestinal enzymes can be treated successfully, chronic infection of the lungs is more difficult to overcome. Masses of staphylococci plug the bronchioles, causing

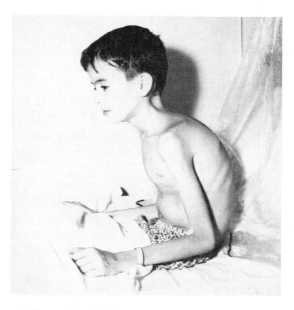

Fig. 24-2. The advanced stages of cystic fibrosis bring wasting, bronchiectasis, emphysema, and cor pulmonale.

repeated bouts of pneumonia, abscess formation, bronchiectasis, emphysema, cor pulmonale, and ultimately death. Prolapse of the rectum is common among younger children having cystic fibrosis, and nasal polyps occur in older children. The nasal polyps often become necrotic and destroy the turbinates and sinuses. Numerous therapeutic and diagnostic procedures must be performed on these children, including colostomy, repair of rectal prolapse, excision of nasal polyps, bronchoscopy, lobectomy, pneumonectomy (Schuster and Schwartz, 1979), tracheostomy, and splenoportal anastomoses for cirrhosis and portal hypertension (Schuster and others, 1977). Because they are sick, coughing thick, heavy, foul-smelling sputum, apprehensive, and often febrile, these children present a miserable picture and a real anesthetic problem. Anesthetic management for pneumonectomy has been described (Chapter 16), and similar considerations apply to the other procedures as well. Patients may be in advanced pulmonary failure as well as severe mental depression, with good reason. In order to prevent further plugging of

airways prior to operation, hydration should be maintained by oral and intravenous routes. Contrary to our previous belief, we have learned that atropine may cause appreciable thickening of the sputum, and it is omitted.

Any operation on patients with cystic fibrosis should be preceded by antibiotic therapy, postural drainage, and maximum pulmonary preparation. Removal of mucopurulent secretions will be essential with whatever agents are used, and one of the prime requisites of anesthetic management is that one must be able to remove airway secretions effectively and quickly at any time. In this regard, it is particularly important to avoid the use of curved endotracheal tubes or adapters. One should take advantage of the opportunity at the end of each anesthetic to clear the trachea and main bronchi while the child is asleep, for the thick secretions are always difficult for the patient to raise and become more dangerous in the postoperative period when they are more tenacious and patients have less ability to cough them out.

There is some difference of opinion regard-

531

ing the best agent to use in advanced cystic fibrosis. If halothane is used, uptake and excretion of the agent are delayed by the presence of secretions and actual pulmonary damage. Unless one is careful to reduce the concentration of halothane or other inhalation agents well before the end of the operation, awakening and return of respiratory control may be considerably delayed. However, if nondepolarizing relaxants are used it is argued that residual weakness may be of greater danger in view of the reduced respiratory function of these patients. One may reasonably infer that intermittent administration of succinylcholine would have increased value. Actually, all of the above approaches may be used safely if the limitations are noted. In addition, individual situations must be borne in mind. If a surgeon wishes to use epinephrine to shrink nasal mucosa during polypectomy, one would naturally use relaxants rather than halothane.

Two anesthetic agents that appear to carry increased risk are thiopental and ketamine. The degree of risk is relatively slight in the case of thiopental, but experience with severe and prolonged airway irritation has convinced us that ketamine is definitely to be avoided in patients with cystic fibrosis.

With such obvious problems related to the lungs of patients with cystic fibrosis, the suggestion to use spinal anesthesia frequently is made. Our experience with spinal anesthesia in three different patients with cystic fibrosis has been uniformly disastrous. The cough reflex of these patients is extremely sensitive, and all three trials were marked by such violent and prolonged coughing that the level of anesthesia reached to the upper thorax or above, none of the patients could tolerate the operation, and none attained prespinal condition for 24 hours.

Tracheobronchial lavage has been tried in patients with cystic fibrosis using instillations of N-acetylcysteine, saline, and other solutions (Hacket and Reas, 1965). Although improvement was noted in some patients, severe exacerbation in others led us to abandon the procedure. The most formidable operations currently undertaken in our institution on patients with cystic fibrosis are pneumonectomy and splenorenal shunts. For additional information, one may refer to Salanitre and associates (1964), Smith (1965), Di Sant' Agnese and Talamo (1967), Doershuk and associates (1972), Brown and associates (1975), and Morris and associates (1978).

METABOLIC DISORDERS
Homocystinuria

Homocystinuria is a rare disorder of amino acid metabolism with urinary excretion of large amounts of homocystine and methionine (Schimke and others, 1965; Brown and others, 1975). Clinical defects consist of mental retardation, hypoglycemia, osteoporosis, arterial and venous thromboses, kyphoscoliosis, and ectopia lentis. Excision of an ectopic lens is the most common indication for operation in these patients. Anesthesia should be designed to avoid dehydration, stress, hypovolemia, and decreased cardiac output in order to reduce the danger of thrombosis. The cause of the hypercoagulability is suspected to be activation of the Hageman factor by homocystine, and aspirin has been used as prophylaxis. The additional defects of hyperinsulinemia and hypoglycemia call for frequent monitoring of blood glucose and suitable correction.

Phenylketonuria

Phenylketonuria (PKU) is a well-documented amino acid (phenylalanine hydroxylase) deficiency that becomes evident in infancy in the form of vomiting, hypertonia, seizures, and mental retardation, all of which can be prevented by early diagnosis and restriction of intake of phenylalanine, but the disease becomes irreversible early in childhood if untreated (Knox, 1972). No specific surgical procedures are indicated, but for incidental surgery, anesthetic management should include continuation of seizure-controlling medication plus light additional sedation and controllable general anesthesia, with care taken to avoid hypoglycemia due to disease or therapy. One should also avoid any anesthetic agent that increases seizure tendency, such as ketamine, enflurane, pentazocine, or phencyclidine, and one should be careful not to traumatize the skin, which may be extremely sensitive.

Glycogen storage diseases

Clinical aspects of a variety of disorders of glucose metabolism were described before their chemical origin was suspected. Following the recognition of an underlying enzymatic defect by Cori, classification was adopted for seven more familiar forms, leaving a great many without name or classification (Stanbury and others, 1966; Hsia, 1966). The different forms all contain inborn defects in glycogen metabolism with resultant reduction of glucose formation and consequent clinical danger of hypoglycemia, acidosis, and related features.

Type I, von Gierke's disease, glucose-6-phosphatase deficiency. Inability to convert glycogen to glucose results in storage of glycogen in the liver with resultant hepatomegaly, hypoglycemia, acidosis, vomiting, weight loss, and convulsions. Therapy consists of maintaining blood glucose level by frequent feeding, which often must be continued through the night. Intravenous feeding was inadequate so surgeons tried portocaval shunts, but simple gastrostomy has been found to be an easy way to introduce glucose on frequent day-and-night schedules (Crigler and Folkman, 1978). Cox (1968) reported anesthetic experiences with 11 type I and 1 type III glycogen storage disease patients. Operations for liver biopsy and tonsillectomy and one open-heart procedure were performed. One death occurred early in the series during tonsillectomy under open-drop ether. Our experience in anesthetizing two children for portocaval shunt and nine (all type I) for gastrostomy has been relatively uneventful. Care must be taken to hydrate the children preoperatively, to maintain blood glucose level within normal range, and to prevent development of ketoacidosis. The relatively brief operations for gastrostomy offered slight challenge, but those for portocaval shunts required greater manipulative control.

Type II, Pompe's disease, acid maltase de-ficiency. The chief clinical symptoms are hypotonia and severe cardiac disease and failure. Glycogen deposits in muscle and death in infancy are outstanding features.

Type III, Forbes' disease. This is clinically similar to type I but less severe, and it should offer no particular anesthetic problems.

Type V, McArdle's disease, muscle glycogen phosphorylase deficiency. This is a rare variety characterized by rapid fatigue of muscles and danger of cardiac failure. No anesthetic experiences have been reported to our knowledge.

Type VI, Hers' disease, liver glycogen phosphorylase deficiency. This is a poorly defined type having a variable hyperglycemic response to epinephrine and glucagon.

Type VII, glycogen synthetase deficiency. These patients have deficient glycogen synthesis with hypoglycemia and starvation in infancy that is amenable to frequent glucose feedings.

Mucopolysaccharidoses

The problem of classifying unusual diseases is apparent in the case of the mucopolysaccharidoses, which have been variously classified as neurologic disorders (Katz and Kadis, 1973), as skeletal disorders and later as carbohydrate disorders (Vaughan and McKay, 1975), and as heritable connective tissue disorders (McKusick, 1972) and have been listed alphabetically (Jones and Pelton, 1976).

The mucopolysaccharides are basic components of connective tissue, occurring in most parts of the body. Consequently, all of the above listings are justifiable. Seven different clinical varieties of abnormal mucopolysaccharide metabolism have been identified, and there are believed to be at least twice that many that are not clearly distinguishable from one another. The seven established varieties are designated as mucopolysaccharidoses I through VII, but several are better known by their pseudonyms, in particular Hurler's, Hunter's, Sanfilippo's, and Morquio's syndromes.

Hurler's syndrome, mucopolysaccharidosis I, gargoylism. Hurler's syndrome is the

For induction and maintenance of anesthesia, one has the choice of local methods, titration with morphine and scopolamine, or use of halothane. Local anesthesia, with elimination of airway encroachment, has priority but has relatively rare indication. The use of small increments of morphine supplemented by sedation with scopolamine, or possibly diazepam, has been extremely valuable. With further addition of topical anesthesia, tracheal intubation may be attempted with greater safety than under most other agents. In our experience with approximately 50 of these children over the past 30 years, halothane has been most useful. To reduce obstruction, induction may be started with the child sitting up, and later he may be positioned on his side. If possible, operation is performed without intubation. An airway, well lubricated with anesthetic gel and inserted as soon as possible, serves to maintain the airway. In several cases, it has been impossible to pass a laryngoscope beyond the base of the tongue, and the uvula could not even be sighted.

Two deaths are known to have occurred because of inability to establish an airway during such cases, and an emergency tracheostomy once barely saved us from a similar experience.

Hunter's syndrome, mucopolysaccharidosis II. As previously noted, Hunter's and Hurler's syndromes are not easily distinguished from each other, but Hunter's syndrome is inherited as an X-linked recessive rather than an autosomal recessive trait and in general is considerably less severe, with patients often living to be 30 or more years old (Leroy and Crocker, 1966).

Sanfilippo's syndrome, mucopolysaccharidosis III. Inherited as an autosomal recessive trait, this disease also is similar to but less severe than Hurler's syndrome, rarely having any of the cardiac defects common in Hurler's but with more marked mental retardation.

Morquio's syndrome, mucopolysaccharidosis IV. Classified as a chondrodystrophy and characterized by multiple crippling deformities of vertebrae and ribs, normal men-

tality, and high incidence of aortic regurgitation, these patients are occasionally seen as candidates for orthopedic support. Kyphosis, airway problems, general weakness, and cardiac defects require gentle and intelligent management. Atlanto-occipital subluxation offers added danger.

The remaining numbered mucopolysaccharidoses, and many unnumbered, vary in mode of inheritance and in chemical and anatomic characteristics, but they are rarely encountered.

Niemann-Pick disease and Gaucher's disease

Niemann-Pick disease (Crocker and Farber, 1958) and Gaucher's disease (Vaughan and McKay, 1975), are disorders of lipid storage in which marked hyperplasia may occur about the mouth and pharynx as well as in the spleen. Niemann-Pick disease is characterized by apathy, pancytopenia, hepatosplenomegaly, emaciation, and death in early childhood. Gaucher's disease is slightly less severe and has both acute and chronic forms. Pancytopenia is absent, but a pseudobulbar syndrome is typical. Muscle hypertonia, laryngeal spasm, and trismus also are present. Both diseases present problems to the anesthesiologist because of severe malnourishment and chronic liver dysfunction. The greatest difficulty is associated with upper airway obstruction due to lymphoid hyperplasia.

Familial dysautonomia (Riley-Day syndrome)

As suggested by its descriptive name, familial dysautonomia is an inherited (autosomal recessive) disease characterized by generalized disturbance of the autonomic nervous system (Riley and others, 1949; Riley and Moore, 1966). Outstanding features include labile blood pressure, absence of sweating, poor temperature control, difficulty in swallowing with frequent aspiration and pneumonitis, lack of response to pain, and emotional instability (Bortels, 1970). Dancis and Smith (1966), Gitlow and associates (1970), and Ziegler and associates

(1976) have demonstrated that there is ineffective circulatory adjustment to standing or exercise, the blood pressure falling appreciably without any compensatory acceleration of heart rate, apparently because of lack of norepinephrine response.

Anesthetic experiences have been reported by McCaughey (1965), Inkster (1971), Meridy and Creighton (1971), and others. Repeated bouts of aspiration pneumonia should call for careful evaluation of lungs before operation, and airway control and ventilation pose particular dangers through the operation. Bronchial secretions are thick, and atropine may best be omitted. Normal responses to hypoxia and hypercarbia are absent, and lack of signs of anesthetic depth adds to the risk. Kadis and associates (1973) warned of the several dangers of apprehension, marked blood pressure and temperature lability, and possible abnormal response to depolarizing muscle relaxants. In our experience, airway control has been of major importance. In addition to several minor procedures, vagotomy and gastroenterostomy have been performed on four patients by Schuster with moderate clinical improvement. Halothane served as the principal agent, and complications were avoided.

Down's syndrome

Children with Down's syndrome (trisomy 21, mongolism) are usually recognizable at a glance because of the combination of round head and face; small, dull, reddened, slanted eyes with epicanthal folds; open mouth; and protruding tongue (Benda, 1969). Regrettable misdiagnoses have been made on the basis of such brief examination of small infants, however, and it is advisable to see what the parents look like and also to examine the child's hands for characteristic simian folds and curled fifth fingers before making any drastic statements. Severe mental retardation, hypotonia, and the presence of endocardial cushion defect or other cardiac lesion should make the diagnosis highly probable, to be definitely confirmed by chromosome analysis (Smith, 1964; Greenwood and Nadas, 1976).

Infants and children with Down's syndrome are familiar to most pediatric anesthesiologists, since the syndrome is frequently seen in infants with tracheoesophageal fistula and other neonatal defects and in larger children presenting for repair of cardiac defects, extensive dental rehabilitation, herniorrhaphy, or other problems.

Anesthetic management is planned to cope with altered mentality, airway problems, and the probability of major cardiac defects. Although these children are characteristically hypotonic, quiet, and friendly, when excited they can go to the opposite extreme. Sedatives have been unpredictable and must be reduced to avoid overaction. Consequently, a resistant child may be intractable and will only be controllable by induction with intravenous thiopental (Fig. 24-4).

Vague warnings concerning the danger of using atropine in Down's syndrome are seen repeatedly in pediatric literature. These refer to findings that patients with Down's syndrome show abnormally great dilation of the pupils in response to atropine eye drops (Berg and others, 1960; Priest, 1960). The reason for this has not yet been determined. In addition, Harris and Goodman (1968) have demonstrated that these patients show significantly greater increase in heart rate in response to repeated doses of atropine.

In clinical management of this group of patients there has been no recognizable complication attributable to atropine, and most anesthesiologists believe it to be especially useful in view of the large tongue and excessive saliva usually encountered.

The characteristic hypotonia of these children has been treated with 5-hydroxytryptamine with some promise.

Mental retardation and epilepsy

Children who are physically normal but mentally retarded respond poorly to attempts at preoperative conditioning. If they are not antagonistic, mild sedation may be successful and should be followed by carefully controlled, light anesthesia. When such children appear antagonistic, they may become excited and unmanageable after barbi-

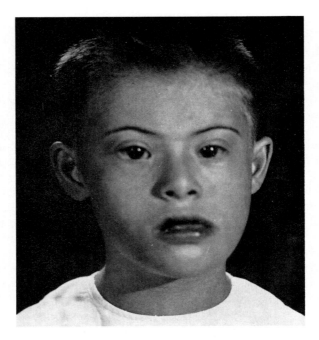

Fig. 24-4. In Down's syndrome, the response to anesthesia is unpredictable.

turate medication. A better approach has been to put them to sleep in their own beds with rectal or intravenous thiopental.

Quite frequently a physician calls in the warning that the child who he is admitting for operation is subject to epileptic seizures, implying that under anesthesia the seizure tendency might be increased. This, of course, is not true, for an epileptic patient usually is benefitted by sedation and general anesthesia and seldom presents any problem to the anesthesiologist from this standpoint. If these patients have been receiving anti-seizure medication, it should not be omitted prior to anesthesia but should be used to bring the child to as near normal condition as possible, after which further sedation should be allowed in order to promote easy, relaxed induction.

ENDOCRINE DISORDERS
Diabetes mellitus

Diabetes mellitus occurring in childhood, or juvenile diabetes, is generally considered to be more severe and more difficult to con-

trol, or brittle, than the disease in older individuals. Childhood diabetics differ in that their hyperglycemia is seldom due to intolerance to insulin, as frequently is the case in older patients, but is due to lack of insulin. They also differ in being dependent on insulin for control, and they seldom can be treated by diet alone. Physically they have a definite tendency to be thin, while the typical adult diabetic has difficulty in preventing obesity (Schwartz, 1971).

The control of juvenile diabetics in the operative period follows the adult pattern more closely. The general aim is to prevent hypoglycemia by changing insulin preparations to short-acting forms, giving half the daily dose before operation, running an infusion of 5% dextrose in ¼% saline solution at a standard rate for metabolic need throughout the operation, and giving the remainder of the insulin at completion of the operation. Blood glucose should be tested before anesthesia is begun and may be tested during long procedures or in critical situations. It usually suffices to test the urine, which should show some excess glucose, as proof that hypoglycemia is not imminent.

The sedative and anesthetic agents currently in use have little effect on insulin or blood glucose as compared with ether. Halothane and other inhalation agents or intravenous combinations may be used. The chief concern is to avoid stressing the patients in any manner or exposing them to danger of infection and also to have them wake up soon after the operation is completed.

Adrenogenital syndrome

It has been our experience that children with adrenogenital syndrome present a markedly increased anesthetic risk. Sudden cardiovascular collapse has occurred during anesthesia in three such children, without any obvious cause. Gross obesity may play a large role, as well as abnormal catechol response (Fig. 24-5). Many of these children, like those with craniopharyngioma, excrete large quantities of salt, and if replacement is neglected during operation, acute salt depletion can cause sudden myocardial depression (Bongiovanni and Root, 1963). Children with adrenogenital syndrome may require operation for excision of tumor or for clitorectomy, a rather uncomplicated procedure, one would expect, but the one that produced all three of the sudden hypotensive episodes just mentioned.

DERMATOLOGIC DISORDERS: EPIDERMOLYSIS BULLOSA

Four varieties of this rare lesion were described by Zackheim and associates (1973). All four consist of the formation of blisters that occur either following mild trauma or spontaneously, and all are genetically determined. The simplex type shows limited distribution of blisters, or bullae, chiefly at points of friction, particularly the hands and feet of crawling infants. The hyperplastic cystrophic and polydysplastic dystrophic forms are both moderately severe, with the bullae often arising spontaneously. Involvement of mucous membranes is a serious feature in this disease, occurring infrequently in the hyperplastic form but almost always in

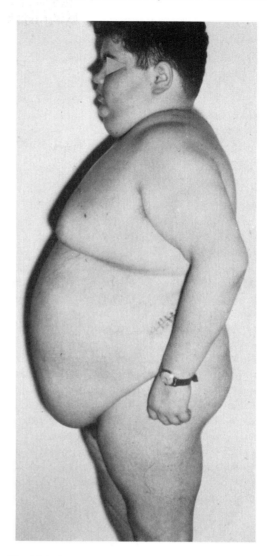

Fig. 24-5. Adrenogenital syndrome may cause obesity, acute salt deficiency, and abnormal catechol response.

the polydysplastic form. The fourth type, justly termed lethalis, virtually strips the skin of affected infants and involves much of their respiratory and digestive tracts as well.

Clinical management of epidermolysis bullosa has been described in several articles concerned with a single case in which the chief concern was that of airway management (Kubota and others, 1961; Marshall, 1963;

Hamann and Cohen, 1971; Reddy and Wong, 1972). In severe forms, this is complicated by the presence of large bullae on the lips and on the inside of cheeks and palate, as well as marked restriction of motion of jaws and neck due to limitation of joint movement and local scar formation. Concern over the danger of more trauma further limits one's attempts to use any kind of pressure in establishing an airway. Unfortunately, abnormal dentition and scar formation in the esophagus often require surgical repair. Injections may initiate more bullae and are avoided when possible. If the patient has a history of bulla formation in the respiratory tract, endotracheal intubation will carry very considerable risk, as would tracheostomy. Operations other than those inside the mouth, including intrathoracic procedures, would be more safely managed with mask technic, the face being carefully protected by layers of moistened pads. Sedatives may include any of the usual agents, including morphine or meperidine, given by mouth, and general anesthesia, if used, would probably be most satisfactory with halothane. In such cases, it would certainly be worth the effort to use hypnosis, and it would be quite reasonable to develop a hypnotic "potential" in patients in preparation for eventual need. In spite of one report recommending ketamine for intraoral procedures on such patients, this agent would appear to be stimulating, would prevent relaxation, and would invite more trauma and airway occlusion.

SEPARATION OF CONJOINED (SIAMESE) TWINS

Now that open-heart surgery is commonplace, the most spectacular operation in pediatric circles probably is the separation of conjoined twins. In 1976, Fournier and associates stated that there had been about 60 reported operations of this nature. According to these authors, the types of fusion best suited for operative separation are:

1. Thoracopagus twins, joined by the thorax, often having a common pericardium (Filler and Crocker, 1979; Towey and others, 1979)

2. Xyphopagus (or omphalopagus) twins, joined by the abdomen and lower thorax, usually having a common liver (Fournier and others, 1976; Filler and Crocker, 1979)
3. Pygopagus twins, joined by the thighs, often having a common anus
4. Ischiopagus twins, joined by the pelvis, usually sharing parts of digestive and genitourinary tracts
5. Craniopagus twins, joined by the skull, sharing meninges and parts of the brain (Grossman and others, 1953; Hall and others, 1957)

When the union is superficial and positioning offers no problems, the situation is easily managed. One anesthesiologist cares for each infant and treats him as an individual. Major difficulties arise, however, when unions involve airway problems, as in the brow-to-brow position or when vital organs are shared (Fig. 24-6). Here the unusual combination of conditions makes it imperative to organize a carefully worked out plan of action, with special attention to reducing the number of bystanders who crowd into every corner of space, adding even greater confusion to the already stressed situation.

In the preoperative care of conjoined twins, the usual laboratory studies are made, and the infants are nursed into optimal condition before operation is undertaken. An important point made by Aird (1954) and stressed by Allen and associates (1959) is the possibility that the adrenal development of one twin may be defective, and death may occur after separation unless provision is made for this by adequate cortisone administration before, during, and after operation.

At the time of operation, infusions are started in both infants, each infant being cared for by an individual anesthesiologist. Endotracheal intubation will be indicated in all but the simplest types of union and may be performed with the patient awake or under anesthesia, depending on the situation (Furman and others, 1971; Filler and Crocker, 1979).

During the operation, monitoring must be particularly well coordinated, with emphasis placed on continuity and moment-to-mo-

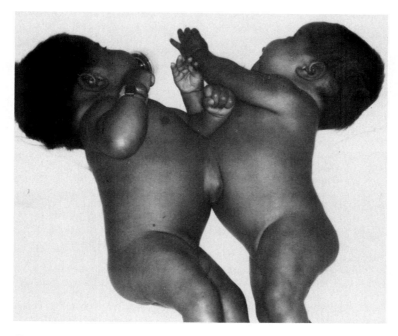

Fig. 24-6. Thoracopagus twins. (Courtesy Dr. Dean Crocker, Boston, Mass.)

ment observation rather than on extensive instrumentation (Simpson and others, 1967). One of the major dangers in these operations lies in the extreme and punishing handling and repositioning of the infants. Maximum danger exists when there is circulatory communication between the two twins, for then it is possible for one infant to "bleed out" into the other. This complication occurred during intubation in the case of Allen and associates (1959) and during operation in an experience described by Bachman (1967). In both cases, the sudden shocklike condition was corrected by rapidly placing the infants beside each other.

BIBLIOGRAPHY

Aird, I.: The conjoined twins of Kano, Br. Med. J. **1:**831, 1954.

Allen, H. L., Metcalf, D. W., and Giering, C.: Anesthesia management for the separation of conjoined twins, Anesth. Analg. (Cleve.) **38:**109, 1959.

Bachman, L.: Personal communication, 1967.

Benda, C. E.: Down's syndrome; mongolism and its management, New York, 1969, Grune & Stratton, Inc.

Berg, J. M., Brandon, M. W. G., and Kirman, B. H.: Atropine in mongolism, Lancet **2:**441, 1960.

Betts, E. K., and Parkin, C. E.: Use of ketamine in an asthmatic child; a case report, Anesth. Analg. (Cleve.) **50:**420, 1971.

Boba, A.: Anesthetic problems in hereditary muscular abnormalities; clinical anesthesia conference, N.Y. State J. Med. **72:**1051, 1972.

Bongiovanni, A. M., and Root, A. W.: The adrenogenital syndrome, N. Engl. J. Med. **268:**1283, 1963.

Bortels, J. M.: Familial dysautonomia, J.A.M.A. **212:** 318, 1970.

Brown, B. R., Jr., Walson, P. D., and Taussig, L. M.: Congenital metabolic diseases of pediatric patients; anesthetic implications, Anesthesiology **43:**197, 1975.

Converse, J. G., and Smotrilla, M. M.: Anesthesia and the asthmatic, Anesth. Analg. (Cleve.) **40:**336, 1961.

Coran, A. G., and Eraklis, A. J.: Inguinal hernia in the Hunter-Hurler syndrome, Surgery **61:**302, 1967.

Cox, J. M.: Anesthesia and glycogen storage disease, Anesthesiology **29:**1221, 1968.

Crigler, J. F., Jr., and Folkman, J.: Glycogen storage disease; new approaches to therapy, Ciba Found. Symp. **55:**331, 1978.

Crocker, A. C.: Personal communication, 1978.

Crocker, A. C., and Farber, S.: Niemann-Pick disease; a review of 18 patients, Medicine **37:**1, 1958.

Dancis, J., and Smith, A. A.: Familial dysautonomia, N. Engl. J. Med. **274:**207, 1966.

Di Sant'Agnese, P. A., and Talamo, R. C.: Pathogenesis and physiopathology of cystic fibrosis of the pancreas, N. Engl. J. Med. **277:**1287, 1344, 1359, 1967.

Doershuk, C. F., Reyes, A. L., Regan, A. G., and others: Anesthesia and surgery in cystic fibrosis, Anesth. Analg. (Cleve.) **51:**413, 1972.

Ellis, F. R.: Neuromuscular disease and anaesthesia, Br. J. Anaesth. **46:**605, 1974.

Filler, R. M., and Crocker, D.: Conjoined twins. In Ravitch, M. M., Welch, K. J., Benson, C. D., and others, editors: Pediatric surgery, ed. 3, Chicago, 1979, Year Book Medical Publishers, Inc.

Fournier, L., Goulet, C., Waugh, R., and Chouinard, R.: Anaesthesia for separation of conjoined twins, Can. Anaesth. Soc. J. **23:**425, 1976.

Furman, A. B., Roman, D. G., Hairabet, J., and others: Management of anesthesia for surgical separation of newborn conjoined twins, Anesthesiology **34:**95, 1971.

Gilbertson, A. A., and Boulton, R. B.: Anaesthesia in difficult situations; influence of disease on pre-op preparation and choice of anaesthetic, Anaesthesia **22:**607, 1967.

Gitlow, S. E., Bertani, L. M., Wilk, E., and others: Catecholamine metabolism in familial dysautonomia, Pediatrics **46:**513, 1970.

Gold, M. I.: Pulmonary mechanics and blood gas tensions during anesthesia in asthmatics, Anesthesiology **27:**216, 1966.

Gold, M. I.: Anesthesia for the asthmatic patient, Anesth. Analg. (Cleve.) **49:**881, 1970.

Greenwood, R. D., and Nadas, A. S.: The clinical course of cardiac disease in Down's syndrome, Pediatrics **58:**893, 1976.

Grossman, H. J., Sugar, O., Greely, T. W., and Sadove, M. S.: Surgical separation in craniopagus, J.A.M.A. **153:**201, 1953.

Hacket, P. R., and Reas, H. W.: A radical approach to therapy for the pulmonary complications of cystic fibrosis, Anesthesiology **26:**248, 1965.

Hall, K. D., Merzig, J., and Norris, F. G., Jr.: Case report; separation of craniopagus, Anesthesiology **18:**908, 1957.

Hamann, R. A., and Cohen, P. J.: Anesthetic management of a patient with epidermolysis bullosa dystrophica, Anesthesiology **34:**389, 1971.

Harris, W. S., and Goodman, P. M.: Hyper-reactivity to atropine in Down's syndrome, N. Engl. J. Med. **279:**407, 1968.

Hirshman, C. A., and Bergman, N. A.: Halothane and enflurane protection against bronchospasm in an asthmatic dog model, Anesth. Analg. (Cleve.) **57:**629, 1978.

Hsia, D. Y.: Inborn errors of metabolism. Part 1. Clinical aspects, ed. 2, Chicago, 1966, Year Book Medical Publishers, Inc.

Inkster, J. S.: Anaesthesia for a patient suffering from familial dysautonomia (Riley-Day syndrome); case report, Br. J. Anaesth. **43:**509, 1971.

Jones, A. E. P., and Pelton, D. A.: An index of syn-dromes and their anaesthetic implications, Can. Anaesth. Soc. J. **23:**207, 1976.

Kadis, L. B., Diaz, P. M., and Lack, J. A.: Neurological disorders, In Katz, J., and Kadis, L. B., editors: Anesthesia and uncommon diseases; pathophysiologic and clinical correlations, Philadelphia, 1973, W. B. Saunders Co.

Katz, J., and Kadis, L. B.: Anesthesia and uncommon diseases; pathophysiologic and clinical correlations, Philadelphia, 1973, W. B. Saunders Co.

Knox, W. E.: Phenylketonuria. In Stanbury, J. B., and others, editors: Metabolic basis of inherited disease, ed. 3, New York, 1972, McGraw-Hill Book Co.

Kubota, Y., Norton, M. L., Goldenberg, S., and Robertazzi, R. W.: Anesthetic management of patients with epidermolysis undergoing surgery, Anesth. Analg. (Cleve.) **40:**244, 1961.

Leroy, J. B., and Crocker, A. C.: Clinical definition of the Hunter-Hurler phenotype, Am. J. Dis. Child. **112:**518, 1966.

Marshall, B. F.: A comment on epidermolysis bullosa and its management in dental operations, Br. J. Anaesth. **35:**724, 1963.

McCaughey, T. J.: Familial dysautonomia as an anaesthetic hazard, Can. Anaesth. Soc. J. **12:**558, 1965.

McKusick, V. A.: Heritable disorders of connective tissue, ed. 4, St. Louis, 1972, The C. V. Mosby Co.

Meridy, H. W., and Creighton, R. E.: General anesthesia in eight patients with familial dysautonomia, Can. Anaesth. Soc. J. **18:**563, 1971.

Morris, L. J., Mascia, A. V., and Farnsworth, P. B.: Cystic fibrosis; making a correction and early diagnosis, J. Fam. Pract. **6:**749, 1978.

Priest, J. G.: Atropine response of the eyes in mongolism, Am. J. Dis. Child. **100:**869, 1960.

Reddy, A. R. R., and Wong, D. H. W.: Epidermolysis bullosa; a review of anaesthetic problems and case reports, Can. Anaesth. Soc. J. **19:**536, 1972.

Riley, C. M., Day, R. L., Greeley, D. M., and Langford, W. S.: Central autonomic dysfunction with defective lacrimation, Pediatrics **3:**468, 1949.

Riley, C. M., and Moore, R. H.: Familial dysautonomia differentiated from related disorders; case reports and discussions of current concepts, Pediatrics **37:**435, 1966.

Salanitre, E., Klonymus, D., and Rackow, H.: Anesthetic experience in children with cystic fibrosis of the pancreas, Anesthesiology **25:**801, 1964.

Schimke, R. N., McKusick, V. A., Huang, T., and others: Homocystinuria, J.A.M.A. **193:**711, 1965.

Schuster, S. R., and Schwartz, M. Z.: Surgical management of the pulmonary complications of cystic fibrosis. In Ravitch, M. M., Welch, K. J., Benson, C. D., and others, editors: Pediatric surgery, ed. 3, Chicago, 1979, Year Book Medical Publishers, Inc.

Schuster, S. R., and Shwachman, H.: Pulmonary surgery in cystic fibrosis, J. Thorac. Cardiovasc. Surg. **48:**750, 1966.

Schuster, S. R., Shwachman, H., Harris, G. B. C., and others: Pulmonary surgery in patients with cystic fibrosis, J. Thorac. Cardiovasc. Surg. **48:**750, 1964.

Schuster, S. R., Shwachman, H., Toyama, W. M., and others: The management of portal hypertension in cystic fibrosis, J. Pediatr. Surg. **12:**201, 1977.

Schwartz, G.: Orthostatic hypotension syndrome of Shy-Drager, Arch. Neurol. **16:**123, 1967.

Schwartz, R.: The critically ill child; diabetic ketoacidosis and coma, Pediatrics **47:**902, 1971.

Shapiro, N. D., and Poe, M. F.: Sickle disease; an anesthesiological problem, Anesthesiology **16:**771, 1955.

Shwachman, H.: Therapy of cystic fibrosis of the pancreas, Pediatrics **25:**155, 1960.

Shwachman, H., Toyama, W. M., Rubino, A., and Khaw, T. K.: The management of portal hypertension in cystic fibrosis, J. Pediatr. Surg. **12:**201, 1977,

Simpson, J. S., Pelton, D. A., and Swyer, P. R.: The importance of monitoring during operations on conjoined twins, Can. Med. Assoc. J. **96:**1463, 1967.

Smith, D.: Autosomal abnormalities, Am. J. Obstet. Gynecol. **90:**1055, 1964.

Smith, R. M.: Anesthetic management of patients with cystic fibrosis, Anesth. Analg. (Cleve.) **44:**143, 1965.

Stanbury, J. B., Wyngaarden, J. B., and Fredrickson, D. S., editors: The metabolic basis of inherited disease, ed. 2, New York, 1966, McGraw-Hill Book Co.

Taussig, L. M., and Landau, L.: Cystic fibrosis. In Kelley, V. C., editor: Practice of pediatrics, ed. 4, New York, 1976, Harper & Row, Publishers, Inc.

Towey, R. M., Kisia, A. K. L., Jacobacci, S., and Muoki, M.: Anaesthesia for the separation of conjoined twins, Anaesthesia **34:**187, 1979.

Vaughan, V. C. II, and McKay, R. J., Jr., editors: Nelson textbook of pediatrics, ed. 10, Philadelphia, 1975, W. B. Saunders Co.

Warkany, J.: Congenital malformations, Chicago, 1971, Year Book Medical Publishers, Inc.

Wilson, R. D., Traber, D. L., Priano, L. L., and others: Anesthetic management of the poor risk anesthetic patient, South. Med. J. **62:**767, 1969.

Woolley, M. V., Morgan, S., and Hays, D. M.: Heritable disorders of connective tissue; surgical and anesthetic problems, J. Pediatr. Surg. **2:**325, 1967.

Zackheim, H. S., Rudzinski, D. J., Katz, J., and Spademan, R. G.: Skin and bone disorders. In Katz, J., and Kadis, L. B., editors: Anesthesia and uncommon diseases, Philadelphia, 1973, W. B. Saunders Co.

Ziegler, M. G., Lake, C. R., and Kopin, I. J.: Deficient sympathetic nervous response in familial dysautonomia, N. Engl. J. Med. **294:**630, 1976.

PART THREE

ALLIED TOPICS

CHAPTER 25

Fluid therapy and blood replacement

BASIC QUESTIONS IN FLUID THERAPY

This chapter is intended to serve as a practical guide that will offer useful advice on how to administer fluids to infants and children under a variety of conditions.

Fluid therapy is primarily a clinical matter and one of great importance. Discussion of the subject is difficult, however. It is easy to become lost in theory and confuse the reader and equally easy to oversimplify and leave nothing but handy guides without adequate documentation; it is also quite difficult to avoid biased interpretation of aspects that have yet to be firmly established.

In an attempt to avoid these pitfalls, keep to the point, be practical, give adequate evidence, and show minimal bias, the approach will be directed toward answering the following questions that are of basic importance:

1. Does fluid therapy need to be complicated?
2. Is there any simple guide for use in uncomplicated cases?
3. What does fluid therapy for sick patients include?
4. What are the indications for fluid therapy? When is an infusion needed?
5. How do children differ from adults in fluid metabolism?
6. How do neonates differ from children?
7. *How do neonates differ from one another?*
8. How do premature infants differ from neonates?
9. What other patients require special fluid management?
10. What preoperative therapy is needed?
11. What intraoperative therapy is needed?
12. What postoperative therapy is needed?
13. What signs and monitors are needed?
14. What are the dangers of inadequate fluid therapy?
15. What are the dangers of excess therapy?

The first two questions, directed toward the same point, can be answered relatively quickly.

Does fluid therapy need to be complicated?

It is evident that children over 2 years old with normal kidneys can tolerate considerable variation in both the type of solution and the amount given. One should have a general understanding of the use of intravenous fluids, but the computation of ions and osmols should not be necessary in all cases.

Is there any simple guide for use in uncomplicated cases?

In the belief that fluid therapy often can be simple, the classic outline of Holliday and Segar (1957) is offered for use in normal children undergoing relatively short and uncomplicated operations. The indications, type of fluid, and amount and rate of administration are considered.

Indications. This approach may often be used for such operations as hernia repair, minor plastic procedures, reduction of fractures, or suturing of lacerations, where there has been minimal dehydration and no blood loss is expected. The chief reason for infusion here may be to have an accessible route for use in administering medication, but one still must choose the type of fluid and the amount to be given.

Type of fluid. Several solutions containing glucose and similar, but not identical, combinations of electrolytes are acceptable for standard use. Our preference is 5% dextrose in ¼-strength saline solution.

Amount and rate of administration. As suggested by Holliday and Segar (1957), Table 25-1 serves as an excellent basic guide for uncomplicated cases.

What does fluid therapy for sick patients include?

When a child is unable to maintain his own fluid metabolism, the scope of supportive therapy includes the following functions:

1. Preoperative replacement of deficits and correction of imbalances in fluid, electrolyte, and hematologic components
2. Intraoperative provision of water for replacement of insensible water loss and maintenance of kidney function
3. Provision of electrolytes for chemical needs and acid-base balance
4. Provision of calories for production of energy
5. Administration of colloids for maintenance of oncotic pressure
6. Replacement of losses incurred during anesthesia and surgery
7. Over prolonged periods, in addition to the above, provision of needed protein, fat, and vitamin components

Indications for fluid therapy: when is an infusion needed?

Because there may be serious differences of opinion as to the indications for intravenous infusion, it should be pointed out that there are two distinctly different reasons for the establishment of an infusion: first, to administer supportive fluids, and second, to have a means of administering drugs. It follows that there will be at least two different

TABLE 25-1. Basic guide for pediatric fluid therapy in uncomplicated cases

Body weight	Amount and rate
0-10 kg	4 ml/kg/hr
10-20 kg	40 ml + 2 ml/kg/hr for each kg over 10
Over 20 kg	60 ml + 1 ml/kg/hr for each kg over 20

From Holliday, M. A., and Segar, W. E.: The maintenance need for water in parenteral fluid therapy, Pediatrics **19**:823, 1957. Copyright American Academy of Pediatrics 1957.

answers to our question. A great many anesthesiologists would say that an infusion is needed in every case, having in mind their preference for a ready route for medication. This seems reasonable if not carried too far, as in multiple attempts at venipuncture in a child about to undergo circumcision.

The indications for actual administration of fluids would be less all-inclusive, because children coming to short procedures while still relatively well hydrated could hardly be said to be in need of supportive fluids. The fact that fluids are given to many patients who do not need them is accepted as a precautionary procedure, but as in the above situation, one is not justified in carrying the practice to the extreme.

At The Children's Hospital Medical Center, it is our belief that if children have prominent, easily accessible veins, one is justified in administering anesthesia for many ambulatory surgical procedures and other minor operations without an infusion.

In most situations, the establishment of an intravenous infusion is definitely preferable, as in the majority of operations of more than an hour's duration, in those starting in midmorning or later, and in patients who are slightly warm or have not been taking fluids. There are many more times when infusion is mandatory, and the operation should not be started until at least one infusion is reliably established. These, of course, include all extensive procedures involving high-risk patients but in addition include several that might not be suspected to involve particular hazard. Foremost among the procedures where an infusion has unrecognized importance are closure of colostomy, anoplasty, and other perineal operations and drainage of a septic hip, all in infants under 2 years of age. Surgeons may deny the need for infusion and scoff at the idea of transfusion, but blood is frequently needed in colostomy closure and perineal repairs. An infected hip joint in an infant usually entails general symptoms of fever, dehydration, and fatigue, the infant usually is a chubby 1-year-old, and the surgeons often will want to open the hip after aspirating the joint.

A discussion of the indications for fluid therapy might also call for a review of the specific signs or measurements that should be recognized as symptoms of fluid need, whether volume, electrolyte, or other components, at any time in the course of the operative procedure. Such signs would include the appearance of marked sweating, temperature elevation, tachycardia, pallor, bleeding, or hypothermia and laboratory findings of hypoglycemia, acidosis, and hemoconcentration.

Why is fluid therapy in infants and children different from that in adults?

1. Body fluids differ with age in respect to anatomy, physiology, and pathology.
2. The relative size of fluid compartments differs in different age groups.
3. Metabolic rate is more variable in young infants.
4. Children change more rapidly, both in outward activity and in physiologic response to stimuli.
5. The added effect of growth distorts the picture.
6. There is more danger of metabolic acidosis, hypothermia, and hypoglycemia in children.
7. The rate of fluid metabolism is two to three times faster in infants than in adults.
8. The degree of maturity of the infant kidney is not well understood.
9. Because of renal immaturity, the margin for error is definitely reduced.
10. Measurements are more difficult to make and errors are magnified because of the infant's small size.

What fluids are needed?

As shown in Table 25-2, commercially available solutions have been prepared to meet the requirements of most types of fluid imbalance as well as the demands of most of the experts in the field.

Essentially healthy children with normal kidneys can accept a fairly wide range of solutions. For short-term support, solutions containing water, glucose, and saline are adequate, and potassium may be added on occasion when there has been loss of gastric fluid or loss by dialysis. Each type of deficit or

Table 25-2. Parenteral solutions for pediatric infusion

Solution	Dextrose (g/L)	Na (mEq/L)	Cl (mEq/L)	K (mEq/L)	Ca (mEq/L)	Mg (mEq/L)	Lactate (mEq/L)	Cal/L	pH	Tonicity	mOsm/L
5% dextrose in water	50	—	—	—	—	—	—	170	5.0	Hypo	253
10% dextrose in water	100	—	—	—	—	—	—	340	4.9	Hyper	505
5% dextrose in ½-strength saline	50	77	77	—	—	—	—	170	4.9	Hyper	407
5% dextrose in ⅓-strength saline	50	51.3	38.5	—	—	—	—	170	4.5	Hyper	355
5% dextrose in ¼-strength saline	50	38.5	38.5	—	—	—	—	170	4.7	Hyper	330
2.5% dextrose in ½-strength Ringer's	25	74	78	2	2	—	28	85	4.8	Iso	281
Ringer's lactate	—	130	109	4	3	—	28	9	6.7	Iso	273
Normosol-R, pH 7.4	—	140	98	5	—	3	—	18	7.4	Iso	295
0.9% saline	—	154	154	—	—	—	—	—	5.7	Iso	308
50% dextrose in water	500	—	—	—	—	—	—	1700	4.2	Hyper	2526
8% sodium bicarbonate	—	952	952	—	—	—	—	—	7.8	Hyper	2000
THAM-E	—	30	35	5	—	—	—	—	10.6	Hyper	—
20% mannitol	—	—	—	—	—	—	—	—	6.2	Hyper	1098

imbalance may require a solution of different composition depending on the type and degree of electrolyte or acid-base disturbance.

For replacement in preoperative problems of dehydration and metabolic acidosis, isotonic balanced electrolyte solutions are generally most reliable.

Several of the less frequently used fluids involve individual drawbacks. Vascular irritation caused by 10% calcium chloride and myocardial depression caused by potassium are undesirable, while excess osmotic pressure following administration of sodium bicarbonate (2000 mOsm/L) may be lethal.

What is the background to current differences in fluid management?

To understand the problems presently met in pediatric fluid therapy, a review of the background may be helpful.

The first use of intravenous fluids in both children and adults was directed toward treatment of acute gastrointestinal infections in which there was severe loss of fluid and electrolyte. During this period, extensive and laborious investigation of fluid metabolism, metabolic activity, and renal function was carried out by physiologists and pediatricians, the work of Gamble (1951, 1954), Darrow and Pratt (1950), Talbot and associates (1955), and McCance (1950) being among the most outstanding.

The initial growth of pediatric surgery, between 1930 and 1950, found pediatricians more experienced than surgeons in the use of fluids. Consequently, pediatricians were called on to manage surgical fluid therapy. Their habitual use of large quantities of fluids led to widespread overdosage, however, and the surgeons took matters into their own hands. Because of the problems of overloading and influenced by reports of McCance and Widdowson (1952) and others concerning the limited excretion of sodium by neonates, the surgeons established a regimen that combined strict limitation of fluid with complete elimination of sodium for neonates, emphasizing the need of large amounts of glucose. Children were given 5% dextrose in water and infants 10% dextrose in water, with additional blood replacement as needed.

This concept of keeping children, and especially infants, "on the dry side" was embraced throughout the field of pediatric surgery for approximately 30 years. During this time, it proved to be practical, and remarkable surgical achievements were recorded. Some credit may have been owed to the fact that children were brought to surgery in good condition, that generous amounts of whole blood were used, and that surgeons made a fetish of getting the child off the operating table as quickly as possible. While the more extensive procedures currently undertaken do require longer operating time, the earlier emphasis on speed undoubtedly reduced third-space losses considerably when compared with the prolonged handling that infant viscera now endure.

During the past 10 years a decidedly different approach to pediatric fluid therapy has been advanced. Proponents of the Shires concept of ample fluid replacement have swept forward, urging the use of generous amounts of both water and saline solution from birth onward (Bennett and others, 1970; Herbert and others, 1971; Berry, 1974; Furman and others, 1975). Backing for this concept is found in the revised estimation of the infant's renal function, with evidence now pointing to maturation of most aspects by the second or third month of life. There is reason to believe, however, that the broad application of increased allowance of fluid would endanger many infants who are in cardiac or respiratory failure. The concept of abundant fluid allowance is open to further criticism because there is little evidence that it has improved clinical results and because infants, unlike adults, rarely develop postoperative renal failure, this complication having been the intial reason for its use in adults. It is the intent in this chapter to point out inadequacies in both approaches and to emphasize the *importance of individualizing therapy* rather than applying one concept to all patients.

For the pediatric anesthesiologist, the body of knowledge having direct application to the supportive management of infants and children has reached enormous proportions, as has the technical sophistication required for its application. Among the new problems that now confront us are open-heart operations on premature infants in cardiac failure, kidney transplants in children in renal failure, 15-hour craniofacial reconstructions where blood loss may double the child's blood volume, and extensive spinal fusions on children whose parents, as Jehovah's Witnesses, forbid the use of all blood products. It is the newborn who still presents the greatest challenge and causes the greatest difference of opinion among anesthesiologists.

In reviewing past experience, one finds that errors have always plagued intravenous therapy in children. Formerly, errors were primarily those of inadequacy, whether in judgment, equipment, or skill. Many of these errors have been eliminated by experience and technical advances. Today our errors tend to be those of commission rather than omission; overhydration, vascular injury, and increased instrumentation are among the worst offenders.

What are the fundamental factors in body fluids, and how do they differ between infants and adults?

The factors that affect fluid control throughout life include *anatomic factors* relating to volume, distribution, and composition of body fluids, *physiologic factors* relating to metabolism, rate of fluid turnover, and requirements for maintenance and growth, and *pathologic factors* relating to abnormal effects of illness, anesthesia, and surgery.

In all aspects of these considerations, a wide degree of variability must be accepted in describing both normal and abnormal conditions. The spread of figures in numerous instances suggests how inaccurate it would be to allow any single figure to represent a biologic variable.

Anatomic factors. The human body is made up of solids and body fluids. The solids include fat, skeletal muscle, and cell solids.

Total body water. Total body water (TBW) consists of extracellular fluid (ECF) and intracellular fluid (ICF). ECF includes plasma volume (PV) and interstitial fluid volume (ISF). Early in fetal existence, 90% of the human body consists of water. Although this proportion is reduced during gestation, infants are born with a high TBW content, variously estimated as between 70% and 84% of their total body weight in contrast to the average of 55% to 60% in adults (Fig. 25-1). This greater proportion of TBW present at birth and in the early months of life constitutes the first major difference between the body fluids of infants and adults.

Several variables may alter the degree of neonatal water content: (1) premature babies can be expected to have proportionately higher total body fluid, (2) infants born by caesarean section retain the fluid that ordinarily would be wrung from them during their passage through the birth canal, and (3) infants allowed a placental transfusion prior to division of the umbilical cord will show a gain of approximately 100 ml according to Strauss and associates (1965).

Infants generally experience natriuresis and loss of considerable fluid during the first days of life and a continuing reduction of the ECF excess throughout the first 6 to 9 months. Adult proportions of fluid to body weight are reached between 9 months and 2 years of life according to several investigators (Friis-Hansen, 1961; Kerrigan, 1963; Rickham, 1979). There is no difference between the TBW of males and that of females until puberty, when females begin to develop a slightly higher body fat content, with a relative reduction of TBW to approximately 55% of body weight as compared with the 60% average of the adult male.

Blood volume. Blood volume represents approximately 10% of TBW. It is usually esti-

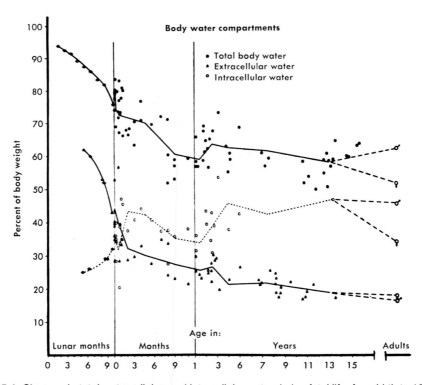

Fig. 25-1. Changes in total, extracellular, and intracellular water during fetal life, from birth to 16 years of age, and extended to corresponding normal values in the adult female and male subject. (From Friis-Hansen, B.: Acta Paediatr. Scand. [Suppl.], vol. 110, 1957.)

mated as changing proportion in ml/kg, as shown in Table 25-3.

Figures for TBW and blood volume are easily confused. In the infant, TBW is calculated as 80% of body weight and would amount to 2000 ml in a 2.5-kg neonate, while blood volume is calculated as 80 ml/kg body weight. In the same 2.5-kg baby this would total 200 ml:

TBW = 80% × 2500 g = 2000 g or 2000 ml
Blood volume = 80 ml × 2.5 kg = 200 ml

Distribution of body fluids. Since most of the excess fluid present at birth (estimated as approximately 500 ml) is carried as ECF, the ECF in neonates equals or exceeds the ICF. This represents the second major difference between the body fluids of infants and adults. Adults retain approximately the same proportion of ICF but show a loss of more than half the original proportion of ECF (Table 25-4). As previously noted, much of this loss occurs in early infancy.

While there is little question as to the relatively larger ECF of the infant, there is considerable disagreement over whether the larger ECF works to his advantage or disadvantage. Kaplan (1969) and others feel that

this fluid acts as available reserve that can be called on to compensate for the rapid losses in infancy, but this concept is contested by others who deny that the "expanded" ECF plays any protective role.

There is considerable discrepancy in the figures reported for ICF and ECF in both infants and adults. This probably reflects both the difficulty in measuring fluid spaces* and the wide variation that actually exists in different individuals.

As shown in Table 25-4, in infants at term, ICF and ECF each usually constitute approximately 40% of body weight, while in adults (male), ICF and ECF would approximate 40% and 20% of body weight, respectively.

Extracellular water is made up of interstitial fluid and plasma. Plasma remains at approximately the same proportion of body weight (5%) throughout life. Consequently, it is the interstitial water that is greater in infancy (35%), declining to 15% and 10% of body weight, respectively, in adult males and females.

Composition of body fluids. There are several minor differences between the composition of the body fluids of infants and adults (Table 25-5). The infant's higher plas-

*NOTE: Although the term *fluid compartments* suggests the existence of bounded spaces, no true boundaries exist. Intracellular water includes all body water inside the cells (including red and white blood corpuscles), while extracellular water includes all fluid outside the cells (including plasma, lymph, spinal fluid, and joint fluid).

Table 25-3. Blood volume related to age and sex

Age and sex	Blood volume (ml/kg)
0-2 yr	80
2-16 yr	70
Adult	
Male	60
Female	55

Table 25-4. Distribution of body fluids in the newborn and adult

	Newborn (% body weight)	Adult (% body weight)
Extracellular		
Interstitial	35	15
Plasma	5	5
Intracellular	40	40
	80	60

Table 25-5. Extracellular chemical elements of newborn infants and adults

	Newborns	Adults
Sodium (mEq/L)	140	140
Potassium (mEq/L)	5.0-6.5	3.8-6.0
Chloride (mEq/L)	107	103
Bicarbonate (mEq/L)	21-24	22-27
Phosphate (mEq/l)	5.0-8.0	2.5-4.5
Protein (g/100 ml)	5	7
Osmotic pressure (mOsm/L)	310	310

Adapted from Bland, J. H.: The clinical use of fluid and electrolyte, Philadelphia, 1952, W. B. Saunders Co.

ma chloride and lower pH and bicarbonate suggest a tendency toward metabolic acidosis and reduced buffering power, while lower protein concentration implies reduced oncotic pressure. The significance initially attributed to these findings now appears exaggerated, for slight acidity at this age favors oxygen release to the tissues, and other compensatory factors may be found that will justify the existence of other seemingly abnormal figures.

Although the concentration of sodium in the neonate's additional 500 ml of ECF remains at 140 mEq/L, thereby showing no evidence of sodium increase, the total sodium content obviously is greater by 70 mEq.

It should be emphasized that although one speaks of the differences between infants and adults, in respect to body fluid characteristics most of the changes to "adult" figures take place in infancy or early childhood.

Physiologic and pathologic factors. Much of the difficulty one finds in pediatric fluid therapy is caused by the changing rates of fluid metabolism in the young infant. While the fluid metabolism in terms of water requirement stays at approximately 1500 ml/m² from early childhood well into adult life, the infant starts below this level and later exceeds it.

Fluid metabolism proceeds slowly during the first 3 or 4 days after birth. Water exchange is chiefly negative because of losses via skin, lungs, and excretions, with little intake. As soon as the baby begins to take feedings, however, fluid metabolism accelerates rapidly, reaching peak level at about 2 years of age. At this time, as impressively shown by Gamble (1954), the 7-kg infant with a 1400-ml ECF takes in and excretes 700 ml of fluid daily, thus showing a 50% turnover of his ECF, while a 70-kg adult with a 14,000-ml ECF has only a 2000-ml, or 14%, ECF turnover. The effect of the more rapid fluid exchange is to expose the infant to more sudden development of either dehydration or overhydration. (It is worth noting here that the danger of dehydration, which has been widely recognized, is reduced by the presence of several natural defense mechanisms that have evolved over millennia, while the danger of overhydration is of modern origin, chiefly due to therapeutic error, and thus there has not been sufficient time for protective responses to evolve.)

PHYSIOLOGIC CONTROL OF FLUID METABOLISM

Differences that exist in the TBW and in the rate of fluid metabolism offer problems, as has been pointed out, but they are measurable and can be overcome with reasonable accuracy.

The factors that control fluid metabolism, on the other hand, are not yet clearly established. Measurement is difficult, and numbers, when obtained, will have little meaning if the response is not developed.

It is in this tangle of developing hormonal and renal physiology that our main problems of water retention and sodium excretion have been snarled and are slowly being extricated. (For excellent coverage of this area, see chapters on The Kidney, by Edelmann and Spitzer, and Endocrinology II by Fisher, both in *The Physiology of the Newborn Infant* [1976] by Smith and Nelson.)

The factors that control fluid metabolism in adult life include the circulation, sympathetic nervous system, endocrine system, and kidneys. It is believed that the same factors are effective from fetal existence, but the relationships are not clear. As outlined in Chapter 2, circulatory and sympathetic nervous systems are well organized at birth. The state of development of endocrine and renal control is the subject of intense study but is less certainly defined. Of chief importance here are the antidiuretic hormone (ADH), aldosterone, the renin-angiotensin system of the kidney, and the various functions of the infant kidney, also described in Chapter 2. Important questions to be considered are: (1) does the infant have normal hormonal output and (2) is the kidney able to respond effectively to hormonal signals?

ADH, or vasopressin, has been studied extensively in the adult, its synthesis in the posterior thalamus being well established. Activated by volume receptors in the chest and by thirst and osmolality centers in the anterior hypothalamus (Strauss, 1957), ADH has as its main function the maintenance of plasma volume (Table 25-6).

There are several conditions that stimulate ADH secretion, among which hypovolemia and hyperosmolality are the most important. Hypovolemia is definitely the stronger of these two. During progressive dehydration in older children and adults, ADH response is first stimulated by thirst and subsequently by hypovolemia. Other ADH stimuli include various stressing conditions such as pain, anxiety, anesthesia, and surgery. Such specific drugs as nicotine and morphine also stimulate ADH secretion. Continuous positive pressure ventilation is believed to have a similar effect (Sladen and others, 1968).

ADH acts by increasing the resorption of water in the distal collecting tubules of the kidney, thereby increasing plasma volume, reducing osmolality, and at the same time depressing aldosterone secretion with resultant increased excretion of sodium. The rate of ADH secretion under normal circumstances in adults is reported to be approximately 0.1 to 0.3 mU/kg/hr (Moore, 1959).

As previously stated in Chapter 2, McCrory (1972) considers the infant's ADH con-

Table 25-6. Antidiuretic hormone (ADH), vasopressin

Normal activity	Inappropriate ADH secretion
Stimuli	Stimuli
Hypovolemia	Hypovolemia
Hyperosmolality	Hypotonicity
Anxiety	Responses
Anesthesia	Water retention
Operation	Continued Na
Nicotine	excretion
Morphine	Result
Positive pressure ventilation	Hypotonic hy-
Responses	pervolemia
Increased plasma volume	Seizures
Increased resorption	Cerebral edema
Reduced urine loss	Death
Reduced serum osmolality	
Depression of aldosterone	
Increased Na excretion	

trol to be comparable with that of older patients, and there is increasing evidence to confirm his conviction. Levina (1968) and Heller and Zaimis (1949) have shown that the neonate's posterior pituitary holds a large quantity of vasopressin at birth (from 4 to 5 units), while the maximal antidiuresis in adults requires only a few milliunits.

During and immediately after birth, considerable amounts of ADH have been found in the infant's circulation, appreciably more in those born by active labor than by caesarean section (means of 113 and 35 μU/ml, respectively) (Hoppenstein and others, 1968). In the neonate, blood levels of ADH are easily demonstrable. Blood levels on the first day average 0.5 μU/ml, and they average 1.3 μU/ml between the first and fourth day (Hoppenstein and others, 1968). Some workers have been unable to detect any ADH in infants between 1 and 3 to 5 months of age (Hradcova and Heller, 1962). However, Ames (1953) and Hoppenstein and associates (1968) have identified low concentrations of ADH throughout the first 3 months, with an initial level of 0.46 μU/ml later rising to 3 μU/ml during the first month. An impressive augmentation of ADH response to stimulation was also demonstrated during the first 3 months (Fig. 25-2).

Fisher (1976) found evidence that the newborn is able to release vasopressin in response to both osmolar and volume stimuli within a few hours after birth and that, on exposure to cold (below 30° C), epinephrine release inhibits ADH and causes diuresis. The presence of vasopressin during the critical period of fluid therapy appears to be established, as are the mechanisms for its release and inhibition. The renal response, as stated by Fisher (1976), is temporarily reduced by developmental limitations of "glomerular filtration rate and concentrating capacity but the resulting limitation in ability of the newborn to conserve free water is minimal."

Inappropriate secretion of ADH

Abnormal ADH activity is seen in several situations, some of which may be due to al-

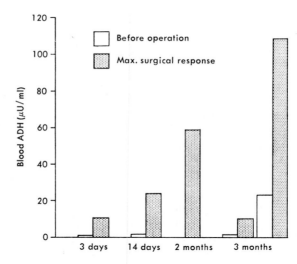

Fig. 25-2. Blood ADH response of infants to operation. (From Hoppenstein, J. M., Miltenberger, F. W., and Moran, W. H., Jr.: Surg. Gynecol. Obstet. **127**:966, 1968. By permission of Surgery, Gynecology & Obstetrics.)

tered conditions peculiar to infants, such as low dietary urea content, high fluid intake, and, according to Winters (1973), inability to handle large water loads. The disturbance known as *inappropriate ADH secretion* (Schwartz and others, 1957) is characterized by an active response of ADH to hypovolemia in spite of the presence of hyponatremia. This is often associated with pediatric operations, disorders of the central nervous system and lungs, tumors, and other strong stimuli. The result is severe *hypotonic hypervolemia*. Diagnosis is confirmed by the finding of hypertonic urine in the presence of hypotonic hypervolemia (Winters, 1973). The relatively frequent postoperative appearance of this syndrome in elderly patients was reported by Deutsch and associates (1966). Its occurrence in infants is well known and may lead to confusion in therapy, because the presence of hyponatremia is easily mistaken for inability of the kidneys to conserve sodium when it is actually due to dilution.

Particular concern has been voiced repeatedly in the last few years about the danger of inappropriate secretion of ADH following hypoxic periods in premature and newborn infants with perinatal asphyxia (Feldman and

others, 1970; Kaplan and Feigin, 1978). Marked cerebral edema rapidly progressing to death has occurred in several cases. Laboratory findings of a typical case reported by Kaplan and Feigin showed the following: serum sodium, 110 mEq/L; weight increase, 230 g in one day; plasma osmolality, 217 mOsm/kg; urine osmolality, 568 mOsm/kg; arginine vasopressin level, 2.5 μU/ml (mean average in children 7 months to 15 years, 0.7 μU/ml).

Aldosterone, the most potent mineralocorticoid synthesized by the adrenal cortex, is easily identifiable from birth onward. Weldon and associates (1967) found a secretion rate of 23 μg/24 hr in neonates, which rises to 72 μg/24 hr in infants from 1 to 12 weeks old. Minick and Conn (1964) reported a higher aldosterone concentration in infants (1.6 μg/kg) than in adults (1.0 μg/kg).

As in adults, hyponatremia is an effective stimulus to the production of aldosterone (Table 25-7), levels of 7, 77, and 303 μg/kg having been found in response to high, medium, and low sodium administration, respectively (Siegel and others, 1974). Bennett and associates (1970, 1971) reported the potent stimulation of aldosterone secretion by hypo-

Table 25-7. Aldosterone

Stimuli	Responses
Low serum sodium	Sodium retention
Increased BUN	Reduction of BUN
Decreased urinary specific gravity	Increased plasma volume
High serum potassium	Potassium excretion

natremia and the less potent direct relationship of aldosterone to blood urea nitrogen (BUN) and urinary specific gravity. As noted by Fisher (1976), however, renal tubules of the infant sometimes do not respond predictably. Some cases have been found where administration of aldosterone either had no effect on sodium excretion or actually caused increased excretion (Greenberg and others, 1967). It has also been found that the young infant may need an increased stimulus to produce an increased aldosterone secretion (Weldon and others, 1971).

Again we find that the substance is present and the basic responses usually occur, but there is reason to suspect that the situation is not exactly the same during early infancy as in later life, and the evidence of sodium control is not convincing.

Other less well understood factors affect renal function, among which the natriuretic hormone, or "third factor," has been found to produce sodium excretion in spite of extensive damage to filtration mechanisms (Bricker, 1967).

Kidneys

The intricate role of the kidneys in fluid metabolism was described in Chapter 2. The main points may be summarized as follows.

There still is widespread belief that (1) the neonatal kidney has limited ability to concentrate urine (maximum osmolality 800 mOsm/L in the neonate as compared with 1400 mOsm/L in the adult), (2) it has limited ability to excrete large water loads rapidly (Davenport, 1950), and (3) it has limited ability to excrete many common compounds that older kidneys excrete easily (Calcagno, 1960, 1967; Cooke, 1968).

It is obvious, however, that the normal infant kidney does an excellent job in managing its large natural load of fluid, and there is increasing evidence that it could more nearly match adult levels of performance if presented with similar conditions (higher dietary urea, decreased preponderance of fluid intake). There is also general agreement that by the end of the second week great changes have taken place and that practically all renal function has reached adult performance levels by the time the normal infant is 9 to 12 months old.

There are still major gaps in our information, points of disagreement and uncertainty, and inadequate consideration of important established information. Whether the neonate is an obligatory salt-loser or whether low serum sodium is due to inappropriate ADH secretion seems uncertain. The answer is important but difficult to determine.

Studies of premature infants carried out by Oh (1976) show that smaller premature infants have relatively greater insensible water loss due to several factors, including relatively greater body surface area, exposure to phototherapy, and increased peripheral blood flow. If this water loss is not replaced, an increased serum sodium level will result, but if only water is replaced, hyponatremia will occur. Further imbalance is caused by treatment involving positive pressure ventilation and/or high humidification. It is becoming increasingly obvious that fluid therapy in the small infant demands meticulous measurement of several variables and that treatment must be highly individualized. The maturity of the infant at birth, the type of ventilatory and supportive treatment required and the presence of congenital cardiac lesions may weigh against increased fluid administration, while the excessive losses of infants with intestinal obstruction or necrotizing enterocolitis will demand greatly increased replacement.

Osmolality

As emphasized by Moore (1959), Finberg (1969, 1977), and Rowe and Marchildon (1976), an understanding of the significance

of the osmolality of blood, urine, therapeutic
fluids, and drugs is essential in clinical management of patients.

Osmolality is defined as the number of particles of solute contained in 1 unit volume
of a liquid. The standard units are millios-
mols/liter (mOsm/L). For direct measurement of osmolality one uses an osmometer,
which works on the principle of freezing
point depression. For clinical practice it is
usually possible to base one's estimate on
serum sodium, which makes up a major portion of serum osmolality. Using twice the
serum sodium measured in mEq/L and
changing the units to mOsm/L will provide
a useful approximation, accounting for all but
the relatively small amount contributed by
colloids, in this case urea and glucose. When
there is marked derangement of BUN or glucose, as in severe burns, peritonitis, lipemia,
or cardiorenal diseases, this simple method
of estimating osmolality would be quite inaccurate, the error being referred to as "the
anion gap" (Oh and Carroll, 1977). For more
precise determination of osmolality in such
situations the following formula is used:

$$\text{Osmolality (mOsm/L)} = 2Na + \frac{BUN}{2.8} + \frac{glucose\ (mg/dl)}{18}$$

Osmolality determines the movement of
fluids within the body; more dilute fluid is
drawn through permeable membranes toward more concentrated fluid. Normal serum
osmolality is considered to vary between 280
and 295 mOsm/L (Table 25-8), although
some extend the upper range to 305 or 310
mOsm/L. The osmolality of urine is roughly
1.5 times that of serum under normal conditions. The reduction of serum osmolality
below 240 mOsm/L entails danger of edema
and convulsions and would be associated
with marked hyponatremia. In pediatric
anesthesia, the greatest danger related to
osmolal derangement lies in excessive use of
sodium bicarbonate (osmolality 2000 mOsm/
L) in attempts to correct metabolic acidosis.
Rapid changes in osmolality increase the
danger greatly, and any rise of more than 25
mOsm/L in less than 24 hours is considered

Table 25-8. Osmolality

	Amount (mOsm/kg)
Normal serum osmolality	270-290
Severe hypotonicity	Under 240
Severe hypertonicity	Over 340
ICF	295
ECF	295
Plasma water	295
Urine (1-1.5 × serum osmolality)	310-450

by Finberg (1967, 1977) to be extremely
hazardous. Because of the danger of inducing
hyperosmolal damage to the brain, the use
of either sodium bicarbonate or tris(hydroxymethyl)aminomethane (THAM) is contraindicated when serum osmolality approaches
320 mOsm/L.

TYPES OF FLUID AND ELECTROLYTE IMBALANCE OCCURRING PREOPERATIVELY

Anesthesiologists are not usually responsible for corrective fluid therapy before patients come to the operating room. However,
they should understand the types of imbalance that occur, know how to correct them,
and know what complications to look for.

In the management of fluid therapy, the
intraoperative replacement of losses and
overall provision of maintenance usually are
much less complicated than the correction of
states of imbalance in patients coming to operation. Disturbances of body fluids may be
described under four headings: water, electrolyte, acid-base, and colloid imbalances
(Table 25-9). Unfortunately, these rarely occur as a single pathologic defect but, except
in milder forms, appear in varying degrees
and numerous combinations. The more severe the situation, the more complex the involvement, with dehydration progressing to
hypertonicity, acidemia, azotemia, and so on.

In general, the descriptions of the more
serious disturbances of fluid balance relate
to nonsurgical patients suffering from acute
diarrhea, prolonged vomiting, extreme fever,

Table 25-9. Types of body fluid imbalance

Water	Electrolyte	Acid-base	Colloid
Overhydration	Excess or deficit of:	Metabolic acidosis	Excess or deficit of:
Dehydration	Sodium	Metabolic alkalosis	Red blood cells
Isotonic	Chloride	Respiratory acidosis	Serum albumin
Hypotonic	Potassium	Respiratory alkalosis	Serum globulin
Hypertonic	Calcium	Mixed acid-base response	Abnormal albumin/globulin ratio
	Magnesium		

or salt poisoning. Infants and children seldom come to operation in the critical state of dehydration or hypernatremia seen on medical wards, but the occasional infant with acute necrotizing enterocolitis or the child with craniopharyngioma may require specific therapy, and other surgical patients make it necessary to understand some of the finer points of fluid balance.

Correction of imbalances can only be accomplished after one has recognized their existence, diagnosed the type, and evaluated the degree of abnormality. Valuable time will be saved if one knows when to expect serious deficits and does not wait until they have become blatantly evident. Certainly one should expect to find metabolic acidosis in cold, hypoxic neonates, metabolic alkalosis in infants with pyloric stenosis, and respiratory acidosis in children with early cystic fibrosis.

Water imbalance

Overhydration. Some degree of dehydration is frequently seen in patients coming to operation and does not necessarily connote underlying pathology. The occasional patient with overhydration is apt to present a more dangerous situation and should arouse immediate concern. Overhydration is most commonly seen in small infants as a result of iatrogenic overloading in the presence of cardiac or renal disease. This is seen more often in the postoperative phase, but if these infants are brought back for reoperation, as frequently happens, the result of postoperative treatment may still be prominent. Other causes of water overload include dilutional hyponatremia, inappropriate ADH secretion, and cardiac or renal failure.

The presence of water overload is easily overlooked. Hypervolemia will first cause venous distension. In small infants an early sign is the disappearance of the tiny creases in their upper eyelids and then the appearance of a bluish sheen in the tissue of the upper lids (Conn, 1978). Ankle edema is rarely seen in young patients, and pulmonary edema is one of the later signs. One should look for overhydration in any patient with suspected cardiac or renal disease, unexplained weight gain, excess intake as compared with output, low urine output, prominent veins, flushed skin, high arterial and central venous blood pressure, reduced pulse rate, and laboratory findings of low hematocrit and low serum sodium and osmolality.

For correction of overhydration in the preoperative patient, one naturally restricts fluid intake. When there is marked overload, operation should be delayed until the patient can be "dried out" by fluid restriction or use of diuretics. Since diuretics may further upset electrolyte balance, electrolytes should be rechecked before operation. Furosemide (Lasix) in intravenous dosage of 0.5 to 1.0 mg/kg is among the most effective agents in current use.

Dehydration. Dehydration is the most common type of fluid disturbance in clinical anesthesia. It is most frequently seen in small children who have been denied food and fluid prior to operation. Since these children usually have been in good condition until this time and the "starvation" is brief, this form of dehydration is generally so mild that it is not clinically detectable. Occasionally more severely dehydrated children come to operation having lost excessive fluid through vomiting, intestinal drainage, infection, or increased metabolism.

Dehydration may occur in any situation where the loss of water exceeds water intake for a significant period. The loss of body water to the outside environment must occur as a loss from the ECF and therefore will represent loss of both water and electrolytes. The resultant type of dehydration is determined by the ratio of water to electrolyte remaining in the ECF; consequently, it may be isotonic, hypotonic, or hypertonic. While differentiation may be neither evident nor essential in milder forms, correct diagnosis is important in advanced stages, since improper treatment can be disastrous.

Because sodium is the principal determinant of serum osmolality, it usually may be assumed that isotonic, hypotonic, and hypertonic forms of dehydration are isonatremic, hyponatremic, and hypernatremic, respectively.

In *isotonic dehydration,* the fluid that is lost contains the same electrolyte concentration as the ECF from which it came, and the osmolality remains unchanged at 275 to 290 mOsm/L. There will therefore be no compensatory replacement of ECF, which, having stood the entire loss, will be significantly reduced, and shock may ensue if the situation is allowed to progress. As seen in the list below, losses of gastrointestinal fluid by vomiting, bowel obstruction, and other visceral effusions often fall into this group (see p. 562 for therapy).

CLINICAL CONDITIONS ASSOCIATED WITH FLUID AND ELECTROLYTE LOSS

Isotonic dehydration (270-290 mOsm/L)
Pyloric obstruction
Upper and lower bowel obstruction
Loss of gastrointestinal secretions via fistulae, drains, and ileostomy

Peritonitis
Starvation
Hypotonic dehydration (less than 270 mOsm/L)
Salt-losing nephritis
Adrenogenital syndrome
Fever
Diarrhea
Starvation
Hypertonic dehydration (more than 290 mOsm/L)
Loss of surface moisture, sweating, fever
Burns
Tracheostomy
Diarrhea

In *hypotonic dehydration,* more electrolyte (Na) is lost than water. This may be caused by starvation and leaves the ECF diluted to an osmolality of less than 275 mOsm/L. The reduced ECF osmolality causes further movement of fluid out of the extracellular space and into the intracellular space, thereby speeding the loss of circulating volume and increasing the danger of shock.

Hypertonic dehydration involves greater loss of water than electrolyte, and the resultant high osmolar concentration of ECF leads to the influx of fluid from surrounding tissues. While the danger of the development of shock is thereby reduced, rapidly developing hypertonic dehydration, as seen in acute diarrhea, introduces other hazards that render this the most dangerous of all forms of dehydration. Fortunately, acute diarrhea is rarely seen as a complicating factor in children coming to operation.

The clinical severity of dehydration depends on two factors: the degree or amount of the disturbance and the rate or speed at which it occurs. The *degree* of dehydration can be estimated with some reliability by the loss of body weight, if the figures are available. The total weight loss is calculated as fluid. Thus, the loss of each kilogram of body weight will be an indication for 1 kilogram, or 1 liter, of replacement fluid:

$$\text{Water deficit} = 1 \text{ L/kg weight loss}$$

If, as often happens, the initial weight is not known, one must estimate the degree of hydration by the child's history, clinical signs, and laboratory findings. It has been observed that the degree of dehydration can be correlated with an estimated percentage weight loss. Pediatricians and physiologists seem to believe unanimously in the concept that clinical signs do not appear until a child has lost 5% of his normal weight, that a 10% weight loss is moderate, that 15% is severe, and that 20% is often fatal. Here again, the more rapid the onset of dehydration, the greater the danger to the child. Evaluation of the degree of dehydration never is simple, and all aids should be used. Dell's chart (Fig. 25-3) and Table 25-10 may help to correlate signs, weight loss, and severity of fluid deficit.

The *rate of development* of dehydration naturally is more rapid in younger patients. Because of relatively greater body surface area and associated elevated metabolic rate, the infant depletes his fluid stores three times faster than the adult. In clinical situations, however, many variables come into play. The age of the child first accelerates the basic time progression a predictable amount, and further increases occur with the superimposition of losses from gastric drainage, fistulae and surgical drains, vomiting, fever, sweating, crying, increased activity, and especially acute diarrhea. Depletion of ECF in adults, which would take 10 days, would be expected to take only 3 days in a normal 1-year-old child and approximately 1 day if this child were acutely ill.

What then is the progression of dehydration of the child awaiting operation? The first sign of dehydration in normal infants is considered to be loss of skin turgor, which may become evident after 15 to 18 hours of starvation. Other early signs of dehydration are seen after about 24 hours, when the infant will first show appreciable (5%) loss of weight. By this time, thirst, drying mucous membranes, and reduced salivary secretions will have induced antidiuretic activity, and the normal rate of urinary excretion is reduced to compensate for reduced intake. During the next 10 to 15 hours the infant will show decreasing urinary output and in-

Table 25-10. Severity of dehydration (isotonic)

Severity	Amount lost	
	Infants	Older children and adults
Mild	50 ml/kg (5%)	30 ml/kg (3%)
Moderate	100 ml/kg (10%)	60 ml/kg (6%)
Severe	150 ml/kg (15%)	90 ml/kg (9%)

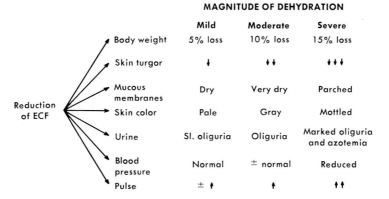

Fig. 25-3. Correlation of the intensity of clinical signs with the magnitude of dehydration. The correlation shown applies to isotonic dehydration in an infant. Modifications are required for hypertonic and hypotonic dehydration as well as for age. (From Dell, R. B.: Pathophysiology of dehydration; normal acid-base regulation. In Winters, R. W., editor: The body fluids in pediatrics, Boston, 1973, Little, Brown & Co.)

creasing blood and urine osmolality, glycogen stores will be burned, and fat metabolism will be evident in developing acidemia and ketonuria, later followed by increasing metabolic acidosis. The compensatory mechanisms for preservation of fluid control are such, even in the newborn, that in spite of absolute deprivation of all intake, these infants show continued activity and cardiorespiratory function for 8 to 10 days. The effective water conservation is shown in mounting azotemia and oliguria progressing to anuria, which, it is surprising to find, is readily reversed by administration of fluid.

While no patient should be exposed to such trials unnecessarily, observations drawn from experience with infants that have incurable brain defects have been valuable and have made it possible to gain better perspective on the overall hazards of dehydration. It is acknowledged that the infant kidney is capable of greater function than once believed. In light of the minimal effect of early dehydration, however, it does not seem reasonable to put infant kidneys to maximum capacity function during surgery.

Treatment (adapted from Graef and Cone, 1974). Regardless of the type of dehydration, two general principles of treatment are: (1) if shock is present, fluid volume should be made up rapidly with whole blood, plasma, albumin, Ringer's lactate, or saline solution and (2) intravascular volume should be restored first, followed by replacement of interstitial volume.

In the presence of severe deficits involving hypotension, deficits should be made up rapidly until blood pressure is restored. In the presence of normotension, both deficit and maintenance fluids are best given slowly in order to prevent (1) sudden cardiovascular overloading, (2) cerebral edema, and (3) hyperglycemia and resultant diuresis.

Although daily allowances will be prescribed here, pediatric intravenous fluids are always prescribed with the definite understanding that all patients will be checked at not more than 4-hour intervals and orders will be revised as needed.

ISOTONIC DEHYDRATION (dehydration with osmolality between 175 and 300 mOsm/L, serum sodium between 135 and 150 mEq/L). The fluid loss is isotonic, and therefore the replacement should be isotonic.

Procedure:
1. Calculate weight loss by direct measurement or by evaluation on the basis of signs. Weight loss in kg (or g) = fluid deficit in L (or ml).
2. Replace deficit with 0.9% saline or Ringer's lactate solution.
3. Provide maintenance fluid with 1500 to 2000 ml/m²/day, or 100 ml/kg/day in infants under 10 kg.

Example: A 10-kg child with dehydration and weight loss of 5%, serum sodium 138 mEq/L.
Fluid deficit = 10 × 0.05 = 0.5 L or 500 ml.
Deficit is made up with 500 ml of 0.9% saline solution.
Maintenance for 24 hours will approximate 1000 ml of 5% dextrose in one-fourth strength saline solution.

HYPOTONIC DEHYDRATION (dehydration with serum osmolality less than 275 mOsm/L, serum sodium less than 130 mEq/L)

Procedure:
1. Fluid deficit is calculated as in isotonic dehydration.
2. Sodium deficit is calculated as follows:
Sodium deficit (mEq) = (Normal value for sodium − present sodium value) × kg body weight × ECF.

Example: A 10-kg infant with weight loss of 5%, serum sodium 110 mEq/L.
Fluid deficit = 10 kg × 0.05 = 0.5 kg or 500 ml.
Sodium deficit = (140 − 130) × 10 kg × 0.6 = 60 mEq.
When 0.9% saline solution with 154 mEq of sodium per L is used, the infant would need 60/154 × 1000 ml = 390 ml of 0.9% saline to make up sodium deficit; the rest of the fluid deficit (110 ml) might be 5% dextrose in ¼% saline solution.

HYPERTONIC DEHYDRATION (dehydration with serum osmolality over 300 mOsm/L, serum sodium over 150 mEq/L). This type of dehydration must be replaced slowly, since there is both extracellular and intracellular loss. Rapid replacement may cause cerebral edema and convulsions. Between 24 and 48 hours are allowed for replacement in severe hypertonic dehydration. Solutions that may be used are 5% dextrose in half-strength saline or 5% dextrose in half-strength Ringer's lactate.

Electrolyte deficits

In addition to sodium, there may be important deficits in chloride and potassium and less frequently in calcium and magnesium (Srouji, 1967). Chloride deficit is characteristically seen in infants with pyloric stenosis who have been vomiting for several days. Potassium deficit may occur in more severely dehydrated infants with pyloric stenosis, but it is more commonly seen as a result of diuretic therapy. Calculation of deficit for each serum electrolyte is made as follows:

Electrolyte deficit (mEq) =
   (Normal serum concentration −
     pathologic serum value) ×
            kg body weight × ECF

EXAMPLE: A 6-kg infant with pyloric stenosis and 10% weight loss, serum chloride 85 mEq/L.

Chloride deficit = (100 − 85) ×
            6 × 0.6 = 54 mEq

Repair is calculated as follows, using 0.9% saline solution:

$$54/154 \times 1000 \text{ ml} = 350 \text{ ml}$$

Potassium imbalance. Serum potassium deficit is uncommon in pediatric patients, occurring chiefly in relation to pyloric stenosis and the use of diuretics. When serum potassium level is less than 3.2 mEq/L, replacement may be indicated but requires great care. Potassium is not replaced until the patient has received enough water to form urine. Then 10 to 20 mEq/L are added to 500 ml of infusion and given over 24 hours (Bush, 1971).

Hyperkalemia (serum K > 5.5 mEq/L) is regarded as a contraindication to anesthesia. This may be reduced preoperatively in children, as in adults, by dialysis or the use of polystyrene sodium sulfonate (Kayexalate), 1 g/kg. Intraoperative hyperkalemia may be treated by rapid infusion of 10% cal-

cium gluconate, 0.5 mg/kg IV (Williams and others, 1973). Intravenous administration of insulin and glucose (adult dose, 10 units of regular insulin with 25 grams of glucose) also may be used for the same purpose. Hyperventilation is advised to reduce serum pH.

Acid-base imbalances

Aberrations in acid-base control are common among pediatric patients and have played a major part in the death of many infants during the operative period. They offer special hazards in young patients because of the rapidity with which they develop, the degree to which they advance, the difficulty in their evaluation, and the hazards of treatment, which is presently a serious problem, particularly overadministration of sodium bicarbonate with resultant hyperosmolal cerebrovascular hemorrhage (Finberg, 1973; Feig and McCurdy, 1978).

An additional encumbrance in acid-base management has been the confusing terminology that has dogged this phase of medicine from the outset. Anions and cations erroneously considered to be acid and base by definition, similar but slightly different terms denoting alkali reserve, carbon dioxide combining power, total CO_2, actual bicarbonate, buffer base, and negative buffer base excess, and other errors have accumulated over the years. Recently, however, they have been subject to attempts at clarification. The simplification by Schwartz and Relman (1963) has been most helpful, enabling us to abandon all but pH, Pco_2, and bicarbonate (HCO_3^-) in calculation of acid-base disorders (see below).

To clarify the terminology further, the terms *acidemia* and *alkalemia* have been introduced to describe actual states of abnormally low pH (less than 7.35) and high pH (more than 7.45), while the terms *acidosis* and *alkalosis* now may designate body fluids that would be acid or alkaline but have been neutralized by compensatory reactions.

Determination of pH, Pco_2, and (HCO_3^-). It is now possible to perform adequate blood gas determination on 0.5 ml of heparinized arterial blood in a few seconds. The normal

563

concentrations of blood gases show only slight differences related to age once the neonate has made the initial adaptation to extra-uterine existence (Table 25-11). The fact that infants show a slight tendency toward more acidotic blood gases is of interest but of questionable significance.

Definition of terms. Definitions of some of the terms related to bicarbonate concentrations may be of help.

standard bicarbonate The plasma bicarbonate concentration after blood has been equilibrated to a Pco_2 of 40 mm Hg. This value is independent of the patient's Pco_2. Unit is mEq/L. Normal value is 24 mEq/L.

buffer base The sum of buffer anions of blood or plasma (not dependent on Pco_2).

total CO_2 The total amount of carbon dioxide that can be liberated from blood or plasma. Normally equal to HCO_3^- plus H_2CO_3 plus 1.27 mEq/L.

actual bicarbonate Total CO_2 minus the carbonic acid and physically dissolved CO_2. Same as alkali reserve.

CO_2 combining power The total CO_2 of the anaerobically separated plasma after equilibrium to a Pco_2 of 40 mm Hg at room temperature. Unit is mmole/L. (Astrup and others, 1966).

standard CO_2 Same as CO_2 combining power.

Estimation and correction of acid-base imbalances. The mechanisms involved in acid-base disturbances in children are similar to those in adults, but several special features

Table 25-11. Normal acid-base values related to age

	Infant	Child	Adult
pH (arterial)	7.38	7.39	7.40
Pa_{CO_2} (mm Hg or torr)	34	37	40
HCO_3^- (mEq/L)	20	22	27
Base excess (mEq/L)	−3.0	−2.0	0

are of significance, and the classic examples of the various types of disturbance are quite different from those representing adult groups (e.g., the 2-kg premature infant with marked metabolic and respiratory acidosis). Table 25-12 shows the principal acid-base disturbances and primary and secondary responses.

Metabolic acidosis. This is commonly seen in sick neonates, especially those who have been exposed to cold and are hypoxic, and those suffering from intestinal lesions. Diaphragmatic hernia, in which both metabolic and respiratory acidosis are often combined, is an outstanding example and presents the problem of whether one should delay operation in order to improve the metabolic situation. This is discussed in Chapter 15.

In the treatment of acid-base disorders, correction of underlying factors plays a major part and should be attempted immediately. Warmth, oxygen, fluids, and corrective surgery have been found to be as effective in correction of metabolic acidosis as definitive hydrogen ion support (Rowe and Uribe, 1971).

When definitive correction of metabolic acidosis is needed, sodium bicarbonate is often advocated. The bicarbonate dosage is calculated by using the following formula:

$$HCO_3^- \text{ (mEq)} = HCO_3^- \text{ deficit} \times \\ \text{kg body weight} \times \text{distribution factor}$$

The distribution factor, or "bicarbonate distribution space," is a relatively new adaptation of the ECF value customarily used in this equation and ranges from 0.4 for infants to 0.2 for adults. It has been shown that in severe metabolic acidosis in which HCO_3^- is reduced to less than 10 mEq/L, more HCO_3^- may be lost than is held in the ECF, and re-

Table 25-12. Primary and secondary responses in acid-base disturbances

	Normal range	Metabolic acidosis	Metabolic alkalosis	Respiratory acidosis	Respiratory alkalosis	Mixed response
pH	7.35-7.45	↓6.80-7.35	↑7.46-7.80	↓6.80-7.35	↑7.46-7.80	7.20-7.50
Pa_{CO_2}	30-40 torr	30-40 torr	30-40 torr	↑41-120 torr	↓5-39 torr	20-60 torr
HCO_3^-	20-24 mEq/L	↓5-19 mEq/L	↑25-35 mEq/L	↑25-35 mEq/L	↓10-19 mEq/L	15-30 mEq/L

placement must be allowed for a larger volume, often termed "the bicarbonate space," which carries values that increase with the degree of acidosis, ranging from 0.6 in infants to 0.4 in adults.

EXAMPLE 1. A 5-kg infant with intestinal obstruction shows an HCO_3^- concentration of 16 mEq/L, a loss of 4 mEq/L from normal neonatal level:

$$HCO_3^- \text{ deficit} = 4 \times 5 \times 0.4 = 8 \text{ mEq}$$

EXAMPLE 2. A similar 5-kg infant lost 12 mEq/L of HCO_3^-, the greater loss changing the calculation as follows:

$$HCO_3^- \text{ deficit} = 12 \times 5 \times 0.6 = 36 \text{ mEq}$$

The deficit is replaced as sodium bicarbonate. Some workers have strong convictions about preoperative correction of metabolic acidosis and advocate aggressive therapy with sodium bicarbonate. In view of its high osmolality (2000 mOsm/L) and the danger of cerebral edema and intracranial hemorrhage in neonates, we side with Finberg (1969), Rowe (1971), and Feig and McCurdy (1978), who favor primary reliance on correction of causative factors and use of bicarbonate as a supplementary agent. Other precautions advised are to attempt correction of the pH derangement only halfway with bicarbonate and the important rule to determine all use of bicarbonate by osmolality and avoid its use if serum sodium exceeds 150 mEq/L or if osmolality exceeds 325 mOsm/L.

THAM has the advantage of not causing CO_2 release, but it carries the same danger of excessive molality. If used, it is given as 3.6% ($\frac{1}{3}$M) in 5% dextrose. For correction of metabolic acidosis the equation would be:

ml THAM = HCO_3^- deficit ×
           kg body weight × distribution factor

Metabolic alkalosis. Bicarbonate excess is figured in the same way as bicarbonate deficit. In patients coming to operation it would rarely be necessary to use an acid to correct metabolic alkalosis, though NH_4Cl may be used when indicated (Kildeberg, 1968; Winters, 1973). Metabolic alkalosis most frequently occurs as the result of pyloric stenosis but also may be caused by potassium depletion and by iatrogenic therapy with citrate, lactate, gluconate, or a diuretic. Therapy consists chiefly of restricting oral intake in patients who are vomiting and of replacing chloride loss with saline solution. Potassium depletion should be calculated and replaced after hydration has been restored. Respiratory compensation for metabolic alkalosis is unpredictable and seldom of appreciable effect. The management of infants undergoing pyloromyotomy is described later.

Respiratory alkalosis. This is seldom encountered in children coming to operation but probably occurs in the majority of patients during and after operation as a result of overzealous passive ventilation. Initial hyperventilation reduces PCO_2 and pH, followed by reduction of HCO_3^- and subsequent compensatory excretion of alkaline urine. Blood gas alterations often vary between pH 7.46 and 7.60 and occasionally reach 7.80 or more.

Treatment of respiratory alkalosis is by reduction of the rate of respiration or the tidal exchange, or both, with serial determination of arterial gases. In unanesthetized patients, hyperventilation caused by anxiety states, hypermetabolism, or neurologic lesions may be aided by treatment with morphine or other sedatives.

Respiratory acidosis. This is caused by any form of ventilatory depression by drugs, disease (cystic fibrosis, airway obstruction), or prematurity. There is initial accumulation of CO_2 (rising PCO_2) and corresponding pH reduction, followed by rising HCO_3^- and subsequent compensation by excretion of acid urine.

When respiratory acidosis is recognized, the first and principal method of treatment should be through increased ventilation. This may require improved airway, increased tidal volume, expansion of atelectatic lung, operative intervention, or relief of external pressures. Recourse to bicarbonate or THAM should be delayed until time has been allowed for effective ventilatory response.

Mixed acid-base response. This refers to situations where two different acid-base disturbances exist simultaneously, either accentuating the pH derangement or reducing it. In contrast to a compensated disturbance, where there is one primary cause and a defensive response to reduce the reaction, in the mixed response there are two primary factors operating at the same time, such as a diabetic child who has ketoacidosis and pneumonia (metabolic and respiratory acidosis). The four possible combinations are metabolic and respiratory acidosis, metabolic and respiratory alkalosis, metabolic acidosis and respiratory alkalosis, and metabolic alkalosis and respiratory acidosis. In the treatment of these patients, it is important to recognize the degree of electrolyte disturbance in those responses that have opposite effect on pH and to correct them simultaneously so that pH will not be severely displaced.

Preoperative correction of colloid and red cell problems

Hypovolemic states. Induction of anesthesia in children with chronic or acute hypervolemia may cause sudden hypotension and hypoxia. In cachectic or shocked patients, the presence of hypovolemia may be obvious, but it is easily overlooked in milder forms. Habitually poor eaters, undernourished, chronically ill children, and those having cleft lip or other defects about the mouth are often found to have reduced plasma volume. Signs that may be useful in diagnosis are general inanition, collapsed veins, sunken fontanelle, and hypotension. Iatrogenic hypovolemia should be suspected in teaching centers, where excessive quantities of blood may be withdrawn for laboratory purposes.

In the presence of acute shock, whole blood is indicated to replace circulating blood volume. The use of albumin and supporting fluids is indicated, as in adult therapy. Anesthesia and surgery are delayed until the child's condition has stabilized and arterial pressure, cardiac output, and renal function have regained satisfactory levels.

Correction of chronic hypovolemic states may require time to determine the cause as well as discretion in the method and rate of therapy. The type of replacement may be guided in part by hematocrit. A hematocrit of less than 25% is an indication for use of blood. Long-standing or severe hypovolemia will present the danger of cardiac failure if replacement is rapid. Consequently, correction should be carried out over a period of 24 hours or more. With less severe states and a hematocrit of more than 25%, circulating volume can be restored with 5% albumin, Ringer's solution, or 5% dextrose in ¼% saline solution.

In correction of hypovolemia there will always be danger of giving too much fluid, or giving it too rapidly, and leaving the child in worse condition than at the outset. Adequate peripheral circulation, moderate filling of veins, return of tissue turgor, and urine output of 0.5 to 1 ml/kg/hr are reliable signs of effective circulating blood volume and indications to slow or stop replacement.

Correction of red blood cell excess. Hemoconcentration, or red cell excess, is seen primarily in patients with congenital cardiac defects involving reduced pulmonary circulation. Hematocrit frequently is in the range of 50% to 65% and may be as high as 80%.

With increasing concentration of red cells, there is relative increase in danger of thrombosis, sludging, and restrictive circulation. These hazards are aggravated by restriction of fluids, cooling, and hypotension. Measures to be considered are maintenance of hydration during preoperative preparation of all patients, replacement of red cells with albumin or crystalloid to reduce hematocrit to a maximum of 65% prior to operation, and maintenance of body temperature.

Correction of red blood cell deficit. As discussed previously, there has been a tradition that patients coming to elective operations should have a hemoglobin level of not less than 10 g/dl or a hematocrit of 30%. As a broad policy, some such rule is commendable, but in practical application there are many situations that alter the ratio of need-to-hazard that must be considered before any blood transfusion. In pediatric age groups there are three general groups of patients to consider: those with so-called anemia of infancy, those with uncomplicated deficits due to blood loss, malnutrition, or defects in red cell production, and those with anemic states in which transfusion carries increased risk or danger of other complicating factors.

Infants presenting with a hematocrit of 27% to 30% and no other signs of illness are familiar to all. If a low hematocrit is noted prior to hospital admission, it is preferable to delay elective procedures until a trial of iron therapy can be completed. If the condition is not found until the child is admitted and ready for operation, it is often reasonable to proceed with hernia repair or other simple operations without transfusion. When the deficit is larger or when more extensive procedures are planned, a transfusion of whole blood or red blood cells has greater value. Since the anemia of infancy with hematocrit 27% to 30% is still believed to cause little impairment of tissue oxygenation, it is regarded with less concern than other types of red cell deficit.

Anemias due to blood loss, malnutrition, and defective production would call for more immediate attempts to regain normal or better than normal hematocrit before operation, especially when children are faced with repeated operation, as in burn or tumor therapy. When there are no additional risks involved in transfusion, the minimal hematocrit of 30% might even be raised to 35%.

A variety of conditions offer arguments against the use of blood in the presence of red cell deficits. These include hemolytic anemia, sickle cell anemia, chronic renal failure, and the children whose parents are Jehovah's Witnesses. It has been found that extensive procedures can be carried out successfully in patients who have carried low hematocrit levels over a sufficient period to allow compensatory development of 2,3-DPG and normal circulating plasma volume. Individual decisions must be made in all such cases, depending not only on the patient and the disease but also on the personnel and facilities available for their care.

Choice and calculation of preoperative blood replacement. When it has been found that blood replacement is needed, one must decide between (1) the use of whole blood, which may be fresh, stored at 4° C, or frozen, and may be stored in acid-citrate-dextrose (ACD) or citrate-phosphate-dextrose (CPD) preservative, and (2) the use of packed (or washed) red blood cells.

Whole blood, when prepared in reliable laboratories, has the advantage of being more readily available, being exposed to fewer hazards of contamination and other handling errors, and carrying full complement of platelets, immune factors, and balanced osmotic properties that might have to be replaced as separate components with a red cell infusion. Whole blood is particularly valuable when both volume and red cells need replacement. A definite contraindication to whole blood transfusion is chronic renal failure, where it is essential to remove white blood cells. When whole blood is used for preoperative replacement of red cell deficits, it carries increased risk of overloading the cardiovascular system. Decisions are made by judgment rather than by rules.

Stored, or bank, blood is satisfactory for transfusion of relatively small volumes, but fresh whole blood is preferable when more than one fourth or one third of the patient's blood volume needs replacement. CPD preservative is superior to ACD in that it is less acid and also maintains a considerably higher concentration of 2,3-DPG during the first 10 to 14 days of storage.

If whole blood is used to make up preoperative deficit, 5 ml/kg is probably the maximum that may be given safely at one time to normal children (Kevy, 1979). When there is severe deficit or danger of cardiac decompensation, it is safer to use red blood cells, with 3 ml/kg the maximum to be given at one time.

There is increasing interest in use of red blood cells for all transfusions, and it appears particularly advantageous in preoperative replacement of red cell deficit, where volume usually is normal. Added advantages of red cell transfusions are reduced danger of conveying hepatitis and of sensitization. A disadvantage of red cell administration is that the greater concentration of the fluid makes it more difficult to infuse into smaller infants.

Among methods of calculating red cell replacement, that of Furman and associates (1975) has been the most widely adopted. They use 80 ml/kg as blood volume and 30% as normal hematocrit:

Estimated blood volume (EBV) =
$$\text{kg body weight} \times 80$$

Estimated red cell mass (ERCM) = EBV × 30

With this formula, the calculation for a 5-kg infant with a hematocrit of 27% would be:

$$\text{EBV} = 5 \times 80 = 400 \text{ ml}$$
ERCM for normal infant of 5 kg =
$$0.30 \times 400 = 120 \text{ ml}$$

ERCM for infant with a hematocrit of 27% =
$$0.27 \times 400 = 108 \text{ ml}$$

The difference, 12 ml, represents the red cell mass deficit to be made up by direct infusion of the same amount of red cells.

Preoperative blood and colloid imbalance: indications for preoperative transfusion of blood. One should bear in mind that the value of transfused blood, whether whole blood or red cells, does not reach maximum for several hours after administration. Thus, if preoperative replacement is to be of intraoperative value, it should be given the night before operation.

Furthermore, in the transfusion of a premature infant, the use of adult blood, which has no fetal hemoglobin, to replace infant blood, which has an appreciable quantity of fetal hemoglobin, will shift the infant's oxyhemoglobin dissociation curve to the right, improving its oxygen delivery to the tissues but at the same time exposing the child to greater hazard of retrolental fibroplasia (Delivoria-Papadopoulas and others, 1971).

INTRAOPERATIVE FLUID THERAPY
Major concerns

Under usual conditions, when patients are brought to surgery with acceptable fluid balance there are two major concerns related to fluid therapy:

1. Provision of maintenance requirements of water, calories, and electrolytes. These include the basic requirements of the resting child, to which alteration must be made for increases due to fever, stress, or other factors. Some allowance also may be made for the period of restricted oral intake preceding operation.
2. Replacement of blood, drainage fluids, and third-space losses incurred during operation.

Major issues or points of dispute

The amount of maintenance fluid to be given is the area in which the major issues are found. As suggested previously, they are related largely to the management of neonates (infants under 2 weeks old). This is an extremely important group for two principal reasons: (1) during the first 2 weeks a large number of major life-threatening conditions require operation and (2) the highest mortality of the entire life span falls within this time.

There are two specific issues:

1. Should neonates be denied water or allowed quantities comparable to those in older children and adults?
2. Should salt be restricted or allowed as in older patients?

In order to provide further background on which to construct the overall picture, management of maintenance fluids for older patients will be discussed first and the problems of neonates and other special patients will be discussed as individual problems.

Estimation of intraoperative needs

Several approaches must be used in estimating intraoperative fluid needs:

1. Maintenance requirements are determined by application of formulas based on decades of investigation by pediatricians and physiologists. Since they are based on average figures, they serve only as guides for initiating therapy.
2. Direct measurements are used where possible to determine the need for therapy as well as the type and amount needed. Indi-

rect guidance by laboratory methods is helpful in many situations.

3. Continued observation of clinical signs will always serve as the deciding factor in the most important decisions.

Development of formulas for maintenance requirements

A great deal of investigation went into the establishment of guides for parenteral fluid and electrolyte administration. The first effort was toward finding the measurable factor most closely related to total fluid metabolism. Plans were developed on three different basic references: body weight, body surface area, and estimated body metabolism. They are briefly summarized as follows:

1. The *body weight* method relies on weight alone for calculation of water and electrolyte requirements. Formulas that depend on weight as a major determinant are subject to considerable error, especially in older children who may be grossly overweight for their age or height.

2. The *body surface area* method is more rationally based on square meters of body surface area, which is definitely related to metabolic rate throughout much of life (approximately 1000 cal/m² body surface area) (Calcagno, 1960). Drawbacks to this method are the necessity of using a nomogram for calculation of body surface area and the fact that the metabolic activity of neonates usually is less than the standard 1000 cal/m² while that of older children usually exceeds it.

3. Use of *estimated metabolic rate,* or *caloric expenditure,* was found to be the most accurate method of determining intravenous fluid and electrolyte requirement. Unfortunately, to apply this method it was first necessary to determine the metabolic rate of the individual patient in question. This problem was greatly simplified by Holliday and Segar (1957), who determined a range of caloric expenditure for different age groups and related these to body weight. The resultant formula is actually based on caloric expenditure, conveniently arrived at indirectly by the relationship of weight to caloric expenditure rather than weight to fluid requirement. The requirements for

fluids are stated as ml/100 cal expended, and the requirements for electrolytes are stated as mEq/100 cal expended. This formula (Table 25-1) has been widely adopted for use in medical and surgical care of pediatric patients and is generally accepted as the standard method in current pediatric anesthesia (Bennett and others, 1970; Bush, 1971; Berry, 1976).

Normal maintenance requirements for water and electrolytes

The amount of water required per day should equal that lost via the totalled components, i.e., insensible loss through lungs and skin plus that lost in sweat, urine, and stools. These are usually stated to equal approximately 115 to 125 ml/100 cal, as shown in Table 25-13. The intravenous replacement is reduced by 15 to 25 ml/100 cal, because this amount is gained from water produced by internal metabolic processes or by oxidation. Thus, in the absence of sweating, the average intravenous requirement in normal adults is approximately 100 ml/100 cal expended.

Normal variation in activity causes considerable change in requirements, while different disease states alter requirements even more, with water requirement occasionally reaching 500 to 600 ml/100 cal and sodium and potassium requirements occasionally reaching 30 mEq/L.

Daily requirements for electrolytes are quoted with remarkable changeability. Values for sodium, potassium, and chloride normally fall between 1 and 5 mEq/100 cal, but individual values vary both in amount and in relation to one another. Thus, one author may give the requirements for Na, K, and Cl as 3.0, 2.5, and 2.5, respectively, whereas

Table 25-13. Basic allowances

	Amount (per 100 cal expended)
Water	100 ml
Sodium	3.0 mEq
Chloride	2.5 mEq
Potassium	2.5 mEq
Glucose	5 g

another may state them as 3.0, 3.0, and 5.0 mEq/100 cal.

Daily requirements of calcium and magnesium are given by Cooke and Levin (1968) as approximately 500 and 100 mg/100 cal, respectively. While calcium is contained in Ringer's solution, neither electrolyte is needed in the average short-term infusion.

It is evident that it would be impossible to estimate the exact requirement under such diverse conditions. The kidneys of infants over 1 month old can adjust for fairly wide discrepancies in volume replacement, but the margin for error is much narrower in the first weeks of life.

In infants over 2 weeks old and other children, the basic allowance of water and electrolytes shown in Table 25-13 has wide application.

Daily caloric expenditure and glucose allowance

Glucose is the primary source of energy replacement for patients receiving intravenous support. Although it would be desirable to replace the entire 100-cal expenditure in order to retain caloric balance, this is not advisable. Because of the high osmolality of glucose solutions, one is limited to using not more than the 5% solution (5% dextrose in ¼% saline = 330 mOsm/kg). In spite of the discrepancy, this amount of glucose is enough to provide an appreciable amount of energy, prevent ketosis, and spare endogenous protein. It has become a widely accepted practice to regard 5 g of glucose/100 cal expended as the standard amount of glucose for intravenous support. The term "requirement," suggesting full caloric replacement, would seem to be a misnomer, since only one fifth of the caloric expenditure is replaced. The term "glucose allowance" is suggested as being less confusing.

Although lactated solutions may be used with the assumption that they will increase caloric support, as shown in Table 25-2 they offer hardly any, and since infants have difficulty metabolizing lactate there is little indication for their use in smaller patients.

Calculation of fluid needs

Step 1: calculation of normal maintenance support. We have now arrived, by the slow route, at the same set of guidelines that are listed at the beginning of the chapter, but hopefully with a better understanding of both their origin and their limitations:

1. Calculation of basic maintenance fluid requirement for a normal infant or child more than 2 weeks old follows the plan of Holliday and Segar (1957) given in Table 25-1.
2. One must determine the basic allowance of electrolyte and calories. By choosing 5% dextrose in ¼% saline as the fluid to be given, one will be giving 5 g of glucose (or 20 calories), 3.8 mEq of sodium, and 3.8 mEq of chloride per 100 ml. This should be an adequate allowance for maintenance requirements but must be altered at the start to suit existing conditions of activity or imbalance and must be adjusted repeatedly as initial conditions change.

EXAMPLE: At the beginning of strabismus correction in an 11-kg boy, an infusion of 5% dextrose in ¼% saline solution is started at a rate of 40 + 2 = 42 ml/hr.

As stated at the beginning of the chapter, this is all that is needed in a multitude of short (under 1 hour), uncomplicated cases such as herniorrhaphy, tonsillectomy, strabismus correction, operation on digits, and removal of small tumors.

It will be seen that the fluid allowance decreases from 4 ml/kg/hr in infants weighing less than 10 kg to 1.8 ml/kg/hr in children weighing 50 kg.

Step 2: consideration of the period of preoperative restriction of oral intake. Although the actual degree of dehydration that is caused by fluid restriction is relatively minor and seldom enough to be clinically detectable, it deserves consideration. When children are in relatively poor condition or when the period of fluid restriction is prolonged, it is reasonable to allow an amount calculated by the product of hourly requirement and hours of restriction. Thus, a 10-kg child who had no oral intake for 8 hours might be given 40 × 8 = 320 ml of standard solution in addition to the maintenance allowance of

40 ml/hr. There is definite danger in giving this too rapidly. It is customary to give half of the makeup solution in the first hour of operation and the remainder over the next 2 hours. Thus, this infant would receive a total of 200, 120, and 120 ml in the first 3 hours of operation. When one is dealing with small infants, possible inability to manage large fluid loads requires particular care, and it is our custom to reduce both the amount and the rate of administration of makeup fluids or to eliminate them altogether.

Step 3: addition of fluid for increased activity. If a child obviously shows more activity than is usual, whether in muscular action, crying, or simply in the work of breathing, an additional 1 to 3 ml/kg/hr may be added to the hourly maintenance.

Step 4: replacement of intraoperative fluid losses other than blood. Intraoperative loss of fluids other than blood includes saliva, respiratory tract moisture, sweat, evaporation from wounds and exposed viscera, drainage from stomach, intestine, and fistulous tracts, edema, and third-space losses. Other imbalances related to fluid that may occur during operation include electrolyte disorders, hypoglycemia, and alterations in acid-base balance as well as in osmotic and oncotic pressures.

Only a few of the above variables are measurable, and one must rely on indirect measurements and a variety of signs. The result of this uncertain situation is a focal point where the most serious errors in fluid therapy are made.

Gastric and intestinal drainage should be measured directly. When appreciable in amount, these fluids should be examined for pH and electrolyte content. The composition of such fluids is variable, and replacement should be made with solutions resembling those lost. Urine is collected by catheter drainage in more extensive cases, the volume is monitored, and specific gravity, osmolality, and electrolyte concentration are measured when indicated.

Saliva and sweat rarely amount to much in infants and children. Loss of moisture from the respiratory tract may be significant if an unhumidified nonrebreathing system is used, but if heavy humidification is employed there may even be retention of fluid, with reduction of water requirement. Evaporation from the open chest or abdomen cannot be measured but should be considered if hot lights are used and the exposed tissues are not kept moistened.

Of greatest importance are third-space losses, loss of peritoneal exudate, and, of course, blood loss. Although these may not occur in many procedures, in situations where they do occur the effect may be critical. Peritoneal exudate, especially when associated with severe peritonitis, will contain large amounts of protein that should be replaced. Third-space losses, estimated to amount to as much as 10 ml/kg in extensive abdominal operations, are impossible to measure and must be estimated by the degree of handling of viscera and the duration of operation (Finlayson, 1972).

Translocation removes fluid from the ECF for a period of several hours and may be of sufficient magnitude to induce shock (Winters, 1973). It is our custom to use additional fluid during such procedures as abdominoperineal repair for Hirschsprung's disease and urinary diversion. A second infusion is started using Ringer's lactate solution, usually at one-half to one-third the rate of the maintenance infusion. For slightly less extensive procedures, it should be sufficient merely to increase the maintenance allowance by 25% to 30% during the early part of the procedure. On the other hand, in the presence of inflammatory lesions of the bowel or in more traumatic surgery, as has been shown by Macbeth and Pope (1968), Hoye and associates (1972), and others, massive amounts of albumin may be lost, with associated loss of plasma volume. With this in mind, it is often wise to use 5% albumin, fresh-frozen plasma, or whole blood, even when blood loss has not been extensive. In all situations, clinical signs must be closely and continuously observed and given precedence over all other forms of evaluation.

As will be discussed later, infants with gastroschisis show marked plasma losses, while those with necrotizing enterocolitis probably have the most severe loss of exudative fluid encountered in pediatric surgery (with the possible exception of burns).

Evaluation of intraoperative changes in fluid balance

Signs of fluid balance during surgery are similar to those of the preoperative phase, but there are several variations. First, the loss of consciousness by itself eliminates one reliable sign of cerebral vascular flow. The effect of anesthetic agents on the vascular system changes other signs. A mild degree of hypovolemia that might have passed unnoticed in the awake, mildly vasoconstricted infant or child will show prompt reduction of blood pressure with the induction of light halothane anesthesia or the administration of d-tubocurarine. Vasodilation plays a part in both cases. With halothane, however, vagal tone may also contribute to hypotension by slowing the heart and reducing cardiac output unless atropine has been used to prevent this action. Since both halothane and atropine will be working to reduce cardiac rate, this will be less responsive to changes in plasma volume.

Other signs of hypovolemia are reduction of CVP and urine output, collapsed veins, decreased peripheral perfusion, sunken fontanelle, drying of the skin and mucous membranes, and increasing hematocrit and urinary specific gravity. Measurement of urinary output is of primary importance during most extensive operations, but one may be misled if light anesthesia stimulates increased secretion of ADH.

Hypovolemia developing during surgery usually is isotonic, but one should consider all possibilities and confirm by monitoring serum electrolytes before using suitable corrective methods as previously outlined (pp. 562 and 671).

In the management of pediatric hydration, there probably is more danger in hypervolemia than hypovolemia, for overloading is more difficult to correct than shock. Caused by water-filled lungs, tachypnea is the first sign of hypervolemia in infants. As hypervolemia progresses one finds a slow, bounding pulse, loud heart sounds, distended veins, flushed skin, puffy eyelids, and increased urine output, followed by moist breath sounds and frothy bronchial secretions that finally fill the lungs and gush out of the endotracheal tube.

Positive pressure ventilation and discontinuation of fluids are the first corrective steps, followed, when indicated, by diuretics (furosemide, 0.5 to 1.0 mg/kg, or mannitol, 200 to 300 mg/kg) and dexamethasone, 0.25 mg/kg, to reduce cerebral edema. Should the overload be enough to endanger the patient, blood may be withdrawn directly from the heart, aorta, or a peripheral vessel, depending on the operation in progress.

Changes in specific elements may be recognized either by measurement or by clinical signs. Obvious peritoneal exudation or prolonged abdominal operations may induce loss of protein. Serum protein below 5.5 g/dl usually calls for administration of 5% albumin, 10 to 20 ml/kg.

Hyperpotassemia, whether a result of chronic renal failure or cardiac failure, is recognizable by high T-wave EKG changes. Anesthesia is believed to be contraindicated with serum potassium levels at 5.0 or 5.5 mEq/L. This is best corrected the night before operation by dialysis, but for more prompt results one may use either polystyrene sodium sulfonate (Kayexalate) or insulin and glucose approaches (West, 1975).

One must be aware of potential iatrogenic complications in relation to fluid therapy. As Bennett (1973) has stressed, solutions containing lactate are not advisable for patients who have hyperosmolar states, metabolic alkalosis, cystic fibrosis, or other forms of sodium depletion.

There is increasing evidence that free recourse to sodium bicarbonate carries considerable danger. Not only may rapid increase in arterial pH induce lethal CSF changes, but the increase in osmolality may cause cerebral hemorrhage. Serum calcium is also affected and may be critically reduced. In general, one should refrain from use of sodium bicarbonate until hyperventilation has been given full trial and then use with the guidance of ECG, serum electrolytes, blood glucose, and osmolality. Calcium may be given, preferably when indicated by ECG changes (high T-wave) or reduced serum calcium levels (total calcium below 9 mEq/L or ionized Ca^{++} below 1.6 mEq/L). Either the gluconate or the chloride may be used. The chloride, containing more ionized substance, is preferable for resuscitation (intracardiac injection of 20 mg/kg), but the less irritating gluconate is recommended for correction of hypocalcemic states (intravenous injection of 60 mg/kg with confirmation of effect).

Intraoperative replacement of blood

Several changes have occurred in concepts of blood replacement, all trending toward more restricted and specialized use of blood. Prior to 1963 there was great emphasis on the importance of the loss of small amounts of blood, and virtually all blood loss was replaced with whole blood (in ACD preservative). In 1963 this enthusiasm was tempered by the report of Davenport and Barr, who suggested that in pediatric surgery, blood replacement could be withheld until the loss reached 10%, was advisable between 10% and 20%, and was mandatory after 20%. This suggestion was widely endorsed. During the next 10 years, blood was not replaced until approximately 10% had been lost, at which point replacement was usually started, again with whole blood.

A major factor in reducing the use of blood has been the general abandonment of sharp surgical dissection in favor of cautery.

Three more changes toward economy in blood replacement are now seen in the increasing use of blood fractions instead of whole blood (Furman, 1977), the use of albumin instead of blood to replace losses of 10% to 20% (Downes, 1976), and the use of hypotensive and hemodilution technics to facilitate surgery and reduce or at least delay blood replacement (Salem and others, 1974; Furman, 1977).

Indications for blood replacement. It has already been emphasized that because of the many variables concerned (and the different concepts just mentioned), one should speak of guides to blood replacement rather than rules.

It is important to plan ahead for blood replacement. Before operation one should consider whether there is any probability of significant blood loss. If so, one next considers the possibility of any contraindication or limiting factor, such as sickle cell anemia or chronic renal failure. One also looks for indications that might favor the use of blood at an earlier stage than usual, such as a low hematocrit.

The concept that blood should be replaced after a 10% loss still is applicable in the majority of cases. For this purpose, it is practical to consider blood volume as 80 ml/kg throughout infancy and childhood.

The anesthesiologist must learn by experience which operations will call for the use of blood. Depending on local situations and individual surgeons, the repair of cleft lip, for instance, may never or may always require blood replacement. Several operations require unexpectedly large amounts of blood, such as repair of craniosynostosis in small infants, where a total of 200 ml usually is needed for operative and postoperative replacement. The scalp, face, tongue, and perineum often bleed profusely. Closure of colostomy has previously been described as a procedure that frequently requires blood replacement.

In some cases experience can be misleading. For many years in our institution, blood was always given to children during division of patent ductus arteriosus and was given in large quantities during repair of coarctation of the aorta. Now, largely because of use of cautery and more deliberate technic, blood is never used with ductus repair and is used sparingly, if at all, with coarctation.

The use of blood fractions preoperatively has already been discussed. Certainly, the use of whole blood has greater merit in intraoperative replacement than in preoperative therapy of anemias, and as losses increase, the value of whole blood becomes more obvious.

The succinct guide of Broennle (1977),

given below, suggests the use of albumin until 10 to 20 ml/kg have been lost, after which blood is recommended.

FLUID AND BLOOD REPLACEMENT
(Philadelphia Children's Hospital)*

Maintenance fluids

5% to 10% dextrose in 0.2% physiologic saline at 4 ml/kg/hr

Plasma replacement

10 to 20 ml/kg 5% albumin (ALB) in lactated Ringer's (LR) solution

Blood replacement

Assume normal blood volume = 80 to 90 ml/kg
Assume normal hematocrit = 40%
Replace 10 to 20 ml/kg with 5% ALB/LR or fresh-frozen plasma
Replace losses over 20 ml/kg with blood to maintain hematocrit at 35% to 40%

Technic

Warm fluids and blood
Use calibrated syringe pump

Estimation of blood loss. Measurement of blood loss is accomplished by several methods, none of which is completely accurate. The weighing of blood accumulated on dry sponges, collection of blood via suction, serial hematocrit determination of mixed venous blood, and visual estimation of blood-soaked sponges are methods commonly used. The combination of gravimetric and suction measurement will give useful assistance in many procedures such as spinal fusion, where large amounts of blood may be lost and where dry sponges are used. During brain surgery, however, where small patties and irrigating fluid are in continual use, and in abdominal surgery, where wet sponges are used, these methods have little value. An exception might be where there is such profuse hemorrhage that suctioned blood reaches massive proportions, in which case its measurement could be of considerable help. Otherwise one must rely on the clinical signs listed opposite or on other methods.

*From Broennle, A. M.: The neonate; intraoperative management, lecture presented at Annual Convention of American Society of Anesthesiologists, New Orleans, 1977.

SIGNS OF BLOOD LOSS IN PEDIATRIC SURGERY

Mild (0% to 10%)

Visible loss
Blood pressure reduction (5% to 15%)
Veins less visible
Reduction in CVP
Reduction in urine output
Decreased conjunctival circulation

Moderate (10% to 20%)

Visible loss
Blood pressure reduction (10% to 25%)
CVP 0
Veins collapsed
Heart sounds less audible
Extremities cooler than body
Increasing relaxation
Decreasing respiratory effort
Hematocrit reduction
Marked reduction in urine output
Increase in urine osmolality, specific gravity
Fontanelle depressed
Conjunctivae pale
Weak peripheral pulse
Decreasing capillary refill

Severe (over 20%)

Visible loss extensive
Severe blood pressure reduction (over 25%)
Decreased heart sounds
Cold fingers and toes
Generalized blanching (except fingertips, with exceptions)
Anuria
No conjunctival circulation visible
Increasing anesthetic depth
Hypothermia
Flaccidity
Shock
Unobtainable pulse
Unobtainable blood pressure
Asystole
Gasping respiration for 2 to 5 minutes
Apnea

Furman (1977) places reliance on serial hematocrits taken from a central venous catheter, and his formulas, published in 1975, have come into common usage. By this method, blood replacement is started when hematocrit falls below 30% or when a 10% loss has been reached.

The signs of blood loss are necessarily much like the signs of dehydration and other types of reduced circulating plasma volume. However, there are additional factors in the assessment of acute blood loss in the anesthetized patient that deserve individual consideration.

Frank hemorrhage is the most easily recognized indication of blood loss, but an equal amount of blood may accumulate in the peritoneum or chest without being observed. Changes in the patient's color may be deceptive. An acidotic child will have bright red lips in spite of blood loss, and the fingertips of an infant may remain pink even with exsanguination. The one site where color change has proved reliable in my experience is the conjunctival circulation. By retracting the lower lid at intervals, one finds early and reliable signs of blood volume. The usual network of bright red capillaries will thin and disappear entirely with advancing blood loss.

Blood pressure, without doubt, is the most valuable sign of reduced blood volume and must be followed assiduously in any case where bleeding is a problem, for shock occurs rapidly in smaller patients. When an infant's blood pressure suddenly becomes unobtainable, it is easy to be misled by the assumption that the apparatus is at fault. In such situations one should check other signs immediately and assume that the child is in shock rather than that the monitor is wrong.

Less obvious signs of blood loss are greater relaxation under the same anesthetic concentration, mottled color, poor capillary return, and peripheral cooling.

Massive blood replacement. The term "massive blood loss" is difficult to define, for it is related to both the amount and the rate of the loss. When a child loses approximately one third of his blood volume in less than 30 minutes, we feel that special therapy is indicated. Greater losses require additional measures.

The use of fresh whole blood is our first concern in order to replace volume, oxygen-carrying power, osmolality, and clotting factors. The use of calcium to counter the possible negative inotropic effects of citrate and/or potassium has been in vogue for a number of years (Bunker, 1955) and probably has merit. We prefer to use the gluconate preparation in order to avoid vascular irritation. The dosage of calcium gluconate is difficult to prescribe with confidence. We use approximately 0.5 mg of calcium gluconate per ml of blood when more than 30% of blood volume is replaced. While it is theoretically preferable to avoid use of the same infusion for calcium and blood, this has been necessary many times and has not caused appreciable harm. As a precaution in such situations, one may inject a bolus of saline solution into the line before and after injecting the calcium.

Maximum danger of complication from blood transfusion occurs with the combination of a large volume given rapidly and administered via the upper extremity. This situation is encountered in operations involving excision of Wilms' and other large abdominal tumors and in hepatic resection or repair, when blood given through saphenous veins could be obstructed. Naturally, the presence of any defect in the blood will be accentuated in proportion to the volume and rate of infusion, and when given via the arm, this blood will be delivered to the heart almost as a bolus, having had little chance to mix with the patient's own blood.

The chief dangers at this time are hypothermia, acidity, and hyperkalemia. The warming of blood is always preferable but is not mandatory when relatively small amounts are given slowly to healthy children. When blood at 4° C is pumped into a child in shock, however, it may cause immediate death. Technics and precautions related to warming of blood for pediatric patients are similar to those for adults.

The use of CPD instead of the traditional ACD raises the pH of bank blood slightly, but the pH of fresh CPD blood seldom exceeds 6.90. Further alkalinization is possible by addition of sodium bicarbonate or THAM. While this may reduce the danger of myocardial depression at the moment of infusion, subsequent metabolism of either agent produces a rebound metabolic alkalosis, and therefore we have discontinued the practice.

The potassium content of stored blood increases rapidly, being drawn into the circulating plasma by increasing acidity. Reduction of 2,3-DPG proceeds more rapidly in

ACD blood during the first 2 weeks of storage, after which there is marked depletion in both ACD and CPD solutions.

When blood loss requires the replacement of three to five times the child's total blood volume, which can happen in repair of ruptured liver, one should test for clotting factors (prothrombin time, partial thromboplastin time) and give fresh-frozen plasma to restore deficits. Because of the higher risk of hepatitis in mixed plasma, one should not give it without indication. An excellent discussion by Kevy on the use of blood in pediatric medical and surgical patients is found in *Pediatric Surgery* (1979) by Ravitch and associates.

A strongly negative inotropic response to plasma also has been seen (in our experience, chiefly during shunt procedures on children with tetralogy of Fallot). This has been controlled by use of intravenous calcium gluconate and is believed to be due to the high citrate content of pooled plasma.

METABOLIC RESPONSE OF INFANTS AND CHILDREN TO STRESS, ANESTHESIA, AND SURGERY

In addition to maintenance requirement and losses of fluids and blood, it is necessary to consider the metabolic effect of preoperative preparation, anesthesia, and surgery on fluid requirements.

Here the waters become very murky, for many of the measurements on which our convictions are based have been affected by iatrogenic factors. Restriction of food and fluid for a considerable period prior to operation and limitation of fluid, electrolytes, and calories during anesthesia, whether reasonable or not, have introduced greater ADH response and alteration of osmolality and acid-base relationships that can be interpreted to the benefit of either side.

Although many careful studies have been carried out by Colle and Paulsen (1964), Knutrud (1965), Calcagno (1967), Rickham and Johnson (1969), and others, Bennett and associates (1977) have justifiably stated that there has been much inconsistency and some

alteration of views concerning the role of the kidneys, the beneficial or harmful effect of electrolytes, and the amount of fluids required. Moore (1962) and others have established some convincing data on the effect of operation on adults, showing that an initial hypermetabolic state causes an anabolic phase with a negative nitrogen balance during operation and for several days afterward. This is followed by an early anabolic and then a late anabolic phase, lasting sometimes as long as 4 to 6 weeks, until normal relationships are restored.

Results have been confusing, but there has been agreement on some items. Infants appear to show less stress reaction to the operative procedure, the catabolic phase being less marked and considerably shorter than that of the adult, and the total period of recovery from the same type of operation is approximately half as long. The gastrointestinal response is reduced, seldom involving ileus, and nausea and vomiting are less troublesome. Whether this is related to the more intense mental reaction of the adult is not known, but it is a definite possibility.

Certain specific differences have been established. The young child, and in particular the infant, has a lower blood glucose level and a greater tendency to develop hypoglycemia. The negative nitrogen balance typical of the adult undergoing surgery is mild or absent in the young child. There is less adrenocortical response, less ADH reaction, and the effect on renal function is slight unless there is extensive surgery. All this suggests that one need be less concerned about the effect of operative stress on the infant kidney, though much is still unknown about the subject.

PATIENTS REQUIRING SPECIAL CONSIDERATION IN FLUID MANAGEMENT

There are several groups of patients who require a departure from the standard approach to fluid management. First, and most controversial, are the neonates, followed by children with cardiac lesions, those with neurosurgical pathology, and those in renal failure. There are many others who call for individual therapy, but those mentioned will be discussed first.

Neonates

There are two features of outstanding importance in respect to fluid management in neonates or in infants under 2 weeks old. The first, which is well recognized, is that *there is great difference between neonates and older patients.* The second, which is rarely mentioned, is that *there is great difference between individual neonates.*

Recognition of the marked variation among neonates with different lesions and emphasis on their different fluid needs would constitute a major advance and would clear up much of the indecision about the choice between restriction of fluid and generous use of fluid in the first weeks of life.

Differences between neonates and older patients. These have been referred to many times already. Some of them have been clearly established. Others, the controversial points, are not firmly established and may be twisted in one direction or another, according to individual bias. Established differences include the relatively greater TBW content of neonates, the difference in composition of their body fluids, their tendency toward acidosis, their increased amount of ECF, and their varying rate of fluid metabolism, which starts slowly and then, in later months, reaches maximum rate of turnover.

The extrarenal factors controlling fluid balance in infants, ADH and aldosterone, have not been documented with certainty, and there is still widespread belief that although the infant kidney functions effectively within 2 to 4 weeks, during the neonatal phase there is glomerulotubular imbalance, reduced glomerular filtration rate, reduced ability to excrete water load promptly, inability to excrete acids, and reduced concentrating power.

The two questions that arouse the most controversy are how rapidly the neonate can excrete sodium and whether he can excrete large loads of water. Those who believe that neonates excrete sodium effectively appear

to be gaining ground, but the presence of hyponatremia, instead of proving that sodium is being excreted, may be evidence of dilution due to inappropriate ADH secretion (Oh, 1976), and the problem remains unsettled.

An even more confusing problem concerns the degree to which various disease states derange the functions of the neonatal and infant kidney. It would seem logical to suspect that many medical defects retard the development of kidney function.

The result of this disagreement is to divide the experts into two factions. Those who believe that infants should be "kept on the dry side" allow neonates 0 to 4 ml/kg/hr of dextrose solutions containing little or no salt, while the "hydrationists," believing that neonatal kidneys can handle both water and salt, prescribe as much as 25 ml/kg/hr for standard use (Berry, 1976).

Although both groups have shown a gradual trend toward moderation, one still gets the impression that each is making the same kind of mistake. While one group believes that all neonates should be kept dry and the other believes that all infants should be well hydrated, both are erroneously assuming that all neonates are basically alike, resemble one another, and are very different from older patients. Rather than the differences between neonates and older individuals being stressed, more emphasis should be placed on the vast differences that occur between different members of a group of neonates and the different fluid requirements that result. Instead of the restrictive group at one extreme and the hydrationists at the other, a concept of greater individualization of management should be adopted, with stress placed on the wide range of required fluid replacement, as discussed below.

Differences between neonates and the allowances that must be made in fluid management. The guide suggested by Holliday and Segar (1957) gives one formula for infants over 10 days old and a different one for neonates in the first 10 days of life. The formula for neonates, shown in Table 25-14, is followed by a great many pediatricians as well

Table 25-14. Intraoperative fluid allowance during the first week of life

Day	ml/kg/hr	ml/kg/24 hr
1	0	0
2, 3	2	50
4, 5, 6	3	75
7	4	100

as many anesthesiologists and surgeons who care for small babies.

While this is definitely a valuable and reasonable guide, one must alter amounts greatly before arriving at the correct total allowance. A basic 4 ml/kg/hr is chosen by many, and standard additions for different types of neonates, usually with allowance for third-space loss in abdominal procedures, amount to 3 to 6 ml/kg/hr.

In order to establish the wide individual differences more clearly, neonatal patients coming to surgery may be divided into at least five separate groups on the basis of their probable fluid requirements:

Group 1. Premature and newborn infants having known cardiac defects, babies of diabetic mothers, those with cystic lung, diaphragmatic hernia, or tracheoesophageal fistula with suspected cardiac anomaly, and those with neurosurgical lesions have little need for added fluid over the minimum of 0 to 2 ml/kg/hr. Furthermore, they carry increased danger of fluid overload. Maintenance fluid should be dextrose-saline solution without lactate or potassium. Additional fluid and electrolytes may be ordered as indicated by specific signs or measurements, but makeup fluid and other formula extras are best avoided.

Group 2. Premature infants without cardiac defects. It has been shown by Oh and Carroll (1977) that because of their relatively large surface area, premature infants suffer more insensible water loss and loss of salt than full-term infants. Hence, these infants might be expected to need more than 4 to 6 ml/kg/hr. The smaller the infant, the more carefully he must be observed. Hypoglycemia must be recognized promptly; blood glucose level should be considered abnormal when under 30 mg/dl in premature infants and when under 40 mg/dl in full-term infants. Treatment with light for hyperbilirubinemia often raises the metab-

olism of these infants appreciably, while high humidity reduces the loss of moisture from the respiratory tract. Both factors should be considered in adjustment of the fluids to the infant's individual needs, which, as usual, can only be determined by repeated reevaluation.

Group 3. Normal neonates having surgical defects without cardiorespiratory or other systemic complications, e.g., inguinal hernia, phimosis, congenital dislocated hip, choanal atresia, cleft lip, cystic hygromas, or extra digits. These infants may receive "standard" regimens of various types with no additional hazard and no need of large added allowances of fluid. Moderate fluid makeup, plus maintenance fluid of 0 to 4 ml/kg/hr as suggested by Holliday and Segar's formula, will do little harm.

Group 4. Neonates having moderate need of additional fluid allowance. This group includes infants with a variety of intestinal defects involving different degrees of obstruction. The initial allowance should be increased to 5 to 9 ml/kg/hr, and one should be ready to add more to ensure normal urine output (0.5 to 1 ml/kg/hr). Additional losses are weighed or measured and returned ml for ml. Blood pressure is maintained and circulating volume supported as required. In this group one will find infants with intestinal atresia, malrotation, meconium ileus, imperforate anus, megacolon, and Hirschsprung's disease. During operation there will be ongoing loss by translocation that must be evaluated by examination of blood and urine as well as by physical signs.

Group 5. Neonates needing maximal fluid support. This group consists chiefly of neonates with gastroschisis, ruptured omphalocele, and necrotizing enterocolitis. Preoperative losses of peritoneal fluid and intestinal exudate may be of massive proportions and require several times the maintenance allowance. These are the infants studied by Jahrig and Margies (1972) and found to need from 15 to 25 ml/kg/hr, and others have confirmed their findings. In addition to dextrose-electrolyte solutions, these infants will require large amounts of albumin to prevent shock.

It is apparent that much more fluid is being administered to small infants than in former years. However, there is good reason why it is better to err on the dry side than to overhydrate an infant. Most will admit that dehydration is easier to correct than overhydration and involves fewer dangers. In addition, pediatric surgeons make one point that is not widely recognized by anesthesiologists, i.e., that with only slight overhydration, the site of anastomosis of the esophagus or other intestinal repairs develops enough edema to interfere with healing and lead to renewed intestinal obstruction.

Children undergoing cardiovascular surgery

Infants and children with cardiac lesions usually fall into two groups: those whose defects lead to heart failure and those whose lesions ultimately lead to hypoxia and hemoconcentration. A neonate with a large patent ductus or coarctation, if not already in failure, can easily be overhydrated, with rapid development of failure. Whether patients of this type are being operated on for correction of the cardiac defect or for some unrelated lesions, the intravenous fluid should be held to a minimum, 1 to 2 ml/kg/hr serving as maintenance. If the ductus is being divided, there is sudden shifting of fluid from pulmonary to systemic circulation at the moment of occlusion of the ductus, and the tendency toward initiation of cardiac failure is even greater (see Chapter 16). Children with atrial and ventricular septal defects share the same danger of overloading (Novak and Feldt, 1972).

The fluid management of patients with cardiac defects that cause hypoxia calls for careful monitoring of hematocrit and administration of enough fluid to keep the hematocrit below 70%. When the hematocrit is in excess of 70% before operation, it is often advisable to reduce it by withdrawing blood and replacing it with albumin, plasma, or electrolyte solution. If plasma is used, one should administer it slowly and add calcium to counteract the negative inotropic effect of the citrate-rich solution, which may also contain high concentrations of potassium. The procedure should be performed with the aid of an ECG and serum electrolyte determinations.

Children undergoing neurosurgery

As with cardiac lesions, the chief danger involved in administration of fluids during pediatric neurosurgery is overhydration. During intracranial operations, the use of excess fluid can distend the cerebral vasculature and cause edema or hemorrhage. It is generally agreed that the maintenance fluids of these patients should be reduced. In his classic text, Matson (1969) advised limitation of fluid to 20 ml/kg/24 hr on the operative day and use of only dextrose in water. Since his death, others have modified this regimen but have not bettered his results. Today there is a general tendency to use dextrose-saline or dextrose-lactate solutions at slightly less than average maintenance allowances (Bennett, 1973; Furman, 1977). We use 2 to 4 ml/kg/hr adjusted to signs, urine output, and brain tension.

When there is brain edema or intraoperative swelling of the brain, correction includes reduction of fluids, hyperventilation, and use of diuretics and dexamethasone, as outlined in Chapter 18.

Operations for correction of myelomeningocele often require blood replacement. Blood loss can be reduced if the infant is positioned to reduce pressure on the abdomen, thus decreasing the return of blood via the valveless vertebral plexus of veins. Following operation, the elimination of the expansile sac often causes increasing CSF pressure with resultant hydrocephalus. While both intracranial and spinal operations are complicated by excess fluid, Matson warned against radical reduction of fluids, emphasizing the need to maintain the child in a narrowed, low-normal fluid balance. As in intracranial operations, we favor reduced allowances of 5% dextrose in ¼-strength saline solution adjusted as indicated by individual situations.

Children with chronic renal failure

Infants and children with renal anomalies and infections present individual problems in fluid management. Heird and Winters (1973) described the progressive course of pathology in obstructive renal failure to include reduction of concentrating ability, acidification mechanism, sodium resorption, and glomerular filtration, with resultant polyuria, hyperchloremic acidosis, hyponatremic dehydration, and azotemia. The restricted tolerance to both water and electrolytes associated with renal failure appears to be very similar to that described by Holliday and Segar (1957) as being characteristic of normal neonates. With decreasing urinary output, one must measure fluid administration with increasing accuracy, allowing just enough to replace insensible loss and measured urine output. While excess water or sodium administration increases the danger of retention, inadequate replacement increases the tendency toward more rapid development of severe lack of water and essential constituents.

In patients receiving dialysis support and in those awaiting the arrival of donor kidneys, serum potassium should be monitored by repeated examination.

Children tolerate dialysis relatively well. Serum potassium climbs gradually with increasing concentration of BUN and creatinine in the intervals between dialysis, and protein and albumin concentration fall. Acidosis and postnephrectomy hypocalcemia are added complications that require attention and correction.

Management of fluids for genitourinary operations not associated with renal failure consists of a basic allowance plus 3 to 4 ml/kg/hr for third-space loss. During parathyroidectomy, shunt procedures, nephrectomy, and similar operations on children in renal failure, 5% dextrose in ¼-strength saline solution is given at 2 ml/kg/hr, and the estimated intraoperative loss of blood and urine is added to this.

Infants with pyloric stenosis

The anesthetic management of infants with hypertrophic pyloric stenosis was described in Chapter 15. Discussion of their fluid management was reserved for this chapter, however, because pyloric stenosis has been used for many years as the prime example of metabolic alkalosis. Times have not changed the disease, but more alert pediatricians now rarely allow the process to reach its classic full-blown stage, and the all-out approach of

2 or 3 days of rehydration prior to operation rarely is necessary. For theoretical purposes, however, one should be thoroughly aware of the entire picture. For this reason, the unusual case of the severely dehydrated infant is described first, followed by discussion of the infant diagnosed in the early stages of the process.

In pyloric stenosis, no material can pass from the duodenum back into the stomach. The vomiting that takes place consists only of gastric contents and consequently is high in hydrochloric acid. With continued failure to retain feedings and vomiting of fluid and hydrochloric acid, isotonic dehydration and metabolic alkalosis are the natural consequences. When no oral intake is retained and normal losses via skin, respiratory tract, and kidneys continue, the development of dehydration may reach a relatively advanced state within 3 or 4 days, with laboratory evidence of metabolic alkalosis appearing in the form of rising serum pH, hyponatremia, and hypochloremia. As reported by Kildeberg (1968) and Winters (1973), the respiratory compensation for metabolic alkalosis is apt to be unpredictable and ineffective as compared with the respiratory compensation for metabolic acidosis, and in such advanced cases, arterial pH often exceeds 7.50 and occasionally 7.60.

An important factor in the electrolyte disturbance of advanced pyloric stenosis is the depletion of serum potassium, which is believed to be caused in part, at least, by the metabolic alkalosis. Potassium is excreted as a cation partner to reduce bicarbonate excess and thus is actually removed from the body. In addition, serum potassium is further reduced by being withdrawn into the intracellular compartment by virtue of its greater affinity for acid media.

The behavior of the kidneys of infants with pyloric stenosis has been a point of special interest. In the early phase of the process, the urine is alkaline, as one would expect, with sodium or potassium being used to enable the kidneys to excrete bicarbonate. Subsequently, however, the urine unexpectedly becomes acid. The explanation for the so-called paradoxical aciduria discovered in this and several parallel situations was found to be that the kidneys, faced with unreplaced deficits of sodium and chloride, must choose between further loss of cations or augmentation of the existing alkalosis. Their apparent choice is to conserve sodium at the expense of increased serum alkalinity, using H^+ ions to facilitate bicarbonate excretion (Winters, 1973).

Treatment. The combination of vomiting, starvation, and dehydration can be fatal in 2 to 3 weeks. Prior to the end stages, infants show marked weight loss (over 20%), hypoproteinemia, and anemia in addition to electrolyte deficits and alkalosis. Laboratory findings may approximate sodium of 100 mEq/L, potassium of 3.0 mEq/L, chloride of 70 mEq/L, hematocrit of 24%, and total serum protein of 4 g/dl. Such an infant might need to be treated for shock first, with albumin and whole blood used to replace circulating volume. Interstitial fluid is next replaced with isotonic solutions containing 2.5% dextrose in ½-strength saline. In severely alkalotic patients, NH_4Cl is believed by some to be more effective. Potassium must be added to correct its deficit and to assist in correction of the alkalosis, but it should not be given until urination has given evidence of initiation of rehydration.

EXAMPLE 1: A 1-month-old baby boy with marked inanition and dehydration. Initial weight, 5 kg; present weight, 4 kg; serum sodium, 100 mEq/L; chloride, 80 mEq/L; potassium, 3.0 mEq/L; pH, 7.5; Pa_{CO_2}, 30 torr; HCO_3^-, 30 mEq/L.

Water deficit = (5 − 4 kg) =
    1 kg, converted to fluid = 1000 ml
Sodium deficit = (140 − 100 mEq) × 5 ×
                0.4 = 80 mEq

With use of 0.9% saline solution (158 mEq of Na/L), the infant would need 500 ml, which would cover Na and Cl deficit, to which one should add the daily allowance of 5 × 4 × 0.4 = 8 ml/hr × 24 = 192 ml, this consisting of 5% dextrose in ¼-strength saline solution. Maintenance allowance to be spread over 24 hours, deficit made up over 72 hours. Potassium, 4 mEq/kg/day, to be added to fluid daily.

EXAMPLE 2: A 1-month-old infant with vomiting

off and on for 4 days; no weight loss or signs of dehydration. Laboratory report negative, mass felt in right hypogastrium. Infant put on "nothing by mouth" regimen. Infusion of 5% dextrose in ¼-strength saline solution started to give estimated daily requirement plus 5 ml/kg/hr to make up for recent lack of intake. Operation should require no more than 20 to 30 minutes without appreciable third-space or other loss.

Standard requirements for long-term maintenance. To supply adequate fluid and nutrition for 2 or 3 days, it is sufficient to add daily needs of potassium, calcium, and vitamins to previously listed items. More prolonged dependence on parenteral feeding will require complete nutritional and growth materials, including protein, fats, and greater quantities of calorie-producing foods than are available in glucose. This is provided by use of total parenteral feeding via a central venous catheter.

APPARATUS AND TECHNICS FOR ADMINISTRATION OF FLUIDS

Regardless of the operation to be performed, the establishment of reliable infusions in small infants remains a real test of skill and patience. It is most important to have suitable equipment for the purpose and to use it to best advantage.

Infusion sets

Fortunately, apparatus for infusions has been refined to acceptable standards and is generally available. Fluids supplied in 500-ml flasks or plastic bags are practical for pediatric use; smaller containers have little advantage. Infusion sets should include a finely calibrated reservoir chamber that holds 100 to 125 ml for small infants or 200 to 250 ml for larger children. A float valve at the outlet of the chamber prevents air from entering the system when the reservoir empties. Under the calibrated chamber there is a visible drip apparatus that enables one to adjust the flow to the number of drops desired per minute, then a length of clear plastic tubing fitted with entry ports and three-way stopcocks for the addition of supplemental drugs, monitoring devices, or blood-pumping apparatus, and finally the plastic adapter for needle or cannula.

Standard filters are used for transfusion of 1 or 2 units of stored blood, but microfilters are used when large amounts of stored blood are given. When fresh blood is administered, filters that remove platelets are avoided. For slow, accurate delivery of fluids, electrically driven pumps are preferable. Warming devices are added for administration of blood to infants and for massive infusion of blood via an arm, when the infused blood reaches the heart with little admixture with the warmer circulating blood of the child.

When blood held in plastic containers is administered, pressure usually is applied by use of an external pneumatic sleeve, and the amount delivered is measured by use of a spring scale from which the bag and pneumatic cuff are suspended. For very small children it frequently is safer to pump blood in small aliquots by use of a syringe. For larger children requiring immediate replacement of massive hemorrhage, a mechanical pumping device is needed. For this purpose, a single rotary pump, such as is mounted on most heart-lung pump-oxygenators, may easily be adapted.

Needles and cannulae

There is a wide and rapidly expanding choice of needles and cannulae available for use in fluid therapy. Hubless steel scalp vein needles frequently are preferable for shorter procedures, for those not involving blood transfusion, and for very small veins. They are easier to insert, less painful, less apt to cause local infection, and less expensive than plastic cannulae. They are available in 19-, 21-, 23-, and 25-gauge sizes. The 19-gauge carries blood with relative ease, the 21-gauge delivers clear fluids easily and blood at moderate rates if under slight pressure, the 23-gauge will serve for fluids other than blood at relatively slow rates, and the shorter and finer 25-gauge is avoided if possible but will serve for clear fluids at a very slow rate. These hubless needles are especially useful for infusions started in conscious children in areas where accessible veins are of limited

length, as on the dorsum of the hand or foot. They are not suitable for use at the internal malleolus of the ankle or near any joint where motion might dislodge them.

Infusion sites and technics

Many variations are acceptable in the technic of infusion. We first attempt to use the dorsum of the child's hand, taking a hubless needle for short, minor cases or a cannula for major procedures. Older children and adolescents may have developed the radial vein, which becomes the best mark in adults. Though it may "roll" badly, this vein travels in a straight subcutaneous line longer than any other and is the largest in the forearm. We generally prefer to have the blood pressure cuff on the right arm and the infusion in the left arm, which allows the patient use of the right hand on awakening.

If veins of the arm fail us, we move to the feet, trying those on the dorsum of the foot with hubless 21-gauge needles or 20-gauge cannulae. The internal saphenous vein is large and ideal for cutdown infusions, but its sudden angulation just above the ankle makes it difficult to cannulate and contraindicates the use of a metal needle. Should none of these attempts succeed, the next step in a small infant would be to use a cutdown infusion at the ankle. In a child of 8 to 10 months, we might inspect the neck for a suitable external jugular vein for percutaneous cannulation, first lowering the head of the table to distend the veins.

When it appears that veins are present but collapsed, hot towels may be used to help them fill, or the limb may be allowed to hang over the side of the operating table. Since halothane is a great help in promoting venous distension, it often helps to induce anesthesia with halothane before starting the infusion.

Plastic cannulae are more suitable for most procedures of moderate extent and for those requiring blood. For premature infants, the 22-gauge cannula may be sufficient, but the 20-gauge cannula is far more valuable and often can be inserted into the dorsum of an infant's hand. The 20-gauge cannula can be used for blood transfusions of moderate amounts if well placed in a major vein. In extensive operations, when the 20-gauge cannula appears insufficient, it often is easier to start another infusion with a 20-gauge cannula than it is to set up an infusion with an 18-gauge cannula. We seldom use an 18-gauge cannula in children less than 5 or 6 years old.

Insertion of cannulae by operative cutdown continues to be a valuable method when others fail. Cannulae are most easily placed in the internal saphenous vein at the ankle or the radial vein at the wrist. When one is faced with a small, fat baby, it frequently is preferable to go ahead with the cutdown before delaying the operation too long. One should be able to cannulate the saphenous vein in 6 to 8 minutes, establishing a foolproof infusion usually at least one size larger than would have been possible with a percutaneous cannula.

There has been increasing enthusiasm for insertion of cannulae via the internal jugular vein (Seldinger, 1953; Rao and others, 1975). The risk of complication is definitely greater here, and it has been our preference to use external jugular or cutdown infusions when standard cannulae cannot be passed.

The volar aspect of the wrist almost always shows one or two clearly visible minute veins that look inviting but that we use only after all others fail, and then only for induction, since extravasation under the carpal sheath is a major concern. In preference, we may start by using a 25-gauge hubless needle in the larger veins of the antecubital space, also for induction only. Small veins in the scalp may serve for induction in infants and may be used throughout the operation if only needed for infusion of clear fluids.

Solutions available for parenteral use

The variety of solutions that have been administered to infants and children gives lasting proof of the miracle of human kidney function, which, under normal conditions, has been able to compensate for intentional and unintentional challenges of the wildest divergence, often correcting excesses or deficits without any evident sign of the physiologic price paid. While it is true that there is considerable latitude in the choice of solution for brief intraoperative maintenance of normal children, errors in type or amount of fluid become increasingly evident in children whose renal function is restricted. Fluids must be chosen carefully here, and the amounts must be determined by close watch and frequent reevaluation. Choice of fluids depends on the needs to be fulfilled. Fluid volume, caloric need, electrolyte replacement, osmolar repair, oncotic pressure, and oxygen-carrying capacity are the factors most often desired. A list of solutions and their composition are given in Table 25-2.

BIBLIOGRAPHY

Ames, R. G.: Urinary water excretion and neurohypophyseal function in full term and premature infants shortly after birth, Pediatrics 12:272, 1953.

Astrup, P. K., Engel, K., Jorgensen, K., and Siggaard-Andersen, O.: Definitions and terminology in blood acid-base chemistry, Ann. N.Y. Acad. Sci. 133:59, 1966.

Bennett, E. J.: Fluids and electrolytes for infants and children, lecture presented at Annual Convention of American Society of Anesthesiologists, San Francisco, 1973.

Bennett, E. J., Bowyer, D. E., and Jenkins, M. T.: Studies in aldosterone excretion of the neonate undergoing anesthesia and surgery, Anesth. Analg. (Cleve.) 50:638, 1971.

Bennett, E. J., Daugherty, M. K., and Jenkins, M. T.: Fluid requirements for neonatal anesthesia and operation, Anesthesiology 32:343, 1970.

Bennett, E. J., Patel, K. P., and Grundy, E. M.: Neonatal temperature and surgery, Anesthesiology 46:303, 1977.

Berry, F. A.: Pediatric fluid and electrolyte therapy, lecture presented at Annual Convention of American Society of Anesthesiologists, Washington, D.C., 1974.

Berry, F. A.: Fluid therapy, lecture presented at Annual Convention of American Society of Anesthesiologists, San Francisco, 1976.

Bland, J. H.: Clinical metabolism of body water and electrolytes, Philadelphia, 1963, W. B. Saunders Co.

Bricker, N. S.: The control of sodium excretion with normal and reduced nephron populations, Am. J. Med. 43:313, 1967.

Broennle, A. M.: The neonate; intraoperative management, lecture presented at Annual Convention of American Society of Anesthesiologists, New Orleans, 1977.

Bunker, J. P.: Citric acid intoxication, J.A.M.A. 157:1361, 1955.

Bush, G. H.: Intravenous fluid therapy in paediatrics, Ann. R. Coll. Surg. Engl. **49:**92, 1971.

Calcagno, P. L.: Parenteral fluid therapy in the pediatric surgical patient, N.Y. J. Med. **60:**1252, 1960.

Calcagno, P. L.: Parenteral and electrolyte fluid therapy. In Gellis, S., and Kagan, B., editors: Current pediatric therapy, Philadelphia, 1967, W. B. Saunders Co.

Colle, E., and Paulsen, E. P.: Fluid therapy in surgical conditions, Pediatr. Clin. North Am. **11:**943, 1964.

Conn, A. W.: Personal communication, 1978.

Cooke, R. E., and Levin, S., editors: The biologic basis of pediatric practice, New York, 1968, McGraw-Hill Book Co.

Darrow, D. C.: Body-fluid physiology; the role of potassium in clinical disorders of body water and electrolytes, N. Engl. J. Med. **242:**978, 1014, 1950.

Darrow, D. C., and Pratt, E. L.: Fluid therapy; relation to tissue composition and expenditure of water and electrolyte, J.A.M.A. **143:**365, 1950.

Davenport, H. T., and Barr, M. N.: Blood loss during pediatric operations, Can. Med. J. **89:**1309, 1963.

Davenport, R. A.: Renal physiology in infancy, Am. J. Med. **9:**229, 1950.

Delivoria-Papadopoulos, M., Morrow, G. III, and Oski, F. A.: Exchange transfusion in the newborn infant with fresh and "old" blood; the role of storage on 2,3-diphosphoglycerate hemoglobin-oxygen affinity and oxygen release, J. Pediatr. **79:**898, 1971.

Dell, R. B.: Pathophysiology of dehydration; normal acid-base regulation. In Winters, R. W., editor: The body fluids in pediatrics, Boston, 1973, Little, Brown & Co.

Deutsch, S., Goldberg, M., and Dripps, R. D.: Postoperative hyponatremia with the inappropriate release of anti-diuretic hormone, Anesthesiology **27:**250, 1966.

Downes, J. J.: Respiratory care in the newborn, lecture presented at Annual Convention of American Society of Anesthesiologists, San Francisco, 1976.

Edelmann, C. M., Jr., and Spitzer, A.: The kidney. In Smith, C. A., and Nelson, M. M., editors: The physiology of the newborn infant, Springfield, Ill., 1976, Charles C Thomas, Publisher.

Feig, P., and McCurdy, D. K.: Physiology in medicine; the hypertonic state, N. Engl. J. Med. **297:**1444, 1978.

Feldman, W., Drummond, K. N., and Klein, M.: Hyponatremia following asphyxia neonatorum, Acta Paediatr. Scand. **59:**52, 1970.

Finberg, L.: Dangers to infants caused by changes in osmolal concentrations, Pediatrics **40:**1031, 1967.

Finberg, L.: Hypernatremic dehydration, Adv. Pediatr. **16:**325, 1969.

Finberg, L.: Diarrheal dehydration. In Winters, R. W., editor: The body fluids in pediatrics, Boston, 1973, Little, Brown & Co.

Finberg, L.: Dehydration secondary to diarrhea. In Smith, C. A., editor: The critically ill child, Philadelphia, 1977, W. B. Saunders Co.

Finlayson, D. C.: Fluid and electrolyte requirements during anesthesia and surgery, Anesth. Analg. (Cleve.) **51:**69, 1972.

Fisher, D. A.: Endocrinology II. In Smith, C. A., and Nelson, M. M., editors: The physiology of the newborn infant, Springfield, Ill., 1976, Charles C Thomas, Publisher.

Friis-Hansen, B.: Changes in body water compartments during growth, Acta Paediatr. Scand. (Suppl.), vol. 110, 1957.

Friis-Hansen, B.: Body water compartments in children, Pediatrics **28:**169, 1961.

Furman, E. B.: Pediatric anesthesia; fluid balance, lecture presented at Annual Convention of American Society of Anesthesiologists, New Orleans, 1977.

Furman, E. B., Roman, D. G., Lemmer, L. A. S., and others: Specific therapy in water, electrolyte and blood volume replacement during pediatric anesthesia, Anesthesia **42:**187, 1975.

Gamble, J. L.: Companionship of water and electrolytes in the organization of body fluids, Lane Medical Lectures, Stanford, 1951, Stanford University Press.

Gamble, J. L.: Chemical anatomy, physiology and pathology of extracellular fluid, ed. 6, Cambridge, Mass., 1954, Harvard University Press.

Graef, J. W., and Cone, T. C., Jr.: Manual of pediatrics, Department of Medicine, The Children's Hospital Medical Center, Boston, 1974, Little, Brown & Co.

Greenberg, A. J., McNamara, H., and McCrory, M. M.: Renal tubular response to aldosterone in normal infants and children with adrenal disorders, J. Clin. Endocrinol. Metab. **27:**1197, 1967.

Heird, W. C., and Winters, R. W.: Fluid therapy for the pediatric surgical patient. In Winters, R. W., editor: The body fluids in pediatrics, Boston, 1973, Little, Brown & Co.

Heller, H., and Zaimis, E. J.: The antidiuretic and oxytoxic hormones in the posterior pituitary glands of the newborn infants and adults, J. Physiol. **109:**162, 1949.

Herbert, W. I., Scott, E. B., and Lewis, G. B.: Fluid management of the pediatric surgical patients, Anesth. Analg. (Cleve.) **50:**376, 1971.

Holliday, M. A., and Segar, W. E.: The maintenance need for water in parenteral fluid therapy, Pediatrics **19:**823, 1957.

Hoppenstein, J. M., Miltenberger, F. W., and Moran, W. H., Jr.: The increase in blood levels of vasopressin in infants during birth and surgical procedures, Surg. Gynecol. Obstet. **127:**966, 1968.

Hoye, R. C., Bennett, S. H., Geelhoed, G. W., and Goschboth, C.: Fluid volume and albumin kinetics occurring with major surgery, J.A.M.A. **222:**1255, 1972.

Hradcova, L., and Heller, J.: Values of antidiuretic activity of the plasma in childhood, Helv. Paediatr. Acta **17:**531, 1962.

Jahrig, K., and Margies, D.: Osmolar clearance of total electrolytes in newborn infants, Biol. Neonate **20:**93, 1972.

Kaplan, S. A.: Fluid and electrolyte therapy; maintenance, abnormal states, methods of administration, Pediatr. Clin. North Am. **16:**581, 1969.

Kaplan, S. A.: Fluid therapy in pediatrics. In Gellis, S. S., and Kagan, B. M., editors: Current pediatric practice, vol. 5, Philadelphia, 1971, W. B. Saunders Co.

Kaplan, S. L., and Feigin, R. D.: Inappropriate secretion of antidiuretic hormone complicating neonatal hypoxic-ischemic encephalopathy, J. Pediatr. **92:** 431, 1978.

Kerrigan, G. A.: In Bland, J. G., editor: Clinical metabolism of body water and electrolytes, Philadelphia, 1963, W. B. Saunders Co.

Kevy, S. V.: Surgical implications of hematologic disorders. In Ravitch, M. M., Welch, K. J., Benson, C. D., and others, editors: Pediatric surgery, ed. 3, Chicago, 1979, Year Book Medical Publishers, Inc.

Kildeberg, J.: Clinical acid-base physiology studies in neonates, infants and young children, Baltimore, 1968, The Williams & Wilkins Co.

Knutrud, O.: The water and electrolyte metabolism in the newborn child after major surgery, Oslo, 1965, Universitetsforlaget.

Levina, S. E.: Endocrine features in development of human hypothalus, hypophysis and placenta, Gen. Comp. Endocrinol. **11:**151, 1968.

Macbeth, W. A., and Pope, G. R.: Effect of abdominal operation upon protein excretion in man, Lancet **1:** 215, 1968.

Matson, D. D.: Neurosurgery of infancy and childhood, Springfield, Ill., 1969, Charles C Thomas, Publisher.

Maxwell, N. H., and Kleeman, C. R., editors: Clinical disorders of fluid and electrolyte metabolism, New York, 1962, McGraw-Hill Book Co.

McCance, R. A.: Renal function in early life, Physiol. Rev. **28:**331, 1948.

McCance, R. A.: Renal physiology in infancy, Am. J. Med. **9:**229, 1950.

McCance, R. A., and Widdowson, E. M.: The correct physiological basis on which to compare infant and adult renal function, Lancet **11:**860, 1952.

McCrory, W. W.: Developmental nephrology, Cambridge, Mass., 1972, Harvard University Press.

Minick, M. C., and Conn, J. W.: Aldosterone excretion from infancy to adult life, Metabolism **3:**681, 1964.

Moore, F. D.: Metabolic care of the surgical patient, Philadelphia, 1959, W. B. Saunders Co.

Moore, F. D.: Regulation of the serum sodium concentration; origin and treatment of tonicity disorders in surgery, Am. J. Surg. **103:**302, 1962.

Novak, L. P., and Feldt, R. H.: Body fluids and electrolytes in infants and children with congenital heart disease, Mayo Clin. Proc. **47:**327, 1972.

Oh, W.: Disorders of fluid and electrolytes in newborn infants, Pediatr. Clin. North Am. **23:**601, 1976.

Oh, W., and Carroll, H. J.: Current concepts; the anion gap, N. Engl. J. Med. **297:**814, 1977.

Rao, T. L., Wong, A. Y., and Salem, M. R.: A new approach to percutaneous internal jugular vein catheterization, paper presented at Annual Convention of American Society of Anesthesiologists, Chicago, October 1975.

Rickham, P. P.: In Ravitch, M. M., Welch, K. J., Benson, C. D., and others, editors: Pediatric surgery, ed. 3, Chicago, 1979, Year Book Medical Publishers, Inc.

Rickham, P. P., and Johnson, J. H.: Neonatal surgery, New York, 1969, Appleton-Century-Crofts.

Rowe, M. I.: The role of serum osmolality measurements in the management of the neonatal surgical patient, Surg. Gynecol. Obstet. **133:**93, 1971.

Rowe, M. I.: Preoperative and postoperative management; the physiologic approach. In Ravitch, M. M., Welch, K. J., Benson, C. D., and others, editors: Pediatric surgery, ed. 3, Chicago, 1979, Year Book Medical Publishers, Inc.

Rowe, M. I., and Marchildon, M. B.: Physiologic considerations in the newborn surgical patient, Surg. Clin. North Am. **56:**245, 1976.

Rowe, M. I., and Uribe, F. L.: Diaphragmatic hernia in the newborn infant; blood gas and pH considerations, Surgery **70:**758, 1971.

Sacks, M. J.: The use of blood and colloids in the newborn, Pediatr. Clin. North Am. **28:**169, 1961

Salem, M. R., Wong, A. Y., Bennett, E. J., and others: Deliberate hypotension in infants and children, Anesth. Analg. (Cleve.) **53:**975, 1974.

Schwartz, W. B., Bennett, W., Curelop, S., and Bartter, F. C.: A syndrome of renal sodium loss and hyponatremia probably resulting from inappropriate secretion of antidiuretic hormones, Am. J. Med. **23:**529, 1957.

Schwartz, W. B., and Relman, A. S.: A critique of the parameters used in acid-base disorders, N. Engl. J. Med. **268:**1382, 1963.

Seldinger, S. I.: Catheter replacement of the needle in percutaneous arteriography, Acta Radiol. **39:**368, 1953.

Shires, G. T., Williams, J., and Brown, F.: Acute changes in extracellular fluids associated with major surgical procedures, Ann. Surg. **154:**803, 1961.

Siegel, S. R., Fisher, D. A., and Oh, W.: Serum aldosterone concentration related to sodium balance in the newborn infant, Pediatrics **53:**410, 1974.

Sladen, A., Laver, M. B., and Pontoppidan, H.: Pulmonary complications and water retention in prolonged mechanical ventilation, N. Engl. J. Med. **279:**448, 1968.

Smith, C. A., and Nelson, N. M., editors: The physiology of the newborn infant, Springfield, Ill., 1976, Charles C Thomas, Publisher.

Srouji, M.: The acid-base status of the surgical neonate on admission to the hospital, Surgery **62:**958, 1967.

Strauss, J., Adamsons, K., Jr., and James, L. W.: Renal function of normal full-term infants in the first hours of extrauterine life, Am. J. Obstet. Gynecol. **91:**286, 1965.

Strauss, M. B.: Body water in man, Boston, 1957, Little, Brown & Co.

Talbot, N. B., Kerrigan, G. A., Crawford, J. D., and others: Application of homeostatic principles to the practice of parenteral fluid therapy, N. Engl. J. Med. **252:**856, 898, 1955.

Weldon, V. V., Kowarski, A., and Migeon, C. J.: Aldosterone secretion rates in normal subjects from infancy to adulthood, Pediatrics **39:**713, 1967.

Weldon, V. V., Kowarski, A., Talbert, J. L., and others: Effect of operation upon sodium metabolism and aldosterone secretion rate in children, Surgery **70:** 433, 1971.

West, C. D.: Parenteral fluid therapy. In Shirkey, H. L., editor: Pediatric therapy, ed. 5, St. Louis, 1975, The C. V. Mosby Co.

Williams, G. S., Klenk, E. L., and Winters, R. W.: Acute renal failure in pediatrics. In Winters, R. W., editor: The body fluids in pediatrics, Boston, 1973, Little, Brown & Co.

Winters, R. W., editor: The body fluids in pediatrics, Boston, 1973, Little, Brown & Co.

Winters, R. W., and Heird, W. C.: Special problems of the pediatric surgical patient. In Winters, R. W., editor: The body fluids in pediatrics, Boston, 1973, Little, Brown & Co.

CHAPTER 26

Anesthetic complications

GENERAL CONSIDERATIONS
Stages in the development and elimination of anesthetic problems

Each anesthetic complication can be traced through several stages of development. In the first stage, the complication exists but is not recognized as an entity. Seven different children died during anesthesia, three from hemorrhage. All are labelled anesthesia deaths, and nothing is learned from the experience. The situation is repeated several times in various institutions before someone notices that the children who died following hemorrhage did not die until large amounts of blood were being pumped back into the exsanguinated but still functioning circulation. It then becomes evident that there is a specific factor in addition to the exsanguination that is responsible for the deaths. Recognition of the problem as a clinical entity is the second stage. Stage three includes a gathering of forces to teach, study, and treat the complication, in this case involving a dispute over the existence of citrate poisoning. While surgeons attempted to improve the situation by reduction of blood loss, clinicians and investigators struggled to define the problem more clearly. In time, the problem became reasonably explained, the onus of death was divided between citrate toxicity

(Bunker, 1955), hyperkalemia (Marshall, 1962), and acidemia and hypothermia (Howland and Schweizer, 1964), and the problem reached the end stages where both treatment and prevention could be accomplished.

Many of the familiar complications of pediatric anesthesia developed in similar fashion. The aspiration of vomitus, certainly the most thoroughly emphasized hazard of all branches of anesthesia, was encountered for many years but dealt with in inadequate methods (Smith, 1948, 1956).

Deaths were commonplace until general recognition and alarm focussed attention on the problem and strict methods of management were adopted. Other complications that may be traced through similar stages, some not to completion, include asystole following administration of succinylcholine to traumatized patients (McCaughey, 1962) and, of course, malignant hyperthermia (Denborough and others, 1962; Denborough, 1978), which has been recognized, widely popularized, and endlessly discussed but for which we still lack understanding, treatment, and even positive methods of diagnosis.

It is not to our credit that anxiety, fright, and lasting psychic disturbances, which are commonplace, rarely are mentioned in discussions of anesthetic complications. They do not appear to have reached the stage of recognition.

Evaluation of comparative importance of anesthetic complications

Before specific complications are discussed, another general recommendation is

pathology. Seizures that occur during recovery or that develop some time thereafter have more serious implications and may suggest posthypoxic damage, hypoglycemia, cerebral edema, or water intoxication. When an episode of hypoxia has been sufficient to cause prolonged defects of any kind, however, there is usually a relatively severe episode of cerebral edema immediately after operation. The child recovers slowly from this, being comatose at first, then having gradual return of consciousness and speech, and occasionally remaining blind for several weeks before gaining the final state of fixed, incomplete recovery (Williams and Spencer, 1958; Strong and Keats, 1967; Kristoffersen and others, 1967).

During past decades, treatment of potentially dangerous hypoxia has alternately involved use of hypothermia and normothermia (Strong and Keats, 1967). Interest has been greatly stimulated by the work of Hägerdal and associates (1978), Michenfelder and associates (1976), Conn and associates (1978), and Bleyaert and associates (1978), who have produced greatly improved survival and reduction of brain damage by combination of heavy barbiturate sedation (pentobarbital blood level of 2.5 to 4 mg/dl) with reduction of temperature (30° C) for 48 to 72 hours or more.

Other complications related to the central nervous system include damage to peripheral nerves caused by pressure or stretching due to faulty positioning, although these appear to occur less frequently among younger patients. Damage to the spinal cord and nerve trunks due to injection of local anesthetics is rare, as would be expected from the infrequent use of these technics in smaller patients. The danger of drug toxicity incurred in relation to local anesthesia administered to the mother for delivery must be considered in treatment of the neonate.

THERMIC COMPLICATIONS
Inadvertent hypothermia

The tendency for infants and small children to lose body heat has been discussed previously in Chapters 2 and 15 and else-

where. Infants' relatively greater body surface area, the ease with which they become exposed prior to operation, and their inadequate defense against cooling often produce temperature responses similar to that shown in Fig. 26-1. The initial fall occurs when the infant is brought into an unprepared operating room and uncovered while anesthesia is started, monitoring devices and infusions are established, the skin is cleansed with cold solutions, and unwarmed intravenous solutions are infused (Smith, 1968, 1968a, 1973; Roe, 1973; Bennett and others, 1977).

With subsequent heating of the operating room, the use of a warming light and water mattress (Goudsouzian and others, 1973), and the effect of draping and reflected body heat of the surgical team (Clark and others, 1954), the infant's temperature may reverse and even exceed normal after 2 or 3 hours. If the child is warm on awakening, the short duration of hypothermia at 34° or 35° C has probably done no harm and could even have been beneficial. If the child is still cold on awakening, however, there will be increased oxygen need, delayed return of activity, and respiratory depression. It is this situation that has often set the stage for sudden cardiorespiratory arrest in the early postoperative period.

Knowledge that neonates can be cooled to 15° C and held in cardiac asystole for 2 hours for open-heart procedures (Chapter 16) may

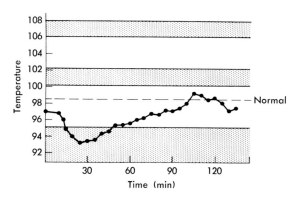

Fig. 26-1. Chart showing typical temperature change in an infant after entering operating room and throughout subsequent operation.

reduce one's concern for the infant who loses 4° to 5° C during lesser procedures. However, the cardiac patients are under a thoroughly controlled system, and the risk is not the same. It is generally believed that when an unprotected infant's temperature falls below 35° C, there is increasing incidence of metabolic acidosis (Hackett and Crosby, 1960; Roe, 1973), hypoglycemia, hypocalcemia, and viscosity of red cells (Marty and others, 1971; Hackel, 1975). Changes of this nature do not reverse promptly upon rewarming, and the infant is left in a weakened condition.

Among older patients, those having cerebral palsy have shown extreme hypothermic responses to general anesthesia and should be monitored with carefully calibrated thermometers.

Treatment. The treatment of both hypothermia and hyperthermia is best planned on a three-phased approach. Phase I, the external approach, includes simple external warming methods, phase II, internal warming methods, and phase III, what may be termed metabolic methods. These are outlined below. One naturally begins with the simpler phase I steps for minor degrees of hypothermia and progresses to phases II and III to treat more profound cooling. External methods will have relatively little effect when cooling has been sufficient to cause significant peripheral vasoconstriction. There is growing evidence that body temperature can be most effectively raised by ventilating the lungs with warmed, humidified air and cooled by use of cool, dry air (or gases) (Tapper and others, 1974; Pflug and others, 1978).

THREE-PHASE APPROACH TO TREATMENT OF INADVERTENT HYPOTHERMIA

Phase I (external approach)
1. Warm operating room
2. Cover body with warmed blankets
3. Apply sheet wadding to limbs
4. Cover head with stockinette cap
5. Use lamp on infant's head
6. Use water blanket

Phase II (internal approach)
1. Infuse warm parenteral fluid

2. Irrigate peritoneum or chest with warm saline solution
3. Ventilate with warm, humidified gases

Phase III (metabolic approach)
1. Reduce rate of ventilation
2. Reduce gas flows, close system
3. Discontinue halothane, relaxants
4. Change to spontaneous ventilation, light anesthetic, preferably ketamine and nitrous oxide

Postoperative shivering has been a matter of some concern, because the increased activity may cause excessive oxygen demand (Harverth and others, 1956). The distinction between excess activity due to the regaining of control of motor function and true shivering is discussed in Chapter 10.

Several drugs have been advocated for control of shivering, including epinephrine, ephedrine, methylphenidate, and calcium gluconate. Among these, Liem and Aldrete (1974) reported best results with methylphenidate (20-mg adult dose), while Bidwai and Stanley (1978) found calcium more effective (3 to 5 mg/kg). At The Children's Hospital Medical Center, neither approach has been impressive in our experience. The work of Pflug and associates (1978) suggests that inhalation of warm, moist gases is the best preventive and the most effective cure for shivering.

Hyperthermia (nonmalignant)

Temperature elevation during anesthesia has been a major source of concern for the past 50 years. It was a relatively common occurrence for children to develop appendicitis, undergo ether anesthesia without preliminary hydration, and suddenly begin to convulse, develop a temperature of 40° to 42° C, and die (Pledger and Buchan, 1969). The exact mechanism of the seizure remained somewhat of a mystery, but metabolic acidosis and hypoxia often made a lethal combination. With elimination of ether and cyclopropane and somewhat better preparation of children for operation, this type of response is rarely seen anymore. Hydration, antibiotics, and nasogastric suction have played an important role in increasing survival.

Temperature elevation still occurs in anesthetized children and may be due to any one of several causes. A heated environment is the most common cause, for operating room temperatures tend to rise on sunny afternoons (Fraser, 1978). Older children who have gone 10 to 12 hours without fluids and are draped from head to foot for a long tympanoplasty quite understandably become hyperthermic. The added effect of atropine in hyperthermia has been disputed. While many anesthesiologists and surgeons feel that atropine does cause temperature elevation, this has been difficult to document, and there is some evidence that it does not affect body temperature, even in a tropical climate.

Underlying infections have often been present in children who suddenly show a spiking temperature during anesthesia (Saidman and others, 1964; Modell, 1966). This has occurred in children during appendectomy and other procedures, and unexpected temperature elevations have occurred so frequently in children undergoing operations on the urinary tract that these procedures are always watched with particular care, since there is an increased tendency for sudden release of pathogens into the general circulation. Temperature elevations of this sort may reach 39° to 40° C but usually are short-lived and have not caused permanent damage in our experience. Transfusion reactions also are commonly accompanied by hyperthermia.

Unexplained temperature elevation has been seen in sporadic groups of patients immediately after spinal fusion and procedures for correction of pectus excavatum. It is possible that this stems from cartilaginous injury (Folkman, 1978), but the inconsistency of the occurrence makes this explanation appear doubtful.

The retention of carbon dioxide due to any one of several factors rates among the most common causes of hyperpyrexia and may play either a primary or a secondary role. Certainly, in the event of any temperature elevation, a heated environment, carbon dioxide retention, dehydration, sepsis, and transfusion reaction should be thought of first (Schweizer and others, 1971) (see list below).

ETIOLOGY OF PERIOPERATIVE HYPERTHERMIA

Environment
　　Warm room; excessive use of blankets, heating devices, surgical lights
Dehydration
Carbon dioxide retention
Bacteremia
Iatrogenic pathogens
Transfusion reaction
Preexisting infection
Malignant hyperthermia
Atropine (?)

While the heat loss that small patients suffer during operations is a natural phenomenon that does not suggest the presence of any pathologic process, temperature elevation has many pathologic causes, and the first sign of an elevation should be regarded with concern. In many situations, hyperthermia shows an actively progressive course, with the temperature rising in an accelerating curve as though stimulating its own rise (Fig. 26-2). This makes it imperative to start action early in the course of the process and not wait until the temperature reaches 43° to 44° C, when it may be impossible to control.

Treatment. Therapy for hyperthermia may effectively be planned along lines that are similar to treatment of hypothermia. The approach is based on three phases: external cooling, internal cooling, and metabolic therapy, as outlined below. One should not assume that every patient whose temperature rises 1 or 2 degrees has malignant hyperthermia, but one should look for stiffness, tachycardia, arrhythmias, and rapidly rising fever in order not to miss the diagnosis and the opportunity to start suitable treatment promptly, in the unlikely chance that one is dealing with malignant hyperthermia.

TREATMENT OF INTRAOPERATIVE NONMALIGNANT HYPERTHERMIA

Phase I (external approach for temperatures 37.5° to 39° C)
　　1. Cool room
　　2. Uncover patient as much as possible
　　3. Apply ice bags to neck, groin, axillae
　　4. Increase air circulation

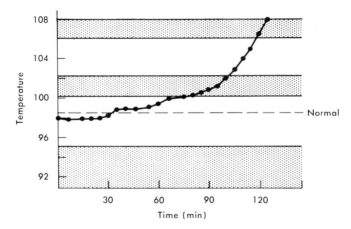

Fig. 26-2. Chart showing gradual start and increasing speed of temperature elevation in hyperthermic patient.

Phase II (internal approach for temperatures 39° to 41° C)

1. Irrigate stomach with iced saline solution
2. Irrigate rectum similarly
3. Irrigate operative site (chest or abdomen)
4. Infuse cold parenteral fluids
5. Apply ECG

Phase III (metabolic approach)

1. Ventilate actively with dry, unwarmed gases
2. Use d-tubocurarine or halothane unless malignant hyperthermia is suspected
3. Measure and correct arterial P_{O_2}, HCO_3, pH
4. Measure and correct electrolytes
5. Use buffer ($NaHCO_3$, 2 to 3 mg/kg), avoid ketamine
6. Use antipyretic agents: chlorpromazine, aspirin, acetaminophen (Tylenol)

Malignant hyperthermia

From the standpoint of frequency of occurrence, malignant hyperthermia stands last. However, its rapid onset and high mortality demand high priority in the minds of anesthesiologists. In normal populations, the incidence of malignant hyperthermia is estimated as between 1 in 20,000 and 1 in 100,000. The syndrome is characterized by sudden appearance of tachycardia and other arrhythmias, followed by temperature elevation to 42° to 44° C within 30 to 45 minutes and death in 60% to 70% of the approximately 1000 cases thus far documented (Britt and Kalow, 1970; Aldrete and Britt, 1978). The syndrome has been associated with the use of almost all the known anesthetic agents. Succinylcholine and halothane have been the outstanding offenders, and the local anesthetic agents mepivacaine (Carbocaine) and lidocaine are also believed to be hazardous (see list below). Agents that have been used successfully also are listed below.

ANESTHETIC AGENTS ASSOCIATED WITH MALIGNANT HYPERTHERMIA*

Halothane (60% of cases)
Succinylcholine (77% of cases)
Nitrous oxide–meperidine
Methoxyflurane
Ether
Ethyl chloride
Trichloroethylene
Cyclopropane
Ethylene
Gallamine
d-Tubocurarine
Isoflurane
Ethrane
Lidocaine (local, regional, or spinal)
Mepivacaine (Carbocaine) (local, regional, or spinal)

ANESTHETIC APPROACHES USED SUCCESSFULLY IN PATIENTS AT RISK OF MALIGNANT HYPERTHERMIA

Innovar (droperidol and fentanyl)
Barbiturates, nitrous oxide, and narcotics

*From Ryan, J. F.: Malignant hyperthermia; recognition, lecture presented at Annual Convention of American Society of Anesthesiologists, Chicago, 1978.

Local anesthetics of ester type
  Cocaine
  Procaine
  Tetracaine
  Chloroprocaine
  Proparacaine
  Piperocaine

In the clinical development of the syndrome, one's first warning may be the appearance of generalized rigidity following administration of succinylcholine. Masseter spasm, without rigidity of the rest of the body, may be encountered when endotracheal intubation is attempted in inadequately relaxed patients and presents a difficult diagnostic problem. Although several patients have been carried on through anesthesia and operation without further incident, we have encountered three whom we became concerned about and stopped the procedure. Subsequent muscle biopsies were termed positive. Although one may adopt a conservative approach and halt all procedures when the jaw appears to be stiff, it is hoped that a better solution will be found.

Many of the early cases of malignant hyperthermia were first noticed when surgeons felt the unusual heat of the viscera and thermometers read 40° to 42° C. Somewhat later, it was noted that prodromal tachycardia and arrhythmias often could be observed. It has been found that there are many variables in the syndrome. Only about half of the patients show stiffness, which initially was believed to be one of the outstanding manifestations. Other signs that usually, but not always, are observed include cyanosis, skin mottling, sweating, and unstable blood pressure. Britt and Kalow (1970) stated that tachycardia is the prime symptom of malignant hyperthermia. It has been postulated that the syndrome of malignant hyperthermia might occur without any elevation of temperature if prodromal signs were observed and prompt treatment forestalled its progress. It has also been reported that in some cases of a fulminant nature, cardiac asystole has occurred before there was any marked temperature elevation (Britt, 1974; Ryan, 1976).

The pathophysiology of malignant hyperthermia has yet to be clearly understood. There is uncertainty as to whether the process is primarily a disease of muscle, a result of neuropathic changes, a result of endocrine disturbances, or a general derangement in membrane structure and function (Rosenberg, 1978). The basic defect appears to be related to the storage of calcium in the sarcoplasmic reticulum of striated muscle and to the mode of release of the calcium into the muscle cells to produce the excitation-contraction coupling necessary for muscular activity (Chidsey, 1972; Nelson, 1978). The demonstration of alteration of this mechanism by halothane and other agents may explain part of the etiology of malignant hyperthermia, but recognition of stress and overactivity as triggering factors suggests a multiplicity of causes.

Predisposing characteristics of susceptible individuals. Individuals with various anatomic and physiologic defects have been reported to show increased susceptibility to malignant hyperthermia. As shown in the list below, many of the defects relate to neuromuscular disorders. Denborough (1977) stated that all individuals who are susceptible to malignant hyperthermia have either a subclinical or a recognizable disease of muscle. In preevaluation of patients, one certainly pays maximum attention to history of intraoperative fever in either patient or relative. There has been a significantly high incidence of myopathies and dystonias in malignant hyperthermia, but warnings concerning children with inguinal hernia, cleft lip, and uncomplicated squint or ptosis seem less convincing.

The importance of the etiologic roles of heavy musculature and nervous tension has also been recognized. Our lesson was a sad one. The death of an 18-year-old college football player alerted us to two unusual features of malignant hyperthermia. This patient developed characteristic, full-blown signs of malignant hyperthermia during induction of anesthesia for open reduction of a fractured lower leg. Operation was halted, and the patient responded to symptomatic treatment.

The next day he tolerated a 4-hour operation under Innovar to relieve arterial occlusion and reduce the fracture. He recovered, spent a normal night, and appeared to be doing well, but he was anxious, and while a group of physicians were discussing his problems at his bedside his anxiety heightened, he trembled and became comatose, and his heart stopped. During the next 4 hours all known forms of therapy were attempted, including bypass perfusion and dantrolene, without success. Increased muscular tension has been observed in other patients who developed malignant hyperthermia and is now considered to be an important warning sign. The possibility that a patient could develop a fatal response when not anesthetized had not been known to us, nor had the importance of keeping the patient completely undisturbed.

MALIGNANT HYPERTHERMIA

Predisposing factors
Family history of occurrence
Neuromuscular defect
Heavy musculature
High-stress response

Diagnostic features
Preinduction tension
Generalized muscle spasm on induction
Tachycardia and arrhythmias
Hyperthermia
Cyanosis
Flushing, sweating, hot skin and body
Hyperventilation
Irregular blood pressure

Treatment
Stop operation
External cooling
  Cool room
  Uncover, apply ice
Internal cooling
  Give cold intravenous infusions
  Perform iced saline irrigation of chest, peritoneum, brain, as situation permits
Metabolic therapy
  Hyperventilate with oxygen
  Correct metabolic acidosis
Monitoring
  Arterial blood gases and pressure
  Temperature
  Acid-base balance
  ECG
  Urethral catheter
  CVP
  Serum potassium, calcium
Specific therapy
  Procaine amide
  Dantrolene
  Cardiopulmonary bypass
  Mannitol

Postoperative considerations
Avoidance of emotional stress
Continuation of intensive care
High-level support

Late complications
Myoglobinuria
Renal failure
Cardiac failure
High emotional tension

Treatment. When symptoms appear suggestive of malignant hyperthermia, a planned course of action should be instituted at once (Fraser and others, 1976; Ryan, 1978). As outlined above, the first step is to alert the surgeons to the situation and abandon the operation as soon as possible. Organization of effective teamwork without causing generalized panic and pandemonium will be a major problem. Six additional helpers should be able to handle the extra work, and others should be asked to leave.

Several approaches are followed at once, including measures to cool the environment, cool the patient externally and internally, correct metabolic imbalance, provide additional monitoring and supportive measures, and provide specific therapy, also outlined above. Several measures are of particular importance. Hyperventilation of the patient with oxygen should be carried out at a greatly increased ratio, since the excessive metabolic rate requires large amounts of oxygen and produces proportionately large amounts of CO_2. Ventilation at three times the normal rate and volume should be a minimum until arterial gases give more accurate guidance.

Establishment of at least two major infusions, one a central venous line, and an arterial monitoring line should be started, and a Foley catheter should be inserted in the bladder.

The temperature is monitored by esophageal and nasal or oral thermistors. It is the cardiac action that determines the life of the patient, however. It has been shown that patients may survive temperatures as high as 44° C (111.2° F) if the circulation can be maintained (Ryan, 1978). For this reason, efforts should be made to monitor with an ECG, direct arterial pressure gauge, and cardiac output determination, to administer inotropic agents as indicated, and to consider the use of a heart-lung oxygenator for patients whose temperature is reaching top levels or whose cardiac output begins to falter (Ryan and others, 1974).

With a Foley catheter in place, one should proceed to administer large quantities of cold glucose (for cardiac support) and saline (for circulating volume). Mannitol (200 to 300 mg/kg) or furosemide (Lasix) (0.5 to 1 mg/kg) should be given to ensure rapid excretion of the water load.

For treatment of the intramuscular disorder, procaine hydrochloride has been given. When first used, the large prescribed dose aroused reasonable concern, but the modified plan of administering 1 gram of procainamide in 500 ml of intravenous solution (adult dose) appears more reasonable (Strobel, 1971).

The muscle relaxant dantrolene sodium has become the drug of choice for specific therapy for malignant hyperthermia (Harrison, 1975; Ryan, 1978). The agent is available in small ampoules as used for muscle soreness. For use in large quantities, bulk powder has some advantage but is of low solubility and requires several minutes to mix. The dose suggested is 10 mg/kg. This drug has appeared to be effective in treating several patients and is now available, but its use has been considered questionable in the light of work by Green and associates (1976).

Management of survivors and those suspected of being susceptible. Practical questions pose some of the most difficult problems. At present, the safest type of anesthesia for patients known or suspected to be at risk for malignant hyperthermia is generally believed to be Innovar or a similar combination of narcotic and sedative. Three forms of drugs have been found to induce muscle contrac-

ture and thereby initiate the development of malignant hyperthermia. These are the cholinergic compounds, including succinylcholine, the neutral anesthetics, including halothane, and the caffeine-type drugs, including procaine (Thorpe and Seeman, 1973).

When a patient has recovered from what was believed to be malignant hyperthermia, one is faced with the question of when it would be safe to attempt anesthesia again. Since there is no available data on the subject, it would seem wisest to postpone any elective operation for several weeks and certainly consider abandoning it completely. If the child has appendicitis, however, and operation is mandatory, Innovar and oxygen, with additional small amounts of morphine given as needed, would be chosen by the majority of anesthesiologists, who also would surround the patient with every safety device imaginable.

What then, do you tell the parents and relatives about the restrictions and limitations to be placed on siblings and more remote relatives after a patient has shown convincing signs of malignant hyperthermia? Our practice in several situations of this type has been to advise muscle biopsies on close relatives who are over 12 or 13 years old and to have the procedures performed under local anesthesia, preferably lidocaine. The information that these tests have given has been equivocal, and better methods are urgently needed. Because of the lack of certainty of present diagnostic methods, small children have not been made to undergo such tests. It is recommended that a letter stating the danger and suggesting that Innovar be used in case of emergency be carried by each child or a guardian.

RESPIRATORY COMPLICATIONS

Critical respiratory complications occur less frequently than in the days of use of ether and spontaneous respiration, but they are still among the most common and most lethal. The origin of these complications varies considerably but basically involves *depression, obstruction, or insufficient oxygen supply*, alone or in any combination. These may occur before, during, or after operation. Regardless of their type or timing, their management consists first of their *prevention,* which is suggested in preceding chapters, while their treatment should consist of three essential steps of *clearing the airway, promoting ventilation, and increasing the oxygen supply* (Smith, 1977).

Respiratory depression

A child's ventilation may be depressed before operation because of illness or preoperative sedation, the latter due either to excessive dosage or to individual hypersensitivity. This should be recognized promptly and the causes assessed. Unless there is question of previously unsuspected central nervous system lesion or other defect, one may proceed with the intended operation using assisted or controlled ventilation and taking added care to see that adequate exchange is present at termination of the procedure.

Depression of respiration during anesthesia usually is intended under current technics and is not considered a complication. Using proper monitoring methods, one should never fail to recognize the presence of respiratory depression, whether induced or pathologic.

Respiratory depression following anesthesia may be caused by failure to eliminate inhalation agents, inadequate reversal of muscle relaxants, functional lesions, pathophysiologic causes, or combinations thereof. Barbiturates characteristically cause slight pupillary constriction and depression of both tidal volume and rate of respiration. Narcotic overdosage shows more marked pupillary constriction and slow rate of respiration with full tidal exchange. Inadequate reversal of muscle relaxants is easily diagnosed by means of a nerve stimulator.

If relaxants have been used, apnea or hypoventilation may be prolonged. Nondepolarizing agents should be reversed with neostigmine (Prostigmin) or glycopyrrolate. Apnea following succinylcholine is more difficult to overcome and usually requires ventilatory assistance and investigation, as described in Chapter 13. After spontaneous respiration begins to return, one must not expect the patient to breathe unassisted until full respiratory function has returned.

Hiccoughs

Hiccoughs most frequently occur during induction of anesthesia, when they often are a side effect of intravenous hexobarbital and somewhat less frequently of other intravenous barbiturates. Hiccoughs may also occur at any time during an anesthetic unless totally controlled ventilation is being used. In addition to being a nuisance to the surgeon, this irregular, spasmodic ventilation may easily lead to hypoxia and hypercarbia. One's first responsibility is to make sure that ventilatory exchange is provided and then attempt to find and correct the cause. Irritation of the diaphragm by gastric overdistension is an initial consideration, and gas or other material is removed by means of nasogastric suction. The attainment of full surgical plane of anesthesia frequently ends the hiccoughs. Otherwise, one may rely on use of a muscle relaxant to control the situation. Unless adequate passive ventilation is carried on during the apneic phase, the hiccoughs may return when the relaxant wears off. Several maneuvers have been used with occasional success, including massage of the carotid sinus, eyeball pressure, and irritation of the nasal mucosa either by insertion of an atraumatic instrument or by induction of sneezing in patients who are awake. For this, snuff or a small bit of pepper works nicely. Methylphenidate has been recommended by Gregory and Way (1969) and hyperinflation of the lungs by Baraka (1969), but during anesthesia, prompt control by means of a muscle relaxant usually is advisable.

Airway obstruction

The causes of airway obstruction are many and varied and may be divided into nonpathologic and pathologic types.

Obstruction by tongue. Although infants are supposed to be nose breathers, ventilation usually is considerably improved by introduction of an oral airway as soon as anesthesia has been induced. When a neonate's mouth is opened, the tongue almost always will be found pressed against the roof of the mouth, entirely blocking any oral exchange. The relatively large tongue of the older infant and child does not cleave to the hard palate in the same way but falls back and obstructs the pharynx during induction and at any time during anesthesia unless the patient is intubated. It is possible to prevent much of this by having the child's head in the "sniffing" position before induction is started. The custom of waiting until the child is half asleep and then abruptly repositioning the head may initiate the trouble that one is trying to prevent. When thiopental is used for induction, the greater incidence of airway spasm makes preliminary head positioning particularly important. Enlarged tonsils and adenoids are equally troublesome.

During induction and maintenance of nonintubated patients, the angle of the chin must be supported to bring the mandible forward. If obstruction occurs early in induction, turning the child's head to one side may suffice until anesthesia is deep enough to allow introduction of an oral airway. Fortunately, young patients appear to tolerate introduction of oral airways during lighter planes of anesthesia than adults.

Excessive secretions. Although respiratory exchange may be obstructed by secretions at any time, this is most likely to occur during induction of anesthesia. Suction apparatus must always be available, but if the secretions appear early in the course of induction, the use of suction will stimulate the child and cause him to awaken. It may be preferable here also to turn the child's head to the side, allowing tongue and secretions to fall forward into the child's cheek until induction has progressed far enough to allow secretions to be removed.

After suction has been used in the pharynx, there still may be sounds of moist airway obstruction. Usually, if a laryngoscope is used to expose the larynx, a few drops of secretions will be seen in the glottis and may easily be removed. Occasionally it is necessary to pass the catheter down into the trachea to clear secretions from the trachea and bronchi.

If the secretions are copious, atropine or scopolamine may be repeated using a slightly reduced dose by intravenous route. It was once believed that such drying agents should not be given if secretions already were present for fear of reducing the secretions to sticky plugs. In our experience this has occurred only in patients with cystic fibrosis.

Glottic obstruction. As induction progresses, one very often notices retraction of the suprasternal or sternal area on inspiration, denoting early glottic obstruction. To correct this, or preferably to prevent it, one should maintain a constant pressure on the breathing bag throughout the entire respiratory cycle. Once allowed to start, obstruction may be extremely difficult to control. While not apt to be of the severity of postanesthetic spasm, infants can develop severe hypoxia with permanent brain injury in such situations.

Stridor. Respiratory stridor, or crowing, may occur before, during, or after operation, with quite different significance. Preoperative stridor suggests inflammation or pathologic process such as paralysis or tumor of the vocal cords (Bennett and others, 1969). During operation, stridor suggests light anesthesia and vagal stimulation, while postoperative stridor suggests irritation due to tracheal intubation, upper respiratory tract infection, or nerve injury. Definitive diagnosis and treatment are indicated. Stridor occurring during anesthesia is controlled by removal of stimulation, deeper anesthesia, or tracheal intubation. Postoperative stridor may call for treatment with oxygen, mist, dexamethasone, and inhalation of racemic epinephrine, as described below with other complications of intubation.

Aspiration of gastric contents. Aspiration of gastric secretions may cause irritation of the trachea and bronchi because of their acidity, while aspiration of large amounts or pieces of food may cause hypoxia and death. These problems are discussed in Chapter 21.

Postoperative atelectasis. Small infants, especially those who have had intrathoracic procedures for tracheoesophageal fistula, diaphragmatic hernia, or cardiac surgery, have an increased incidence of lobar or total lung atelectasis. Positioning them with the collapsed lung up and giving chest therapy every hour may be enough to clear the collapse. However, exposing the glottis, passing an endotracheal catheter, and alternately suctioning and expanding the lung may be more effective. In so doing, one should be sure that the infant's stomach is empty and that atropine has been given (0.02 mg/kg) to prevent vagal sensitivity. Instillation of 1.5 to 2.0 ml of saline solution prior to suction may help to loosen thickened secretions or aspirated milk curds.

COMPLICATIONS OF ENDOTRACHEAL INTUBATION

A full chapter could be devoted to the discussion of complications of endotracheal intubation alone. It seems apparent that the airway is the most critical single feature in pediatric anesthesia, that it remains of moment-to-moment importance throughout the entire course of anesthesia and recovery, and that the endotracheal tube, which serves as the essential means of maintaining the airway, has caused an astonishing variety of complications previously unknown.

Reports of complications relating to endotracheal intubation have appeared in the anesthesia literature less frequently as technics have improved. In general medical journals, however, and more particularly in those of otolaryngologists, pediatricians, neonatologists, and pathologists, reports of trauma, gross errors, and widespread pathology are rampant and place the endotracheal tube in the role of one of the major threats of modern medicine. The reasons for the difference and the true nature of the situation are brought into slightly better focus by examination of some of the facts.

The number and variety of complications related to endotracheal intubation certainly are impressive. The sites at which they may occur start with the external surface of the face, which may suffer from irritation or actual laceration related to fixation of the tube, and then, progressing down the airway, include ulceration and scarring of the nares, obstruction of the nostril, tearing of the nasal mucosa, and penetration of the posterior pharyngeal mucosa, with continued mishaps extending well beyond the carina (see list below). Several varieties of complication may occur in addition to simple trauma, including hypoxic pathology of different degrees resulting from problems of intubation or extubation, the hazards of misplaced, kinked, or obstructed tubes, and problems of postoperative irritation from various causes that will be discussed below.

COMPLICATIONS OF ENDOTRACHEAL INTUBATION

Traumatic

Irritation and laceration of surface of the face
Ulceration and scarring of nares (Hyman and Pederson, 1969; Jung and Thomas, 1974; Baxter and others, 1975)
Laceration, perforation, and hemorrhage of nasal septum, turbinates, mucosa of pharynx, glottis, or trachea (Hyman and Pederson, 1969; Blanc and Tremblay, 1974; Serlin and Daily, 1975)
Perforation of hard palate with formation of cleft (Duke and others, 1976)
Damage, displacement, and aspiration of teeth, disturbance of dental development (Boice and others, 1976)
Ulceration and granuloma formation of vocal cords
Sloughing of hyoid bone
Postoperative laryngotracheitis (Striker and others, 1967; Stetson, 1970)
Dislocation of jaw
Dislocation of cervical vertebrae with damage to spine
Sloughing of vocal cords, tracheal mucosa, epiglottis (Joshi and others, 1972)
Histologic trauma (Farmati and others, 1967; Rasche and Kuhns, 1972)

Hypoxic

Induced apnea followed by difficult intubation
Spasm of vocal cords on intubation or extubation
Excessive suctioning (Boutros, 1970)
Obstruction of endotracheal tube (Stoelting and Procter, 1968; Karis, 1973)
  Adenoidal or other tissue, blood
  Kinked tube
  Defective cuff occluding trachea below tube
  External compression by cuff (Jacobson, 1969; Patel and others, 1978)
  Defective tube made with lumen occluded
Intragastric or endobronchial intubation

Postoperative
  Stridor, hoarseness, sore throat (Koka and others, 1977)
  Acute airway obstruction, with reintubation or tracheostomy
  Laryngotracheitis (Jordan and others, 1970; Adair and others, 1971; Westley and others, 1978)
  Subglottic stenosis (Hatch, 1968; Fishman, 1969; Steward, 1970; Holinger and others, 1976)

Other
  Accidental extubation, recognized
  Accidental extubation, unrecognized
  Separation of tube and adapter with aspiration or swallowing of tube (Tahir, 1972; Flynn and Lowe, 1973; Mitchell and others, 1978)
  Gastric distension
  Pneumothorax
  Atelectasis

Upon first inspecting the array of complications shown above, anesthesiologists might cry out in disbelief, immediately assuming that they are being charged with all the gross errors and acts of violence listed. While the findings undoubtedly are reported with reasonable accuracy, anesthesiologists probably are less guilty than such data would suggest.

Anesthesia journals carry fewer reports of intubation errors not because of anesthesiologists' fear of self-incrimination, but because there are many reasons why they seldom make the more traumatic mistakes. Intubation of the trachea, which we practice daily and continually study, is the most important maneuver in our profession. Not only do we have the advantage of having ample equipment available, but most of our patients are reasonably healthy, with effective blood pressure, and at the time of intubation are well oxygenated and fully relaxed. It is also to our great advantage that our patients seldom remain intubated for prolonged periods.

Anesthesiologists are no longer the only group to perform tracheal intubation. Neonatologists and pediatricians now practice the art, but under definite disadvantages. Neither group has the opportunity to spend adequate time in learning the technic nor to use it frequently. Neonatologists also have to deal with the worst possible patients—sick premature infants who must be intubated while awake and then maintained for prolonged periods with ventilatory support—

while pediatricians, with even fewer opportunities, face only emergencies where anoxic children must be intubated and resuscitated under all sorts of inadequate conditions. If an endotracheal tube enters the esophagus instead of the trachea or if teeth are dislodged at such times, it is hardly surprising.

The reports of airway damage found by otolaryngologists must be read with some concern, for they undoubtedly come across many subclinical lesions that anesthesiologists do not recognize. The mild subglottic stricture or the glottic web that is found several months after operation by a consultant laryngologist may well be caused by mild trauma or use of a slightly oversized tracheal tube. Again, anesthesiologists no longer need assume that they are responsible for all the lesions reported by the laryngologist.

One more point of reassurance for the concerned anesthesiologist deals with the reported findings of pathologists. It is striking to learn that deep ulceration and necrosis of glottis and trachea are found in 60% to 70% of autopsied patients who had been intubated for 48 to 72 hours! This is at odds with the incidence of sick patients who recover after days and weeks of intubation without any appreciable airway damage. It seems highly probable that the ulceration and necrosis have little to do with the technic of intubation but occur in the last few hours before death, when failing circulation can no longer supply the areas on which the endotracheal tube presses, even quite lightly.

Now that the anesthesiologist has been exonerated of many of the more gross misdeeds, there are several areas that still deserve attention. Advances have been made in reducing trauma by development of better technic, more suitable equipment, and provision of adequate relaxation—in other words, by carrying out all the details discussed in Chapter 8. Figures are not available to show how often children are allowed to become mildly or severely hypoxic at intubation, either because of a delay in the procedure or because of occlusive spasm. Numerous errors are made, including endobronchial intubation, laceration of the mucosal lining of the pharynx, accidental extubation, and other mistakes that may or may not lead to more serious problems.

During the surgeon's preparation of the child for operation, changing the position of the head or the whole body always carries the risk of displacing the endotracheal tube, and throughout maintenance of anesthesia there is continual danger because of the delicate structure of the tube and the forces that may be applied to it.

After years of insistence on use of a tube with maximum allowable lumen, it has been shown that the most important way to avoid postoperative tracheitis is to use a tube that is not airtight (Fig. 26-3) but allows a slight leak (Conn, 1977; Koka and others, 1977). For further protection, placing children in mist tents with 50% oxygen and administering dexamethasone (0.1 mg/kg), followed, if necessary, by inhalation of racemic epinephrine (Adair and others, 1971), should keep the incidence of tracheitis to a minimum. The incidence at our hospital has been 1.0% of 7685 intubated children (Koka and others, 1977).

The presence of an endotracheal tube does not exclude the possibility of airway obstruc-tion. The tube may become kinked, may be filled with secretions or blood, or may have been obstructed before insertion because of faulty construction or the presence of foreign bodies or dried secretions in previously used tubes. Either bronchus may be occluded if the tube is passed beyond the carina, or the tube itself may be obstructed by an overin-flated cuff.

If it is difficult to inflate the patient's chest and the endotracheal tube appears to be pa-tent and properly placed, bronchospasm may be present, and one may try atropine or aminophylline for relief. Bronchospasm is rare, however, and one usually does better to remove the tube in such cases, for a kink or improper insertion is more apt to be the problem.

Glottic spasm after tracheal extubation and after operations about the head and neck has been one of our most frequent complications. Although halothane is recognized as the least irritant anesthetic for induction, it is associated with postanesthetic glottic spasm more than most of the other agents. To prevent this dangerous complication, some believe that extubation during deep anesthesia is essential, while others favor extubation in a

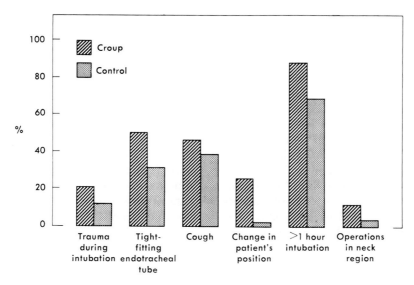

Fig. 26-3. Traumatic factors in the development of postintubation croup. (From Koka, B. V., Jecn, I. S., Andre, J. M., and others: Anesth. Analg. [Cleve.] **56**:501, 1977.)

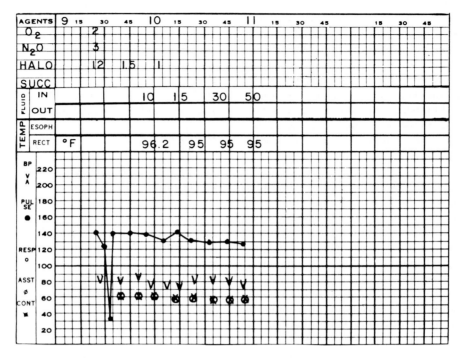

Fig. 26-4. Anesthesia chart showing severe bradycardia following intravenous administration of suc-cinylcholine to an infant receiving halothane without atropine protection.

Arrhythmias

Smith and Wiley (1957), Gold and Smith (1957), and Soule and Mazuzan (1969) studied ECG findings in pediatric patients during cardiac procedures, tonsillectomy, and general surgery. More commonly seen arrhythmias included atrioventricular nodal rhythms, premature ventricular contractions, bigeminy or coupling, ST deviation, and wandering pacemaker.

There has been an increasing tendency to use lidocaine or propranolol for immediate control or intraoperative arrhythmias or to change the anesthetic agent. Since drugs used for treatment of cardiac arrhythmias usually produce appreciable myocardial depression and changing agents in the middle of an operation may be upsetting, we prefer to start with other approaches. As noted by

Morrow and Logic (1969) in relation to adults, few of the arrhythmias seen during anesthesia have great significance. This appears to be equally true in the pediatric age group, and we feel that an arrhythmia that causes neither bradycardia nor hypotension calls for conservative methods rather than premature pharmacologic depression.

Our first response is to hyperventilate the child to make sure that there is neither hypoxia nor hypercarbia. At the same time, we ask the surgeon to refrain from manipulating any sensitive areas, and if these steps are not effective, a bolus of 0.2 to 0.4 mg of atropine is given intravenously. These measures have been successful in a great majority of situations. If arrhythmias persist and blood pressure remains stable, it often is permissible to proceed without further change for 10 to

15 minutes. If there is continuing arrhythmia of a disturbing nature, our next step would be to discontinue all halogenated agents and change to balanced technic. Our last choice would be the intravenous administration of lidocaine, 0.5 to 1.0 mg/kg, or propranolol, 0.03 to 0.06 mg/kg, or the supportive use of isoproterenol and/or digitalis, depending on analysis of the situation.

The current rather free use of lidocaine has given some evidence of its effectiveness. Our hesitance is based in part on views of local pediatric cardiologists, supported by knowledge of the death of a healthy 2-year-old following successive doses of lidocaine and propranolol for treatment of simple tachycardia during herniorrhaphy.

Unexpected cardiac asystole (cardiovascular collapse, cardiac arrest)

Prior to 1950, hearts that ceased to beat during operation rarely ever beat again, and most of these incidents were recorded as anesthetic deaths. With slightly improved methods of resuscitation, some patients were restored to life, and the term "cardiac arrest" was used to describe the incident. It was a convenient term, for it implied no reason for the incident, and instead of pointing to the error that usually caused the complication, it gave the impression of being an act of God, an intensely interesting experience, and definitely a status symbol for the person who gave the anesthesia.

As early as 1955, Jacoby and associates deplored the use of the term, which by that time had come into general use. Unfortunately, a more accurate one has yet to be found to represent a situation where a patient's heart, from any one of several possible causes, ceases to beat and subsequently may or may not resume action. Between 1950 and 1975, numerous articles described groups of patients who suffered "cardiac arrest" from such a wide diversity of causes that one gains little more than a feeling of relief that most of the gross errors described are behind us. Failure to reverse muscle relaxants, "crash" intubation of infants with gastric distension, errors in fluid therapy, and administration of succinylcholine to traumatized children were among the complications reported by Snyder and associates (1953), Rackow and associates (1961), Greenberg (1965), and Salem and associates (1975). Estimates of the frequency of cardiac arrest in such reports are of interest, but it is doubtful that they should stand as representative figures because of the dissimilarity of the underlying etiology and attendant situations. It does seem probable that unexpected cardiac asystole occurs more frequently during the course of pediatric anesthesia than during adult anesthesia and that the reason for this is related both to greater susceptibility of younger patients and to less skilled management. Fortunately, children appear to have far greater recuperative power, and the incidence of recovery is relatively high.

Anesthesiologist's role in treatment of cardiac asystole. The excitement that immediately follows recognition of cardiac asystole may cause utter confusion unless surgeon and anesthesiologist act according to an organized, predetermined plan (Singer, 1977; Schoonmaker, 1978).

Upon failure to obtain the pulse or heart beat, the anesthesiologist can make several important moves *within a very few seconds*. He looks at the clock to be able to measure duration of arrest, flushes out the anesthetic, ventilates the child with oxygen repeatedly, again checks the heart by carotid pulse, auscultation, and ECG, and calls for a check of blood measurements and for rapid infusion, if indicated. In the meantime, the surgeons have stopped operating, removed all large instruments, and returned all displaced viscera to their proper locations, and all members of the team attempt to find the cause of the asystole. The most common factors have been hypoxia, hyperactive vagal responses, blood loss, airway obstruction, overdosage, and overinfusion.

If an endotracheal tube is in place when asystole occurs, the patient is ventilated immediately with 100% oxygen. If the patient is not intubated, it is still preferable to oxygenate first by mask and then intubate, thus avoiding additional seconds of hypoxia in the process of intubation.

The execution of both ventilation and cardiac compression is of critical importance, for each must be adequate but not excessive. Inadequate ventilation obviously will not provide sufficient oxygen, while overzealous expansion of the chest will retard venous return, which is seriously reduced in most situations of this nature. One should not have the surgeon interrupt cardiac compression to allow for ventilation, as once believed, for it is essential for him to provide continuous support of the circulation. Ventilation should be delivered in quick, effective bursts, monitored by precordial stethoscope or direct visualization of the open chest, at rates of 40 to 80 per minute in smaller patients, with complete bag relaxation between breaths.

Because of hurried tracheal intubation in such emergencies, whether in the operating room or elsewhere, incorrect placement of the endotracheal tube (endobronchial or esophageal) or use of too small a tube with excessive leak may produce inadequate expansion and prevent resuscitation. Both sides of the chest should be auscultated, and *both sides of the upper rib cage should be seen to expand on inflation of the chest if the tracheal tube is correctly placed and ventilation is effective.*

The surgeon also follows a planned approach. If working in the chest, he observes the action of the heart and can tell at once whether it is beating weakly, fibrillating, or still. Ventricular fibrillation is unusual in such cases among infants and children. In any of these situations, direct manual compression is applied at once, with quick, effective force and at a rate of 160 to 180 per minute in small infants or 120 to 140 per minute in older children. As with ventilation, full relaxation should be allowed between each cardiac compression to allow cardiac refill. As previously noted, massage should not be interrupted for ventilation.

Adequacy of compression may be estimated by palpation of a peripheral pulse. ECG observation is useful to see if there is any spontaneous nervous impulse but gives no measure of its effect. A normal tracing may be seen when cardiac output is completely ineffective. The return of pupils to normal size is an indication that cerebral circulation has been restored, but continued presence of dilated pupils may be caused by either hypoxia or the effect of atropine and/or epinephrine. Blood pressure should be measured by direct or indirect method as soon as cardiac action returns.

If the disaster occurs during an abdominal procedure, the surgeon can perform slightly less effective cardiac massage without opening the diaphragm but should open the diaphragm if the heart does not respond promptly. Compression of the abdominal aorta is a useful maneuver at this time, increasing the distribution of blood to essential organs.

External cardiac massage is used when neither chest nor abdomen is open. In small infants, pressure is applied at midsternum rather than at the lower third, as in adults. If the infant is on a firm table or bed, adequate effect may be gained by pressing on the sternum with three fingers, but this will be unsatisfactory if the chest is not supported. It is more effective to grasp the child's chest in the hands, with thumbs at midsternum, and compress the chest to slightly more than half its normal anteroposterior depth (Fig. 26-5, A).

Several deaths have occurred because of compression and rupture of the liver and stomach during this technic of massage. This danger may be averted by reversing one's position so that the hands encircle the chest rather than the abdomen (Fig. 26-5, B). In order to increase the venous return in larger patients, it is advisable to elevate the child's legs on a pillow or rolled-up sheets. If cardiac action does not return at once, further diagnostic and therapeutic action is indicated. Medications for cardiac resuscitation are shown in Table 26-3.

Direct intracardiac injection of calcium and epinephrine has been used for resuscitation of patients during asystole, but needling the chest at the nipple line easily punctures the lung, especially during attempted hyper-

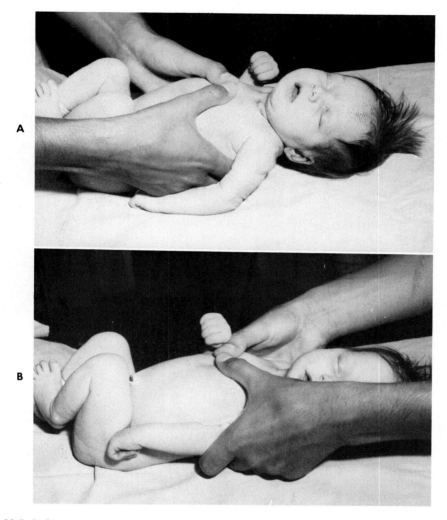

Fig. 26-5. A, Closed chest massage. Thumbs are properly placed at midsternum, but hands may compress and rupture descending liver and stomach. **B,** Preferred method of producing the same cardiac compression but allowing free descent of diaphragm.

Table 26-3. Medications for cardiac resuscitation

Drug	Concentration	Dose	Route	Interval
Atropine	0.04 mg/ml	Neonate 0.15 mg Infant 0.2 mg Child 0.4 mg	IV or IM	20 min, or as needed
Calcium chloride and calcium gluconate	10%, 1000 mg in 10-ml ampoule	20 mg/kg (chloride), 60 mg/kg (gluconate)	IV or IC	10 min, or as indicated by serum Ca^{++}
Epinephrine	1 ml 1:1000	Dilute to 10 ml and give 0.1 ml/kg	IV or IC	5-10 min
Isoproterenol (Isuprel)	0.2 mg/ml 1:5000	1 mg in 250 ml 5% D/W = 4 μg/ml Give 0.1-0.5 μg/kg/min (titrate for effect)	IV	Constant

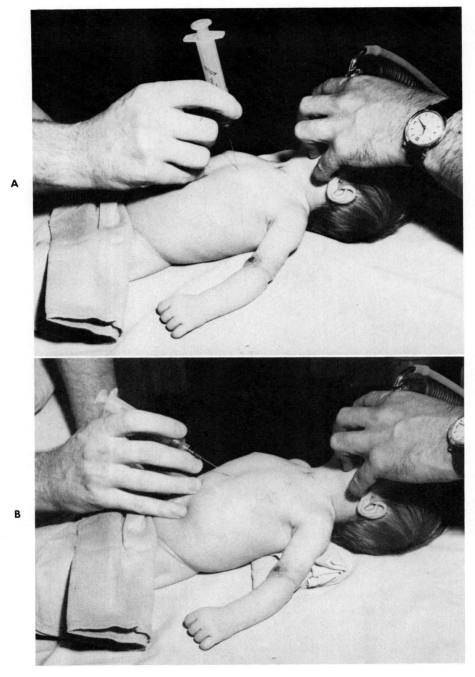

Fig. 26-6. A, Intracardiac injection via the intercostal space may injure the lung. **B,** Substernal route provides greater safety.

ventilation. If the anesthesiologist does not inflate the lung at this time, the danger is reduced. However, the substernal approach avoids this hazard entirely (Fig. 26-6).

If a freely running infusion is available and effective cardiac massage is being carried out, administering drugs by intravenous route would seem a reasonable, and probably a better, method.

The first drug given may be atropine, in a full-strength dose of 0.2 to 0.6 mg in order to remove any vagal component. Calcium and epinephrine are valuable inotropic agents that should be available for immediate use. Both calcium chloride and calcium gluconate are effective. The chloride, being more potent, is favored for treatment of asystole (20 mg/kg). The gluconate should produce comparable results in slightly greater dosage (60 mg/kg). Because it causes less vascular irritation than the chloride, it is preferable for prophylactic use.

The effect of calcium and other drugs should be observed on the ECG. If possible, the serum ionized calcium is measured before administration is repeated. Normal concentration of ionized calcium is 2.5 to 4.0 mEq/L.

The use of epinephrine is no longer universal but still is popular. Intracardiac or intravenous injection of 0.1 ml of 1:10,000 solution per kg is a reasonable amount to try. Infants and children tolerate epinephrine extremely well, and acidotic subjects require considerably higher doses than normal patients.

If the heart is severely depressed for more than 2 to 3 minutes, correction of metabolic acidosis will be in order. For this, sodium bicarbonate is customarily advised in initial dosage of 3 mEq/L. Because of the hyperosmolality of sodium bicarbonate (2000 mOsm/L), this drug should not be given repeatedly without knowledge of the patient's approximate serum osmolality. We consider a concentration of 325 mEq/L to be a questionable contraindication and a concentration of 350 mEq/L or over a definite contraindication to sodium bicarbonate.

In addition to treatment of hypovolemia and myocardial depression, it is important to think of hypoglycemia and hypothermia during such catastrophes. Intravenous solutions should be warmed, and the child should be either covered or warmed by a portable heating lamp during attempts at resuscitation. Defibrillation and cardiac pacing may be required in cases that are unresponsive, and supported infusion of isoproterenol and/or dopamine has become of primary value (Tables 26-4 and 26-5).

HEPATORENAL COMPLICATIONS
Halothane hepatitis: result of survey

The subject of hepatitis following halothane anesthesia was discussed at length in Chapter 5, but details of a survey referred to were withheld for listing among other anesthetic complications in this chapter.

In an attempt to validate the concept that children rarely develop halothane hepatitis, a search was made of American and European literature of the past 15 years to find documented cases and a questionnaire was addressed to major centers throughout North America to find suspected cases that had not been reported. Because of the impossibility of sorting out the numerous complicating features in patients who survived varying degrees of postoperative liver involvement, only patients who died of what appeared to be a liver death were taken into consideration. It was estimated that the survey involved approximately 1.5 million halothane anesthetics administered to patients between birth and 20 years of age.

In our survey of the literature, we found only two reports of deaths related to halothane hepatitis in children under 10 years of age and five more in patients from 10 to 20 years of age. The questionnaire revealed four more under 10 years and three more between 10 to 20 years, giving totals of six children under 10 and eight children between 10 and 20 years of age.

The information on most of these patients is incomplete, but there is enough to show that there were many complicating factors, making a clear case against halothane impossible in nearly all instances. The principal

609

Table 26-4. Dopamine dosage chart

Infusion rate (ml/hr)	Dose* (μg/min)—concentration						
	0.5 mg/ml	1.0 mg/ml	2.0 mg/ml	3.0 mg/ml	4.0 mg/ml	5.0 mg/ml	6.0 mg/ml
0.93	7.7	15.5	31.0	46.5	62.0	77.5	93.0
1.3	10.8	21.1	43.3	65.0	86.7	108.0	130.0
1.8	15.0	30.0	60.0	90.0	120.0	150.0	180.0
2.5	20.8	41.7	83.3	125.0	167.0	208.0	250.0
3.6	30.0	60.0	120.0	180.0	240.0	300.0	360.0
5.0	41.7	83.3	167.0	250.0	333.0	417.0	500.0
7.0	58.3	117.0	233.0	350.0	467.0	583.0	700.0
9.8	81.7	163.0	327.0	490.0	653.0	817.0	980.0
14.0	117.0	233.0	467.0	700.0	933.0	1167.0	1400.0
19.0	158.0	317.0	633.0	950.0	1267.0	1583.0	1900.0
27.0	225.0	450.0	900.0	1350.0	1800.0	2250.0	2700.0

Concentration desired (mg/ml)	Dopamine (ml)	D_5W (ml)	Total volume (ml)
0.5	0.5	39.5	
1.0	1.0	39.0	
2.0	2.0	38.0	40
3.0	3.0	37.0	
4.0	4.0	36.0	
5.0	5.0	35.0	

*Usual effective dose, 4 to 20 μg/kg/min.

Table 26-5. Isoproterenol (Isuprel) dosage chart

Infusion rate (ml/hr)	Dose (μg/min)—concentration				
	0.25 mg/dl	0.5 mg/dl	1.0 mg/dl	2.0 mg/dl	4.0 mg/dl
0.93	0.04	0.08	0.15	0.31	0.62
1.3	0.05	0.11	0.22	0.43	0.87
1.8	0.07	0.15	0.30	0.60	1.2
2.5	0.10	0.21	0.42	0.83	1.7
3.6	0.15	0.30	0.60	1.2	2.4
5.0	0.21	0.42	0.83	1.7	3.3
7.0	0.29	0.58	1.2	2.3	4.7
9.8	0.41	0.82	1.6	3.3	6.5
14.0	0.58	1.2	2.3	4.7	9.3
19.0	0.79	1.6	3.2	6.3	12.7
27.0	1.1	2.2	4.5	9.0	18.0

features of each case are summarized below.

Deaths in which halothane was the principal suspect

1. An 8-year-old boy with diagnosis of primary hepatoma underwent liver biopsy and 5 days later showed acute fulminating hepatic failure. Liver enzymes elevated, preoperative bilirubin 3.5. Death in 5 days. (Unreported case of W. S. Jordan.)

2. A 12-year-old boy had biopsy of mass on right arm and excision of mass 2 days later, both operations under halothane. Vomiting and delirium 72 hours later, death shortly afterward. (Unreported case of J. K. Rosales.)

3. An 11-year-old girl was operated on three times in 6 weeks for osteolytic lesions of femur and pelvis. All three operations under very stable halothane anesthesia lasting 4, 2, and 4 hours. Temperature rose to 103° F 7 hours after last operation, and child developed jaundice, tender liver, and coma. She had six exchange transfusions but went on to have massive bleeding that became uncontrollable and ended in death 20 days after the last operation. (Included in review of Carney and Van Dyke, 1972.)

4. A 12-year-old boy treated for hematuria had pyelogram and dorsal slit on first exposure to halothane, pyeloplasty 2 days later, and prolonged retropelvic procedure for high undescended testis 6 weeks after that. Three days after last operation, all under halothane, he developed progressive picture of acute hepatic failure ending in coma and death. (Unreported case of H. Rackow.)

5. A 16-year-old girl who fell through a glass door and sustained a deep laceration of right wrist required a 4-hour operation (under halothane) to repair eight tendons and median nerve. On ninth postoperative day, she developed nausea, vomiting, fever, and lethargy; no mass or jaundice, but died 14 days after operation. Autopsy showed acute massive necrosis of liver and severe nephrosis. (Reported, Case 98, National Halothane Study, Bunker, 1969.)

Deaths following halothane in patients who had preexisting diseases

6. A 9-year-old boy who was believed to have Rendu-Osler-Weber disease, or hereditary hemorrhagic telangiectasia, because of recurrent nosebleeds, underwent halothane anesthesia for dental restorative surgery. During the next 8 days he travelled from Milwaukee to New Mexico and back, and his mother developed flulike symptoms on the trip. On the eighth day the child developed fever and vomiting, became delirious, later incoherent and comatose. Other signs included enlarged liver, elevated SGOT, SGPT, LDH, and blood ammonia (67 μg/dl). On the fifteenth postoperative day he developed seizures and shock and could not be resuscitated. (Unreported case of F. Vladny.)

7. A 13-year-old girl had repair of atrial septal defect under total cardiopulmonary bypass and hypothermia. Heart fibrillated during most of the repair. On the first postoperative day she was transiently hypotensive to 60/40. On the second day she started to have convulsions originating in the left upper extremity. After 1.5 hours of this,

she had cardiac arrest from which she could not be resuscitated. Details of urine volume are not clear. She was never jaundiced. She died 2 days after surgery. Necropsy findings: interatrial septal defect, repaired; pulmonary edema; hemorrhagic centrilobular necrosis of the liver; acute tubular necrosis of the kidneys. (Reported, Case 609, National Halothane Study, Bunker, 1969.)

8. A 14-year-old black male with early onset juvenile rheumatic arthritis underwent a 6-hour halothane anesthesia for release of a 6-mm mandibular opening. The first abnormal signs were chills and temperature of 102° F on second postoperative day, followed by return to normal, and patient was discharged on seventh day. On ninth day the temperature rose to 103° F, and 2 days later the child had anorexia, jaundice, and ankylosis of joints of hands, wrists, left knee and hip, several ribs, and cervical vertebrae. The liver and spleen became enlarged and tender. Laboratory values included SGOT 2699, SGPT 4045, and markedly prolonged PT and PTT. There were seizures followed by cardiac arrest and death, which occurred on the thirteenth day after operation. (Case published by Campbell and associates, 1977. The article contains an interesting discussion of the hepatitis seen with juvenile arthritis, with and without aspirin therapy [Schaller and others, 1970; Rich and Johnson, 1973].)

9. A 16-year-old boy with Fanconi syndrome underwent five halothane anesthetics for orthopedic procedures. Low-grade fever and jaundice with abdominal pain and tenderness followed the third operation, and fever without other signs followed the fourth. Five days after the fifth operation, a tibial osteotomy, the patient again developed fever, abdominal pain and tenderness, jaundice, and elevation of bilirubin and enzymes, and subsequently coma and death occurred 1 month after surgery. Anesthesiologists believed the patient died from hepatic hypersensitivity following repeated halothane administration. (Unreported case of G. B. Lewis and D. Leigh.)

Deaths following halothane complicated by additional perioperative factors

10. A 5-month-old infant was operated on for pyloric stenosis. The operation was uneventful, and recovery was normal for the first 3 postoperative days. Signs of toxicity progressed from the third day onward, with fever, jaundice, and hepatosplenomegaly. Hemolytic anemia developed, the hemoglobin falling from 19 g/dl on the first postoperative day to 6.8 g/dl on the eighth

postoperative day, on which day the infant died. It was thought that the picture resembled a liver dystrophy rather than halothane toxicity, but it was difficult to be sure. (Case from Germany, reported by Schneider, 1965.)

11. A 9-month-old infant girl who had severe tetralogy of Fallot required a Waterston shunt, two subsequent revisions of the shunt, and multiple anesthetics for dilations secondary to a tracheostomy, most of the procedures having been done under halothane. Her life was complicated also by several episodes of hypoglycemia. Halothane hepatitis was suggested as a possible diagnosis on the basis of total liver destruction found at autopsy. (Unreported case of S. Austin.)

12. A complicated case of an infant born with tracheoesophageal fistula who had multiple operations, the last, at $2^{10}/12$ years, a colonic replacement of the esophagus. The course of the last procedure was entirely uncomplicated. The liver was seen to be normal on inspection and palpation. An hour after operation a pneumothorax developed on the left side but was immediately drained by underwater seal. The child awoke and talked, appearing quite normal until 8 hours after the operation when he became listless, sweaty, and 2 hours later convulsed and died. Postmortem examination showed a pale yellow liver, smaller than normal. Halothane hepatitis, hypoglycemia, and viral hepatitis were considered, without final decision. (Case from Israel, reported by Lernau and others, 1970.)

13. A 2-year-old child whose record could not be located but who was remembered to have undergone multiple abdominal procedures under halothane, died with typical findings of acute hepatic necrosis. (Unreported case of H. L. Zauder.)

14. A small, cyanotic 10-year-old girl had cardiac catheterization at 7 months and was found to have tetralogy of Fallot. Her condition had been deteriorating during the 2 years before her final operation. Operation consisted of repair of ventricular septal defect and plastic enlargement of the right ventricular outflow tract under total cardiopulmonary bypass. The enlargement of the right outflow tract was inadequate. At the end of the operation she remained dependent on a pacemaker because of complete heart block. She remained hypotensive and died on the first postoperative day, never having been jaundiced, but acute massive congestion of the liver was found, with central lobular degeneration. (Reported, Case 657, National Halothane Study, Bunker, 1969.)

A survey of this type is unreliable and tends to put excessive blame on halogen, since a similar investigation of several other drugs, when given in comparable quantities and under similar conditions, might have been associated with as many complications and deaths. From the information gathered, it might be said that infants and children appear to have hepatic necrosis very rarely and that it is possible that underlying diseases and pathologic conditions may reduce the child's resistance to this complication.

BIBLIOGRAPHY

Adair, J. C., Ring, W. H., Jordan, W. S., and others: Ten-year experience with IPPB in the treatment of acute laryngotracheobronchitis, Anesth. Analg. (Cleve.) **50:**649, 1971.

Aldrete, J. A., and Britt, B. A., editors: Second International Symposium on Malignant Hyperthermia, New York, 1978, Grune & Stratton, Inc.

Baraka, A.: Inhibition of hiccups by pulmonary inflation, Anesthesiology **32:**271, 1969.

Baraka, A.: Intravenous lidocaine controls extubation laryngospasm in children, Anesth. Analg. (Cleve.) **57:**506, 1978.

Baxter, R. J., Johnson, J. D., Goetzman, B. W., and Hackel, A.: Cosmetic nasal deformities complicating prolonged nasotracheal intubation in critically ill newborn infants, Pediatrics **55:**884, 1975.

Bennett, E. J., Patel, K. P., and Grundy, E. M.: Neonatal temperature and surgery, Anesthesiology **46:**303, 1977.

Bennett, E. J., Tsuchiya, T., and Stephen, C. R.: Stridor and upper airway obstruction in infants, Anesth. Analg. (Cleve.) **48:**75, 1969.

Bidwai, A. V., and Stanley, T. H.: Intravenous calcium terminates spinal anesthesia induced shivering in obstetric patients, abstracts of scientific papers, annual meeting of American Society of Anesthesiologists, Chicago, 1978, p. 169.

Blanc, V. F., and Tremblay, N. A. G.: The complications of tracheal intubation; a new classification with a review of the literature, Anesth. Analg. (Cleve.) **53:**202, 1974.

Bleyaert, A. L., Nemoto, E. M., Safar, P., and others: Thiopental amelioration of brain damage after global ischaemia in monkeys, Anaesthesia **49:**390, 1978.

Boice, J. B., Krous, H. F., and Foley, J. M.: Gingival and dental complications of orotracheal intubation, J.A.M.A. **236:**957, 1976.

Boutros, A. R.: Arterial blood oxygenation during and after endotracheal suctioning in the apneic patient, Anesthesiology **32:**114, 1970.

Britt, B. A.: Malignant hyperthermia; a pharmacogenetic disease of skeletal and cardiac muscle, editorial, N. Engl. J. Med. **290:**1140, 1974.

Britt, B. A., and Kalow, W.: Malignant hyperthermia; a statistical review, Can. Anaesth. Soc. J. **17:**293, 1970.

Bunker, J. P.: Citric acid intoxication, J.A.M.A. **157:** 1361, 1955.

Bunker, J. P., editor: The national halothane study, Bethesda, Md., 1969, National Institutes of Health.

Campbell, R. L., Small, E. W., Lesesne, H. R., and others: Fatal hepatic necrosis after halothane anesthesia in a patient with juvenile rheumatoid arthritis, Anesth. Analg. (Cleve.) **56:**589, 1977.

Carney, F. M. T., and Van Dyke, R. A.: Halothane hepatitis; a critical review, Anesth. Analg. (Cleve.) **51:**135, 1972.

Carruthers, H. C., and Graves, H. B.: The complications of endotracheal anaesthesia, Can. Anaesth. Soc. J. **3:**244, 1956.

Chidsey, C. A. III: Calcium metabolism in the failing heart, Hosp. Pract. **7:**8, 1972.

Clark, R. E., Orkin, L. R., and Rovenstine, E. A.: Body temperature studies in anesthetized man; effect of environmental temperature, humidity, and anesthesia system, J.A.M.A. **154:**311, 1954.

Conn, A. W.: Personal communication, 1977.

Conn, A. W., Edmonds, J. F., and Barker, G. D.: Near-drowning in cold fresh water; current treatment regimen, Can. Anaesth. Soc. J. **25:**259, 1978.

Cooper, J. B., Newbower, R. S., Long, C. D., and McPeek, B.: Preventable anesthesia mishaps; a study of human factors, Anesthesiology **49:**399, 1978.

Denborough, M. A.: Foreword. In Aldrete, J. A., and Britt, B. A., editors: Second International Symposium on Malignant Hyperthermia, New York, 1978, Grune & Stratton, Inc.

Denborough, M. A., Forster, J. E., Lovell, R. H., and others: Anesthetic deaths in a family, Br. J. Anaesth. **34:**395, 1962.

Duke, P. M. Coulson, J. D., Santos, J. I., and Johnson, J. D.: Cleft palate associated with prolonged orotracheal intubation in infancy, J. Pediatr. **89:**990, 1976.

Eckenhoff, J. E.: Relationship of anesthesia to postoperative personality changes in children, Am. J. Dis. Child. **86:**587, 1953.

Farmati, O., Quinn, J. R., and Fennell, R. H., Jr.: Exfoliative cytology of the intubated larynx in children, Can. Anaesth. Soc. J. **14:**321, 1967.

Fink, B. R.: The etiology and treatment of laryngeal spasm, Anesthesiology **17:**569, 1956.

Fink, B. R.: The human larynx; a functional study, New York, 1975, Raven Press.

Fishman, N. H.: Post-intubation tracheal stenosis, Ann. Thorac. Surg. **8:**47, 1969.

Flynn, A. L., and Lowe, A. R.: Endotracheal tube swallowed by a neonate, Med. J. Aust. **1:**62, 1973.

Folkman, J.: Personal communication, 1978.

Fox, E. J., Sklar, G. S., Hill, C. H., and others: Complications related to the pressor response to endotracheal intubation, Anesthesiology **47:**524, 1977.

Fraser, J. G.: Iatrogenic benign hyperthermia in children, Anesthesiology **48:**375, 1978.

Fraser, J. G., Crumrine, R. S., and Izant, R. J., Jr.:

A preplanned treatment for malignant hyperpyrexia, Anesth. Analg. (Cleve.) **55:**713, 1976.

Gitlow, S. E., Bertani, L. M., Wilk, E., and others: Catecholamine metabolism in familial dysautonomia, Pediatrics **46:**513, 1970.

Gold, S. M., and Smith, R. M.: Repeated cardiac arrhythmia during ether anesthesia, Am. Heart J. **54:** 448, 1957.

Goudsouzian, N. G., Morris, R. H., and Ryan, J. F.: The effects of a warming blanket on the maintenance of body temperatures in anesthetized infants and children, Anesthesiology **39:**351, 1973.

Green, R. A., Heffron, J. J. A., and Mitchell, G.: Effects of potassium, procaine, and dantrolene on the calcium-dependent and "basal" ATPase activities of sarcoplasmic reticulum of skeletal muscle, Gen. Pharmacol. **7:**361, 1976.

Greenberg, H. B.: Cardiac arrest in 20 infants and children; causes and results of resuscitation, Dis. Chest **47:**42, 1965.

Gregory, G. A., and Way, W. L.: Methylphenidate for the treatment of hiccoughs during anesthesia, Anesthesiology **31:**89, 1969.

Hackett, P. R., and Crosby, R. M. N.: Some effects of inadvertent hypothermia in infant neurosurgery, Anesthesiology **21:**356, 1960.

Hägerdal, M., Welsh, F. A., Keykhah, M., and Harp, J. R.: The protective effects of a combination of hypothermia and barbiturates in cerebral hypoxia, Crit. Care Med. **6**(2):110, 1978.

Harrison, G. G.: Control of the malignant hyperpyrexic syndrome in MHS swine by dantrolene sodium, Br. J. Anaesth. **47:**62, 1975.

Harverth, S. M., Spurr, G. B., Hutt, B. K., and Hamilton, L. H.: Metabolic cost of shivering, J. Appl. Physiol. **8:**595, 1956.

Hatch, D. J.: Prolonged nasotracheal intubation in infants and children, Lancet **1:**1272, 1968.

Holinger, P. H., Schild, J. A., Kutnick, S. L., and Holinger, L. D.: Subglottic stenosis in infants and children, Ann. Otol. Rhinol. Laryngol. **85:**591, 1976.

Howland, W. S., and Schweizer, O.: Acid-base lesion of bank blood, Anesthesiology **25:**102, 1964.

Hyman, A. I., and Pederson, H.: Nasopharyngeal stenosis, Anesthesiology **31:**480, 1969.

Jackson, K.: Psychologic preparation as a method of reducing the emotional trauma of anesthesia in children, Anesthesiology **12:**293, 1951.

Jacobson, J.: A hazard of armored endotracheal tubes, Anesth. Analg. (Cleve.) **48:**37, 1969.

Jacoby, J. J., Flory, F. A., Ziegler, C. H., and Hamelberg, W.: Safety in surgery, Anesth. Analg. (Cleve.) **34:**346, 1955.

Jordan, W. S., Graves, C. L., and Elwyn, R. A.: New therapy for postintubation laryngeal edema and tracheitis in children, J.A.M.A. **212:**585, 1970.

Joshi, V. V., Mandavia, S. G., Stern, L., and others: Acute lesions induced by endotracheal intubation, Am. J. Dis. Child. **124:**646, 1972.

Jung, A. L., and Thomas, G. K.: Stricture of the nasal

vestibule; a complication of nasotracheal intubation in newborn infants, J. Pediatr. **85**:412, 1974.

Karis, J. H.: Misadventure during endotracheal anesthesia, J.A.M.A. **226**:676, 1973.

King, J. O., and Denborough, N. A.: Anesthetic-induced malignant hyperpyrexia in children, J. Pediatr. **83**:37, 1973.

Koka, B. V., Jeon, I. S., Andre, J. M., and others: Postintubation croup in children, Anesth. Analg. (Cleve.) **56**:501, 1977.

Korsch, B. M.: The child and the operating room, Anesthesiology **43**:251, 1975.

Kristoffersen, M. B., Battenborg, C. C., and Holaday, D. A.: Asphyxial death; the roles of acute anoxia, hypercarbia and acidosis, Anesthesiology **28**:488, 1967.

Lernau, O. Z., Levy, E., Path, F. R., and others: Early postoperative death of a child after repeated halothane anesthesia, Anesthesiology **32**:467, 1970.

Liem, S. T., and Aldrete, J. A.: Control of post-anaesthetic shivering, Can. Soc. Anaesth. J. **21**:506, 1974.

Marmer, M. J.: Iatrogenesis in anesthesiology, Anesth. Analg. (Cleve.) **48**:612, 1969.

Marshall, M.: Potassium intoxication from blood and plasma transfusions, Anaesthesia **17**:145, 1962.

Marty, A. T., Eraklis, A. J., Pelletier, G. A., and Merrill, E. W.: The rheologic effects of hypothermia on blood with high hematocrit values, J. Thorac. Cardiovasc. Surg. **61**:735, 1971.

McCaughey, T. J.: Hazards of anesthesia for the burned child, Can. Anaesth. Soc. J. **9**:220, 1962.

Michenfelder, J. D., Milde, J., and Sundt, T.: Cerebral protection by barbiturate anesthesia, Arch. Neurol. **33**:345, 1976.

Mitchell, S. A., Shoults, D. L., Herron, A. L., and Benumof, J. L.: Deglutition of an endotracheal tube; case report, Anesth. Analg. (Cleve.) **57**:590, 1978.

Modell, J. H.: Septicemia as a cause of immediate postoperative hyperthermia, Anesthesiology **27**:329, 1966.

Morrow, D. H., and Logic, J. R.: Management of cardiac arrhythmias during anesthesia, Anesth. Analg. (Cleve.) **48**:748, 1969.

Nelson, T. E.: Excitation-contraction coupling; a common etiologic pathway for malignant hyperthermia susceptible muscle. In Aldrete, J. A., and Britt, B. A., editors: Second International Symposium on Malignant Hyperthermia, New York, 1978, Grune & Stratton, Inc.

Owen-Thomas, J. B.: A follow-up of children treated by prolonged nasal intubation, Can. Anaesth. Soc. J. **14**:543, 1967.

Patel, K., Teviotdale, B., and Dalal, F.: Internal herniation of a Murphy endotracheal tube, Anesthesiol. Rev. **5**(4):60, 1978.

Pflug, A. E., Aasheim, G. M., Foster, C., and Martin, R. W.: Prevention of post-anaesthesia shivering, Can. Anaesth. Soc. J. **25**:43, 1978.

Pledger, H. G., and Buchan, R.: Deaths in children with acute appendicitis, Br. Med. J. **4**:466, 1969.

Rackow, H., Salanitre, E., and Green, L. T.: Frequency

of cardiac arrest associated with anesthesia in infants and children, Pediatrics **28**:697, 1961.

Rasche, R. F. H., and Kuhns, L. R.: Histopathologic changes in airway mucosa of infants after endotracheal intubation, Pediatrics **50**:632, 1972.

Rex, M. A. E.: A review of the structural and functional basis of laryngospasm and a discussion of the nerve pathways involved in the reflex and its clinical significance in man and animals, Br. J. Anaesth. **42**:891, 1970.

Rich, R. R., and Johnson, J. S.: Salicylate hepatotoxicity in patients with juvenile rheumatoid arthritis, Arthritis Rheum. **16**:1, 1973.

Roe, C. F.: Temperature regulation and therapy metabolism in surgical patients, Prog. Surg. **12**:96, 1973.

Rosenberg, H.: Malignant hyperthermia; etiology, lecture presented at Annual Convention of American Society of Anesthesiologists, Chicago, 1978.

Ryan, J. F.: Malignant hyperpyrexia; etiology and treatment, lecture presented at Annual Convention of American Society of Anesthesiologists, San Francisco, 1976.

Ryan, J. F.: Malignant hyperthermia; recognition, lecture presented at Annual Convention of American Society of Anesthesiologists, Chicago, 1978.

Ryan, J. F., Conlon, J. V., Malt, R. A., and others: Cardiopulmonary bypass in the treatment of malignant hyperthermia, N. Engl. J. Med. **290**:1121, 1974.

Saidman, L. J., Havard, E. S., Eger, E. I. II: Hyperthermia during anesthesia, J.A.M.A. **190**:73, 1964.

Salem, M. R., Bennett, E. J., Schweiss, J. F., and others: Cardiac arrest related to anesthesia; contributing factors in infants and children, J.A.M.A. **233**:238, 1975.

Schaller, J., Beckwith, B., and Wedgewood, R. J.: Hepatic involvement in juvenile rheumatoid arthritis, J. Pediatr. **77**:203, 1970.

Schneider, I.: Akute Leberdystrophie bei einem Säugling nach Halothan-Narkose, Dtsch. Gesundheitsw. **20**:465, 1965.

Schoonmaker, G. W.: Axioms on cardiac arrest, Hosp. Med. **14**(10):6, 1978.

Schweizer, O., Howland, W. S., Ryan, G., and Goldiner, P. L.: Hyperpyrexia in the operative and immediate postoperative period, Anesth. Analg. (Cleve.) **50**:906, 1971.

Serlin, S. P., and Daily, W. J. R.: Tracheal preformation in the neonate, J. Pediatr. **86**:596, 1975.

Singer, J. J.: Cardiac arrests in children, J. Am. Coll. Emer. Phys. **6**(5): 198, 1977.

Smith, R. M.: Complications of anesthesia in pediatrics, Anesth. Analg. (Cleve.) **27**:227, 1948.

Smith, R. M.: Some reasons for the high mortality in pediatric anesthesia, N.Y. State J. Med. **56**:2212, 1956.

Smith, R. M.: The management of airway emergencies. In Green, M., and Haggerty, R. J., editors: Ambulatory pediatrics, Philadelphia, 1968, W. B. Saunders Co.

Smith, R. M.: Thermic emergencies in anesthesia, Hosp. Pract. 3:68, 1968a.

Smith, R. M.: Temperature monitoring and regulation. In Gans, S. L., editor: Surgical pediatrics, New York, 1973, Grune & Stratton, Inc.

Smith, R. M.: The pediatric anesthetist, 1950-1975, Anesthesiology 43:144, 1975.

Smith, R. M.: Respiratory arrest and its sequelae. In Smith, C. A., editor: The critically ill child, ed. 2, Philadelphia, 1977, W. B. Saunders Co.

Smith, R. M.: Pediatric anesthesia in perspective, Anesth. Analg. (Cleve.) 57:634, 1978.

Smith, R. M., and Wiley, H. P.: Evaluation of electrocardiography during congenital heart surgery, Anesthesiology 18:398, 1957.

Snow, J. C., Kripke, B. J., Norton, M. L., and others: Corneal injuries during general anesthesia, Anesth. Analg. (Cleve.) 54:465, 1975.

Snyder, W. H., Snyder, M. H., and Chaffin, L.: Cardiac arrest in infants and children; report of 66 original cases, Arch. Surg. 66:714, 1953.

Soule, A. B., and Mazuzan, J. E., Jr.: Cardiac arrhythmias in the pediatric surgical patient, paper presented at Annual Convention of American Medical Association, New York, 1969.

Stetson, J. B.: Prolonged tracheal intubation, Int. Anesthesiol. Clin. 8:969, 1970.

Steward, D. J.: Post-intubation stenosis, Can. Anaesth. Soc. J. 17:388, 1970.

Stoelting, R. K., and Proctor, J.: Acute laryngeal obstruction after endotracheal anesthesia, J.A.M.A. 206:1558, 1968.

Striker, T. W., Stool, S., and Downes, J. J.: Prolonged nasotracheal intubation in infants and children, Arch. Otolaryngol. 85:210, 1967.

Strobel, G. E.: Treatment of anesthetic-produced malignant hyperpyrexia, Lancet 1:40, 1971.

Strong, J. M., and Keats, A. S.: Medical intelligence; induced hypothermia following cerebral anoxia, Anesthesiology 28:920, 1967.

Tahir, A. H.: Endotracheal tube lost in the trachea, J.A.M.A. 222:1061, 1972.

Tapper, D., Arensman, R., Johnson, C. G., and Folkman, J.: The effect of helium-gas-oxygen mixtures on body temperature, J. Pediatr. Surg. 9:597, 1974.

Thorpe, W., and Seeman, P.: Drug-induced contracture of muscle. In Gordon, R. A., Britt, B. A., and Kalow, W., editors: International Symposium on Malignant Hyperthermia, Springfield, Ill., 1973, Charles C Thomas, Publisher.

Thurlow, A. C.: Cardiac dysrhythmias in out-patient dental anaesthesia in children; the effect of prophylactic intravenous atropine, Anaesthesia 27:429, 1972.

Waltermath, C. L.: The febrile patient; pathologic physiology and anesthetic management, Anesth. Analg. (Cleve.) 48:795, 1969.

Westley, C. R., Cotton, E. K., and Brooks, J. G.: Nebulized racemic epinephrine by IPPB for the treatment of croup, Am. J. Dis. Child. 132:484, 1978.

Williams, C. R., and Spencer, F. C.: The clinical use of hypothermia following cardiac arrest, Ann. Surg. 148:462, 1958.

Wilson, R. D., Traber, D. L., Priano, L. L., and Evans, B. L.: Anesthetic management of the poor-risk pediatric patient, South Med. J. 62:767, 1969.

Wilson, W. E.: Preoperative anxiety and anesthesia; their relation, Anesth. Analg. (Cleve.) 48:605, 1969.

CHAPTER 27

Respiratory insufficiency and pediatric intensive care

ETSURO K. MOTOYAMA, DAVID R. COOK, and TAE H. OH

Pathophysiology of respiratory insufficiency
Diagnosis of respiratory insufficiency
Management of respiratory insufficiency
Intensive care of common respiratory
    problems

Management of respiratory insufficiency in infants and children has improved dramatically within the last decade. Such progress in intensive care has been brought about by a number of factors, including (1) improved technology and availability of blood gas and pH apparatus, (2) ever-increasing understanding of problems associated with long-term intubation, such as humidification and oxygen concentration of inspired gas, (3) improved quality and routine sterilization of endotracheal tubes, respirators, and humidifiers, (4) organization of respiratory (inhalation) therapy as a paramedical specialty, (5) development of intensive care units for neonates, infants, and children, and (6) a multidisciplinary approach to the care of the acutely ill. It is difficult to judge the relative contribution of these factors to the progress of respiratory intensive care, since advances in these areas have occurred interdependently. One of the significant catalytic factors of this progress has been the emergence of anesthesiologists as specialists and coordinators of medical and surgical subspecialties in the intensive care unit, with a more aggressive approach to the management of respiratory

failure. On the other hand, progress in respiratory intensive care of infants and children has created new problems, such as subglottic stenosis following prolonged intubation, chronic lung disease caused by oxygen toxicity and possibly by mechanical ventilation, and infection from contaminated equipment.

In this chapter we shall review briefly the pathophysiology of respiratory insufficiency in infants and children and outline the general approaches to the management of the acutely ill. We shall then assess various procedures and therapy commonly utilized in the management of respiratory failure. Finally, we shall describe the current treatment of respiratory insufficiency caused by various diseases commonly seen in the pediatric and neonatal intensive care units. There are several review articles on this subject in the recent literature (Downes and Raphaely, 1975; Pontoppidan and others, 1972; Robin and others, 1973). The reader is also referred to Chapter 3 for a review of basic respiratory physiology.

PATHOPHYSIOLOGY OF RESPIRATORY INSUFFICIENCY

Respiratory insufficiency or failure is an impairment of alveolar ventilation and pulmonary gas exchange characterized by an inability to maintain arterial P_{CO_2} and P_{O_2} within the range compatible with life. Respiratory insufficiency is often the consequence of a lung disease, such as bronchiolitis, status asthmaticus, or viral pneumonia, but also arises from a variety of nonpulmonary organ disorders, particularly circulatory failure and central nervous system dysfunction. In either case, the dominant clinical features are those of respiratory failure: hypoventilation (hypercapnia), restriction of the lung, upper or lower airway obstruction, or their combinations, resulting in ventilation-perfusion imbalance, right-to-left shunt, and hypoxemia. Functional classification of respiratory insufficiency and its common causes in infants and children are shown in Table 27-1.

Neurogenic disorders

Failure of the central nervous system, whether caused by trauma, infection, or poisoning, is a frequent cause of immediate respiratory emergency, since depression of the central nervous system is frequently accompanied by hypoventilation or apnea. Furthermore, cortical and brainstem depression abolishes protective upper airway reflexes, increases the risk of gastric regurgitation and aspiration, and further complicates the clinical picture of respiratory insufficiency.

In addition, head injuries, particularly those involving the hypothalamus, are often the cause of acute pulmonary edema. Clinical and experimental observations suggest that neurogenic pulmonary edema may be caused by massive sympathetic discharge and increased capillary permeability (Theodore and Robin, 1976).

Peripheral nerve and neuromuscular disorders such as Guillain-Barré syndrome (polyneuritis), myasthenia gravis, and improper use of curariform drugs can also lead to acute respiratory insufficiency in infants and children by a reduction of ventilation, loss of ability to cough, and impairment of upper airway reflexes.

Obstructive pulmonary disorders

Upper airway obstruction. Life-threatening upper airway obstruction is relatively common in neonates and older infants for a number of reasons. First, the upper airways in infants are small in absolute size and are

Table 27-1. Functional classification of respiratory insufficiency in infants and children

Disorders	Examples
Neurogenic	
Central depression and increased intracranial pressure	Apnea of prematurity
	Head trauma
	Cerebral edema, hemorrhage
	Encephalitis
	Reye's syndrome
	Hydrocephalus
	Status epilepticus
	Drug overdosage
Peripheral or neuromuscular disorders	Myasthenia gravis
	Polyneuritis (Guillain-Barré)
	Tetanus
	Misuse of curariform drugs
Pulmonary obstruction	
Upper airway obstruction	Choanal atresia
	Macroglossia
	Epiglottitis
	Subglottic croup
	Subglottic stenosis
	Vascular ring
	Tracheomalacia
	Foreign body
Lower airway obstruction	Bronchiolitis
	Status asthmaticus
	Bronchopneumonia
	Cystic fibrosis
Pulmonary restriction	
Parenchymal (pulmonary)	IRDS
	Wilson-Mikity syndrome
	Pneumonia (infections, aspiration)
	Pulmonary edema, hemorrhage
	Congestive heart failure
	Pulmonary fibrosis
	Oxygen toxicity
	Atelectasis
Extrapulmonary	Diaphragmatic hernia
	Pneumothorax
	Hemothorax
	Empyema
	Abdominal distension
	Obesity
	Kyphoscoliosis

subject to disproportionately severe obstruction with secretions, inflammation, and foreign bodies. Second, the relatively large head of the infant tends to overflex the neck and to obstruct the upper airways, particularly when the infant is asleep or depressed. Since the newborn, and especially the premature infant, responds to hypoxia with respiratory depression rather than stimulation (Rigatto and others, 1975), a benign obstruction of the upper airway, which causes only snoring in adults, could become a major catastrophe in young infants. Third, newborns are obligatory nose-breathers; nasal obstruction such as bilateral choanal atresia often causes acute respiratory distress. Other congenital anomalies of newborns, such as micrognathia as seen in Pierre Robin and Treacher Collins syndromes, may cause acute upper airway obstruction. When micrognathia is coupled with glossoptosis, life-threatening airway obstruction may occur when the infant is sedated or recovering from general anesthesia. The supine position should be avoided at all times lest the tongue fall over the posterior wall of the pharynx and cause complete airway obstruction. Aspiration of feeding with resultant pneumonitis is common because of inability to swallow properly. Suturing of the tongue to the floor of the mouth or, in severe cases, nasotracheal intubation may be required.

A vascular ring formed by an anomalous aortic arch or major arteries may produce severe obstruction of the trachea. Signs and symptoms of airway obstruction exacerbated by feeding often start in the newborn nursery. On examination, the chest may be over-inflated. Expiratory wheezes and rhonchi are heard. Chest radiograph may show hyperinflation, atelectasis, and pneumonia.

By far the most life-threatening emergency of older infants is acute epiglottitis, which may cause complete upper airway obstruction within hours. Subglottic croup (laryngotracheobronchitis) is another frequent respiratory emergency in the same age group. Management of these diseases is discussed later in this chapter.

Lower airway obstruction. Lower airway disease occurs more frequently in infants than in older children and young adults (Glezen and Denny, 1973). The compliance of the lung and thorax is exceptionally high and elastic recoil pressure is low in infants

(Motoyama, 1977) and young children (Zapletal and others, 1976). There is a tendency toward premature closure of small airways comparable with that seen in older adults with emphysema (Mansell and others, 1972). These unusual features of the lung in infants and young children, together with the small absolute (not relative) size of the lower airways, account for the picture of severe lower airway obstruction, as seen in infants with bronchiolitis, status asthmaticus, and congestive heart failure. In addition to inflammation and spasm of small airways, viscous secretions, if not cleared promptly, would further increase lower airway obstruction. Poor response to bronchodilator therapy in patients in status asthmaticus may indicate that the main pathophysiology is not bronchiolar spasm but the plugging of small airways with mucus (Levison and others, 1974).

Congenital heart disease with a large left-to-right shunt and increased pulmonary blood flow increases lower airway resistance, probably through compression of small airways by engorged pulmonary and bronchiolar vessels that surround the airways, with or without interstitial edema (Motoyama and others, 1978; Ganeshananthan and others, 1975). Patients with pulmonary venous hypertension with mitral or aortic valvular disease exhibit increased extravascular lung water and interstitial edema that could further occlude small airways by compression (Staub and others, 1967). Such occlusion results in reduction of airspace, right-to-left shunt of blood, disturbance of alveolar ventilation–pulmonary perfusion ($\dot{V}_A/\dot{Q}$) balance, and hypoxemia unless proper treatment is instituted.

Restrictive pulmonary disorders

Pulmonary parenchymal disorders. Pulmonary parenchymal insufficiency may be the manifestation of pulmonary diseases per se but may also be the consequence of other organic or systemic disorders. A unique and frequent cause of pulmonary parenchymal insufficiency in infants is the idiopathic respiratory distress syndrome of the newborn

(IRDS or RDS). This disease occurs mostly in premature infants whose lungs are still immature and have an insufficient surfactant system to maintain aeration of small airspaces (see Chapter 3 and below). The use of continuous positive airway pressure (CPAP-CPPB) prevents alveolar collapse at the end of each ventilatory cycle and has significantly reduced the morbidity and mortality of this disease (Gregory and others, 1971). The necessity for oxygen therapy in these infants often leads to acute and chronic manifestations of pulmonary oxygen toxicity (bronchopulmonary dysplasia) characterized by stiff lung (pulmonary edema and fibrosis), ventilatory failure, and hypoxia (Northway and others, 1967).

There is another form of acute respiratory insufficiency that results from pulmonary infection, left-heart failure, open-heart surgery, or other acute insults to the lung parenchyma. This type of respiratory insufficiency is often referred to as acute respiratory failure (ARF) in adult patients (Wilson and Pontoppidan, 1974). It is also referred to by a variety of names such as "shock lung," "postperfusion (pump) lung," "wet lung" or "adult respiratory distress syndrome" (ARDS) (Pontoppidan and others, 1972) to distinguish it from RDS of the newborn. In ARF the clinical as well as the pathophysiologic picture is rather nonspecific despite the wide variety of etiologic factors. A patient in acute pulmonary parenchymal insufficiency is usually hypoxic and dyspneic unless cerebrocortical function is severely obtunded. Chest radiograph often shows diffuse density or infiltrates, but it is often difficult to distinguish pulmonary edema from pneumonia, even with the aid of other clinical information. Collapse of alveoli and terminal airspaces in ARF may be secondary to loss of pulmonary surfactant or the consequence of small-airway closure as a result of an inflammatory process, secretions, or interstitial edema, with subsequent absorption of trapped gas behind the closed airway. If the patient is ventilated with 100% oxygen, or without an inert gas, so-called resorption atelectasis occurs more rapidly (Fahri, 1964).

General anesthesia or the use of depressant drugs reduces the resting lung volume, or functional residual capacity (FRC), by 25% or more (Westbrook and others, 1973). Such reduction in FRC further promotes airway closure. As already mentioned, infants and young children, not unlike older patients with emphysema, are more prone to the closure of small airways because of unusually low elastic recoil pressure of the lung and thorax (Motoyama, 1977).

Accumulation of fluid in the extravascular space in the lung may occur with pulmonary venous hypertension resulting from fluid overload, left-heart failure, or, more frequently, injury to pulmonary capillary endothelial cells and increased permeability. Altered capillary permeability and resulting interstitial edema have been described as occurring from viral pneumonia; inhalation of such toxic agents as ozone, phosgene, and 100% oxygen; endotoxin; liberation of vasoactive materials such as histamine, kinins, and serotonin; disseminated intravascular coagulation triggered by amniotic-fluid embolism, eclampsia, and fat embolism; open-heart surgery; idiosyncratic reactions to drugs such as sulfonamides, hydralazine, and methotrexate; radiation and uremic pneumonitis; aspiration pneumonia; near-drowning; smoke inhalation; and shock and head trauma (Robin and others, 1973; Wilson and Pontoppidan, 1974; Theodore and Robin, 1976). The immediate treatment should be directed not only toward the prevention of hypoxemia but also toward the cause of pulmonary edema per se, whether it is primarily left-heart failure, pulmonary hypertension, infection, or increased capillary permeability due to other causes.

Extrapulmonary restriction. Respiratory insufficiency can also be brought about by extrapulmonary restriction of the lung. Pneumothorax and pneumomediastinum are common causes of acute respiratory emergency in patients with "stiff" lungs, as in RDS. In the newborn period, congenital anomalies such as diaphragmatic hernia and eventration of the diaphragm cause severe restriction of lung expansion. The lungs under these conditions are often hypoplastic and prone to rupture when positive pressure breathing is attempted. Moreover, gases introduced by positive pressure into the herniated gastro-intestinal tract in the thorax can result in fatality by further restricting lung expansion. Generally, air enters the stomach and accumulates easily in infants with respiratory distress. Frequent emptying of the stomach in these patients is mandatory, since abdominal distension in infants severely compromises ventilation by pushing the diaphragm cephalad.

Summary

Acute respiratory insufficiency in infants and children may be caused by a number of pulmonary and nonpulmonary disorders. Central and peripheral nervous dysfunction may cause hypoventilation, loss of protective mechanisms against aspiration of gastric contents, and even pulmonary edema, possibly via sympathetic stimulation. Severe upper airway obstruction is a unique yet common respiratory emergency in this age group. Lower airway obstruction is particularly severe in infants, probably because of the low elastic recoil of the lung and the small caliber of airways, which are more susceptible to obstruction. Closure of small airways is one of the important contributing factors in the process of parenchymal insufficiency of the lung. Pulmonary parenchymal insufficiency may be caused not only by primary pulmonary disorders, such as pneumonia, RDS of the newborn, oxygen toxicity, and pulmonary hemorrhage, but also by other systemic disorders in the form of pulmonary interstitial edema collectively called wet lung syndrome or ARDS. Extrapulmonary restrictions of the lung are additional important clinical factors modifying the outcome of respiratory insufficiency.

DIAGNOSIS OF RESPIRATORY INSUFFICIENCY

Artificial airways and ventilatory support may be required in infants and children with impaired ventilation and gas exchange of various etiology. The criteria for diagnosing respiratory insufficiency vary considerably, depending on the nature of underlying disorders, and will be outlined later under specific disease categories.

In general, the diagnosis of respiratory insufficiency should be made based on clinical observations together with laboratory examinations, such as arterial blood gas analysis, and bedside assessment of ventilatory function. Clinical criteria for respiratory insufficiency include one or more of the following: (1) severe retractions and the use of accessory muscles of respiration, (2) diminished or absent breath sounds on auscultation, (3) decreased or absent peripheral blood pressure, (4) decreased levels of consciousness and response to painful stimuli, (5) irregular respiration or apneic spells, and (6) loss of muscle tone. The laboratory criteria include (1) hypercapnia (Pa_{CO_2} >60 torr), (2) increased alveolar-arterial P_{O_2} gradient (A-aD_{O_2}) or hypoxemia (Pa_{O_2} <100 torr in 100% inspired O_2 [$F_{I_{O_2}}$ = 1.0] or Pa_{O_2} <50 torr in $F_{I_{O_2}}$ = 0.4), and (3) persistent and severe metabolic acidosis.

A Pa_{CO_2} greater than 60 torr is clear evidence of greatly diminished alveolar ventilation, whether it is due to airway obstruction, central depression, or muscle weakness, and, in general, is an indication for mechanical ventilation. Comatose patients, particularly those with head injury or intracranial hypertension, with a rapidly rising Pa_{CO_2} of greater than 45 torr may be candidates for ventilatory assistance (Gordon, 1971). Severe hypoxemia with increased A-aD_{O_2} may be due to small-airway obstruction and atelectasis, resulting in right-to-left shunt and ventilation-perfusion imbalance. Oxygen and ventilatory support with a ventilator or with CPPB or CPAP is required. Persistent and severe metabolic acidosis (i.e., pH <7.25) that cannot be corrected with a single therapeutic dose of sodium bicarbonate and the maintenance of adequate blood gases is an indication of low cardiac output and circulatory failure. These patients may require circulatory support as well as mechanical ventilation.

Although many cardiopulmonary and neuromuscular conditions may ultimately require mechanical ventilation to provide adequate alveolar ventilation and oxygenation, some interim steps, e.g., oxygen therapy and bronchodilator and IPPB treatment, sometimes improve the condition of some patients at least temporarily. However, unrealistic insistence on conservative treatment is poor medical judgment, since it may deny the benefit of ventilatory support until the child becomes moribund.

Assessment of ventilatory function in acutely ill patients in the pediatric intensive care unit is limited because they are too ill or too young to cooperate with the procedure. Alveolar ventilation can be assessed by the measurement of arterial P_{CO_2} or by an end-tidal CO_2 analyzer. A simple but most useful test of ventilatory function is the measurement of the maximum expiratory flow-volume (MEFV) curve during forced vital capacity with a bedside portable unit (see Chapter 3). With this unit, both large- and small-airway function can be assessed by determining peak expiratory flow rate (PEFR), forced expiratory volume or forced vital capacity at 1 second ($FEV_{1.0}$), and maximum expiratory flow rates ($\dot{V}_{max}$) at low lung volumes. All of these values can be determined in a few seconds. We have found such a device to be quite useful in the pediatric intensive care unit in assessing the degree of obstruction and the efficacy of treatment during illness in patients with status asthmaticus. Inspiratory and expiratory force with airway occlusion at FRC is a useful means of assessing ventilatory capacity, particularly the ability to cough effectively. Inability to generate a pressure of more than ± 20 cm H_2O is an indication of respiratory insufficiency and shows the need for ventilatory support. The dead space to tidal volume (V_D/V_T) ratio is fairly constant (0.3) from infancy to adulthood and can be measured easily at the bedside with a mask, one-way valve, and a weather balloon or a Douglas bag. It is crucial that there be no leak around the airway (or mask) and the one-way valve, since such a leak could make the ratio erroneously high. A V_D/V_T ratio of over 0.5 usually is a sign of respiratory insufficiency.

MANAGEMENT OF RESPIRATORY INSUFFICIENCY
Resuscitation

As soon as respiratory insufficiency is suspected, several basic steps should immediately be taken to restore ventilation and improve pulmonary gas exchange. Clear airways must be established without delay by removing excessive secretions or vomitus in the pharynx. Positive pressure ventilation with oxygen should be started with a bag and mask (or by mouth-to-mouth if equipment is not available). In case of cardiorespiratory failure due to profound hypoxia accompanied by bradyarrhythmia and hypotension, 100% oxygen should be used to ventilate the patient while closed chest cardiac massage is given to restore cardiac function. Heart and breath sounds should be monitored with a precordial stethoscope by the person ventilating the patient, and continuous ECG monitoring should be started. An intravenous line should be secured with a percutaneous plastic cannula or cutdown. Pulmonary hyperventilation should be maintained with a mask and bag until the initial arterial blood gas and pH values are known. In case of circulatory arrest, intravenous sodium bicarbonate (2 mEq/kg) may be given to treat excessive base deficit without waiting for the blood gas results.

Before an artificial endotracheal airway is established, evaluation should be made as to whether certain drug therapies to improve the underlying pathophysiology are feasible under the circumstances. For example, inhalation of racemic epinephrine mist in acute subglottic croup, intravenous aminophylline, isoproterenol, and glucocorticoids in status asthmaticus, or diuretics and digitalis in congestive heart failure may rapidly improve the respiratory status and prevent further development of respiratory insufficiency. Endotracheal intubation should be an elective procedure preceded by ventilation and oxygenation of the patient. Attempts by inexperienced unsupervised persons should be strongly discouraged.

Endotracheal intubation

In emergency situations, orotracheal intubation, rather than nasotracheal intubation, is used to provide a secure airway without delay and to facilitate oxygenation. When artificial airway support is necessary beyond 12 to 24 hours, an orotracheal tube is electively replaced by a nasotracheal tube. The latter provides greater patient comfort and easier fixation and stabilization, particularly when the patient is on a ventilator. Moreover, there is less chance of accidental extubation, less pharyngeal secretions, and easier access to the mouth and pharynx. In addition, nasotracheal tubes produce less arytenoid ulceration, because they assume a more acute curve in the pharynx (Lindholm, 1969). In infants and children under 6 to 8 years of age, an endotracheal tube of the same size used for orotracheal intubation can usually be passed nasally. Sinusitis from nasal intubation reported in adults has not been a frequent problem in infants and children. Tracheobronchial toilet, however, is occasionally more difficult because of the increased length and more acute curve of the tube.

Sterile, disposable plastic endotracheal tubes that are implant-tested should be used. To minimize irritation of the glottis and the subglottic region, the endotracheal tube selected for prolonged intubation should be one size smaller than usual to allow a small leak with positive airway pressure of 20 to 30 cm H_2O. Cuffed endotracheal tubes are not commonly used in children below the age of 8 years, because the diameter of a cuffed tube is too small and flow resistance becomes too high for spontaneous breathing in infants. However, when a very high pressure is needed to ventilate a stiff lung, as in status asthmaticus and bronchiolitis, a tube with a soft, low-pressure, large-volume cuff has been used successfully. Suction, bag and mask, intubating forceps, and oxygen, as well

as at least three different sizes of endotracheal tubes, must be available for all intubations.

It is possible to intubate young infants without muscle relaxants while the head is held in "sniffing" position by an assistant. In older patients, intravenous succinylcholine (1 mg/kg) may be needed. In either case, patients should be given atropine (0.02 to 0.04 mg/kg) intravenously and be oxygenated before intubation. Depending on the reason for intubation and the condition of the patient, amnesia and/or sleep may be induced with a short-acting barbiturate or diazepam. The endotracheal tube should be placed not more than few centimeters below the glottis in infants to prevent endobronchial intubation. Inspection of the chest bilaterally for uniform expansion during inspiration and careful auscultation for equal breath sounds prior to initial fixation of the tube are mandatory. Tincture of benzoin is applied lightly to the exposed endotracheal tube, upper lip, and cheek after the area is dried. One limb of bivalved adhesive tape is first laid across the cheek and upper lip on the side of the tube. The other limb is then fitted securely to the endotracheal tube. A similar piece is fitted from the other side. Careful fixation of the tube as well as restraint of the arms and hands will avoid disastrous accidental extubation. In order to prevent necrosis of the nasal ala, the nasotracheal tube should not be angulated upward.

Radiographic confirmation of the position of the tube should be done routinely, since auscultation of the chest alone may not detect accidental endobronchial intubation in infants. On the radiograph, the tip of the endotracheal tube should be at the level of the second thoracic vertebra.

The greater length of the nasal tube over the oral tube slightly increases airway resistance but is usually of no clinical significance, since the internal diameter rather than the length of the endotracheal tube is the major determinant of the flow resistance. Partial obstruction of the smaller lumen of pediatric endotracheal tubes by a mucous plug or secretions is not uncommon but can be prevented by proper humidification of inspired gases. A nasogastric tube should be inserted following intubation to prevent gastric and small-bowel distension from aerophagia.

Prolonged intubation, especially with the use of a ventilator, has been associated with laryngeal edema, ulceration, glottic granulomas, and subglottic stenosis. Subglottic stenosis is seen in 2% to 8% of patients surviving conditions requiring endotracheal intubation for more than 24 hours (Abbott, 1968; Allen and Stevens, 1965). It is difficult to predict how long an endotracheal tube may be kept safely in place. The patient's age, duration of intubation, number of tube changes, relative tube size, use of mechanical ventilation, effective fixation of the tube, nasal or oral intubation, type and material of the tube, and presence and type of cuff are all contributing variables. In their extensive prospective study involving 7875 children under 17 years postoperatively, Koka and associates (1977) found the incidence of postintubation stridor or retraction to be about 1%. A tight-fitting endotracheal tube was suspected in one half of these cases. Other factors contributing to the laryngeal trauma included trauma related to intubation, duration of intubation, and movement of the neck during anesthesia and surgery.

The incidence of subglottic complications following long-term intubation is highest in patients between 1 and 4 years of age, especially in those intubated for over a week. The highest incidence of postintubation stridor or retraction following short-term intubation for anesthesia is also in this age group (Koka and others, 1977). The infant under 6 months of age appears to tolerate long-term intubation better than the older infant. Marked subglottic granulation tissue, cord erosion, and late fusion of the cords have frequently been observed in infants intubated for over 1 month (Rees and Owen-Thomas, 1966).

Tracheostomy

Tracheostomy should be considered in infants and children when the need for intubation exceeds 1 week or when copious tenacious secretions or bleeding are problems.

In this age group, tracheostomy cannot safely be performed without an endotracheal tube in place to provide an airway and adequate oxygenation. All tracheostomies should be performed in the operating room under controlled sterile conditions. We prefer tracheostomies to be done between the second and third tracheal rings when possible. Low tracheostomies, particularly in the infant, increase the incidence of pneumothorax and endobronchial cannulation. A longitudinal tracheal incision without a wedge-shaped flag is used. Stay sutures are placed in both sides of the tracheostomy site (Stool and others, 1968). In children under 10 years, "Great Ormond Street" soft plastic uncuffed tracheostomy tubes are most commonly used. In older children, low-pressure, high-volume cuffed tubes are used. Double-swivel adapters permit greater flexibility of movement and less traction on the trachea.

Mortality following tracheostomy in infants, especially in inexperienced hands, has been high. This high mortality and the frequent difficulties in decannulating patients with tracheal stenosis at the tracheostomy site (McDonald and Stocks, 1965; Teplitz and others, 1964) have led to a reluctance to do early tracheostomies on infants. The incidence of obstruction of tracheostomy tubes or accidental decannulation, however, decreases as experience is gained in caring for tracheostomies in children (Aberdeen, 1965).

Airway care

Optimum airway care is of utmost importance in infants and children with artificial airways, since it is by far the most crucial factor for the successful outcome of respiratory insufficiency (Young and Crocker, 1976).

Humidification. Humidification of inspired gases through an artificial airway is indispensable for several reasons. When the nose and pharynx have been bypassed by a tracheostomy or endotracheal tube, the natural humidifying function for the respiratory tract is lost. Ciliary function and mucous flow cease when relative humidity in the airway falls below 70% at 37° C. The biophysical mechanisms and problems involved in the inspiration of dry gases have been elaborated by Déry (1971). Inspiration of dry gases causes thickening of secretions, which block natural air passages or indwelling tubes. Finally, energy in the form of heat and body fluids is lost in the process of warming and humidifying the dry inspired gases in the lung. Heated humidifiers are most commonly used, since they are efficient and spare the small patient heat and energy losses. Inspired gases saturated with water vapor at 32° C provide about 70% relative humidity when they reach body temperature in the lung, sufficient humidity to prevent cellular damage of the upper airways (Forbes, 1973). Mobilization of secretions is further facilitated by hourly instillation of small quantities of sterile saline solution at the time of postural drainage and endotracheal suction.

Some unheated nebulizers can provide adequate water content, but body heat is still required to vaporize the particulate water. Of these, ultrasonic nebulizers are the most efficient but must be used with caution, since they may deliver as much as 2 g of water/kg/hr (Cox, 1973). Thus, daily fluid requirements may be exceeded and lead to water intoxication, particularly in small infants. With provision of adequate humidification, insensible water loss from the lungs is negligible. Therefore, maintenance fluid volume must be reduced about 20%. It should be pointed out, however, that the use of radiant-heat warming devices, commonly used for infants in respiratory insufficiency, increases skin temperature and insensible water loss; in premature infants under fluorescent lights, it amounts to as much as 3 g/kg/hr (Yeh and others, 1975).

When heated humidifiers are used, the temperature of the inspired gases should be monitored at the endotracheal tube. Malfunctioning heaters can heat gases excessively, cause unwanted heat gain, or even cause damage to the respiratory mucosa (Klein and Graves, 1974). Inspired gas temperatures should not exceed 35° C.

Removal of secretions. Endotracheal suction combined with hyperinflation of the lung is routinely required hourly or at least every 2 hours. Obviously, in patients in whom secretions are a primary problem, endotracheal suction must be more frequent. Sterile polyvinyl catheters are used. A one–gloved hand "no touch" technic minimizes contamination of the upper airways. Hand-washing immediately prior to and following airway care is mandatory to prevent cross-contamination. The amount of suction (negative pressure) is adjusted by variable occlusion of the open limb of a T-connector. Sterile in-line suction traps permit collection of sputum for bacterial cultures. Small amounts (0.2 to 2 ml, depending on the size of the patient) of sterile saline solution are instilled through the endotracheal tube to facilitate the removal of secretions. Postural drainage with changing body positions facilitated by chest physiotherapy with mechanical vibration or percussion by hand should be tried at 1- to 2-hour intervals to mobilize secretions from smaller airways into the trachea (Safar, 1969). Artificial coughing by inflation of the lung with a self-inflating bag or a modified Jackson-Rees setup followed by manual compression of the thorax may be of help.

Interruption of ventilation and oxygen delivery to the patient for prolonged periods during or following endotracheal suction may lead to hypoxia (Brandstater and Muallem, 1969). In order to minimize the danger of lung collapse during suction, the size of the catheter should be sufficiently small in comparison with the diameter of the endotracheal tube. The lumen of the catheter should be occluded during insertion unless there is a wide-bore T-connector opening to vent negative pressure. Endotracheal suction should always be preceded by oxygen administration and hyperventilation. Reexpansion of alveoli and reoxygenation are imperative after each pass of the suction catheter and are accomplished by repeatedly hyperinflating the lung to near total lung capacity at least six times. A separate oxygen line with a device for reexpansion of the lung should be available at each bedside.

Continuous positive pressure therapy

Recent reintroduction of continuous positive pressure (CPP) therapy to critical care medicine has dramatically improved the management of patients with respiratory insufficiency. Kumar and associates (1970) first reported the efficacy of CPP ventilation (CPPV), or positive end-expiratory pressure (PEEP), in reducing venous admixture in adult patients on mechanical ventilators. Gregory and associates (1971), on the other hand, initiated the use of CPAP, or CPPB, in spontaneously breathing neonates with IRDS, which resulted in dramatic improvements in arterial P_{O_2} as well as in the survival of these infants.

In patients with pulmonary insufficiency from small-airway and/or parenchymal disorders, increased venous admixture is common as a result of small-airway closure, miliary atelectasis, loss of pulmonary surfactant, interstitial edema, or alveolar edema and consolidation. These patients exhibit decreased FRC, decreased lung compliance, and $\dot{V}_A/\dot{Q}$ imbalance. The CPP therapy has been effective in these patients, with or without mechanical ventilation, in improving FRC, lung compliance, and pulmonary gas exchange, presumably by preventing airway closure, recruiting previously collapsed alveoli, and reducing further accumulation of alveolar edema (Ashbaugh and Petty, 1973; Suter and others, 1975). Anesthesia and muscle relaxants in patients in supine position reduce FRC by 25% or more, even in individuals with normal lungs (Westbrook and others, 1973). Thus, a low level of CPP (2 to 4 cm H_2O) may be beneficial in these patients to maintain normal FRC and prevent small-airway closure.

On the other hand, CPP therapy above 5 cm H_2O should not be used in patients with low compliance from pulmonary fibrosis whose alveolar surface activity is intact, in those with emphysema and asthma in whom FRC is increased, in those with hypovolemic and cardiogenic shock, and in those with normal lungs. In these patients, positive airway pressure may push FRC too high, increase the work of breathing, interfere with venous return, and decrease cardiac output. Especially in the hypovolemic patients, hypotension may occur as the airway pressure level is raised. Therefore, frequent accurate determination of blood pressure and blood gases by means of an indwelling intra-arterial cannula is mandatory. Volume expansion with blood, colloid, or crystalloid may be needed in these patients, particularly when the lung pathophysiology calls for CPP therapy.

Spontaneous breathing with CPP (CPPB, CPAP). Since Gregory and associates (1971) first reported successful use of CPAP, it has been adopted extensively for the treatment of IRDS as well as other pulmonary insufficiencies in infants. CPAP may be applied in a patient whose Pa_{O_2} is less than 100 torr with 100% inspired oxygen ($F_{I_{O_2}} = 1.0$) or whose Pa_{O_2} is less than 50 torr with $F_{I_{O_2}}$ above 0.40 and when hypercapnia is not present. Initially, CPP of 4 to 6 cm H_2O is applied, and its effect on arterial blood gases is evaluated within 20 to 30 minutes. The level of CPP is usually raised in increments of 2 cm H_2O until a marked increase in Pa_{O_2} is seen.

There are several ways in which CPAP can be maintained without an endotracheal tube in place. Enclosure of the infant's head in a tight-fitting head box or a soft plastic bag has been tried with some success, but high noise level is a problem (Hoffman and others, 1972; Gregory, 1972). In addition, it is difficult in such a device to gain access to the patient for tracheal toilet. Since the newborn is an obligatory nose breather, nasal prongs or catheters with inflow of fresh gas in tandem with an exhalation valve can maintain CPAP up to 6 to 8 cm H_2O (Hamilton and Singer, 1974). CPAP is lost, however, if the infant cries. Orogastric tubes serve to prevent gastric distension, which would be a serious complication for CPAP without endotracheal tubes. Continuous negative pressure (CNP) has been applied about the chest to achieve continuous expansion of the lung without an endotracheal tube with some success (Chernick, 1973). One problem of this method is maintenance of normal body temperature in infants, since their ambient air tends to cool by dilution from the room air.

If the initial Pa_{O_2} is less than 50 torr with $F_{I_{O_2}}$ of 0.80, or if CPAP at 8 cm H_2O fails to improve Pa_{O_2} significantly, endotracheal intubation may be indicated to achieve higher levels of CPAP. Hypercapnia (Pa_{CO_2} >50 torr) and apneic spells are the indicators for mechanical ventilation. PEEP may be added to the ventilator.

There has been no simple way to determine the optimal level of CPAP in infants other than by the trial and error method, with repeated arterial blood gas determinations as the level of CPP is raised. What interpleural pressure changes are generated by CPAP is not known, although because of stiff lungs, CPAP is not readily transmitted to the pleural space as it is in patients with normal compliant lungs. However, if CPAP exceeds its optimal level, overdistension of small airspaces would decrease lung compliance and cardiac output, increase the physiologic dead space, and possibly lead to lung rupture. Indeed, pneumomediastinum and pneumothorax are not uncommon in patients during CPAP therapy.

In adult ARF, Suter and associates (1975) found that the maximum total respiratory compliance with PEEP coincided with the maximum oxygen transport and the lowest V_D/V_T ratio.

A simple and reliable method of estimating pleural pressure and the optimal levels of CPAP in infants is to monitor end-expiratory pressure with a small water-filled feeding tube in the lower third of the esophagus and a pressure transducer connected to the proximal end. Bonta and associates (1977) reported that below the optimal CPAP levels, esophageal pressure did not change significantly when the level of CPAP was raised. When the optimal airway pressure was reached there was a marked increase in esophageal pressure coinciding with a significant increase in Pa_{O_2}.

Mechanical ventilation

If the patient in acute respiratory insufficiency does not respond rapidly to con-

servative treatment, including topical or systemic drug therapies, endotracheal suction of secretions, or CPAP, mechanical ventilation is required to restore his oxygenation and acid-base balance. Mechanical ventilation is most commonly achieved with an intermittent positive pressure ventilator. A tank-type negative pressure ventilator is rarely used in the modern intensive care unit because of its multiple functional limitations.

In acute respiratory insufficiency, airway resistance is almost always increased and dynamic compliance of the respiratory system decreased. Mechanical ventilators therefore must be capable of accommodating altered and unstable respiratory mechanics. Under these circumstances, volume-controlled ventilators are definitely superior to pressure-controlled ventilators. It is important to choose the endotracheal tube appropriate for each patient, since the advantages of volume-controlled ventilators are lost with the presence of large air leaks around the endotracheal tube or tracheostomy cannula.

Most of the ventilators are provided with an assist mode in which mechanical ventilation is triggered by the negative airway pressure generated by the patient's inspiratory effort against airway occlusion. In the assist mode, the inspiratory force necessary to trigger the ventilator varies greatly from one ventilator to another and may exceed the ability of a sick infant. In addition, the response time is often too slow to be synchronized with the infant's own inspiratory effort (Epstein, 1971). Furthermore, the use of so-called intermittent mandatory ventilation (IMV) practically eliminates the need for the assist mode during the weaning process (p. 627). For these reasons, assisted ventilation in infants and children is of minimal clinical value today.

In volume-controlled ventilators, part of the stroke volume fails to reach the patient because of (1) compression of gas within the system as the pressure is raised above ambient (compression volume loss) and (2) distensibility of delivery tubing (compliance volume loss) (Mushin and others, 1969;

Okmian, 1963). The internal volume of the ventilator in relation to the lung volume of the patient influences to a large degree the compression volume losses. In the adult, these losses are relatively small; in the infant, who has much smaller lung volumes, these losses assume much greater significance. The use of relatively noncompliant tubing reduces compliance volume losses to a minimum. As the patient's compliance decreases or airway resistance increases with resultant increases in the inflation pressure, compliance and compression volume losses increase. The sum of compression and compliance losses is referred to as "effective internal compliance" (ml/cm H_2O) of a ventilator. The tidal volume setting of a ventilator should be increased to compensate for the volume loss due to the internal compliance.

Control of ventilation with a mechanical ventilator can often be accomplished on the awake patient with minimal sedation and without neuromuscular blockade by simply eliminating asphyxia and by providing adequate oxygenation and acid-base balance. In others, adequate sedation and depression of respiratory drive can be produced by intravenous diazepam (0.1 mg/kg) or morphine (0.1 mg/kg) in repeated doses or continuous infusion (Downes and Raphaely, 1975). However, narcotics do not adequately suppress reflex tachypnea resulting from lower respiratory tract infection such as pneumonia, bronchiolitis, or status asthmaticus. In these patients, nondepolarizing muscle relaxants are needed in addition to sedatives. d-Tubocurarine (0.3 mg/kg) or pancuronium (0.06 mg/kg), as initial doses, usually permit control of mechanical ventilation. Doses of relaxant may be repeated as necessary to maintain adequate ventilation. Rarely will d-tubocurarine at this dose cause hypotension. Bronchospasm from histamine release is a theoretical possibility with d-tubocurarine, although the drug has frequently been used without difficulty, even in asthmatics. Hypertension and tachycardia may be seen with higher doses of pancuronium. Oxygenation may suffer because of reduction in FRC secondary to paralysis of the diaphragm and intercostal muscles (Froese and Bryan, 1974). In these patients, low levels of PEEP (3 cm H_2O) should always be added to restore FRC and prevent the closure of small airspaces. It is true that the partially paralyzed cannot breathe if disconnected from the ventilator. However, the use of disconnect alarms on ventilators and one-to-one nursing care in the intensive care unit should prevent such problems.

Intermittent mandatory ventilation. Many ventilators can be modified with low-resistance, one-way valves to provide a fresh gas supply if the patient breathes out of phase with the ventilator. With this device, periodic mechanical hyperinflation at variable preset intervals is possible. These superimposed machine breaths are not patient triggered but are preset by time, hence the term "intermittent mandatory ventilation." The Baby-Bird Ventilator was specifically designed to accomplish this. This feature allows a gradual withdrawal from controlled ventilation to spontaneous respiration without having to shift to the assist mode or to a new apparatus such as a T-piece. In essence, weaning is accomplished on the same ventilator.

IMV has practically eliminated the use of the assist mode of ventilation. It has also obviated the need for hyperventilation, sedatives or analgesics, and muscle paralysis to achieve complete control of ventilation with time-cycled volume ventilators. The incidence of respiratory alkalosis, with its possible detrimental effects on cardiac output, brain blood flow, and renal blood flow, is therefore decreased (Downs and others, 1973; Breivik and others, 1973; Philbin and others, 1970). However, with relatively high IMV rates the patient may still breathe out of phase with the ventilator, and respiratory distress may result. A possible hazard of IMV devices may be that a ventilator cycling coincident with the end-inspiratory phase of a patient's own breath may lead to overdistension of the lung. This would be especially true if the IMV volume were set too high. Continuous monitoring of esophageal pressure is a simple and effective means of evaluating the synchrony of the patient's breath and readjusting IMV rates with the ventilator.

Mechanical ventilators for infants and children

The difference in tidal volume and respiratory rate between infants and older children makes it difficult to use the same ventilator for all age groups. In some instances, one may modify an adult ventilator for infants. On the other hand, a ventilator used exclusively for infants may be unsatisfactory for older children.

An ideal pediatric ventilator should allow accurate control of a wide range of tidal volumes with small internal compliance, inspiratory and expiratory times, inspiratory flow rate, and inspired oxygen concentration. Adequate humidification must be provided. An adjustable high-pressure relief valve should be included. There should be access to the exhalation valve to provide PEEP. In addition, there should be a mechanism to allow the patient to inspire out of phase with the mechanical ventilator (IMV, see p. 627).

In order to meet such demands, volume-controlled ventilators and flow generator–time cycled ventilators have been developed exclusively for infants. Several such infant ventilators are now available. However, the choice of ventilators in any one neonatal or pediatric intensive care unit probably should not exceed two or three types. This limitation permits technicians, nurses, and physicians to become thoroughly familiar with their use and idiosyncrasies, thus improving troubleshooting.

There are several monitoring devices that are built into the ventilator to assure its proper function and the safety of the patient. The inflation pressure generated by the ventilator should be monitored. Changes in the patient's lung compliance will be reflected by this pressure. Pressure alarms must be added to all ventilators to warn if pressure limits are exceeded or if minimal pressure is not reached in a definite time. The latter then serves as a disconnect alarm.

Although the use of oxygen-air blenders has decreased the problems of controlling inspired oxygen concentration, in-line monitoring should be performed frequently or continuously to ensure their accuracy.

The temperature of the inspired gas mixture should be monitored routinely near the endotracheal tube when a heated humidifier is used. As mentioned previously, inspired gas temperature should not exceed 35° C.

A comparison of mechanical ventilators commonly used for infants and children is shown in Table 27-2. Several of them are discussed in more detail below.

Bourns ventilator.* The Bourns volume ventilator is specifically designed for infants weighing less than 5 kg. It is a piston-driven, volume-controlled, pressure-limited ventilator with variable inspiratory flow rates. Inspiratory to expiratory time ratio (I/E) is determined by adjusting the inspiratory flow. It has a separate tidal volume control (5 to 150 ml). This ventilator gives a square wave pressure pattern. The inspired oxygen concentration can be regulated with a blender or with a mixing chamber in older models. Humidification of inspired gas is achieved by the DeVilbis ultrasonic nebulizer, which has been modified to limit its output to prevent water intoxication in infants.

In the control mode, respiratory rate ranges between 20 and 80 per minute; in the newer models, the rate can be decreased to 5 per minute or below, which is useful for setting IMV during the weaning period. There is an expiratory valve to provide up to 15 cm H_2O of PEEP. On the assist mode, this ventilator has the shortest response time to the patient's inspiratory effort to trigger the ventilatory cycle, although the benefit of assisted ventilation is limited. Artificial sigh is produced by two quick successions of tidal volume with the expiratory valve closed but is totally ineffective. Effective internal compliance of this ventilator is 0.5 to 1.2 ml/cm H_2O (Binda and others, 1976).

In general, we set the ventilator tidal volume at approximately 20 ml/kg, with a high airway pressure limit of 30 cm H_2O and a frequency between 30 and 60 per minute, de-

*Bourns Inc., Riverside, Calif.

Table 27-2. Comparison of commonly used ventilators for infants and children

	Amsterdam	Baby-Bird	Bourns (volume)	Bennett MA-1	Emerson (pediatric)
Mode	Time-cycled constant flow	Time-cycled constant flow	Volume-cycled variable flow	Volume-cycled variable flow	Volume-cycled variable flow
Power source	Electric/pneumatic	Pneumatic	Electric	Electric	Electric
Respiratory rate (CPM*)	2-50	5-100	5†-80	6-100	6-50
Stroke volume (ml)	5-300	5-300	5-150	5‡-2200	5-1000
"Internal compliance" (ml/cm H_2O)	NA§	2-4	0.5-1.2	3-4	3-5
Controls					
Volume	−	−	+	+	+
Inspiratory flow	+	+	+	+	−
Inspiratory time	+	+	−	−	+
IMV	−	+	+	+	+
PEEP/CPAP	+	+	+	+	+
Automatic O_2 blender	−	+	−	+	+
Humidifier	Heated humidifier	Unheated jet nebulizer	Unheated ultrasonic nebulizer	Heated humidifier	Heated humidifier

*CPM, cycles per minute.
†0.5 CPM in the new model.
‡With the neonatal adapter (see text).
§NA, data not available.

pending on the nature of the respiratory insufficiency, and aim for an effective tidal volume of approximately 10 ml/kg. Ventilator settings should be adjusted as indicated with the aid of inspection and auscultation of the chest as well as blood gas determination. Patients with stiff lungs, such as those with IRDS, may require an inspiratory pressure as high as 50 to 60 cm H_2O to maintain adequate alveolar ventilation.

Emerson ventilator.* The Emerson ventilator, modified with a pediatric cylinder, is the most versatile ventilator available for infants and children of all sizes. It is particularly useful for older infants who are oversized for the ventilators designed for neonates. It is a piston-driven, volume-controlled ventilator with variable inspiratory and expiratory times and variable tidal volume (5 to 1000 ml). The inspiratory flow is determined by the combination of tidal volume and sine-wave inspiratory time. A heated humidifier is provided. The corrugated delivery tubes are relatively

*J. H. Emerson Co., Cambridge, Mass.

noncompliant and are equipped with heating coils to reduce the accumulation of water droplets. The inspired oxygen concentration can be varied either by an air-oxygen blender or by controlling the oxygen flow into the gas inlet. PEEP can easily be added to the expiratory valve. Effective sighs can be given with a built-in pressure-limited flow generator in the older model. The Emerson ventilator has recently been modified to allow the patient to breathe from a continuous flow of fresh gas on the IMV mode. In the older model, the volume loss due to effective internal compliance is linear at about 3.0 ml/cm H_2O up to a pressure of 40 cm H_2O. A nomogram has been developed to aid in resetting the ventilator as inflation pressure rises (Robbins and others, 1967). The water level of the humidifier affects the internal volume and therefore compression losses (Haddad and Richards, 1968).

As a first approximation, we set the ventilator stroke volume at twice the tidal volume of the patient, as estimated by Radford's nomogram (Radford and others, 1954; see

Chapter 3), or approximately 15 ml/kg body weight, in order to accommodate increased dead space and air leaks around the endotracheal tube. Following auscultation of the patient's chest, the ventilator can be readjusted. Arterial blood gas measurements are necessary to accurately determine the proper subsequent settings.

Bennett MA-1 ventilator. * This is a volume-controlled ventilator commonly used in the adult as well as in the child. By use of a small, less compliant tube assembly, it can also be adapted to neonates and young infants as a time-cycled, pressure-limited ventilator (Jaegar and others, 1972). Inspired oxygen concentration can be adjusted accurately with a built-in oxygen blender. A heated Bennett Cascade humidifier is incorporated in the circuit, with a thermometer near the endotracheal tube to monitor and adjust gas temperature. It has separate inspiratory flow and expiratory time controls as well as variable "inspiratory hold" time that gives an end-inspiratory plateau to facilitate gas distribution in the lung. This ventilator delivers a sine-wave pressure pattern with adjustable respiratory rates (6 to 100 per minute) and tidal volumes (10 to 2200 ml). An effective sigh mechanism with adjustable volumes is available. There is a built-in PEEP mechanism up to 10 cm H_2O in this ventilator. IMV can be added with optional attachments and an oxygen blender. Effective internal compliance with regular tubing is approximately 3 ml/cm H_2O. Effective internal compliance with the infant tube assembly is not known. A major drawback of this and other adult ventilators is the fact that even the lowest setting of inspiratory flow rate is much too high to provide a pressure pattern for optimal distribution of ventilation in a small child.

Baby-Bird ventilator. † The Baby-Bird ventilator is designed specifically for neonates and infants. It provides a constant flow of fresh gas; a time-cycled pneumatic mechanism intermittently occludes a modified Ayre T-piece. The delivered volume is related to the flow rate and the inspiratory time. The peak inspiratory pressure can be adjusted to provide a pressure limit to this time-cycled ventilator. This ventilator is not patient triggered. It is equipped with an air-oxygen blender, unheated nebulizer, PEEP valve, and variable pressure relief valve. The inspiratory and expiratory times and the flow rate are variable. Using a lung simulator, Binda and associates (1976) determined the effective internal compliance of this ventilator with changes in lung compliance and resistance. The effective compliance of the Baby-Bird ventilator with decreases in lung compliance is approximately 2 ml/cm H_2O; with increases in airway resistance, the volume lost by the effective compliance is doubled.

For controlled ventilation of infants, we adjust the initial inspiratory time to about 1 second, the rate to about 30 per minute, and the initial flow rate to 1 L/kg. Tidal volume is increased by increasing the flow rate. A continuous flow of fresh gas allows the patient to breathe safely in between the set rate of the ventilator. The machine rate can be slowed to about 6 breaths per minute to permit IMV. The machine cycling can be stopped and the patient allowed to breathe spontaneously on a T-piece without disconnecting the patient from the ventilator. In older children, this ventilator is less efficient because of the high gas flow required to obtain adequate tidal volumes. A CPAP and PEEP mechanism is added to the exhalation valve. Similar flow generator–time cycled ventilators are also available that appear to be just as effective as the Baby-Bird ventilator (Bourns Pressure Ventilator; Bio-Med Ventilator*).

Amsterdam ventilator. This is a simple, time-cycled constant-flow generator for neonates and young infants. It is electrically driven but can also be operated pneumatically. The tidal volume is determined by inspiratory time and flow rate and ranges from minimal to 300 ml. Respiratory rate ranges between 20 and 50 per minute. PEEP can be added up to 10 cm H_2O, but there is no

---

*Ohio Medical Products, Madison, Wis.
†Bird Corporation, Palm Springs, Calif.

*Bio-Med Device, Inc., Stamford, Conn.

mechanism to allow the infant to breathe out of phase with the ventilator (IMV). The concentration of inspired oxygen is determined by the flow ratio of oxygen and air. There is a heated humidifier, but the effectiveness is questionable. Although available features are limited, this ventilator has the advantages of being small, simple, and portable for the transportation of sick infants in an ambulance.

Patient monitoring

In all patients on ventilators, the ECG is monitored and displayed on an oscilloscope continuously for detection of arrhythmias, tachycardia, or bradycardia, which may be early signs of hypercapnia, hypoxia, or heart failure.

Blood pressure must be monitored accurately, especially in those patients requiring high inflation pressures or PEEP. Transcutaneous Doppler ultrasound allows accurate blood pressure measurement even in small infants, including those with poor peripheral circulation (Kirby and others, 1969). Chest radiographs should be obtained when indicated. As a matter of practicality, daily films are usually recommended in patients admitted to the pediatric intensive care unit.

Body temperature must be monitored and neutral thermal environment maintained for infants (Oliver, 1965). An open bed warmed with radiant heat is much easier to use than a closed incubator for removal of secretions, physiotherapy, and general care of infants on ventilators. However, conductive heat losses are more difficult to control with an open bed. In addition, the use of a radiant heat device increases skin temperature and insensible water loss through the skin. The maintenance fluid volume must be increased to cover such losses.

Frequent determinations of arterial blood gases are essential in the management of patients on ventilators. Intermittent samples can be obtained even in the premature infant with the use of 25-gauge needles. The radial and temporal arteries are the most common sites. These arteries allow preductal gases to be obtained in infants who may be shunting through the patent ductus arteriosus. The femoral artery should be avoided, especially in infants, because of the remote possibility of loss of circulation in the leg and because accidental puncture of the joint capsule of the hip may lead to septic arthritis.

Arterial cannulation. Arterial cannulation for frequent sampling of blood gases and continuous monitoring of blood pressure is essential in critically ill patients with rapidly changing conditions. Umbilical artery, temporal artery, and radial artery catheters are commonly used for these purposes.

Umbilical artery catheters may be passed via the internal iliac artery into the aorta. The optimal position is controversial. Weaver and Ahlgren (1971) suggest that the tip be in the lower thoracic aorta, opposite T-6 and T-10. The potential danger of an improperly placed umbilical artery catheter is grave. Placement near the celiac, renal, or mesenteric arteries may lead to thrombosis, and catastrophe may result. Radiographic confirmation of the catheter position therefore is mandatory. The incidence of serious complications, predominantly thrombosis, following umbilical artery catheterization is about 2% (Cochran and others, 1968; Neal and others, 1972).

Radial artery cannulation is feasible in infants and children of all ages. Thrombosis at the site of cannulation is common (Ryan and others, 1973), but the majority of thrombosed vessels eventually recanalize, usually within 2 weeks (Miyasaka and others, 1976). Integrity of the ulnar collateral circulation to the hand should be checked, since about 3% of the population have incomplete palmar arches with no collateral circulation from the ulnar artery. Percutaneous radial catheters can be introduced relatively easily, except in smaller infants in whom the catheters can be placed under direct vision through a small cutdown. Nontapered 22-gauge Teflon catheters are ideal for small infants. The use of Teflon catheters of this type has reduced the incidence of thrombosis, embolization, and occlusion (Ryan and others, 1973). Continuous irrigation with heparinized Ringer's lactate solution at low flow rates prolongs catheter integrity. Ringer's solution may be superior to normal saline, since its pH is more physiologic than that of commercially available saline. The fluid volume from continuous flush technics must be considered in the fluid balance of small infants. High-pressure, intermittent flushing may embolize small air bubbles to the head (Lowenstein and others, 1971) and may damage small arteries in the distribution of the radial artery.

Arterial P_{O_2}, P_{CO_2}, and pH. Except in rare instances, hyperoxia from high inspired oxygen concentration is of no specific benefit and carries several hazards. Pa_{O_2} of greater than 80 to 100 torr for brief periods has resulted in retinal artery vasospasm in premature infants. Prolonged Pa_{O_2} at greater than these tensions may lead to retrolental fibroplasia and blindness (James and Lanman, 1976). In patients with patent ductus arteriosus, preductal oxygen tensions must be measured to ascertain what oxygen tension the eye is being exposed to. Oxygen toxicity to the lung appears to be related to the inspired concentration, the Pa_{O_2} achieved, and the duration of exposure (Clark and Lambertsen, 1971; Winter and Smith, 1972). In the neonate, Pa_{O_2} between 50 and 70 torr is acceptable. If there is persistent or increasing metabolic acidosis, treatment should be directed toward restoring circulation and tissue perfusion rather than increasing P_{O_2}, since oxygen saturation is high in this age group because of a high concentration of fetal hemoglobin. In the older infant or child, one should use the lowest possible inspired oxygen concentration that will achieve a Pa_{O_2} of 70 to 80 torr. Lower levels of Pa_{O_2} (i.e., 60 to 70) are acceptable if the patient is stable and does not develop metabolic acidosis.

Pa_{CO_2} may decrease rapidly when mechanical ventilation is instituted in a patient with acute respiratory insufficiency. Moderate hypocapnia may lower Pa_{O_2}, impair release of oxygen from hemoglobin, induce hypokalemia and arrhythmias, reduce cardiac output, increase oxygen consumption, and decrease cerebral blood flow (Prys-Roberts and others, 1968). Addition of dead space to the ventilator tubing or of carbon dioxide to the inspired gas mixture to restore Pa_{CO_2} to normal tends to alleviate these problems (Breivik and others, 1973). Keeping Pa_{CO_2} near normal or allowing it to rise prior to weaning will reestablish carbon dioxide stores in the body and facilitate weaning by restoring the central and peripheral chemoreceptor responses to CO_2.

Transcutaneous measurements of oxygen tension and saturation. The technic for transcutaneous measurements of blood oxygen tensions with surface electrodes has developed in recent years. Pa_{O_2} is measured polarographically over the arterialized peripheral capillary region; oxygen molecules diffuse from the superficial capillaries through the skin to the electrodes (Huch and others, 1973). The temperature of a Clark-type P_{O_2} electrode is maintained at 44° C for premature infants and 45° C for older patients, resulting in a skin temperature of 42° to 43° C.

This transcutaneous method has demonstrated good correlation with simultaneously measured arterial P_{O_2} (Huch and others, 1976; Duc and others, 1975). This noninvasive technic has great potential, particularly in the neonatal intensive care unit, since it will eliminate technical difficulties of arterial puncture in small patients as well as a number of complications resulting from frequent arterial punctures or indwelling catheters. However, there are many questions to be answered before routine use of this technic is accepted. These questions include the possibility of localized dermal burn due to the high temperature of the electrode, the safety of the simultaneous use of this technic and other electric monitoring devices in intensive care units and operating rooms, and the reliability of the P_{O_2} values obtained from patients with hypovolemia, hypothermia, or profound shock.

Ear oximetry has been available for over 40 years as a noninvasive method of assessing the oxygenation of arterial blood. However, with the exception of its use in cardiac catheterization laboratories, this technic has never gained wide clinical use. The reason for this failure includes distrust of the principle of the method, reservations concerning its stability and accuracy, and difficulties in operating and maintaining the instrument (Nilsson, 1960). Recent technical advances have led to the development of instruments that are robust, easy to use, and accurately reflect arterial oxygen saturation (Sa_{O_2}) during a condition of rapidly changing oxygenation of patients (Saunders and others, 1976).

Monitoring of central circulation. Recent development in multilumen balloon floatation catheters has greatly improved our capacity to monitor central hemodynamics with relative ease (Swan and others, 1970). Percutaneous internal jugular vein puncture is used most successfully with a margin of safety (Civetta and Gabel, 1972). With such a catheter it is possible to continuously or intermittently monitor right atrial (central venous) pressure, pulmonary artery systolic and diastolic pressures, and, by inflation of the balloon, pulmonary capillary wedge pressure. The measurement of the pulmonary capillary wedge pressure is particularly important, since it has high correlation with the left atrial pressure and reflects left ventricular function (Lappas and others, 1973). Since left-heart failure and pulmonary venous hypertension in infants and children are often associated with severe small-airway obstruction and respiratory failure (Motoyama and others, 1978), the monitoring of central circulation is most valuable in the management of pulmonary parenchymal insufficiency. In addition, P_{O_2}, P_{CO_2}, and O_2 content of mixed venous blood samples obtained from the pulmonary artery catheter accurately reflect cardiac output and adequacy or inadequacy (i.e., mixed venous P_{O_2} <35 torr) of tissue oxygenation.

Bedside assessment of pulmonary function. Assessment of ventilatory function is difficult even in older, conscious children when they are in mild to moderate respiratory distress. It is possible, however, to measure tidal volume and vital capacity (VC) using a simple flow meter. Portable devices for obtaining MEFV curves during forced expiration (see Chapter 3) are available and are quite useful in assessing lower airway ob-

struction in older children above 7 to 8 years.

Measurements of pleural pressure oscillation during the respiratory cycle by means of esophageal pressure monitoring provide useful information on the degree of airway obstruction. Increases in negative esophageal pressure during inspiratory effort reflect increases in airway resistance and work of breathing and/or decreases in dynamic lung compliance.

In a patient who is mechanically ventilated, changes in dynamic compliance of the respiratory system can be measured from the ratio of actual tidal volume and the difference between end-inspiratory and resting airway pressures. Such measurements are also useful in determining the optimal level of PEEP at which the total dynamic compliance is the highest (Suter and others, 1975).

With a special device, MEFV curves may be obtained during forced deflation of the lung in infants and children in respiratory insufficiency who are mechanically ventilated (Motoyama, 1977). Examination of such deflation flow-volume curves is helpful in determining the degree of lower airway obstruction and the efficacy of various forms of treatment in the intensive care unit.

Psychologic aspects of ventilator care

Many children requiring intubation and mechanical ventilation are awake. They feel, see, and hear what is happening not only to themselves but also to other children in the intensive care unit. Witnessing intubations, insertion of chest tubes, etc. can lead to fear, distortion, and fantasy. The children have a simple understanding of the function of airway equipment, although they find it uncomfortable. Often, to avoid repeated endotracheal suction, they try to breathe deeply and to cough. One should realize that the child attempts to communicate his needs in spite of endotracheal tubes (Barnes, 1975). In addition to the fear and stress from the environment of the intensive care unit, physical separation from the parents, especially in the preschool child, can aggravate anxiety.

A kind, honest approach to children is of utmost importance to lessen their anxiety. A preoperative teaching program for both the child having cardiac surgery and his parents has helped decrease the fear of the unknown for both parties. Such a program permits the parents to help support the child (Reinhart and others, 1973). Obviously, in acute illnesses the psychologic aspects of fear and anxiety are markedly increased in the parents as well as the child, and the nursing staff must be extra supportive. Liberalized visiting privileges help the child tolerate ventilator care. In addition, for the more alert child, play therapy can keep him involved with his environment (Reinhart and others, 1973).

As in adults, sleeplessness due to constant therapy and noise may lead to hallucinations (Kiely, 1974). Many children become withdrawn. The ability to distinguish day from night and to see a clock has helped the older child to remain well oriented.

The young infant needs physical contact in order to develop psychologically. We have encouraged mothers to become involved in the simple care of these infants. In lieu of maternal contact, such maternallike contact can be provided by nurses. We have held and rocked infants still requiring mechanical ventilation.

Sedation. Most, but not all, children who are restless, agitated, and breathe asynchronously with the ventilator are found to be hypoxic, acidotic, or hypercapneic. If these factors are not the cause of the agitation, the judicious use of sedatives or narcotics can greatly facilitate ventilator care in children. Obviously, sedatives or narcotics may be dangerous in the spontaneously breathing patient in borderline respiratory failure. Diazepam given in small divided doses (0.1 mg/kg) can provide sedation without cardiovascular depression. Morphine, again in small divided doses (0.1 mg/kg), can provide analgesia and sedation. Because of its central respiratory depressant effect, morphine can facilitate control of ventilation. In supine normovolemic patients it has little effect on cardiac output.

Weaning from mechanical ventilation

The decision to change from controlled ventilation to spontaneous ventilation with an endotracheal tube in place and then to subsequent extubation depends on improvement in the disease condition that necessitated ventilatory assistance. Such improvement is usually a gradual one; weaning may be a protracted process. Patient evaluation of alertness, cardiovascular stability, neuromuscular strength, and tests of pulmonary gas exchange must be considered.

Cardiovascular stability is important before weaning. Gross hemorrhage, hypotension from hypovolemia, low cardiac output state, and arrhythmias must be corrected before extubation is comtemplated. Patients with severe anemia and decreased oxygen-carrying capacity may be stressed or decompensated by the increased metabolic demands of spontaneous ventilation. In these patients, packed red blood cells are indicated as an adjunct to successful weaning (Vidyasagar and Wai, 1975). We maintain hematocrit above 35% before weaning the patient from a ventilator, particularly in young infants below 3 months of age, when oxygen affinity of hemoglobin is still high and oxygen unloading at the tissue level is low. Conditions associated with unusual increases in metabolic rate, such as fever, shivering, and thyrotoxicosis, should be under control before extubation. Adequacy of cardiac output and oxygen uptake should be evaluated by examination of the stability of acid-base balance or mixed venous P_{O_2} ($P\bar{v}_{O_2}$ >35 torr) or by direct measurements of cardiac output if a central vascular catheter is in place (Swan and others, 1970).

The ability of the lung to perform adequate gas exchange must be carefully evaluated before the patient is weaned from mechanical ventilation. Patients without cyanotic heart disease who require CPAP to maintain Pa_{O_2} above 50 torr with FI_{O_2} of 0.4 are not ready for extubation, although they may be weaned from mechanical ventilation gradually. Patients with an A-aD_{O_2} less than 300 torr on 100% oxygen or with a shunt fraction ($\dot{Q}s/\dot{Q}t$) of less than 20% can be considered for weaning (Hodgkin and others, 1974). A-aDo$_2$ can easily be obtained after the patient has breathed 100% O$_2$ for 20 minutes. Estimation of shunt fraction is much more accurate when mixed venous blood samples from the pulmonary artery catheter are available to measure arterial–mixed venous O$_2$ content difference. Patients with V$_D$/V$_T$ ratio of above 0.55 have marked difficulty in maintaining the high minute ventilation needed for adequate alveolar ventilation.

Good gas exchange while on a ventilator does not predict whether the patient has the mechanical ability to breathe for himself. In older children, tidal volume, VC, and inspiratory and expiratory forces against airway occlusion can be measured at the bedside using a simple flow meter and a pressure gauge. A VC of 20 ml/kg appears to be a minimum requirement to cough and sigh adequately. Those patients with VCs of 10 to 20 ml/kg may be weaned from mechanical ventilation but are not candidates for extubation. The inspiratory and expiratory forces (occlusion pressure at FRC) can be measured in even the smallest child or the most uncooperative patient. The patient should be ventilated with increased inspiratory oxygen for several minutes before this test is performed in order to prevent hypoxemia. A T-piece is connected to the endotracheal tube. One limb leads to an aneroid manometer; the other limb is occluded at FRC. If the patient can generate at least −20 to −25 cm H$_2$O, he is a candidate for weaning to spontaneous ventilation, although the pressure alone does not guarantee his ability to breathe adequately. If the inspiratory force generated is −30 cm H$_2$O or better, the patient can be considered for extubation, provided that his VC is adequate.

When the patient is weaned from controlled ventilation to spontaneous respiration on a T-piece, close observation at the bedside is mandatory. Inspired oxygen concentration should be increased by 10% until the blood gas values on spontaneous breathing are available. A low level of CPP (3 cm H$_2$O) should be maintained in all patients who are breathing spontaneously through an endo-

tracheal tube in order to compensate for the lack of a normal physiologic mechanism by the glottis to maintain positive airway pressure during the expiratory phase of tidal ventilation and to prevent premature closure of small airways. Anxiety, struggling, sweating, and tachycardia most frequently are signs of respiratory insufficiency. It is mandatory to sit with the patient when he is first disconnected from the ventilator. The length of time the patient can tolerate spontaneous ventilation is variable. It is highly desirable, if not essential, to have an indwelling arterial line in place and to determine arterial blood gases at 15, 30, and 60 minutes and every 1 to 3 hours thereafter if the patient appears stable or as frequently as required. A stable Pa$_{CO_2}$ of less than 45 torr without acidosis may be considered as a sign of adequate alveolar ventilation. In the patient who has been hyperventilated for a long time, it is important to restore CO$_2$ depletion by decreasing alveolar ventilation for a while before weaning is attempted. If the patient can tolerate at least 12 to 24 hours off the ventilator without any sign of distress, has maintained satisfactory blood gases, still maintains good motor strength as evidenced by adequate VC, and has stable chest radiographs, he may be considered for extubation. Clinical and laboratory criteria for extubation are listed in Table 27-3.

Table 27-3. Criteria for extubation

Clinical	Laboratory
Conscious and alert	Pa$_{O_2}$ >50 torr; Fi$_{O_2}$ = 0.4
Stable cardiovascular function	P$\bar{v}_{O_2}$ >35 torr
No sign of distress on spontaneous ventilation	A-aDo$_2$ <300 torr; Fi$_{O_2}$ = 1.0
No need of CPPB (CPAP)	Pa$_{CO_2}$ <45 torr, stable
Minimal secretions	pH >7.30, stable Hematocrit >35%
Satisfactory chest radiograph	Balanced electrolytes
Nutrition under control	VC >20 ml/kg
Satisfactory fluid balance	V$_D$/V$_T$ <0.50
Stable temperature	Inspiratory force (at FRC) ≤ −30 cm H$_2$O

Redesign of various ventilators to permit IMV has simplified weaning. As gas exchange improves and the patient begins breathing, the number of controlled breaths from the ventilator can be decreased. Pa_{CO_2} can be allowed to rise gradually toward normal.

Extubation should be preceded by chest physiotherapy, removal of endobronchial secretions, and hyperinflation of the lung with high concentrations of oxygen.

Following extubation, humidified 40% oxygen is given by mask or in an oxygen tent for at least 24 hours to prevent dryness of the larynx and trachea, which might have been traumatized by the endotracheal tube. In children below 5 years of age, racemic epinephrine (2.25% solution diluted with saline 1:6) may be nebulized for 5 minutes every 1 to 2 hours up to 12 hours as indicated in an attempt to prevent local swelling (Jordan, 1970). Corticosteroids are not given in our institutions, since there is no convincing evidence of their beneficial effects (Goddard and others, 1967). Chest physiotherapy and postural drainage are maintained frequently for at least 2 days after extubation or as long as .they are indicated.

IPPB may be given to the patient for a few minutes every 1 to 2 hours with nebulized saline solution or a bronchodilator as indicated to expand the lung and to facilitate coughing and removal of secretions. In spite of the wide use of IPPB in patients with acute and chronic pulmonary disease, data for the clinical efficacies of IPPB treatment have been limited (Hyatt, 1974; Baker, 1974).

Summary

Significant progress has been made in the management of respiratory insufficiency during the past decade. Once the diagnosis is made, whether it is pulmonary or nonpulmonary in origin, prompt action should be taken to restore patent airways and proper gas exchange. In most situations, endotracheal intubation should be performed electively after ventilation and oxygenation with a mask and bag have been established. Frequent measurements of arterial blood gas tensions and pH are required to determine the optimal F_{IO_2} and ventilator settings. Once mechanical ventilation is established, adequate levels of sedation and muscle relaxation may be required if the patient's own ventilatory effort is out of phase with the ventilator cycle. A low level of CPP should be maintained at all times to prevent premature airway closure. There are, however, specific indications and contraindications for higher levels of PEEP above 5 cm H_2O, depending on the nature of the pulmonary disease. Optimal airway care is of particular importance in infants and children, with adequate humidification of inspired gas and frequent removal of secretions. Finally, weaning of the patient from the ventilator and extubation may be a protracted process during the period of recovery from respiratory insufficiency. The decision for weaning should be made rationally based on laboratory and clinical findings.

INTENSIVE CARE OF COMMON RESPIRATORY PROBLEMS
Idiopathic respiratory distress syndrome of the newborn

IRDS, or hyaline membrane disease (HMD), is a disorder of prematurity, particularly of the lung with insufficient surface-active material lining the terminal airspaces. IRDS is usually limited to prematurely born infants and is seen more frequently following intrauterine distress. It is characterized by early postnatal onset of increasing respiratory difficulty with tachypnea, grunting and marked retractions, progressive hypoxemia, and metabolic acidosis; a diffuse reticulogranular pattern, with an air-filled tracheobronchial tree, is clearly visible on a chest radiograph (Peterson and Pendleton, 1955; Weller, 1973). Pathophysiologically, decreased lung compliance and alveolar collapse result in abnormally low FRC. Progressive hypoxemia is caused by increased right-to-left intrapulmonary shunting, pulmonary hypoperfusion, and shunting through the foramen ovale and ductus arteriosus. In the United States, approximately 15% of neonates weighing less than 2500 grams develop IRDS, with an estimated mortality of

30% as of 1968 (Wood and Farrell, 1974).

Management. As in any other respiratory failure, the improvement of oxygenation and its maintenance at adequate levels are of utmost importance. Pa_{O_2} between 50 and 70 torr should be maintained with increased F_{IO_2} and/or ventilatory support with or without the use of a ventilator. Pa_{O_2} above this level in premature infants should be avoided lest retrolental fibroplasia and toxicity to the lung result. Frequent determinations of arterial blood gases and pH are essential in these infants to avoid both hypoxemia and hyperoxemia. Except in mild cases of IRDS that do not require CPP treatment, an indwelling arterial catheter should be inserted for continuous monitoring of blood pressure as well as for blood samples. Either the temporal or radial artery is preferred over the umbilical artery, since there may be a substantial P_{O_2} difference above and below the ductus arteriosus. Effort should be made to keep the arterial pH at or above 7.30 by maintaining adequate oxygenation and tissue perfusion. A neutral thermal environment (Brück and others, 1962) should be maintained to minimize unnecessary chemical thermogenesis and oxygen consumption. In case of metabolic acidosis with large base deficit, sodium bicarbonate should be used, but with caution, since excessive sodium and serum osmolality levels may result in cerebral edema and hemorrhage (Finberg, 1967).

Since Gregory and associates (1971) first described successful application of CPPB-CPAP for the treatment of IRDS, it has been adopted widely with impressive results. As described already, CPAP may initially be applied with nasal prongs or a head box without endotracheal intubation. Starting from a CPAP of 6 cm H_2O, 2-cm H_2O increments of CPAP are added until it reaches the optimal level, where Pa_{O_2} increases markedly. Excessive pressure should be avoided, since it would decrease cardiac output as well as net oxygen transport to the tissues (Downes, 1976).

Endotracheal intubation is necessary if an initial F_{IO_2} above 0.80 is required to maintain a Pa_{O_2} of 50 torr or if CPAP higher than 8 cm H_2O is required. Hypercapnia, severe metabolic acidosis, or apneic spells are the indications for mechanical ventilation with CPP (CPPV, PEEP).

Once the optimal level of CPAP or PEEP is established, F_{IO_2} is reduced to adjust the Pa_{O_2} to 50 to 70 torr without changing the airway pressure. During the recovery phase in the succeeding days, when Pa_{O_2} is further increased and stable with F_{IO_2} at or below 0.40, the level of CPAP may be decreased step by step until it reaches 3 to 4 cm H_2O before extubation is contemplated.

Originally CPAP therapy was initiated only after A-aD_{O_2} increased considerably (i.e., Pa_{O_2} <50 torr, F_{IO_2} = 0.60). The current trend, however, is to start CPAP treatment earlier once the diagnosis of IRDS is established. The rationale for this trend is that, by definition, IRDS is expected to worsen if untreated and that the benefit of early application outweighs the risk of CPAP treatment. Indeed, Krouskop and associates (1975) reported that infants with IRDS who were treated early required lower F_{IO_2} and had a less severe clinical course than those in whom CPAP treatment was started at a conventional or later stage of the disease.

In addition to IRDS, a syndrome of acute pulmonary insufficiency with interstitial and alveolar edema and loss of surfactant, which is generally referred to as "wet (shock) lung syndrome" or "adult respiratory distress syndrome," also occurs in infants and children, although the incidence in this age group is not as frequent as in adults. ARDS in infants and children may occur from a variety of causes, including toxic viral or bacterial pneumonia, aspiration pneumonia, oxygen toxicity, endotoxins from pancreatitis, near-drowning, burn, smoke inhalation, open-heart surgery, shock, and head trauma. Although etiologic factors vary widely, the clinical picture of pulmonary insufficiency is not dissimilar. The treatment of ARDS is basically similar to that of IRDS.

Meconium aspiration syndrome

Aspiration of meconium occurs in about 5% of newborns as a result of asphyxia and premature onset of deep inspiration or gasping in pre- and perinatal periods (Gregory and others, 1974). It is a relatively common cause of neonatal respiratory distress, with wide variations in the severity of the clinical picture ranging from mild or no respiratory symptoms to severe respiratory failure with hypoxia, hypercapnia, and combined acidosis requiring ventilatory support. Chest radiographs show focal or generalized areas of diminished aeration. About one third of these patients may develop pneumothorax or pneumomediastinum. Gooding and Gregory (1971) found abnormal chest radiographs in some of these infants who had no meconium in the trachea and were not sick enough to require supplemental oxygen. On the other hand, those with endotracheal meconium had a high incidence of abnormal chest radiographs, and 70% were clinically ill, requiring oxygen or ventilatory support.

The clinical picture of respiratory insufficiency varies, depending on the amount of aspiration and the time course of the syndrome. At birth there may be total occlusion of the larynx and trachea with large meconium plugs, resulting in acute hypoxia and asphyxia. Dissemination of small particles into lower airways after the onset of breathing may produce regional atelectasis, hyperinflation, and maldistribution of ventilation, resulting in right-to-left shunting, ventilation-perfusion imbalance, hypoxemia, and hypercapnia (Vidyasagar and others, 1975). Secondary pulmonary infection may further compromise respiratory insufficiency and the clinical course of the disease. The chemical irritation of meconium on the tracheobronchial mucosa is not well understood. Since the pH of meconium ranges between 5.5 and 7.0, it is less likely to cause severe chemical pneumonitis than that which is seen following aspiration of gastric contents. The efficacy of corticosteroid administration is questionable (Orr and others, 1974).

Management. When meconium aspiration is suspected at delivery it is imperative to do direct laryngoscopy and clear the upper airway before the onset of breathing. If the glottis is meconium-stained, the infant should be intubated immediately and suction applied directly to the tube. There is little danger of atelectasis, since the lung is fluid-filled at this stage. The upper airway may be lavaged quickly with saline solution, if indicated, followed immediately by ventilation with oxygen. This maneuver will diminish dissemination of meconium into the lower airways after the onset of breathing (Gooding and Gregory, 1971) and improve the clinical course of these infants (Burke-Strickland and Edwards, 1973; Gregory and others, 1974).

If hypercapnia or hypoxemia persists, ventilatory support should be started with controlled ventilation or IMV setup. Unlike infants with IRDS, dynamic compliance is relatively high in neonates with meconium aspiration syndrome. Metabolic acidosis is corrected with the administration of sodium bicarbonate.

The use of CPAP or PEEP is recommended, whether the patient is breathing spontaneously or on a ventilator, since a PEEP of 4 to 7 cm H_2O decreases A-aDo_2 (Fox and others, 1975). Antibiotics are given to all infants for the first 24 hours of life; they are discontinued if cultures are negative.

Subglottic croup (croup, laryngotracheobronchitis)

Croup is a condition resulting from acute and severe obstruction of the larynx due to infection, edema, foreign body, or neoplasm and is characterized by stridor, hoarseness, or barking cough. Unfortunately, the term "croup" has been used to describe several unrelated pathophysiologic conditions or disease categories such as subglottic croup, acute epiglottitis, and postintubation stridor. Without further definition, the term has become meaningless.

Subglottic croup, usually viral in origin, may involve the larynx, trachea, bronchi, and even lower airways. Therefore, laryngotracheobronchitis is probably a better term. Myxovirus is the most common etiologic agent. However, adenovirus, *Hemophilus parainfluenzae* 1, 2, and 3, and *Hemophilus influenzae* A2 and B have occasionally been isolated.

Subglottic croup occurs most frequently in infants between the ages of 6 months and 3 years. There is a 2:1 predilection for boys over girls. Generally there is no allergic history. Recurrence is common. The usual history is that of a child with upper respiratory tract infection for several days who then develops inspiratory stridor and a harsh barking cough. Inspiratory supra- and substernal retractions may be present. The patient has a low fever, if any. Rhonchi, rales, and wheezing may be present. There are varying degrees of pharyngeal inflammation with red and swollen vocal cords.

Laryngotracheobronchitis must be distinguished from epiglottitis (see below) or aspiration of foreign bodies without delay (Table 27-4). The history usually gives a clue to the diagnosis of foreign body aspiration. Radiographs of the chest or neck may show opaque objects of art—pins, tacks, or coins. In cases of subglottic croup, lateral radiographs of the neck usually reveal the subglottic portion of the tracheal lumen narrowed by edematous mucosa.

Management. The management of laryngotracheobronchitis depends on the severity of the signs and symptoms. Agitation of the child may increase respiratory flow resistance and aggravate the stridor and retractions.

In the child with severe airway obstruction evidenced by stridor and retractions and accompanied by rhonchi, wheezes, or rales, administration of oxygen to prevent hypoxemia and to meet increased metabolic demand is important. Hypoxemia may or may not be manifested by cyanosis. It is therefore important to determine arterial blood gases to guide oxygen therapy as it becomes necessary and to detect impending respiratory insufficiency. However, whether blood gas determinations should be done in every child with subglottic croup is debatable.

Both nebulized water and warmed humidified air seem to offer relief in a number of cases. Most of the particulate water in the spontaneously breathing patient will be deposited in the upper airway without distribution deeper in the smaller airways (Wolfsdorf and others, 1969). Thus, mist tent therapy has no value for the treatment of lower airways disorders (Motoyama and others, 1972), although it may possibly have beneficial effects in the upper airways by preventing mucosal dehydration. Systemic hydration may also provide some relief in the dehydrated child.

The efficacy of steroids in subglottic croup has not been clearly defined. Children with an allergic history (eczema, asthma, or hay fever) may have significant improvement (Eden and others, 1967). In other children there is no strong evidence that steroids are of benefit.

In 1966 Jordan reported dramatic improvement in the signs and symptoms of laryngotracheobronchitis with the use of nebulized racemic epinephrine. Since the original

Table 27-4. Differential diagnosis of "croup"

	Acute epiglottitis	Subglottic croup	Inhaled foreign body
Age	2-8 yr	3 yr or younger	Mostly less than 5 yr
Onset	Acute	Gradual	Immediate
Organism	*H. influenzae* mostly	Virus	None
Coughing	Rare	Barking	Occasional
Hoarseness	Rare	Moderate to severe	Occasional
Dyspnea	Severe	Mild to moderate	Severe
Stridor	Moderate to severe	Mild to moderate	Occasional
Fever	High	None or mild	None initially
Drooling	Severe	None	Occasional
Laryngoscopy	Cherry-red swollen epiglottis	Normal to mild edema	Normal
Lateral neck radiograph	Large epiglottis	Subglottic narrowing	Normal, or foreign body

report, the incidence of tracheostomy in this disorder has been reduced to nearly zero in his institution (Adair and others, 1971). These authors used 0.5 ml of 2.25% racemic epinephrine diluted with 3 ml of water or saline solution and nebulized with intermittent positive pressure apparatus with oxygen. Unlike its use in asthma, racemic epinephrine is given for its vasoconstrictor rather than its bronchodilator effect. Only the *l*-isomer of epinephrine is pharmacologically active. Therefore, the smaller incidence of cardiac effects with the racemic mixture as opposed to the active *l*-isomer may be related to the dilution.

In relatively mild cases of subglottic croup, which do not respond to simple humidification of inspired air, it is our practice to first give racemic epinephrine, 0.5 ml (2.25%), in 3 ml of saline solution via aerosol. If there is no improvement, the same dose is then repeated by nebulizer and intermittent positive pressure flow generator (IPPB). We prefer this graded approach to therapy, since in many mild cases the child can be spared the discomfort of IPPB, including the possibility of gastric distension.

Recently the beneficial effect of racemic epinephrine solution has been attributed to the nebulization of the saline solution (Gardner and others, 1973; Taussig and others, 1975). On the other hand, Westley and associates (1976) in their double-blind studies have shown a significant difference in efficacy between racemic epinephrine and saline nebulization by IPPB.

If the patient's signs and symptoms worsen in spite of humidification, hydration, steroids, and racemic epinephrine, tracheostomy is considered. All such tracheostomies should be done in the operating room under optimal control. There the patient must be oxygenated and intubated, with or without general anesthesia, in an orderly, controlled manner.

Long-term nasal intubation for croup has led to an extremely high incidence of subglottic stenosis (Downes and others, 1966). Several of these patients subsequently required tracheostomy. Use of endotracheal tubes in the edematous glottis and trachea presumably contributed to this high incidence of complications. More recently, however, Schuller and Birck (1975) reported the use of long-term nasotracheal intubation for subglottic croup with encouraging results that may be attributable to many factors, such as use of smaller endotracheal tubes and improvement of tube material as well as general airway care of these patients.

Acute epiglottitis

In contrast to laryngotracheobronchitis, epiglottitis is an acute illness involving the supraglottic region. In the majority of cases, *Hemophilus influenzae* type B is the causative organism, although in rare instances β-hemolytic streptococci are isolated. The epiglottis, aryepiglottic folds, and arytenoids are principally involved, with little or no involvement of the subglottic area.

Preschool children, ages 3 to 6, have the highest incidence of epiglottitis, although it occurs in younger infants as well as in older children and occasionally in adults. The highest number of cases are reported in the spring and fall, with only sporadic cases in other seasons. The condition usually begins with complaints of sore throat associated with dysphagia and a thick muffled voice. Rarely is there a "croupy" or barking cough. The child looks toxic and has a high fever. Most of the patients with this disease are admitted to the hospital within 12 hours of the onset of illness. The disease progresses very rapidly and may be fatal unless immediate steps are taken to restore the patient's upper airways. Classically, the child is sitting up with the mouth open and drooling. The inspiratory phase is slow, with stridor and retraction; the expiratory phase is unobstructed. The inspiratory sound has been compared to that of a quacking duck.

Management. As soon as acute epiglottitis is suspected in the emergency room, a senior anesthesiologist and otolaryngologist should be called immediately. The child should never be left unattended by one of these physicians, since the disease may progress so rapidly that complete upper airway obstruction may ensue within minutes. The patient should be kept in a sitting or tripod position; supine position makes the obstruction worse. In our institutions, the child is transferred to the operating room without delay, accompanied by an anesthesiologist and an otolaryngologist. A laryngoscope with several blades, bronchoscope, self-inflating bag with face mask and oxygen, and endotracheal tubes with stylets must be ready and near the patient for emergency intubation. Throat examination or direct laryngoscopy should not be attempted in the emergency room, particularly by inexperienced persons, since the risk of complete airway obstruction is great; we prefer to perform direct laryngoscopy in the operating room under optimal conditions and under general anesthesia.

If the child's condition permits, a lateral radiograph of the neck is taken during inspiration and reveals a swollen epiglottis in the majority of patients (Rapkin, 1972).

Direct laryngoscopy without anesthesia is possible by skilled hands. It is not recommended, except in emergency situations, since the examination on a struggling child is difficult and may unnecessarily endanger the life of a child. In the operating room, we induce anesthesia with halothane and oxygen in a sitting position and use an ECG monitor and a precordial stethoscope. Nitrous oxide may be added if the child's condition permits. The use of muscle relaxants is contraindicated, since it often results in complete obstruction of the larynx, and frantic attempts to ventilate the child may result in nothing but gastric dilation, regurgitation, and asphyxia. Before laryngoscopy, atropine (0.02 mg/kg) is given.

Visualization of the bright "cherry red" epiglottis under direct laryngoscopy confirms the diagnosis. In some cases, the picture may be atypical or only a part of the epiglottis may be inflamed or swollen. Throat and blood cultures taken at the time of laryngoscopy have been positive for *Hemophilus influenzae* in most of these cases.

As soon as the diagnosis is made, these patients require immediate establishment of an artificial airway with an endotracheal tube to bypass the swollen epiglottis (Myers, 1973). Whether the child is managed with tracheostomy or long-term nasotracheal intubation is probably best decided on an individual basis, depending on the availability of otolaryngologists experienced in infants, a pediatric intensive care unit, and resident and nursing staffs. However, since acute rapid airway obstruction is the cause of death, these children must have an artificial airway established. Most of the deaths reported from epiglottitis have occurred in patients treated only with fluids, antibiotics, and observation. Failure to establish an artificial airway led to acute and complete obstruction that could not be relieved (Rapkin, 1973).

There is a growing preference to insert nasotracheal tubes under general anesthesia for long-term airway management rather than to perform tracheostomies (Sweeney and others, 1973; Milko and others, 1974; Weber and others, 1976; Oh and Motoyama, 1977). A polyvinyl nasotracheal tube, one size smaller than usual, serves to provide a safe airway. However, such patients must be carefully watched in an intensive care unit. Sedation is rarely required in these patients following nasotracheal intubation. Accidental extubation or self-extubation is a potentially disastrous complication. It can be prevented by proper restraint of the elbows and hands. Antibiotics (ampicillin or chloramphenicol) should be started after throat and blood cultures are obtained. Fluid deficits, if any, should be corrected parenterally.

Usually it is possible to extubate these patients in 2 to 3 days, but decannulation of a tracheostomy tube takes a few days longer. Subglottic stenosis, frequently seen following long-term nasal intubation for laryngotracheobronchitis, does not seem to be a problem in epiglottitis. Thus, nasotracheal intubation for epiglottitis appears to be less invasive than tracheostomy, with shorter duration of intubation and hospitalization (Oh and Motoyama, 1977).

Bronchiolitis

Bronchiolitis, an acute viral infection, is most commonly caused by respiratory syncytium virus or parainfluenza 3 virus. It is manifested by widespread inflammation of bronchiolar and interstitial cells with edema, which obstructs the small air passages. Plugging of the bronchiolar lumen with mucus and cellular debris further exaggerates the clinical symptoms of small-airway obstruction. Bronchiolar spasm does not appear to be a major component of this disease.

It is usually associated with little or no fever. Its peak incidence occurs at 3 to 4 months of age, but it may occasionally be seen in infants up to 2 years of age. It is twice as common in boys as in girls. In about half of the children there is an allergic family history, usually of asthma. In spite of severe symptoms, mortality is relatively low (2% to 7%). On physical examination, the chest is barrel-shaped and hyperresonant. Breath sounds are greatly diminished or absent. The chest radiograph typically shows increased radiolucency and flattened bilateral hemidiaphragms.

Pathophysiologically, the main characteristic of this disease is severe small-airway obstruction (Motoyama, 1977). The increase in expiratory resistance is more severe than that in inspiratory resistance (Wohl and others, 1969). There is a marked increase in trapped air; dynamic compliance is decreased (Phelan and others, 1968). The work of breathing may be increased as much as three to six times that of normal (Krieger and Whitten, 1964; Downes and others, 1968). Hypoxia in room air is common; A-aDo$_2$ is markedly elevated. A V_D/V_T ratio as high as 0.76 has been noted (Downes and others, 1968). Clinically, absent breath sounds or severe retractions are indications for mechanical ventilation, since Pa$_{CO_2}$ is often greatly increased (Downes and others, 1968).

Management. In severe cases, an indwelling arterial catheter is necessary to follow the arterial blood gases closely. We consider intubation and mechanical ventilation when Pa$_{CO_2}$ is elevated above 55 torr over 1 hour with acidosis and decreasing Pa$_{O_2}$. Nasotracheal intubation is preferred, since mechanical ventilation, without major complications such as pneumonia, is required on the aver-

age of 3 days (Downes and others, 1968). Morphine (0.1 mg/kg) or diazepam (0.1 mg/kg) may be given as needed to sedate the patient. Paralysis with nondepolarizing muscle relaxants may facilitate controlled ventilation.

Respiratory rate should be slow in order to facilitate the distribution of ventilation and exhalation. A low level of PEEP (3 cm H$_2$O) appears beneficial to prevent closure of airways, but higher levels of PEEP are detrimental to the patient because they cause an even higher FRC. Bronchodilator drugs are not usually effective, probably because the airway obstruction is primarily caused by obliteration of small airways by edema, mucus, and sloughed epithelial cell debris rather than bronchiolar spasm (Phelan and Williams, 1969). Corticosteroids are not effective (Leer and others, 1969).

Blood gases usually improve rapidly once mechanical ventilation is established, although small-airway obstruction persists for several days. The time for weaning the patient from the ventilator may be evaluated by recording inspiratory airway pressure or dynamic total respiratory compliance and by observing its improvement. Daily chest radiograph is also useful to determine improvements in airway obstruction.

Daily fluid intake should be decreased by 20%, since the humidified gas mixture from the ventilator decreases insensible water loss. Antibiotics are not administered unless there is secondary bacterial infection.

Status asthmaticus

Asthma is episodic bronchial obstruction caused by bronchospasm, secretions, and edema. Acute respiratory insufficiency from asthma usually responds promptly to treatment with bronchodilators, clearing of secretions, and control of respiratory tract infections. Because of a better understanding of the pharmacokinetics of theophylline in children in recent years, this drug has been used widely and more effectively for the treatment of bronchial asthma (Rangsithienchai and Newcomb, 1977; Godfrey, 1977). However, in severe cases, death from status asthmaticus is not uncommon.

Status asthmaticus may be defined as diffuse, bronchodilator-resistant wheezing with signs of hypoxia. In children and young adults, status asthmaticus is usually a combination of severe bronchospasm, marked edema and congestion of the bronchial and bronchiolar mucosa, and profuse secretions. Obstruction of small airways by mucous plugs is the main factor impairing pulmonary ventilation and gas exchange (Levison and others, 1974).

Management. Management of status asthmaticus is a continuum of therapeutic measures with the patient's signs and symptoms used as guidelines. Measurement of arterial blood gases must be made frequently to assess the changing condition of patients. In the early stages, these patients hyperventilate and are hypocapneic because of anxiety and respiratory drive, probably in response to stimulation of pulmonary receptors as well as to hypoxia. As the disease worsens and is prolonged, they become exhausted, and P_{CO_2} may rise rapidly to critical levels.

Adequate oxygenation of the patient's arterial blood must be of primary importance. Continuous spontaneous inhalation of at least 40% humidified oxygen via aerosol face mask is the first step. Small children who will not tolerate a face mask can receive humidified oxygen in a mist tent. In status asthmaticus there is little danger that oxygen inhalation will induce further hypoventilation and CO_2 narcosis (Downes and others, 1968a). If the use of oxygen should result in hypoventilation, ventilatory assistance is indicated.

An initial dose of aminophylline, 6 mg/kg, may be given over 20 minutes. This is followed by continuous infusion of 1 mg/kg/hr (Piafsky and Ogilvie, 1975). The plasma level of aminophylline should be determined repeatedly to achieve optimum therapeutic levels (10 to 20 μg/ml), since the rate of metabolism varies in each individual, particularly in children (Walson and others, 1977). In some patients, higher doses are required to maintain therapeutic levels.

Current understanding of the pathogenesis of asthma indicates that bronchial smooth-muscle tone is regulated primarily by the level of intracellular cyclic adenosine monophosphate (AMP). Adenyl cyclase at the cell membrane is stimulated by β-adrenergic agonists while the intracellular degradation of cyclic AMP by phosphodiesterase is inhibited by theophylline (Walker, 1976). Thus, on theoretical grounds one might expect to see an additive effect of a β-agonist and theophylline.

Intravenous isoproterenol infusion has been found to be effective in reducing the need for mechanical ventilation in status asthmaticus (Downes and others, 1973). Isoproterenol is normally diluted to 5 μg/ml and is given at an initial rate of 0.1 μg/kg/min. The rate is increased as necessary by 0.1 μg/kg/min (using a precision syringe pump) every 15 minutes until a tachycardia of greater than 190 occurs or the maximum dose of 1.5 μg/kg/min is reached. It is imperative to monitor and display the arterial blood pressure continuously by pressure transducer whenever continuous intravenous infusion of isoproterenol is given. Aerosol therapy with isoproterenol is not necessarily beneficial to these patients in improving regional ventilation-perfusion imbalance, since aerosol particles deposit primarily in well-ventilated airways. Its beneficial effect probably occurs after isoproterenol is absorbed into the pulmonary circulation by the upper airway mucous membranes (Knudson and Constantine, 1967).

β_2-Agonists have theoretical advantages over isoproterenol since they have a limited effect on the heart. Isoetharine (1% solution) may be diluted with saline solution four to five times for aerosol treatment, particularly before endotracheal suction.

Intravenous administration of sodium bicarbonate is effective in maintaining a near-normal arterial pH in spite of rising Pa_{CO_2}. A normal range of pH often restores bronchodilator effectiveness to both aminophylline and epinephrine and thus decreases the need for intubation and mechanical ventilation (Kampschulte and others, 1973). Correction of acidosis with sodium bicarbonate is best managed by following arterial blood gases and pH. The extracellular base deficit is corrected using 20% to 25% of body weight as the assumed extracellular fluid volume. If severe bronchospasm is present, 2 mEq/kg may be given empirically over several minutes. Persistent metabolic acidosis is a sign of poor perfusion and tissue hypoxia. In these cases, circulatory status and fluid balance should be evaluated rather than sodium bicarbonate being used indiscriminately. It should be emphasized that the reason for administering an alkalinizing solution in status asthmaticus is to restore the responsiveness of the bronchial tree to sympathomimetic amines and to improve circulatory status, not to correct respiratory acidosis.

Corticosteroids may be administered intravenously in large doses (hydrocortisone, 12 mg/kg/day, or synthetic glucocorticoids such as dexamethasone, 0.3 mg/kg/day, and methylprednisolone, 1 to 2 mg/kg/day) every 6 hours for the first 24 hours. Subsequently the doses are tapered, and steroid medication is discontinued when the asthmatic attack is under control, unless the patient has been receiving maintenance steroids prior to the attack. Patients who have been receiving corticosteroids prior to an episode of status asthmaticus may need even larger doses. The use of steroid aerosols in status asthmaticus is worthless.

In some patients, sedation may help alleviate anxiety. Such treatment should not be tried unless blood gases are monitored frequently to rule out hypoxic agitation. Sedation in these patients may induce a rapid deterioration from compensated respiratory insufficiency. The slightest depression of respiratory drive in these patients may result in CO_2 retention, somnolence, apnea, and death.

Other supportive therapy includes administration of intravenous fluids and electrolytes to correct dehydration and electrolyte disturbances. Fluid deficits are frequently large, on the order of 5% to 10% dehydration. Sodium, chloride, potassium, bicarbonate, hematocrit, and serum osmolality determinations should guide fluid therapy.

Broad-spectrum antibiotic therapy is advisable to counteract secondary infection with mixed gram-positive and gram-negative organisms. Sputum should be obtained for culture with the first tracheal suction. A chest radiograph should be obtained to evaluate the status of the lungs every day.

Intubation and artificial ventilation are indicated only when conventional measures fail to prevent a progressive deterioration in the clinical picture and blood gases. A rise of Pa_{CO_2} from below normal to above 45 torr, particularly if it is rapid, signals ventilatory deterioration. We recommend intubating and ventilating the patient when Pa_{CO_2} starts to rise. Pa_{CO_2} of more than 65 torr in the face of wheezing is considered as "dangerous" hypoventilation and is the absolute indication for mechanical ventilation. Clinically, the patient becomes weak or somnolent, and inspiratory breath sounds diminish while expiratory wheeze increases. This state is usually associated with a Pa_{O_2} of less than 60 torr ($F_{I_{O_2}} = 1.0$) (Downes and others, 1968a).

Since long-term intubation may be required, nasotracheal intubation is preferred over orotracheal. Intubation is more easily accomplished with short-acting muscle relaxants as well as sedation. Neuromuscular blockade usually is necessary to avoid "bucking," which augments bronchial obstruction and asphyxia. Both pancuronium and d-tubocurarine, in spite of the theoretical disadvantages of the latter, have been used successfully for this purpose.

Controlled ventilation is best started by manual bag compression followed by use of a volume-cycled ventilator. If Pa_{CO_2} was markedly elevated before intubation, effort should be made to decrease Pa_{CO_2} gradually in order to avoid hypotension, arrhythmia, and cerebral anoxemia secondary to hypocapnia and severe alkalemia. During prolonged mechanical ventilation, the patient may be kept amnesic by intravenous diazepam (0.1 mg/kg every 3 to 6 hours). Morphine (0.1 mg/kg every 1 to 3 hours) has also been used successfully, although it is known to release histamine. Satisfactory control of ventilation is assured by frequent arterial blood gas measurements and readjustment of ventilator settings accordingly.

The patient remains paralyzed, intubated, and artificially ventilated until the lungs become wheeze-free. When there is improvement in dynamic compliance and blood gases, the patient is weaned gradually with the aid of IMV and then allowed to breathe spontaneously. Extubation is accomplished when arterial pH and P_{CO_2} give objective evidence of adequate spontaneous ventilation and oxygenation.

Congenital heart diseases

The respiratory care of the infant or child with congenital heart disease is often a continuum, beginning in the preoperative period and extending through surgery and into the postoperative period. Congenital cardiac anomalies in infants under 1 year of age are frequently manifested by the signs and symptoms of heart failure. In infants, the incidence of postoperative respiratory failure with profound hypoxemia, metabolic acidosis, or hypercapnia following cardiovascular surgery varies between 20% and 40% (Downes and others, 1970).

Left-sided obstructive lesions, such as mitral and aortic valvular disease or coarctation of the aorta, may produce early left-heart failure due to excessive work. Increased pulmonary blood flow from large left-to-right shunts at the ventricular or ductal levels also produces high-output left-heart failure. Pulmonary edema may develop with left atrial pressures as low as 15 torr (Rudolph, 1970). Pulmonary congestion may be associated with severe lower airway obstruction, decreased lung compliance, increased physiologic dead space, and intrapulmonary shunting (Talner and others, 1965; Lees and others, 1967).

Infants and older children with left-to-right shunts and without heart failure may also have impairment of lung function. In particular, those with increased pulmonary artery pressure may have significant lower airway obstruction (Motoyama and others, 1978). Increased pulmonary venous pressure is associated with increased pulmonary blood volume and increased pulmonary extravascular water (Laver and others, 1970). Engorgement of the peribronchiolar tissues and interstitial edema may compress small airways and airspaces. These changes appear to be reversible after corrective surgery (Ganeshananthan and others, 1975).

In addition to these preoperative factors, operative procedures and anesthetic technics may contribute to postoperative respiratory problems (Brown and others, 1966). Residual narcotics or general anesthetics may contribute to central nervous system depression. Occasionally, cerebral air embolism or hypoperfusion during cardiopulmonary bypass may produce delay in awakening. The residual effects of muscle relaxants will result in weakness and inability to breathe adequately.

Cardiopulmonary bypass alters pulmonary blood volume and extravascular water. Cellular debris and platelet aggregation may occlude pulmonary circulation. However, there is little clinical evidence that cardiopulmonary bypass per se has a specific detrimental effect on lung function (Laver and others, 1970). In large part, the pulmonary dysfunction seen following cardiopulmonary bypass reflects the severity of the underlying preoperative pulmonary dysfunction as aggravated by ineffective cardiac performance. Metabolic derangements and myocardial damage from the bypass may contribute to decreases in myocardial contractility and inadequate cardiac output.

Postoperative management. To measure blood pressure directly and to facilitate blood gas determinations, direct arterial cannulation is mandatory. A CVP catheter and a pulmonary artery catheter are helpful in the management of patients with complex lesions. These lines are most often placed intraoperatively. In patients with chronic pulmonary hypertension from, for example, ventricular septal defect with increased left-to-right shunt, weaning from ventilatory support has been a protracted process (Park and others, 1969). In these patients, the nasotracheal tube is left in place to facilitate ventilatory support while the neuromuscular blockade is not reversed. Partial paralysis permits controlled ventilation in the immediate postoperative period. The purpose of postoperative ventilation is to ensure optimal gas exchange and to reduce the work cost of breathing (Wilson and others, 1973). This in turn permits stabilization of cardiac output. It allows for an orderly evaluation of passive gas exchange and lung mechanics and for gradual weaning from controlled ventilation to spontaneous ventilation.

We ventilate each patient with 100% oxygen for a short period to determine the A-a gradient and to estimate the shunt fraction. The ventilator is adjusted to provide a Pa_{CO_2} between 32 and 40 torr. The FI_{O_2} is lowered in steps of 0.10 to 0.20 to provide a Pa_{O_2} of about 80 torr. Initial base deficit associated with a pH of less than 7.30 is corrected with sodium bicarbonate, provided that plasma sodium level and osmolality are not elevated.

In supine position, particularly with muscle paralysis, FRC is significantly decreased (Westbrook and others, 1973). Such effect may be more pronounced in infants, particularly after thoracotomy, and may result in small-airway closure. A low level of PEEP (3 cm H_2O) should therefore be beneficial in all patients who are intubated and ventilated mechanically.

If the A-a gradient is large, PEEP is increased in 2-cm H_2O increments. In most cases this will allow the FI_{O_2} to be lowered. Infants with severe cardiac disease and preoperative respiratory insufficiency who have had total correction of their heart lesions frequently require prolonged ventilatory support. Some of these patients require ventilatory support for more than a month.

The use of IMV has somewhat simplified the management of postoperative cardiac patients, especially infants, making the transition from total mechanical ventilation to spontaneous ventilation smoother. As the patient's ventilation and gas exchange improve, the inspired oxygen concentration and/or the amount of machine-assisted ventilation can be decreased.

Stewart and associates (1973) have suggested spontaneous breathing with CPAP as an alternative way of providing adequate oxygenation postoperatively in infants. They reverse the neuromuscular blocking agents and begin with spontaneous breathing with CPAP.

Gregory and associates (1975) observed marked decreases in FRC in infants less than 3 months of age following cardiac surgery. CPP of 5 cm H_2O was associated with significant increases toward normal in FRC and Pa_{O_2}. Hatch and associates (1973) also noted that CPAP significantly increased oxygenation of infants with preoperative pulmonary hypertension in whom static pulmonary compliance was low. There was no significant benefit from CPAP in those infants whose compliance was normal.

General criteria for weaning from machine-assisted to spontaneous ventilation have been discussed previously.

Neurogenic disorders

Unlike the patient with respiratory insufficiency caused by intrinsic lung disease, patients in ventilatory decompensation with progressive neuromuscular disease or coma usually have normal lungs initially. The goal of respiratory support in these patients is to relieve upper airway obstruction, to protect the lung from aspiration or regurgitation of gastric contents or salivary secretions, and to provide a means for sighing and removal of secretions. In the absence of upper airway obstruction, gas exchange may initially be normal in these patients.

Guillain-Barré syndrome. Guillain-Barré syndrome is an example of a progressive neuromuscular disease. This syndrome, acute progressive polyneuritis, often follows a nonspecific viral illness. It probably represents a hypersensitivity neural reaction. The disease strikes all age groups. Early symptoms are paresthesias, pain, and weakness. The muscle weakness is progressive and usually ascending in nature; cranial nerves may be involved (Markland and Riley, 1967; McFarland and Heller, 1966).

In those patients with rapidly ascending weakness, respiratory insufficiency is common. Paralysis of the phrenic nerve and bulbar involvement usually follow significant arm weakness. Restlessness and anxiety are early symptoms of respiratory insufficiency. Serial VC or peak expiratory flow measurements are useful in following the course of the respiratory muscle weakness. VC below 20 ml/kg will not allow sufficient respiratory reserve to cough. These patients also have increased risk of aspiration because of depressed swallowing mechanisms and depressed laryngeal reflexes. Arterial blood gases may show progressive hypercapnia.

Management. These patients require endotracheal intubation to protect the airway from aspiration of secretions or gastric contents, to provide assisted or controlled ventilation, and to provide a means for artificial coughing and sighing. Return of muscular function may occur within several days to weeks following the progressive muscular weakness. We begin with insertion of nasotracheal tubes and provide a tracheostomy for airway care in those who show no rapid improvement. Unless pneumonia or aspiration occurs, there are no problems with gas exchange. Aseptic airway care is important to avoid superimposed infection.

Reye's syndrome. Reye's syndrome is a metabolic encephalopathy associated with liver failure that was originally described independently by Reye and associates (1963) and Johnson and associates (1963). It occurs in children of all ages. The syndrome may appear sporadically or in epidemic fashion in association with outbreaks of *Hemophilus influenzae* A and B or varicella. The pathogenic mechanisms and prognostic parameters have not been identified. Pernicious vomiting invariably occurs during recovery from the prodromal infection. Huttenlocher (1972) divided the disease process into four stages. More recently, Lovejoy and associates (1974) proposed the clinical staging of the depth of cerebral dysfunction as follows: stage I, *lethargy* and sleepiness with vomiting; stage II, *disorientation*, delirium and agitation, hyperventilation, and hyperactive reflexes but appropriate response to noxious stimuli; stage III, *coma*, obtundent, hyperventilation, decorticate rigidity, nonpurposeful avoidance

movements to noxious stimuli, and intact pupillary reflexes; stage IV, *decerebrate rigidity*, deepening coma, large fixed pupils, spontaneous breathing, and decerebrate posturing with strong noxious stimuli; stage V, *apnea*, seizures, loss of deep tendon reflexes, and flaccidity. Hypoglycemia, increased ammonia, abnormal liver function, especially prolonged prothrombin time, and elevated SGOT are common. Jaundice is rare. Extreme central hyperventilation is common. Increased intracranial pressure (ICP) with brain herniation appears to be the major cause of death.

Management. Until recently, a variety of treatment protocols, including exchange transfusion and peritoneal dialysis, have been advocated. The superiority of such specific treatment protocols over supportive therapy has not been demonstrated, and mortality remains between 30% and 100%, with most deaths occuring within 2 to 3 days following the onset of cerebral symptoms. Supportive measures have included airway management, a hepatic coma regimen of vitamin K, neomycin, and saline enemas, maintenance of blood glucose level at about 100 mg/dl, and attempts to establish and maintain euthermia in the febrile patient.

In those patients with rapid deterioration or in clinical stage IV (i.e., coma with decerebrate posturing), increased intracranial pressure (ICP) should be presumed. ICP monitoring can make the treatment of intracranial hypertension more rational. Clinical evaluation is unreliable both in detecting increased ICP and in determining the effectiveness of therapy to control ICP. An intraventricular cannula can be inserted under local anesthesia through a small burr hole into the anterior horn of the lateral ventricle of the nondominant hemisphere. Similarly, a subdural catheter for pressure monitoring can be inserted under local anesthesia. Cerebrospinal fluid sampling and drainage are possible with an intraventricular line. Sustained ICP of greater than 15 torr or cerebral perfusion pressure of less than 50 torr indicates the need for more aggressive therapy (Mickell and others, 1976).

Mild elevations of ICP may reduce tissue perfusion severely once the brain loses its ability to compensate for acute changes in intracranial volume. Moreover, mild elevations of ICP may reflect only a fraction of elevations in brain interstitial pressure in regions remote from the ventricles. Therefore, it seems reasonable to treat mildly elevated ICP in the injured brain.

Reduction of ICP can be attempted by a combination of measures. Phenobarbital may be administered to maintain an effective blood level (30 $\mu g/ml$). Hyperventilation to a Pa_{CO_2} of about 20 torr may dramatically lower ICP early in the course of intracranial hypertension. Osmotherapy (mannitol, 0.25 to 1 g/kg) may be used to redistribute brain water into the vascular compartment. Fluid balance must be frequently reassessed to prevent progressive dehydration and serum hyperosmolarity greater than 350 mOsm/L. Small volumes of cerebrospinal fluid can be withdrawn from the intraventricular cannula as long as there is an adequate reservoir of fluid. Finally, therapeutic hypothermia of 30° to 32° C can be instituted in those patients in whom ICP cannot be controlled. In our institution, more aggressive treatment with continuous monitoring of ICP through an intraventricular cannula, of pulmonary artery pressure with a flow-directed catheter (Swan-Ganz), and of radial artery pressure has resulted in a significant improvement in mortality and morbidity since 1975. Out of 29 cases, 24 were in stage III coma and required ICP monitoring. Twenty-seven children (93%) survived; in three of the survivors (10%), significant neurologic residua remained (Schaywitz, and others, 1979).

BIBLIOGRAPHY

Abbott, T. R.: Complications of prolonged nasotracheal intubation in children, Br. J. Anaesth. **40**:347, 1968.

Aberdeen, E.: Mechanical pulmonary ventilation in infants; tracheostomy and tracheostomy care in infants, Proc. R. Soc. Med. **58**:900, 1965.

Adair, J. C., Ring, W. H., Jordan, W. S., and Elwyn, R. A.: Ten-year experience with IPPB in the treatment of acute laryngotracheobronchitis, Anesth. Analg. (Cleve.) **50**:649, 1971.

Allen, T. H., and Stevens, I. M.: Prolonged endotracheal intubation in infants and children, Br. J. Anaesth. **37**:566, 1965.

Ashbaugh, D. G., and Petty, T. L.: Positive end-expiratory pressure, J. Thorac, Cardiovasc. Surg. **65**:165, 1973.

Baker, J. P.: Magnitude of usage of intermittent positive pressure breathing, Am. Rev. Respir. Dis. **110**:170, 1974.

Barnes, C. M.: Levels of consciousness indicated by response of children to phenomena in the intensive care unit, Ph.D. dissertation, Pittsburgh, 1975, University of Pittsburgh, Dissertation Abstracts International, vol. 35, no. 11.

Binda, R., Fischer, C. G., and Cook, D. R.: Advantages of infant ventilators over adapted adult ventilators in pediatrics, Anesth. Analg. (Cleve.) **55**:769, 1976.

Bonta, B. W., Uauy, R., Warshaw, J. B., and Motoyama, E. K.: Determination of optimal airway pressure for the treatment of IRDS by measurement of esophageal pressure, J. Pediatr. **91**:449, 1977.

Brandstater, B., and Muallem, M.: Atelectasis following tracheal suction in infants, Anesthesiology **31**:468, 1969.

Breivik, H., Grenvik, A., Millen, E., and Safar, P.: Normalizing low arterial CO_2 tension during mechanical ventilation, Chest **63**:525, 1973.

Brown, K., Johnston, A. E., and Conn, A. W.: Respiratory insufficiency and its treatment following pediatric cardiovascular surgery, Can. Anaesth. Soc. J. **13**:342, 1966.

Brück, K., Parmelee, H., Jr., and Brück, M.: Neutral temperature range and range of "thermal comfort" in premature infants, Biol. Neonate **4**:32, 1962.

Burke-Strickland, M., and Edwards, N. B.: Meconium aspiration in the newborn, Minn. Med. **56**:1031, 1973.

Chernick, V.: Continuous negative chest wall pressure therapy for hyaline membrane disease, Pediatr. Clin. North Am. **20**:407, 1973.

Civetta, J. M., and Gabel, J. C.: Flow directed–pulmonary artery catheterization in surgical patients; indications and modifications of technic, Ann. Surg. **176**:753, 1972.

Clark, J. M., and Lambertsen, C. J.: Pulmonary oxygen toxicity; a review, Pharmacol. Rev. **23**:37, 1971.

Cochran, W. D., Davis, H. T., and Smith, C. A.: Advantages and complications of umbilical artery catheterization in the newborn, Pediatrics **42**:769, 1968.

Cox, J. M. R.: Prolonged pediatric ventilatory assistance and related problems, Crit. Care Med. **1**:158, 1973.

Déry, R.: Humidity in anesthesiology. IV. Determination of the alveolar humidity and temperature in the dog, Can. Anaesth. Soc. J. **18**:145, 1971.

Downes, J. J.: CPAP and PEEP—a Perspective, Anesthesiology **44**:1, 1976.

Downes, J. J., Nicodemus, H. F., Pierce, W. S., and Waldhausen, J. A.: Acute respiratory failure in infants following cardiovascular surgery, J. Thorac. Cardiovasc. Surg. **59**:21, 1970.

Downes, J. J., and Raphaely, R. C.: Pediatric intensive care, Anesthesiology **43**:238, 1975.

Downes, J. J., Striker, T. W., and Stool, S.: Complications of nasotracheal intubation in children with croup, N. Engl. J. Med. 274:226, 1966.

Downes, J. J., Wood, D. W., Harwood, I., and others: Effects of intravenous isoproterenol infusion in children with severe hypercapnia due to status asthmaticus, Crit. Care Med. 1:63, 1973.

Downes, J. J., Wood, D. W., Striker, T. W., and Haddad, C.: Acute respiratory failure in infants with bronchiolitis, Anesthesiology 29:426, 1968.

Downes, J. J., Wood, D. W., Striker, T. W., and Pittman, P. C.: Arterial blood gas and acid-base disorders in infants and children with status asthmaticus, Pediatrics 42:238, 1968a.

Downs, J. B., Klein, E. F., Desantels, D., and others: Intermittent mandatory ventilation; a new approach to weaning patients from mechanical ventilators, Chest 64:331, 1973.

Duc, G., Bucher, H. U., and Micheli, J. L.: Is transcutaneous PO_2 reliable for arterial oxygen monitoring in newborn infants? Pediatrics 55:566, 1975.

Eden, A. N., Kaufman, A., and Yu, R.: Corticosteroids and croup, J.A.M.A. 200:403, 1967.

Epstein, R. A.: The sensitivity and response times of ventilatory assistors, Anesthesiology 34:321, 1971.

Fahri, L. E.: Atmospheric nitrogen and its role in modern medicine, J.A.M.A. 188:984, 1964.

Finberg, L.: Danger to infants caused by changes in osmolal concentration, Pediatrics 40:1031, 1967.

Forbes, A. R.: Humidification and mucus flow in the intubated trachea, Br. J. Anaesth. 45:874, 1973.

Fox, W. W., Berman, L. S., Downes, J. J., Jr., and Peckham, G. J.: The therapeutic application of end-expiratory pressure in the meconium aspiration syndrome, Pediatrics 56:214, 1975.

Froese, A. B., and Bryan, A. C.: Effects of anesthesia and paralysis on diaphragmatic mechanics in man, Anesthesiology 41:242, 1974.

Ganeshananthan, M., Goto, H., and Motoyama, E. K.: Reversibility of obstructive lung disease in children with heart disease, Am. Rev. Respir. Dis. 111:937, 1975.

Gardner, H. G., Powell, K. R., Roden, V. J., and Cherry, J. D.: The evaluation of racemic epinephrine in the treatment of infectious croup, Pediatrics 52:52, 1973.

Glezen, W. P., and Denny, F. W.: Epidemiology of acute lower respiratory disease in children, N. Engl. J. Med. 288:498, 1973.

Goddard, J. E., Jr., Phillips, O. C., and Marcy, J. H.: Betamethasone for prophylaxis of postintubation inflammation; a double-blind study, Anesth. Analg. (Cleve.) 46:348, 1967.

Godfrey, S.: Childhood asthma. In Clark, T. J. H., and Godfrey, S., editors: Asthma, Philadelphia, 1977, W. B. Saunders Co.

Gooding, C. A., and Gregory, G. A.: Roentgenographic analysis of meconium aspiration of the newborn, Radiology 100:131, 1971.

Gordon, E.: The acid-balance and oxygen tension of the cerebrospinal fluid, and their implications for the treatment of patients with brain lesions, Acta Anaesthesiol. Scand. (Suppl.) 39:1, 1971.

Gregory, G. A.: Noise levels in pressure boxes, N. Engl. J. Med. 287:617, 1972.

Gregory, G. A., Edmunds, L. H., Jr., Kitterman, J. A., and others: Continuous positive airway pressure and pulmonary and circulatory function after cardiac surgery in infants less than three months of age, Anesthesiology 43:426, 1975.

Gregory, G. A., Gooding, C. A., Phibbs, R. H., and Tooley, W. H.: Meconium aspiration in infants; a prospective study, J. Pediatr. 85:848, 1974.

Gregory, G. A., Kitterman, J. A., Phibbs, R. H., and others: Treatment of the idiopathic respiratory-distress syndrome with continuous positive airway pressure, N. Engl. J. Med. 284:1333, 1971.

Haddad, C., and Richards, C. C.: Mechanical ventilation of infants; significance and elimination of ventilator compression volume, Anesthesiology 29:365, 1968.

Hamilton, F. N., and Singer, M. M.: A breathing circuit for continuous positive airway pressure, Crit. Care Med. 2:86, 1974.

Hatch, D. J., Taylor, B. W., Glover, W. J., and others: Continuous positive-airway pressure after open-heart operations in infancy, Lancet 2:469, 1973.

Hodgkin, J. E., Bowser, M. A., and Burton, G. G.: Respiratory weaning, Crit. Care Med. 2:96, 1974.

Hoffman, L. I., Caspe, W. B., Gagliardi, J. V., and Campbell, A. G. M.: Noise levels in pressure boxes, N. Engl. J. Med. 287:617, 1972.

Huch, R., Huch, A., Albani, M., and others: Transcutaneous PO_2 monitoring in routine management of infants and children with cardiorespiratory problems, Pediatrics 57:681, 1976.

Huch, R., Huch, A., and Lubbers, D. W.: Transcutaneous measurement of blood PO_2; method and application in perinatal medicine, J. Perinat. Med. 1:183, 1973.

Huttenlocher, P. R.: Reye's syndrome; relation of outcome to therapy, J. Pediatr. 80:845, 1972.

Hyatt, R. E.: Intermittent positive breathing therapy, Am. Rev. Respir. Dis. 110:169, 1974.

Jaegar, J. G., Smith, R. M., and Crocker, D.: Modification of an adult ventilator to an infant ventilator, Can. Anaesth. Soc. J. 19:567, 1972.

James, L. S., and Lanman, J. T.: History of oxygen therapy and retrolental fibroplasia, Pediatrics 57:591, 1976.

Johnson, G. M., Scurletis, T. D., and Carroll, N. B.: A study of sixteen fatal cases of encephalitis-like disease in North Carolina children, N.C. Med. J. 24:464, 1963.

Jordan, W. S.: Laryngotracheobronchitis; evaluation of new therapeutic approaches, Rocky Mt. Med. J. 63:69, 1966.

Jordan, W. S.: New therapy for postintubation laryngeal edema and tracheitis in children, J.A.M.A. 212:585, 1970.

Weaver, R. L., and Ahlgren, E. W.: Umbilical artery catheterization in neonates, Am. J. Dis. Child. **122:** 499, 1971.

Weber, M. L., Desjardins, R., Perreault, G., and others: Acute epiglottitis in children—treatment with nasotracheal intubation; report of 14 consecutive cases, Pediatrics **57:**152, 1976.

Weller, M. H.: The roentgenographic course and complications of hyaline membrane disease, Pediatr. Clin. North Am. **20:**381, 1973.

Westbrook, P. R., Stubbs, S. E., Sessler, A. D., and others: Effects of anesthesia and muscle paralysis on respiratory mechanics in normal man, J. Appl. Physiol. **34:**81, 1973.

Westley, C. R., Brooks, J. G., and Cotton, E. K.: Nebulized racemic epinephrine administered by intermittent positive pressure breathing more effective than nebulized saline by IPPB in the treatment of croup, Pediatr. Res. **10:**470, 1976.

Wilson, R. S., and Pontoppidan, H.: Acute respiratory failure; diagnostic and therapeutic criteria, Crit. Care Med. **2:**293, 1974.

Wilson, R. S., Sullivan, S. F., Malm, J. R., and Bowman, F. O.: The oxygen cost of breathing following anesthesia and cardiac surgery, Anesthesiology **39:** 387, 1973.

Winter, P. M., and Smith, G.: The toxicity of oxygen, Anesthesiology **37:**210, 1972.

Wohl, M. E. B., Stigol, L. C., and Mead, J.: Resistance of total respiratory system in healthy infants and infants with bronchiolitis, Pediatrics **43:**495, 1969.

Wolfsdorf, J., Swift, D. L., and Avery, M. E.: Mist therapy reconsidered; an evaluation of the respiratory deposition of labelled water aerosols produced by jet and ultrasonic nebulizers, Pediatrics **43:**799, 1969.

Wood, R. E., and Farrell, P. M.: Epidemiology of respiratory distress syndrome (RDS), Pediatr. Res. **8:** 452, 1974.

Yeh, T. F., Vidyasagar, D., and Pildes, R. S.: Critical care problems of the newborn; insensible water loss in small premature infants, Crit. Care Med. **3:**238, 1975.

Young, J. A., and Crocker, D.: Principles and practice of respiratory therapy, Chicago, 1976, Year Book Medical Publishers, Inc.

Zapletal, A., Motoyama, E. K., Gibson, L. E., and Bouhuys, A.: Pulmonary mechanics in asthma and cystic fibrosis, Pediatrics **48:**64, 1971.

Zapletal, A., Paul, T., and Samanek, M.: Pulmonary elasticity in children and adolescents, J. Appl. Physiol. **40:**953, 1976.

CHAPTER 28

Mortality in pediatric surgery and anesthesia

Review of literature
Mortality statistics at The Children's Hospital
Medical Center

Although there are many aspects of pediatric anesthesia, one might expect mortality figures to give final evidence of the adequacy of our efforts, comparing present data of pediatric anesthesia with those of previous years as well as with current mortality figures of adult anesthesia.

Unfortunately, it has been extremely difficult to establish mortality figures with any accuracy for either pediatric or adult anesthesia. However, the subject is an important one and definitely deserves discussion.

There have been many reports containing statistics of anesthetic mortality, particularly from Madison, Wis., thanks to Waters and Gillespie (1944), who initiated painstaking studies of all imaginable factors, to Dornette and Orth (1956), and to a series of subsequent reports continued by Siebecker and Bamforth. Extensive studies of the total anesthetic production of a single hospital have been made, as have studies of hospital groups, including the well-known Beecher-Todd study of 1954 and those of Edwards and associates (1956) of Britain and Kok and Mullan (1969) of Praetoria. In spite of the fastidious detail followed in many of these studies, there are several reasons why few, if any, of the figures can serve as established criteria.

One outstanding reason is that it is extremely difficult to define the term "anesthetic death," as is evident in the variety of interpretations used in papers that have been published on the subject (Keats, 1979). The simple matter of the time of death has caused considerable difficulty. Some writers have included only patients who died during operation; many have included deaths that occurred within 24 hours of operation; others made 48 hours the time limit; and still others have extended the time limit to 2 weeks after operation, but there has been no set standard. Since a patient could suffer severe hypoxic brain damage during anesthesia and not die for weeks or months afterward, any short time limit would be inaccurate. When large numbers are being dealt with, the accuracy is not affected if a few are missed in the count, but in recent studies involving only one or two deaths in several thousand anesthetics, the difference could be great.

Several other factors reduce the value of mortality figures currently available. The age of patients, although of less importance than once assumed, should be considered if different studies are to be compared. Of much greater importance is the physical status of patients in any study, since records of a center for terminal cancer could hardly be compared with those of a suburban community hospital dealing with incidental surgical procedures. In the same category, difference in the type of operation must be taken into account, for statistics on death occurring in relation to circumcision and dental extraction could hardly be compared with those related to open-heart procedures.

One critical variable in the incidence of perioperative deaths is the type of overall care. This, of course, is what anesthetic death incidence is supposed to measure, but there are several factors that underlie this aspect in addition to the person at the head of the table.

The surgeon obviously is accountable as a factor in operative morbidity and mortality (Moyer and Key, 1956). It should be emphasized, however, that his pedigree as professor and writer may be deceiving, for speed can be of greater importance to the survival of the patient. One of the very important problems of modern anesthesia is the fact that in teaching hospitals, major operations often take two or three times as long as the same procedure performed by a skilled operator not imbued with the desire to lecture while operating. As emphasized in Chapter 9 and recently documented by Cooper and associates (1978), anesthesiologist fatigue is a significant factor in the etiology of anesthetic complications. Methods should be developed to overcome the dangers related to the effect of prolonged procedures on anesthetic care.

As mentioned in Chapter 15, the weakest link in perioperative care of pediatric patients may be in early postoperative care, which requires an expert around-the-clock team of intensive care and recovery nurses and physicians as well as anesthesiologists and surgeons. Because many so-called anesthetic deaths are now related to early postoperative management, the comparable adequacy of care must be a consideration in overall statistical evaluation.

The above features are only minor reasons why anesthetic mortality standards have been difficult to establish. By far the greatest problem has been that of determining the actual pathologic cause of death in many surgical patients. There are a few that leave little doubt that the cause was anesthetic. Included here would be an anesthetic explosion and the death of a previously healthy patient due to local anesthetic reaction, to aspiration of vomitus or other types of airway occlusion such as obstructed endotracheal tube or neglected pack left in a patient's pharynx, and to malignant hyperthermia. Usually the death of a patient who is anesthetized but dies before surgery begins may be assumed to be due to anesthesia, but it is hardly fair to term this an anesthetic death, with the attendant implications, if the patient was one who had been moribund and was hurried to the operating room for a terminal attempt at salvage.

The "attendant implications" mentioned above refer to the fact that there is an unwarranted assumption that an anesthetic death means a preventable death and one involving error or negligence on the part of the anesthesiologist. This will be discussed in more detail in Chapter 29.

There are several situations in which anesthesia definitely is not implicated in perioperative death, as when the surgeon opens the aorta on dividing the sternum or when an infant with left-heart insufficiency cannot maintain flow after open-heart repair. Unfortunately, the majority of deaths in the operative period involve patients whose illness reduces them to high-risk status before operation, and postoperative demise, even when due to cardiac failure, infection, or ileus, may have been precipitated by unrecognized effects of drug interaction or usually tolerable degrees of hypotension. Among the most difficult to diagnose accurately have been deaths due to pathology, such as hepatitis, that have several known but indistinguishable causes.

REVIEW OF LITERATURE

One may pick out ten or twenty reports on anesthetic mortality that have been based on work within the past 2 or 3 decades. It is interesting to find how the problems just mentioned have been handled in each report. The interpretation of the term "anesthetic death" comes up at once. Few writers have included a precise definition, but in the Beecher-Todd report it is stated that a death that could not be explained on any other basis would be tallied as an anesthetic death. Most of the more recent studies designate a principal cause, when possible, and contributing causes, thereby including several and dividing the responsibility.

Data of the University of Wisconsin (1954 to 1962), Beecher and Todd (1954), and Kok and Mullan (1969) were basically alike in placing the incidence of anesthetic death in adults at approximately 1 per 1500. In these reports, as was customary at that time, age groups were broken down into decades, but no further. It appeared from these reports that the incidence of anesthetic deaths was distinctly higher in the first decade, probably in the vicinity of 1 per 1000 throughout the entire decade, and higher than any other until the seventh decade was reached. The impression gained was that all children under 10 should be considered greater anesthetic risks than the average patient. This stimulated greater caution in some but also was used as an excuse for many preventable complications and fatalities actually due to inadequate equipment, poor patient preparation, aspiration, and lack of monitoring and/or fluid therapy (Smith, 1956; Graff and others, 1964; Wilson and others, 1969).

The study of Edwards and associates (1956), covering 1000 deaths associated with anesthesia in Britain between 1950 and 1955, points out characteristic errors of that time, recording fourteen sudden intraoperative deaths that occurred in children, several of whom were being anesthetized with unsuitable adult equipment. Aspiration of vomitus is mentioned repeatedly in death reports prior to 1960 and claimed the lives of many children anesthetized for trifling procedures such as reduction of Colles' fracture or dental extraction. With improved management of this problem as well as attempts to perform more extensive operations, intraoperative hemorrhage became the outstanding cause of death, attended by complications associated with rapid blood replacement or the lack of it (Boyan, 1964).

The report of Pledger and Buchan (1969) concerning deaths of children undergoing appendectomy in Britain between 1962 and 1967 gives more insight into our problems. A total of 146 deaths occurred, among whom 54 were believed to have had inadequate fluids, 19 developed temperatures of 40.5° C or more, 13 convulsed, and 10 had major hypoxic episodes. Although this report brings us up to relatively recent time, it is to be hoped that most of these errors have become obsolete.

Impressive statistics were presented by Wilson and associates (1969), who first estimated that 5 million pediatric anesthetics were administered in this country annually, quoted anesthetic death rates for all ages as 3.8 per 10,000 operations and for children as 12.8 per 10,000 operations, and, among other calculations, postulated that there would be one anesthetic death in every 303 anesthetics administered to children in A.S.A. Physical Status Categories 3, 4, and 5. A higher incidence of postoperative death will naturally be expected in poor-risk patients (Elwyn, 1978), but the incidence of anesthetic deaths may still be maintained at a near-zero level under favorable circumstances of personnel and equipment.

The report of Wilson and associates was of further interest in that it dealt chiefly with severely burned children and the resultant problems of extreme heat loss, complications of massive blood loss at skin grafting, and postoperative psychologic problems.

At this time, the establishment of reliable data on overall anesthetic mortality still appears to be difficult. However, by indirect approaches to the problem, enough evidence has been gathered to alter our traditional views rather drastically. Since one of our major problems has been to decide which deaths should be listed as anesthetic, it has been helpful to look for groups of operations in which there were no deaths at all, thereby eliminating the need to decide the cause of death. The widespread popularity of tonsillectomy over the past decades has provided an opportunity to examine results of treatment in comparatively well-controlled groups and also to bear witness to what can be accomplished without mortality.

The excellent achievements reported by several teams seem hardly believable after one reads the estimates of pediatric mortality. Naturally, some of the less successful records have not been documented. A review by Davies (1964) includes the following accomplishments of British surgeons and anesthetists in their management of tonsillectomies:

Author	Opera-tions	Total deaths	Anesthetic deaths
Martin (1922) and Minnitt and Gillies (1948)	23,900	8	3
Campbell and Smith (1955)	12,038	0	0
Welsh (1959)	35,000	0	0
Finer and Stahle (1961)	30,000	0	0
Davies (1964)	21,000	5	1

To these figures should be added the 1974 record of Petruscak and associates of the Pittsburgh Eye and Ear Hospital: no deaths from any cause in 37,000 tonsillectomies.

From figures such as these, it becomes evident that tonsillectomy, even in children, does not carry an obligatory or expected mortality and that the death of any child, whether due to surgery or anesthesia, calls for some explanation. The lesson learned from these data applies broadly to normal children undergoing elective surgical procedures.

No other surgical procedures have amassed such vast totals or can be judged so assuredly as tonsillectomy, but data on specific types of procedures that present limited variables provide valuable examples of what can be accomplished under favorable conditions. Such records include those of Koop and associates (1974), who reported 50 consecutive survivals of neonates operated on for uncomplicated tracheoesophageal fistula, Welch of The Children's Hospital Medical Center, who has corrected over 900 pectus excavatus deformities without mortality, and MacCollum and Gifford, also at our hospital, who have repaired over 4500 cleft lips and palates without mortality. It should be emphasized that such examples cannot be set up at this time as standards that all must attain in order to be considered competent. These records do stand as evidence of the potential viability of pediatric patients as well as the improved capability of surgeons and anesthesiologists.

To return to the problem of reporting overall figures for the entire surgical activity of an institution, this calls for scrupulous collection of all available data and discussion by a group of involved and uninvolved physicians. Such an undertaking has been accomplished by Elwyn (1978), who reported a total of 29,101 anesthetics with only one anesthetic death. His study included all of the anesthetics administered to children under 11 years of age at Primary Children's Hospital in Salt Lake City between 1970 and 1975. His summary includes the following information: a total of 127 deaths occurred, 62.2% were thoracic, 15% were neurosurgical, and 15% were abdominal cases; 48 deaths, or 42%, occurred in the first week of life, and 79 deaths, or 71%, occurred in the first 12 months.

Downes and Raphaely (1979) reported an anesthetic mortality of 0.2 per 10,000 (50,000 patients) at Philadelphia Children's Hospital. This study included deaths that occurred within 24 hours after operation.

MORTALITY STATISTICS AT THE CHILDREN'S HOSPITAL MEDICAL CENTER

In earlier editions of this book, attempts were made to present a variety of figures representing the number of operations performed, the age of patients, their physical status, the total number of deaths occurring within a year following operation, and the number of deaths believed to be due to anesthesia. A brief summary of the principal findings in the data from 1956 through 1960 and from 1962 through 1966 is shown below.

Patients anesthetized under 1 year of age	11,817
Patients under 1 year of age who died within 1 year after operation	495 (4.1%)
Deaths due primarily to anesthesia	3 (1:3700)
Patients anesthetized between 1 and 10 years of age	42,920
Patients between 1 and 10 years of age who died	354 (0.82%)

Deaths due primarily to anesthesia   4 (1:10,700)

Total patients anesthetized between 0 and 10 years of age   54,737

Total deaths, 0 to 10 years old   849 (1.5%)

Deaths due primarily to anesthesia   7 (1:7800)

From the information gained in the earlier data, it appeared obvious that there was a great difference in the perioperative mortality in the first year of life, where 495 of 11,817 infants died (mortality of 4.0%) as compared with 354 deaths that occurred in a total of 42,920 anesthetics administered to all children between 1 and 10 years of age (mortality of 0.82%). These figures suggested that while the infant under 1 year old was definitely a higher operative risk, children beyond that age should prove to be the best possible candidates for anesthesia.

By use of criteria then current, 11 deaths were attributed to anesthesia. Thus, the total of 11 deaths in 54,737 anesthetics gave an incidence of two anesthetic deaths per 10,000 anesthetics in patients under 10 years of age, or one death per 5000. This was far better than the assumed incidence for children (1 per 1000) and also better than the accepted anesthetic death rate for adults (1 per 1500).

Data concerning the years 1968 through 1978 have been added to those previously reported, arriving at a total of 116,784 patients under 10 years of age, of whom 1534 were known to have died (mortality of 1.4%). The number of deaths ascribed to anesthesia for the entire 116,784 was 15. These figures, and those related to an additional 50,000 patients over 10 years of age, are shown in Table 28-1. In this table it may be seen that there is a gradual increase in the total num-

Table 28-1. Anesthetic and surgical statistics, The Children's Hospital Medical Center, Boston

| Year | 0-10 yr | | | | 10-20 yr | | | | Total 0-20 yr |
	Operations	Deaths	Per-cent	Anesthetic deaths	Operations	Deaths	Per-cent	Anesthetic deaths	
1954	3516	67	1.9	0	684	6	0.9	0	4200
1955	3424	58	1.7	2	633	3	0.5	0	4057
1956	4013	54	1.3	2	867	3	0.3	0	4880
1957	4013	70	1.7	1	1455	6	0.4	0	5468
1958	4301	83	1.9	2	1462	13	0.9	0	5763
1959	4419	85	1.9	1	1036	23	2.2	0	5455
1960	4512	78	1.7	1	1024	25	2.4	0	5536
1962	4340	69	1.6	0	1335	21	1.6	0	5675
1963	4874	71	1.5	0	1491	9	0.6	0	6355
1964	5098	74	1.5	1	1724	10	0.6	0	6822
1965	5627	71	1.3	0	1760	14	0.7	0	7387
1966	5969	69	1.1	0	1946	15	0.8	0	7915
1968	6745	69	1.0	0	2451	12	0.5	0	9196
1969	6440	75	1.2	0	2141	13	0.6	0	8581
1970	6225	57	0.9	0	2578	15	0.6	0	8803
1971	5675	65	1.1	2	3301	31	0.9	1	8976
1972	6257	68	1.1	0	2815	16	0.6	0	9072
1973	6351	76	1.2	0	2703	23	0.9	0	9054
1974	5220	66	1.3	1	3464	25	0.7	0	8684
1975	4828	41	0.8	1	4148	17	0.4	0	8976
1976	4952	52	1.0	0	3462	19	0.5	2	8414
1977	5074	56	1.1	0	4228	16	0.4	0	9302
1978	4911	60	1.2	0	3460	21	0.6	0	8371
TOTAL	116,784	1534	1.3	14	50,168	356	0.6	3	166,942

ber of children under 10 years of age and a much more rapid increase in the older group. The incidence of death from all causes remains remarkably constant in the younger group, while the incidence in the older group first is lower, then higher, and finally approximately the same as the younger group. These changes are caused by different trends in the types of surgery performed.

Tables 28-2 and 28-3 show a breakdown of patients under 10 years in respect to age, physical status, and incidence of death. The comparable data of 1956 and 1971 shows considerable similarity in spite of the 15-year difference.

Summarized below is information on the anesthetic deaths incurred.

FIRST SERIES: 1956 THROUGH 1960 AND 1962 THROUGH 1966
Children 0 to 10 years of age

1. **Age:** Newborn. **Diagnosis:** Diaphragmatic hernia. **Status:** ASA 4.
   Postanesthetic death caused by bilateral pneumothorax. Attempt to expand lungs during operation believed to be cause of pneumothoraces, though this complication is common following any management of diaphragmatic hernia. (1956)
2. **Age:** 1 month. **Diagnosis:** Coarctation of the aorta, hypoplastic left arch. **Status:** ASA 4.

To-and-fro cyclopropane anesthesia was tolerated until the chest and pericardium were opened. Complete atrioventricular block occurred and could not be controlled with pacemaker or cardiotonic drugs. Excessive depth of anesthesia suspected. (1959)

3. **Age:** 3 months. **Diagnosis:** Lung abscess, failure to thrive. **Status:** ASA 4.
   Failure to maintain airway in presence of copious thick pus. Pneumonectomy followed by death 1 hour after operation. Continued hypoxemia suspected as major cause. (1959)
4. **Age:** $1^{11}/_{12}$ years. **Diagnosis:** Coarctation of aorta, mitral stenosis, pulmonary hypertension, tricuspid atresia, endocardial sclerosis, and asthma. **Status:** ASA 4.
   Induction under cyclopropane and ether was prolonged, and vomiting occurred, followed by tugging, irregular respiration. The operation progressed to the point of clamping the aorta, at which time the child's heart stopped and could not be resuscitated. Respiratory acidosis and hypoxemia suspected. (1958)
5. **Age:** $2^{5}/_{12}$ years. **Diagnosis:** Patent ductus arteriosus. **Status:** ASA 2.
   Prolonged induction and difficulty with intubation were followed by inadequate ventilation due to a leak in apparatus. There was postoperative convulsion, the temperature rose to 104° F, and the child died 48 hours later. (1958)
6. **Age:** 5 years. **Diagnosis:** Omphalocele, postrepair by skin closure. **Status:** ASA 4.
   A cachectic child with huge mass protruding

Table 28-2. Breakdown of 1956 statistics by age, physical status, and death

Age	Condition										Total
	1	1E	2	2E	3	3E	4	4E	5	5E	
0-7 days	4	1	8	0	12	14	2	35	2	2	80
7 days-1 mo	40	5	20	7	18	10	4	4		3	111
1 mo-6 mo	318	7	137	5	49	8	11	6		1	542
6 mo-1 yr	144	5	66	4	24	7	5	5	1		261
1-2 yr	259	15	106	8	38	6	6	4	2		444
2-3 yr	206	13	102	7	42	3	4	2			379
3-4 yr	206	15	124	8	34	4	7	3			401
4-5 yr	223	9	103	6	26	2	4	1			374
5-6 yr	228	16	117	12	24	8	6	3			414
6-7 yr	145	14	100	5	20	2	5	1			292
7-8 yr	131	12	66	6	17	2	4				238
8-9 yr	151	18	52	8	18	6	2	2	1		258
9-10 yr	118	17	63	6	12	1	1	1		1	219
TOTAL	2173	147	1064	82	334	73	61	67	6	6	4013

from abdomen and containing liver, spleen, and other viscera, all anterior to unyielding rectus muscles. The repair was attempted under endotracheal cyclopropane. During completion of the operation, relatively deep anesthesia was needed for closure. Sudden irreversible collapse occurred, believed to have been caused by depth of anesthesia plus obstructed vena caval flow. (1964)

7. **Age:** 6 years. **Diagnosis:** Acute glomerular nephritis and uremia (NPN 273 mg/dl). **Status:** ASA 5E.

The child was to be dialyzed, but it was decided best to rule out an obstructive renal lesion by cystoscopy beforehand. Since he was semicomatose, light nitrous oxide anesthesia was chosen. After 15 minutes of anesthesia an arrhythmia was noted, followed by cessation of action. The chest was opened, and the heart was found to be in fibrillation. Initial resuscitation appeared successful, but the child died an hour later. Although the child had been considered moribund, it was believed that the anesthesia had precipitated the death. (1964)

SECOND SERIES: 1968 THROUGH 1978
Children 0 to 10 years of age

1. **Age:** 5 years. **Diagnosis:** Acute lymphatic leukemia in remission, Down's syndrome. **Status:** ASA 3.

A 2-minute period of cardiorespiratory collapse occurred during a brief nitrous oxide–halothane–oxygen anesthetic for performance of sternal marrow biopsy. The child appeared to recover promptly but 8 hours later suddenly developed pulmonary edema and died. It was learned subsequently that the child had received doxorubicin (Adriamycin) (a total of 475 mg/m²), an antileukemic agent known to have marked cardiotoxic potential. The anesthesia, in the presence of this drug, was believed to be the reason for the collapse. (1975)

2. **Age:** 5 years. **Diagnosis:** Paroxysmal tachycardia with pacemaker failure. **Status:** ASA 4E. Cardioversion was planned, but induction of anesthesia in the absence of a temporary pacemaker, plus turning the patient, initiated arrest that proved to be terminal. Use of an intravenous pacemaker, suggested by the anesthesiologist but discouraged by the cardiologist, would have prevented this accident. (1974)

3. **Age:** 6 years. **Diagnosis:** Scoliosis and tetralogy of Fallot. **Status:** ASA 4.

This child was moderately handicapped and definitely cyanotic. Induction with oxygen, thiopental, and succinylcholine followed by endotracheal intubation seemed uneventful. Cardiorespiratory arrest occurred 5 minutes after the child had been turned to the prone position, the reason unknown. It is possible that the endotracheal tube was displaced by turning, but this did not appear to be the case. Since the intended spinal fusion had not been started, anesthesia was the apparent initiating factor. (1971)

Table 28-3. Comparable figures for 1971

Age	Condition										Total
	1	1E	2	2E	3	3E	4	4E	5	5E	
0-7 days	8	15	12	12	12	11	9	18	0	1	98
7 days - 1 mo	30	6	25	7	16	9	6	7	1	0	107
1 mo-6 mo	270	29	99	13	49	9	17	3	—	—	489
6 mo-1 yr	152	8	144	13	22	7	5	4	1	3	359
1-2 yr	291	23	91	13	30	5	5	—	—	2	460
2-3 yr	330	30	74	8	37	6	4	4	—	—	493
3-4 yr	360	36	66	23	38	1	5	3	1	—	533
4-5 yr	370	21	99	21	19	8	5	3	—	—	546
5-6 yr	380	25	67	2	26	1	9	1	—	—	511
6-7 yr	385	25	105	17	44	8	9	3	—	1	597
7-8 yr	360	30	91	4	34	1	15	3	1	—	539
8-9 yr	266	26	102	11	24	8	8	4	1	—	450
9-10 yr	287	38	105	12	36	3	6	5	—	1	493
									TOTAL		5675

4. **Age:** 8 years. **Diagnosis:** Myelomeningocele. **Status:** ASA 3.

This child had undergone many operations but was able to communicate and had adapted to his lot rather well. On the occasion of this operation, a revision of his loop colostomy, it was believed that the child was given more halothane than necessary. The child did not awaken as expected and showed progressive signs of brain damage followed by death. (1971)

Patients 10 to 20 years of age

1. **Age:** 12 years. **Diagnosis:** Chronic renal failure, for kidney transplant. **Status:** ASA 3.

A successful renal transplant was performed, but the child was held at a relatively light plane of anesthesia with halothane, nitrous oxide, and *d*-tubocurarine, and there was active motion several times during the operation. The child was extubated rather soon after completion of the procedure and developed considerable airway obstruction, which called for more suction and manipulation and reintubation. Severe difficulty with the airway continued, however, and the child died, with anesthesia the probable primary cause. (1971)

2. **Age:** 18 years. **Diagnosis:** Compound fracture of both bones of the left lower leg. **Status:** ASA 4E.

A 200-pound college football linebacker with shattered left tibia and fibula was anesthetized for reduction of fracture on the day following injury. Induction with thiopental and halothane was followed by sudden temperature elevation to 108° F and typical signs of malignant hyperthermia. He was treated successfully with internal and external cooling devices and appeared to recover completely, but no operation had been performed. Loss of circulation to the foot called for operation the next day, and a 4-hour repair was performed under Innovar without incident. After an uneventful night, he was talking with a group of nurses and doctors around his bed when he suddenly became agitated, had a severe chill and temperature elevation, and progressed rapidly from coma to standstill. He was rushed from the recovery room to the nearest operating room, and for the next 4 hours resuscitation was attempted using coolants, dantrolene, and cardiopulmonary bypass, but without success.

BIBLIOGRAPHY

Alexander, D. W., Graff, T. D., and Kelley, E.: Factors in tonsillectomy mortality, Arch. Otolaryngol. **82**:409, 1965.

Beecher, H. K., and Todd, D. P.: A study of deaths associated with anaesthesia and surgery, Springfield, Ill., 1954, Charles C Thomas, Publisher.

Boba, A.: Death in the operating room, Springfield, Ill., 1965, Charles C Thomas, Publisher.

Boyan, C. P.: Cold or warmed blood for massive transfusion? Ann. Surg. **160**:282, 1964.

Campbell, J. C., and Smith, D. H.: Guillotine tonsillectomy and curettage of adenoids under ethyl chloride anaesthesia, Br. J. Anaesth. **1**:1451, 1955.

Clifton, B. S., and Hotten, W. I. T.: Deaths associated with anaesthesia, Br. J. Anaesth. **35**:250, 1963.

Cooper, J. B., Newbower, R. S., Long, C. D., and McPeek, B.: Preventable anesthesia mishaps; a study of human factors, Anesthesiology **49**:399, 1978.

Davenport, H. T.: Paediatric anaesthesia, Philadelphia, 1967, Lea & Febiger.

Davies, D. D.: Anaesthetic mortality in tonsillectomy and adenoidectomy, Br. J. Anaesth. **36**:110, 1964.

Dornette, W. H. L., and Orth, O. S.: Death in the operating room, Anesth. Analg. (Cleve.) **35**:545, 1956.

Downes, J. J., and Raphaely, R. C.: Anesthesia and intensive care. In Ravitch, M. M., Welch, K. J., Benson, C. D., and others, editors: Pediatric surgery, ed. 3, Chicago, 1979, Year Book Medical Publishers, Inc.

Downs, T. M.: Carotid sinus as etiological factor in sudden death, Ann. Surg. **99**:974, 1934.

Edwards, G., Morton, H. J. V., Pask, E. A., and Wylie, W. D.: Deaths associated with anaesthesia; a report on 1000 cases, Anaesthesia **11**:194, 1956.

Elwyn, A. R.: Perioperative pediatric mortality; A five year study, Postgraduate Symposium on Pediatric Anesthesia, Salt Lake City, 1978.

Finer, B., and Stahle, J.: Anaesthesia in adenoidectomy, Nord. Med. **66**:963, 1961.

Gebbie, D.: Anaesthesia and death, Can. Anaesth. Soc. J. **13**:390, 1966.

Graff, T. D., Phillips, O. C., Benson, D. W., and Kelly, E.: Baltimore anesthesia study committee; factors in pediatric anesthesia mortality. Anesth. Analg. (Cleve.) **43**:407, 1964.

Jacoby, J., Lutsky, I. I., Henschel, E. O., and Green, R. E.: Fatalities erroneously attributed to anesthesia, Anesth. Analg. (Cleve.) **44**:53, 1965.

Keats, A. S.: What do we know about anesthetic mortality? Anesthesiology **50**:387, 1979.

Kok, O. V. S., and Mullan, B. S.: Deaths associated with anaesthesia and surgery; a review of 1,573 cases, medical proceedings, Mediese Bydraes **15**:31, 1969.

Koop, C. E., Schnaufer, L., and Broennle, A. M.: Esophageal atresia and tracheoesophageal atresia; supportive measures that affect survival, Pediatrics **54**:558, 1974.

Martin, G. E.: Complications following removal of the tonsils, J. Laryngol. Otol. **37**:80, 1922.

Marx, G. F., Mateo, C. V., and Larkin, L. R.: Computer analysis of postanesthetic deaths, Anesthesiology **39:**54, 1973.

Minnitt, R. J., and Gillies, J.: Textbook of anaesthetics, ed. 7, Edinburgh, 1948, E. & S. Livingstone.

Minuck, M.: Death in the operating room, Can. Anaesth. Soc. J. **14:**197, 1967.

Moyer, C. A., and Key, J. A.: Estimation of operative risk in 1955, J.A.M.A. **160:**854, 1956.

Petruscak, J., Smith, R. N., and Breslin, P.: Mortality related to ophthalmological surgery, Surv. Anesthesiol. **18:**87, 1974.

Pledger, H. G., and Buchan, R.: Deaths in children with acute appendicitis, Br. Med. J. **4:**466, 1969.

Saklad, M.: Grading patients for surgical procedures, Anesthesiology **2:**281, 1941.

Smith, R. M.: Some reasons for the high mortality in pediatric anesthesia, N.Y. State J. Med. **56:**2212, 1956.

Trent, J. C., and Gaster, E.: Anesthetic deaths in 54,128 consecutive cases, Ann. Surg. **119:**954, 1944.

Waters, R. M., and Gillespie, N. A.: Death in the operating room, Anesthesiology **5:**113, 1944.

Welsh, F.: Death from tonsillectomy (correspondence), Lancet **1:**944, 1959.

Wilson, R. D., Traber, D. L., Priano, L. L., and Evans, B. L.: Anesthetic management of the poor risk patient, South. Med. J. **62:**767, 1969.

Young, W. G., Sealy, W. C., Harris, J., and Botwin, A.: Effects of hypercapnia and hypoxia in response of heart to vagal stimulation, Surg. Gynecol. Obstet. **93:**51, 1951.

CHAPTER 29

Legal aspects of pediatric anesthesia

Interrelationship of law and medicine
Anesthesiologist's defense against legal
    action

Anesthesiologists must be increasingly aware of the possibility that they may be involved in legal suits, whether to defend themselves, to help wronged patients obtain just settlements, or to assist in the defense of a colleague. There are many factors in the practice of medicine and many specific details in the specialty of pediatric anesthesiology that one should bear in mind because of the interrelationships of law and medicine, some of which are beneficial, others necessary, and a few that impose unwelcome burdens or appear to threaten the unwary physician.

INTERRELATIONSHIP OF LAW AND MEDICINE

Exorbitant claims made for relatively minor medical misadventures and the increasing difficulty in obtaining insurance coverage at any price have given many physicians the feeling that the law stands beside them as a grim specter and that all members of the legal profession are natural enemies of the physician. Many also feel that if they are fortunate enough to avoid court action for their own defense, nothing will induce them to participate in suits in defense of a patient or colleague.

It has been enlightening to find that in addition to those lawyers who appear to live by preying on physicians, there are excellent attorneys who devote their entire practice to the defense of physicians. It also seems evident that patients must have some means of securing fair representation and reasonable retribution when there is gross and obvious harm done to them. It is difficult to imagine how either patient or colleague can be fairly defended if the only physicians willing to appear in court are a few who do so at the risk of losing the respect of their associates (Shister, 1976).

ANESTHESIOLOGIST'S DEFENSE AGAINST LEGAL ACTION

There are innumerable details in the practice of medicine that must be properly attended to in order to appear correct in the eyes of the opposing attorney. One should bear in mind at the outset that *what is written* is viewed with greater reverence in legal matters than in medicine. This applies first of all to what is or is not entered in the patient's record by the anesthesiologist and second to statements or opinions of individuals of supposed authority in various fields of medicine. It is to be expected that a patient's chart should contain full information, clearly documented, as to history and physical and laboratory findings plus a standard consent form signed by a child's parent and a witness (Wasmuth and Oleck, 1957). It is also to be expected that any unusual form of therapy will be explained to the parents of the child and will be considered by institutional committees bearing such responsibility. Above all, physicians will be expected to enter in writing motives or explanations for action that is a departure from what is considered to be "accepted" under similar circumstances. Clearly written documentation will be the greatest safeguard that any physician can provide in a courtroom. Prior to this, of course, the best way to avoid any courtroom procedure is to explain such reasoning to patients and parents and have an understanding with all parties concerned of the risk, the possibility of failure, or the cost in emotional or physical duress.

The problem of "informed consent" is particularly difficult in the practice of pediatric surgery and anesthesia. If one were to tell a parent of a fraction of the complications described in Chapter 26, few would leave their children in the hospital overnight. Parents who ask "what is the risk?" may be told with some assurance that the risk of fatality for a normal child undergoing an uncomplicated operation is less than it is when the child is sitting beside them in a moving car. Statistics in recent studies confirm this with sufficient accuracy.

There has been considerable difficulty in dealing with parents who belong to the group calling themselves Jehovah's Witnesses and much discussion among surgical teams as to whether one should give a child blood in spite of parental insistence against use of all blood products. It has been shown that a great many operations may be performed without the use of blood but that when one is faced with such a problem, it is advisable to refrain, if at all possible, from directly counteracting the parents' dictates. Instead one may attempt to persuade the parents to allow such use as is deemed necessary, obtain a court order to act according to medical indications, or refer the case to a team having greater experience in managing such procedures without the use of blood.

In the care of patients during the perioperative period, one must take particular pains to write narcotic orders clearly and to pay extra attention to the protection of patients under sedation who may be either unable to protect themselves normally or subject to injury due to hyperactivity. Any form of external heating device must be used with extreme caution and with full realization that a patient with reduced circulation will be more easily traumatized by both heat and pressure (Scott, 1967).

Damage to teeth and dental appliances is known to occur during endotracheal intubation and has been the basis for suit. When teeth are broken or dislodged during anesthesia, it has been ruled that such risk must be accepted as being one of the necessary risks of anesthesia (Graves, 1957). However, if a tooth has been dislodged, the anesthesiologist must locate it. If it has been swallowed, it may be allowed to pass through the digestive tract, but if it has been aspirated, steps must be taken for its immediate recovery. A ruling has also been made absolving anesthesiologists of responsibility for the postoperative appearance of vocal cord granulomas (Barton, 1958).

Among the precautions of increased importance in dealing with pediatric patients one includes special care to avoid placement of intravenous needles near joints, where they are more apt to become dislodged. The volar aspect of the wrist also is best avoided if possible, except for brief use for induction of anesthesia. The use of invasive monitoring devices has introduced new patient risks (Fig. 29-1), particularly in relation to air embolism and vascular injury (Camps, 1955; Miyasaka and others, 1976).

It has become increasingly important for the anesthesiologist to stay with pediatric patients until recovery from anesthesia has progressed to a suitably stable level or until reliable personnel have taken over.

In an earlier edition of this book, a statement was made to the effect that the term "anesthetic death" signified a death caused by error in judgment or technic of the anesthesiologist. This statement should be corrected, for there are definite situations where death may be related to anesthesia without error or misjudgment. A variety of unusual patient responses to customary treatment, such as malignant hyperthermia, are known that may not give appreciable forewarning and may lead to intraoperative or postoperative death. This point has recently been emphasized by Keats (1979) and refuted by Hamilton (1979).

A most fervent appeal to all anesthesiologists is to go to the extreme in document-

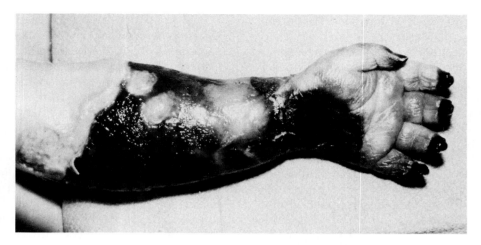

Fig. 29-1. Necrosis of forearm following iatrogenic arterial injury in a 6-month-old infant.

ing any mishap that may occur during operation (Dillon, 1957). Attorneys place unbelievable stress on the anesthesia chart and expect explicit reporting of the timing of each incident, each drug administered, and every act of resuscitation. Such charting is virtually impossible to accomplish in times of real danger unless one has an assistant to act as recorder. Such a practice is used in our institution and is definitely encouraged. It is equally important to refrain from changing anything previously entered on an important chart unless such a change is duly witnessed.

Once again, the patient and the parents provide the best protection against court action. If a mishap has occurred, one's first move is to go to the family and state the situation openly. Misunderstanding and lack of communication cause more lawsuits than malpractice. Patients with real or imagined grievances often may be satisfied by reasonable discussion with the physician. Lacking such, they more easily turn to legal action. Lawyers, taking the plaintiff's case, then set about to build a case on instances where it appears that the physician has committed or omitted some form of treatment that suggests either negligence or an "unaccepted" form

of management. One of the difficulties in the legal defense of a physician is that few lawyers and even fewer jurors realize the relative value of many of the details of medical practice. It is upsetting to find that one may be as closely questioned and as severely criticized for the manner in which one applied a blood pressure cuff as for one's failure to recognize hyperthermia before the temperature reached 106° F. Greater willingness of lawyers and physicians to communicate should improve conditions of this nature.

BIBLIOGRAPHY

Barton, R. T.: Medicolegal aspects of intubation granuloma, J.A.M.A. **166**:1821, 1958.

Camps, F. E.: Medicolegal investigations of some deaths occurring during anesthesia, N. Engl. J. Med. **253**: 643, 1955.

Dillon, J. B.: The prevention of claims for medical malpractice, Anesthesiology **18**:294, 1957.

Graves, H. B.: The medicolegal responsibilities of the anesthetist, Can. Anaesth. Soc. J. **4**:428, 1957.

Hamilton, W. K.: Editorial views; unexpected deaths during anesthesia; wherein lies the cause? Anesthesiology **50**:381, 1979.

Keats, A. S.: What do we know about anesthetic mortality? Anesthesiology **50**:387, 1979.

Miyasaka, K., Edmonds, J. F., and Conn, A. W.: Complications of radial artery lines in the pediatric patient, Can. Anaesth. Soc. J. **23:**9, 1976.

Overton, P. R.: Rule of "respondeat superior," J.A.M.A. **163:**847, 1957.

Scott, S. M.: Thermal blanket injury in the operating room, Arch, Surg. **94:**181, 1967.

Shister, N.: The M.D. expert witness; malpractice's thriving sideline, Hosp. Phys. **6:**12, 1976.

Stetler, C. J., and Moritz, A. R.: Doctor and patient and the law, ed. 4, St. Louis, 1962, The C. V. Mosby Co.

Tarrow, A. B.: Medicolegal aspects of anesthesiology, Anesth. Analg. (Cleve.) **36:**64, 1957.

Wasmuth, C. E., and Oleck, H. L.: The privilege of consent, Anesth. Analg. (Cleve.) **36:**51, 1957.

APPENDIX

PEDIATRIC DOSAGE FORMULAS

Bastedo:

$$\text{Child dose} = \frac{\text{Adult dose} \times \text{child's age (yr)} + 3}{30}$$

Clark:

$$\text{Child dose} = \frac{\text{Child's weight (lb)}}{150} \times \text{adult dose}$$

Cowling:

$$\text{Child dose} = \frac{\text{Child's age at next birthday}}{24} \times \text{adult dose}$$

Young:

$$\text{Child dose} = \frac{\text{Child's age (yr)}}{\text{Child's age} + 12} \times \text{adult dose}$$

Body surface area rule:

$$\text{Child dose} = \frac{\text{BSA (m}^2)}{1.7} \times \text{adult dose}$$

PHARMACOLOGIC AGENTS OF SPECIAL VALUE IN PEDIATRIC PATIENTS
Analgesics

Acetylsalicylic acid (aspirin)	10 mg/kg PO, PR
Codeine	1.5 mg/kg IM
Fentanyl (Sublimaze)	1st dose 0.5-2 μg/kg IV, IM Maintenance 0.5-2 μg/kg/hr IV
Meperidine (Demerol)	1st dose 0.5-2 mg/kg IV, IM Maintenance 0.5-2 mg/kg/hr IV
Morphine	1st dose 0.05-0.2 mg/kg IV, IM Maintenance 0.05-0.2 mg/kg/hr IV
Demerol compound (25 mg meperidine, 6.25 mg chlorpromazine, 6.25 mg promethazine in 1 ml)	1 ml/15 kg IM, not to exceed 2 ml

Narcotic antagonist

Naloxone (Narcan)	0.01 mg/kg IV, IM

Anticholinergics

Atropine	0.1-0.6 mg IV, IM
Glycopyrrolate	0.02-0.1 mg IV, IM
Hyoscine	0.1-0.6 mg IV, IM

Antiemetic

Chlorpromazine	0.5 mg/kg IM

Antihistaminics

Diphenhydramine (Benadryl)	0.2-0.5 mg/kg IV
Hydroxyzine (Atarax, Vistaril)	1-3 mg/kg PO
Promethazine (Phenergan)	0.5 mg/kg

Antipyretics

Acetylsalicylic acid (aspirin)	60 mg/yr of age every 4 hr PO or by suppository
Acetaminophen (Tylenol)	5-10 mg/kg every 6 hr

Cardiovascular reagents

Cardiotonic drugs

Epinephrine (1:200,000) (5 μg/ml)	1-10 μg/kg, may repeat in 10 min
Phenylephrine (Neosynephrine)	0.1-1.0 μg/kg/min
Calcium chloride	10 mg/kg IC, IV
Calcium gluconate	60 mg/kg IC, IV
Digoxin	
Digitalizing dose	0.01 mg/kg every 4 hr × 4
Maintenance	0.01 mg/kg every 6-12 hr
Glucose (50%)	1 ml/kg
Glucagon	40 μg/kg/hr drip
Dopamine	1-10 μg/kg/min
Hydralazine	0.2 mg/kg/6 hr IM
Isoproterenol	0.1-1.0 μg/kg/min

Antiarrhythmic and antihypertensive agents

Atropine	0.2-0.6 mg IV, IM
Edrophonium	0.2 mg/kg IV
Lidocaine (1%)	0.5-1.0 mg/kg IV
Propranolol	0.05-0.1 mg/kg IV
Phentolamine (Regitine)	0.125 mg/kg IV, IM
Reserpine	0.07 mg/kg PO, IM

Cholinesterase inhibitors

Edrophonium (Tensilon)	0.2 mg/kg IV
Neostigmine (Prostigmin)	0.06 mg/kg IV

Diuretics

Chlorothiazide	2-3.5 mg/kg PO
Ethacrynic acid	1 mg/kg PO, IV, IM
Furosemide (Lasix)	0.5-1 mg/kg IV slowly
Mannitol (20%)	Test dose 0.5 g/kg and infuse up to 2 g/kg as needed

General anesthetics and muscle relaxants (Initial Dose)

Ketamine	2 mg/kg IV, 5-8 mg/kg IM
Methohexital (Brevital) (induction)	1-2 mg/kg IV, 10-15 mg/kg PR
Thiopental (Pentothal) (induction)	2-4 mg/kg IV, 20-30 mg/kg PR
Innovar (containing droperidol, 2.5 mg/ml, and fentanyl, 0.05 mg/ml)	0.1 ml/kg IV
Succinylcholine	1.5 mg/kg IV, IM
Gallamine	0.5 mg/kg IV
Metocurine	0.15-0.25 mg/kg IV
d-Tubocurarine	0.3-0.5 mg/kg
Pancuronium	0.05-0.1 mg/kg

Relaxant reversal

Atropine	0.02 mg/kg (or glycopyrrolate 0.004 mg/kg)
Neostigmine	0.06 mg/kg

Sedatives (refer also to Chapter 4)

Chloral hydrate	8-10 mg/kg PO
Chlorpromazine	0.5 mg/kg PO, IM
Diazepam (Valium)	0.1-0.3 mg/kg PO
Droperidol	0.1 mg/kg IM, IV
Flurazepam (Dalmane)	0.2 mg/kg PO
Hydroxyzine (Atarax, Vistaril)	1-3 mg/kg PO
Pentobarbital (Nembutal)	2-6 mg/kg PO, PR, IV
Phenobarbital	2-6 mg/kg PO, IV
Phenytoin	2 mg/kg PO, IM
Promethazine (Phenergan)	0.5-1.0 mg/kg PO
Triclofos	50-90 mg/kg PO
Trimeprazine (Temaril)	1-2 mg/kg PO

Blood chemistry

Constituent	Range
Ammonia (whole blood)	30-70 μg/dl
In newborn	90-150 μg/dl
Base (total fixed cation)	150-155 mEq/L
Bicarbonate (CO_2 capacity or combining power)	22-30 mEq/L
Bilirubin (serum)	
2-4 days	Mean peak 7 mg/dl, range 2-12 mg/dl
After newborn period	<0.8 mg/dl total
Calcium	
(Serum)	9.0-11.5 mg/dl
(Ionized)	1.6-2.6 mg/dl
Chloride (serum)	94-106 mEq/L
Creatinine (serum)	0.9-1.5 mg/dl
Fatty acids (serum)	380-465 mg/dl
Fibrinogen (plasma)	200-400 mg/dl
Globulin (serum)	1.3-2.7 g/dl
Glucose (fasting)	60-90 mg/dl
In newborn	20-80 mg/dl
Lactic acid (fasting)	6-16 mg/dl
Magnesium (serum)	1.5-2.5 mEq/L
Osmolality, serum	285-295 mOsm/L
pH (arterial whole blood)	7.35-7.45 (0.03 lower in venous blood)
P_{CO_2} (arterial)	35-45 mm Hg
P_{O_2} (arterial)	85-100 mm Hg
Phenylalanine (serum)	0.7-4 mg/dl
Phosphatase, acid	1.0-5.0 King-Armstrong units
Phosphatase, alkaline	
Infants	10-20 King-Armstrong units
Adults	4-13 King-Armstrong units
Phosphorus, inorganic (serum)	
1st year	4-7 mg/dl
1-12 years	5-6 mg/dl
Adult	3-4 mg/dl
Potassium (serum)	
0-10 days	Up to 7 mEq/L
Thereafter	4.1-5.6 mEq/L
Proteins, total	6-8 g/dl
Albumin	4.0-5.7 g/dl
Globulin	1.3-2.7 g/dl
Sodium (serum)	134-145 mEq/L
Transaminases (serum)	*SGOT units* *SGPT units*
1st week	10-120 10-90
Thereafter	5-45 5-45
Urea nitrogen (whole blood)	5-20 mg/dl (1st year)
Nonprotein nitrogen	22-40 mg/dl

Adapted from Cooke, R. E., and Levin, S., editors: The biologic basis of pediatric practice, New York, 1968, McGraw-Hill Book Co.

Coagulation factors

Determination	Specimen*	Age/sex	Normal value
Activated clotting time (ACT)	Plasma		<2.16 min
Bleeding time (Ivy)	Whole blood	Premature	1-8 min
		Newborn	1-5 min
		Thereafter	1-6 min
Clot retraction	Whole blood		Complete at 4 hr
Clotting time	Whole blood		
2 tubes			5-8 min
3 tubes			5-15 min
Fibrinogen	Plasma	Newborn	150-300 mg/dl
		Thereafter	200-400 mg/dl
Fibrinolysin (plasminogen)	Plasma		Lysis of clot
Partial thromboplastin time	Plasma	Premature	<120 sec
(PTT)		Newborn	< 90 sec
		Thereafter	< 60 sec
Prothrombin time, one stage	Plasma	Premature	12-21 sec
(PT)		Newborn/neonatal	12-20 sec
		Thereafter	12-14 sec
Thromboplastin generation	Plasma	Premature	8-24 sec at 6 min tube
test (TGT)		Newborn	8-20 sec at 6 min tube
		Thereafter	8-16 sec at 6 min tube

From Vaughan, V. C. II, and McKay, R. J., Jr., editors: Nelson textbook of pediatrics, ed. 10, Philadelphia, 1975, W. B. Saunders Co.
*Anticoagulants and collection instructions vary for individual laboratories.

DEFINITIONS AND TERMINOLOGY RELATED TO USE OF SOLUTIONS

The terms employed in preparation of intravenous fluids can be confusing; consequently, a brief review of the fundamentals is offered for reference.

atomic weight The weight of an element compared with oxygen as a standard, atomic weight of oxygen being fixed as 8. Na = 23, Cl = 35.5.
molecular weight The weight of the total constituent atoms of a substance. O_2 = 16, NaCl = 58.5.
mol, gram molecule, or gram molecular weight Molecular weight expressed in grams. O_2 = 16 g, NaCl = 58.5 g.
molar solution One in which a gram molecular weight of a substance is dissolved in sufficient solvent to make 1 liter of solution. 1M NaCl = 58.5 g in 1 L.
equivalent weight An equivalent weight is equal to the molecular weight divided by the valence.
normal solution One in which one equivalent weight of a substance is dissolved in sufficient solvent to make 1 liter of solution. 1N NaCl = 58.5 g in 1 L.
isotonic solution One in which the osmolality approaches that of extracellular fluid (290 to 300 mOsm/L).

NOTE: The terms "normal saline," "isotonic saline," and "physiologic saline" frequently are used interchangeably to denote a solution containing 900 mg or 0.9 g/dl. This is a 0.9% solution. It is not a "normal" solution nor even a 0.9% "normal" solution.

CONVERSION FORMULAS FOR MILLIEQUIVALENTS AND MILLIOSMOLS

$$\text{Milliequivalents} = \frac{\text{Milligrams} \times \text{valence}}{\text{Atomic weight}}$$

$$\text{Milliosmols (per liter)} = \frac{\text{Milligrams (per liter)}}{\text{Atomic weight}}$$

Body composition and distribution of water (as percentage of body weight)

	Premature infant	Full-term infant	Infant 1-12 months	Adult
TBW	83	79	72-60	58
ECW	50	43.9	32.2-27.4	18.7
ICW	33	35.1	34.3-33	39.3
ECW/ICW	1.5	1.25	1.14-0.83	0.48

Composition of fluids in the body compartments

	Plasma	Interstitial fluid	Intracellular fluid
Cation (mEq/L)			
Na^+	140	138	9
K^+	5	8	155
Ca^{++}	5	8	4
Mg^{++}	4	6	32
	154	160	200
Anion (mEq/L)			
Cl^-	100	119	5
HCO_3^-	26	26	10
Protein	19	7	65
Organic acid	6	6	—
HPO_4	2	1	95
SO_4	1	1	25
	154	160	200

The relatively larger body surface area (BSA) in the young subject is shown by the decrease in the body surface area : body weight ratio

Body weight (kg)	BSA (m^2)	BSA: weight
2	0.15	0.075
3	0.20	0.066
5	0.25	0.05
10	0.45	0.045
20	0.80	0.04
50	1.5	0.03
70	1.75	0.025

Approximate expenditure of calories per kilogram during fasting

Weight (kg)	Cal/kg
2-3	45-50
3-10	60-80*
10-15	45-65*
15-25	40-50
25-35	35-40
35-60	30-35

From Darrow, D. C.: The physiologic basis for estimating requirements for parenteral fluids, Pediatr. Clin. North Am. **6:**29, 1959.

*Metabolism of the growing child is greatest between 6 months and 2 years of age.

Clinical features in electrolyte imbalance*

Diagnostic problem	Urinary value	Primary diagnostic possibilities
Volume depletion	Na$^+$, 0-10 mEq/L	Extrarenal sodium loss
	Na$^+$, >10 mEq/L	"Renal salt wasting" or adrenal insufficiency
Acute oliguria	Na$^+$, 0-10 mEq/L	Prerenal azotemia
	Na$^+$, >30 mEq/L	Acute tubular necrosis
Hyponatremia	Na$^+$, 0-10 mEq/L	Severe volume depletion; edematous states
	Na$^+$, ≥dietary intake	Inappropriate antidiuretic hormone (ADH) secretion; adrenal insufficiency
Hypokalemia	K$^+$, 0-10 mEq/L	Extrarenal potassium loss
	K$^+$, >10 mEq/L	Renal potassium loss
Metabolic alkalosis	Cl$^-$, 0-10 mEq/L	Chloride-responsive alkalosis
	Cl$^-$, ≅ dietary intake	Chloride-resistant alkalosis

Reprinted, by permission, from Harrington, J. T., and Cohen, J. J.: Measurement of urinary electrolytes—indications and limitations, N. Engl. J. Med. **293**:1241, 1975.
*For purposes of this table, it is assumed the patient is not receiving diuretics.

Equivalent glucocorticoid effects of various corticosteroids

Drug	Dose
Cortisone	100 mg
Hydrocortisone	80 mg
Prednisone	20 mg
Prednisolone	16 mg
Triamcinolone	9 mg
9α-fluorocortisol	5 mg
Dexamethasone	2 mg

From Graef, J. W., and Cone, T. E., Jr., editors: Manual of pediatric therapeutics, Boston, 1974, Little, Brown & Co.

Temperature equivalents*

Centigrade	Fahrenheit	Centigrade	Fahrenheit
20	68.0	33	91.4
21	69.8	34	93.2
22	71.6	35	95.0
23	73.4	36	96.8
24	75.2	37	98.6
25	77.0	38	100.4
26	78.8	39	102.2
27	80.6	40	104.0
28	82.4	41	105.8
29	84.2	42	107.6
30	86.0	43	109.4
31	87.8	44	111.2
32	89.6	45	113.0

*$(9/5 \times °C) + 32 = °F$
$(°F - 32) \times 5/9 = °C$

Index

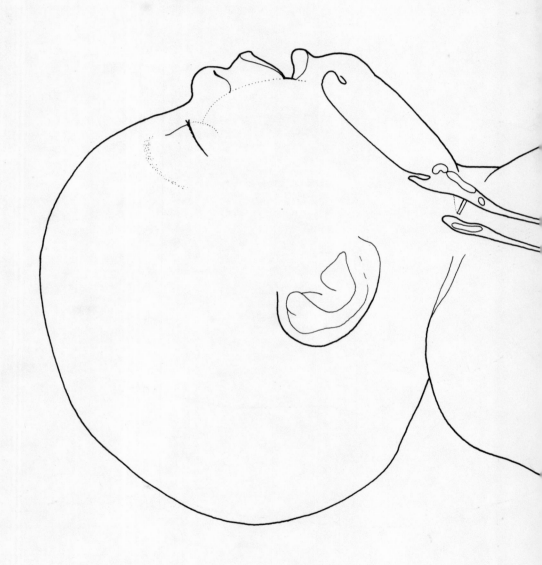